Non-Neoplastic Diseases of the Head and Neck

ATLAS OF NONTUMOR PATHOLOGY

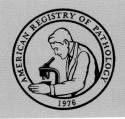 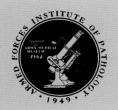

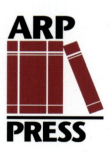

Editorial Director: Mirlinda Q. Caton
Production Editor: Dian S. Thomas
Editorial Assistant: Magdalena C. Silva
Editorial Assistant: Alana N. Black
Copyeditor: Audrey Kahn

ATLAS OF NONTUMOR PATHOLOGY

First Series
Fascicle 11

Non-Neoplastic Diseases of the Head and Neck

Bruce M. Wenig, MD
Esther L. B. Childers, MD
Mary S. Richardson, MD, DDS
Raja R. Seethala, MD
Lester D. R. Thompson, MD

Published by the
American Registry of Pathology
in collaboration with the
Armed Forces Institute of Pathology
Washington, DC

2017

ATLAS OF NONTUMOR PATHOLOGY

EDITOR
Donald West King, MD

ASSOCIATE EDITORS
Ronald A. DeLellis, MD
Leslie H. Sobin, MD
J. Thomas Stocker, MD
Bernard Wagner, MD

EDITORIAL ADVISORY BOARD
Ivan Damjanov, MD
Cecilia M. Fenoglio-Preiser, MD
Fred Gorstein, MD
Daniel Knowles, MD
Virginia A. LiVolsi, MD
Florabel G. Mullick, MD
Juan Rosai, MD
Fred Silva, MD
Steven G. Silverberg, MD

Manuscript Reviewed by:
Ronald A. DeLellis, MD
John G. Batsakis, MD

Available from the American Registry of Pathology
Washington, DC 20006
ISBN: 1-933477-37-7
978-1-933477-37-4

Printed in South Korea

Copyright © 2017 The American Registry of Pathology

All rights reserved. No part of this publication may be reproduced or transmitted in
any form or by any means: electronic, mechanical, photocopy, recording, or any other
information storage and retrieval system without the written permission of the publisher.

INTRODUCTION TO SERIES

This is the eleventh Fascicle of the Atlas of Nontumor Pathology, a complementary series to the Armed Forces Institute of Pathology (AFIP) Atlas of Tumor Pathology, first published in 1949.

Various individuals in the pathology community had suggested the formation of a new series of monographs concentrating on this particular area. In 1998, an Editorial Board was appointed and outstanding authors chosen shortly thereafter.

The purpose of the atlas is to provide surgical pathologists with ready expert reference material most helpful in their daily practice. The lesions described relate principally to medical non-neoplastic conditions. Many of these lesions represent complex entities and, when appropriate, we have included contributions from internists, radiologists, and surgeons. This has led to some increase in the size of the monographs, but the emphasis remains on diagnosis by the surgical pathologist.

Our goal is to continue to provide expert information at the lowest possible cost. Therefore, marked reductions in pricing are available to residents and fellows as well as to pathology faculty and other staff members purchasing the Fascicles on a subscription basis.

We believe that the Atlas of Nontumor Pathology will serve as an outstanding reference for surgical pathologists as well as an important contribution to the literature of other medical specialties.

Donald West King, MD
Ronald A. DeLellis, MD
Leslie H. Sobin, MD
J. Thomas Stocker, MD
Bernard Wagner, MD

PREFACE AND ACKNOWLEDGMENTS

We would like to thank Drs. Donald West King, Ronald A. DeLellis, and Fred Gorstein, as well as the entire Editorial Board for the honor and opportunity to contribute this book to the Atlas of Nontumor Pathology series.

This Fascicle on non-neoplastic head and neck diseases is a broad overview of the spectrum of diseases involving the sinonasal tract, oral cavity, pharynx, larynx, neck, salivary glands, and ear and temporal bone. Even with the best of intentions, no single text can possibly cover all diseases affecting the head and neck. Our approach was to focus primarily on the more common non-neoplastic head and neck diseases that the surgical pathologist will confront in their daily practice. It is our sincere hope that we have accomplished this goal providing the reader with a useful and practical text supplemented with high-quality illustrations with which to diagnose non-neoplastic head and neck diseases.

There are many individuals who have collectively mentored us through our careers offering sage advice and guidance. Some of these individuals included Drs. Vincent J. Hyams and John G. Batsakis, arguably the "godfathers" of head and neck pathology, as well as Dr. Leon Barnes. Special appreciation is made to Dennis K. Heffner, CAPT, USN, MC, the former Chair of Otorhinolaryngic-Head and Neck Pathology at the Armed Forces Institute of Pathology.

Bruce M. Wenig, MD
Senior Member, Anatomic Pathology
Section Head, Head and Neck, and Endocrine Pathology
Moffitt Cancer Center
Professor of Oncologic Sciences
University of South Florida
Tampa, FL

Esther L. B. Childers, DDS
Chair and Professor, Department of Oral and Maxillofacial Pathology
College of Dentistry
Howard University
Washington, DC

Mary S. Richardson MD, DDS
Director of Surgical Pathology
Professor of Pathology and Laboratory Medicine
Medical University of South Carolina
Charleston, SC

Raja R. Seethala, MD
Section Director, Head and Neck, and Endocrine Pathology
Department of Pathology and Laboratory Medicine
University of Pittsburgh Medical Center
Professor of Pathology and Otolaryngology
University of Pittsburgh
Pittsburgh, PA

Lester D. R. Thompson, MD
Consultant Pathologist
Southern California Permanente Medical Group
Woodland Hills, CA

Dedications

To my husband and daughter, for their support and love.
To the many mentors in my career, who have helped me along the way.
Esther L. B. Childers

To my mother, Gladys Cavanaugh (1924-2016) for all her encouragement
and to my husband, David for his never ending support and patience.
Mary S. Richardson

To my wife, Keren, for supporting me throughout my career.
Raja R. Seethala

When I write, I attempt to leave a small part of myself behind, but
try to remember this quote stuck on my wife's computer monitor:
"Will it be important a year from now?"
A true legacy is written by those who love and support you.
Lester D. R. Thompson

To my wife Ana Maria and our children Sarah,
Eli, and Jake; the loves of my life.
Bruce M. Wenig

Permission to use copyrighted images has been granted by:

American Medical Association
Arch Otolaryngol 1971;94:352-353. For figures 1-10 and 1-13.

Elsevier
Atlas of head and neck pathology, 3rd ed. Philadelphia: Elsevier; 2016:719-1095. For table 5-2 and figure 7-17.

Lippincott
Bailey's head and neck surgery: otolaryngology, 5th ed. Philadelphia: Lippincott Williams & Wilkins;2014:692-695. For figures 6-1 and 6-2.
Histology for pathologists, 4th ed. Philadelphia: Lippincott Williams & Wilkins 2012;404. For figure 7-5.

Taylor and Francis
Barnes L, ed. Surgical pathology of the head and neck, 3rd ed. New York: Informa Healthcare; 2009:137. For figure 5-1.
Acta Otolaryngol 1968;66:182. For figure 7-4.

CONTENTS

1. **Nasal Cavity and Paranasal Sinuses** 1
   - Embryology, Anatomy, and Histology of the Nasal Cavity 1
     - Embryology 1
     - Anatomic Borders 1
     - Histology 1
   - Embryology, Anatomy, and Histology of the Paranasal Sinuses 5
     - Embryology 5
     - Anatomic Borders 5
     - Histology 7
   - Classification 7
   - Developmental Lesions 8
     - Heterotopic Central Nervous System (Glial) Tissue 8
     - Encephaloceles 11
     - Nasal Dermoid Sinus and Cyst 15
     - Primary Ciliary Dyskinesia 16
     - Noninfectious Inflammatory and Tumor-Like Processes 19
     - Sinonasal Inflammatory Polyps 19
     - Paranasal Sinus Mucocele 27
   - Sinonasal Hamartomas 30
     - Respiratory Epithelial Adenomatoid Hamartoma 32
     - Seromucinous Hamartoma 35
     - Chondro-osseous and Respiratory Epithelial Hamartomas 39
     - Nasal Chondromesenchymal Hamartoma 40
     - Granulomatosis with Polyangiitis 40
     - Myospherulosis 49
     - Extranodal Sinus Histiocytosis with Massive Lymphadenopathy ... 51
     - Necrotizing Sialometaplasia 54
     - Eosinophilic Angiocentric Fibrosis 54
     - Sarcoidosis 55
     - Rhinophyma 55
     - Relapsing Polychondritis 56
     - Pyogenic Granuloma/Lobular Capillary Hemangioma 57
   - Fungal Diseases 61
     - Fungal Rhinosinusitis 61
     - Noninvasive Fungal Rhinosinusitis: Allergic Fungal Rhinosinusitis ... 61
     - Fungus Ball 65

Invasive Fungal Rhinosinusitis: Acute Invasive FRS. 66
Chronic Invasive and Chronic Granulomatous FRS 67
Sinonasal Mucormycosis 69
Rhinosporidiosis. 72
Other Fungi. 74
Bacterial Diseases 76
Bacterial Rhinoscleroma 76
Sinonasal Botryomycosis 82
Miscellaneous Sinonasal Bacterial Infections. 84
Protozoal Diseases. 85
Mucocutaneous Leishmaniasis. 85
Amebiasis 87
Viral Diseases. 87
Rhinosinusitis. 87
Allergic Rhinosinusitis 90
Infectious Rhinosinusitis 90
Viral Rhinosinusitis. 90
Bacterial Sinusitis 90
Atrophic Rhinosinusitis 90
Aspirin Intolerance or Aspirin-Exacerbated Respiratory Disease 91
Nonallergic Rhinosinusitis with Eosinophilia Syndrome and Eosinophilic
Chronic Rhinosinusitis Syndrome 91
2. Oral Cavity and Jaw 103
Embryology, Anatomy, and Histology 103
Embryology. 103
Anatomy 103
Histology 105
Classification 108
Developmental Lesions. 108
Heterotopias (Choristomas) and Hamartomas. 108
Fordyce Granules 108
Ectopic Thyroid Tissue and Lingual Thyroid 109
Oral Choristoma. 111
Tori and Exostoses 112
Oral Cavity Cysts 113
Oral Lymphoepithelial Cyst 113
Nasopalatine Duct Cyst 114
Infectious Diseases of the Oral Cavity 116
Fungal Disease: Candidiasis 116

Other Fungi	117
Viruses	118
Human Papillomavirus	119
Epstein-Barr Virus	120
Cytomegalovirus	120
Herpes Virus	120
Bacteria and Spirochetes	120
Gonorrhea	121
Syphilis	121
Epithelial Inflammatory or Tumor-Like Processes: Reactive Epithelial and Epithelial-Related Proliferations	122
Verruca Vulgaris	122
Condyloma Acuminatum	122
Oral Mucosal Condyloma Acuminatum	122
Focal Epithelial Hyperplasia	124
Oral Hairy Leukoplakia	125
Verruciform Xanthoma	126
Inflammatory Papillary Hyperplasia	129
Pseudoepitheliomatous Hyperplasia	129
Proliferative Verrucous Leukoplakia	132
Mesenchymal Lesions	134
Peripheral Ossifying Fibroma	134
Peripheral Odontogenic Fibroma	138
Irritation Fibroma	139
Giant Cell Fibroma	142
Giant Cell Lesions	144
Central and Peripheral Giant Cell Granulomas	144
Oral Fibrosing Lesions	152
Oral Submucous Fibrosis	152
Gingival Fibromatosis	152
Vascular Lesions	157
Pyogenic Granuloma (Lobular Capillary Hemangioma)	157
Congenital Epulis (Congenital Granular Cell Tumor)	160
Benign Fibro-osseous Lesions of Craniofacial Bones	161
Fibrous Dysplasia	161
Cemento-Osseous Dysplasia	169
Pigmented Lesions	169
Exogenous Pigmentations	170
Endogenous Pigmentations	172

        Black Hairy Tongue.. 174
        Myospherulosis... 177
    Odontogenic Cysts.. 178
        Dentigerous Cyst... 178
        Eruption Cyst.. 185
        Glandular Odontogenic Cyst... 185
        Lateral Periodontal Cyst... 186
        Periapical Cyst... 187
    Selective Autoimmune, Allergic, Systemic, and Cutaneous-Type Diseases
        Affecting the Oral Cavity.. 189
        Granulomatosis with Polyangiitis... 189
        Lichen Planus.. 189
        Aphthous Stomatitis... 190
    Radiation-Associated Changes.. 192

3. Pharynx... 207
    Embryology, Anatomy, and Histology... 207
        Embryology.. 207
        Anatomy... 207
        Anatomic Borders... 207
        Histology.. 209
    Classification.. 212
    Developmental Cystic Lesions: Nasopharyngeal Cysts...................... 212
        Rathke Pouch Cyst.. 215
        Thornwaldt Cyst.. 216
    Pharyngeal Hamartomas, Choristomas, and Teratomatous Lesions.......... 219
        Nasopharyngeal Hamartomas... 219
        Pharyngeal/Nasopharyngeal Central Nervous System Heterotopias..... 219
        Nasoharyngeal Dermoid, or Teratoid, Lesions............................ 219
        Lymphangiomatous Polyp of the Tonsil.................................. 222
        Salivary Gland Anlage Tumor... 224
    Infectious Diseases... 224
        Tonsillitis.. 224
        Peritonsillar Abscess.. 228
        Lemierre Disease/Syndrome.. 230
        EBV-Related Diseases and Infectious Mononucleosis..................... 230
        Human Papillomavirus.. 235
        Human Immunodeficiency Virus Infection and Acquired Immunodeficiency
            Syndrome... 235
        HIV-Related Lymphoid Changes of Nasopharyngeal and Palatine Tonsils...... 237

	AIDS-Related Opportunistic Infectious Diseases	245
	Cytomegalovirus	245
	Herpes Simplex Virus	245
	Measles Infection	248
	Fungus Infections	248
	Bacteria and Spirochetes	248
Reactive, Inflammatory, and Tumor-Like Lesions		250
	Tangier Disease	250

4. Neck ... 263
    Anatomy ... 263
    Classification ... 263
    Cystic (Non-neoplastic Lesions of the Neck) ... 264
        Branchial Anomalies ... 264
        First Branchial Anomalies ... 267
        Second Branchial Anomalies ... 269
        Third Branchial Anomalies ... 279
        Fourth Branchial Anomalies ... 280
        Thyroglossal Duct Cyst ... 280
        Cervical Thymic Cyst ... 285
        Bronchogenic Cysts ... 287
        Dermoid Cyst ... 292
    Infectious Diseases ... 292
        Mycobacterial Tuberculosis Infection ... 292
        Scrofula ... 294
        Mycobacterial Spindle Cell Pseudotumor ... 297
        Actinomycosis ... 298
        Cat Scratch Disease ... 300
        Bacillary Angiomatosis ... 302
        Other Infectious Diseases ... 305
    Inflammatory and Tumor-Like Lesions ... 306
        Sarcoidosis ... 306

5. Larynx and Trachea ... 319
    Embryology, Anatomy, and Histology: Larynx ... 319
        Embryology ... 319
        Anatomy ... 319
        Histology ... 320
        Laryngeal Cartilages ... 322
    Embryology, Anatomy, and Histology: Trachea ... 324
        Embryology ... 324

Anatomy	324
Histology	324
Classification	324
Developmental Lesions	324
Laryngomalacia	324
Tracheopathia Osteochondroplastica	325
Hamartomas, Choristomas, and Ectopias	327
Infectious Diseases	328
Granulomatous Laryngopharyngitis	329
Viruses	330
Bacteria	331
Fungi	333
Protozoa	334
Noninfectious Inflammatory Diseases	334
Angioedema/Allergic Laryngitis	334
Sarcoidosis	335
Autoimmune Diseases	335
Granulomatosis with Polyangiitis	335
Relapsing Polychondritis	338
Tumor-Like Processes	339
Vocal Cord Nodules and Polyps	339
Laryngocele and Saccular Cyst	340
Other Laryngeal Cysts	342
Contact Ulcer of the Larynx	342
Necrotizing Sialometaplasia	345
Laryngeal Amyloidosis	347
Subglottic Stenosis	349
Rheumatoid Nodule	351
Teflon Granuloma	351
Reactive Epithelial Changes	354
Radiation-Associated Changes	357
Laryngeal Manifestations of Dermatologic Disorders	360
Epidermolysis Bullosa	360
Pemphigus	360
Mucous Membrane Pemphigoid	360
6. Salivary Glands	369
Embryology, Anatomy, and Histology	369
Embryology	369
Anatomy	369

  Histology.. 371
 Classification.. 375
 Developmental Lesions.. 375
  Accessory Parotid Glands.. 375
  Salivary Gland Heterotopia (Ectopias, Choristomas).. 375
  Salivary Gland Hamartomas and Adenomatoid Hyperplasia 377
 Salivary Cysts 377
  Salivary Duct Cyst and Mucous Retention Cyst 377
  Mucus Extravasation Phenomenon (Extravasation Mucocele) 379
  Ranula.. 380
  Lymphoepithelial Cysts 381
  Polycystic (Dysgenetic) Disease 382
 Metaplasia and Hyperplasia 382
  Oncocytic Metaplasia and Oncocytosis 382
  Sialadenosis.. 385
 Infectious, Inflammatory, and Reactive Diseases 386
  Acute Sialadenitis and Viral Parotitis (Mumps) 386
  Chronic Nonautoimmune Sialadenitis 386
  Human Immunodeficiency Virus Salivary Gland Disease 387
  Lymphoepithelial Sialadenitis 390
  Sjögren Syndrome.. 390
  IgG4-Related Sialadenitis 394
  Sarcoidosis.. 396
 Tumor-Like Lesions 398
  Necrotizing Sialometaplasia 398
  Subacute Necrotizing Sialadenitis.. 399
  Extranodal Sinus Histiocytosis with Massive Lymphadenopathy (Rosai-Dorfman Disease).. 400
  Intercalated Duct Lesion.. 401
7. Ear and Temporal Bone.. 413
 Embryology, Anatomy, and Histology 413
  Embryology.. 413
  Anatomy.. 414
  Histology.. 417
  Classification.. 420
 Congenital Abnormalities.. 420
  Accessory Tragus.. 420
  Branchial Cleft Anomalies 421

Tumor-Like Lesions of the External Ear Region 421
    Keloid 421
    Chondrodermatitis Nodularis Chronicus Helicis 425
    Idiopathic Cystic Chondromalacia of the Auricular Cartilage 426
    Exostosis 429
    Synovial Chondromatosis of the Temporomandibular Joint 430
    Kimura Disease and Epithelioid Hemangioma 433
Infectious Diseases of the External Ear 436
    Necrotizing External Otitis 436
Infectious and Inflammatory Lesions of the Middle Ear and Temporal Lobe 438
    Otitis Media 438
    Otic (Aural) Polyp 444
    Cholesteatoma 446
    Langerhans Cell Histiocytosis 450
Heterotopias of the Middle Ear and Mastoid 453
    Middle Ear Salivary Gland Heterotopia 453
    Middle Ear Neuroglial Heterotopia 454
    Acquired Encephalocele 454
Autoimmune, Degenerative, and Systemic Diseases 455
    Relapsing Polychondritis 455
    Granulomatosis with Polyangiitis 457
    Tophaceous Gout 458
    Tophaceous Pseudogout 459
    Osteosclerosis 461
    Paget Disease of Bone 463
    Ménière Disease 463
Developmental Defects of the Middle Ear and Temporal Bone 464
Index 477

1 NASAL CAVITY AND PARANASAL SINUSES

By Dr. Bruce M. Wenig

EMBRYOLOGY, ANATOMY, AND HISTOLOGY OF THE NASAL CAVITY

Embryology

The facial prominences (frontonasal, maxillary, and mandibular) appear around the 4th week of gestation and give rise to the boundaries and structures of the face (1). The nasal placodes, bilateral thickenings of the surface ectoderm along the frontonasal prominence, form the nasal pits, which, by growth of the surrounding mesenchyme, become progressively depressed along their length, giving rise to the primitive nasal sacs, the forerunners of the nasal cavities. The anterior portion of the nasal cavity is the vestibule, the epithelium of which is ectodermally derived and represents the internal extension of the integument of the external nose (1). The epithelium lining the nasal cavities proper (Schneiderian membrane) is also ectodermally derived (1). The nasal septum develops from the merged medial nasal prominences.

The regions of continuity between the nasal and oral cavities following rupture of the oronasal membrane develop into the choanae. The conchae (turbinates) develop as elevations along the lateral wall of each nasal cavity. The olfactory epithelia develop in the superiposterior portion of each nasal cavity and differentiate from cells in the ectodermally derived nasal cavity epithelium.

Anatomic Borders

The nasal cavity is divided into right and left halves by the septum; each half opens onto the face via the nares, or nostrils, and communicates behind with the nasopharynx through the posterior nasal apertures, or the choanae (2,3). Each half of the nasal cavity has the following borders (walls) (figs. 1-1, 1-2): 1) the superior aspect, or the roof, slopes downward in front and back and is horizontal in its middle; the frontal and nasal bones form the anterior sloping part; the cribriform plate of the ethmoid bone forms the horizontal part and separates the nasal cavity from the anterior cranial fossa (medial part of floor). This area represents the deepest part of the cavity. The body of the sphenoid bone forms the posterior sloping part; 2) the inferior aspect (floor) is formed by the palatine processes of the maxillary bone, which represents the majority (75 percent) of the floor and, thereby, intervenes between the oral and nasal cavities; the remainder of the floor is formed by the horizontal process of the palatine bone; 3) the lateral aspect is formed mostly by the nasal surface of the maxilla below and in front, posteriorly by the perpendicular plate of the palatine bone, and above by the nasal surface of the ethmoidal labyrinth separating the nasal cavity from the orbit. Along the lateral wall of each nasal cavity are three horizontal bony projections: the superior, middle, and inferior conchae; occasionally a small fourth concha is identified above the superior concha and is called the supreme concha (3). The air spaces or meatuses (superior, middle, and inferior) lie beneath and lateral to the conchae and are named according to the concha immediately above it; and 4) the medial aspect is the bony nasal septum entirely formed by the vomer and the perpendicular plate of the ethmoid; the anterior portion of the nasal septum represents the septal cartilage (2).

Histology

The nasal vestibule is a cutaneous structure composed of keratinizing squamous epithelium and underlying subcutaneous tissue, with cutaneous adnexal structures (hair follicles, sebaceous glands, and sweat glands) (4). The mucocutaneous junction (limen nasi) is approximately 1 to 2 cm posterior to the nares and represents the point at which the epithelial surface changes from keratinizing squamous epithelium to ciliated pseudostratified columnar (respiratory) epithelium, the latter lining the entire nasal cavity (fig. 1-3) and, as previously

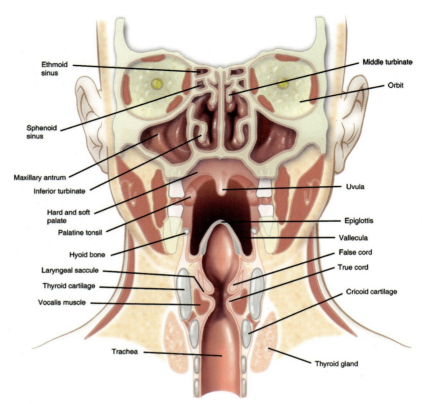

Figure 1-1

ANATOMY OF THE SINONASAL TRACT

A coronal section through the head at the level of the molar teeth displays the anatomy of the nasal cavity, as well as the pharynx, larynx, and some of the paranasal sinuses.

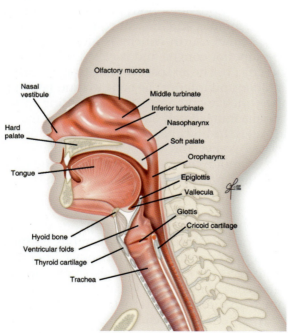

Figure 1-2

SAGITTAL VIEW OF THE UPPER RESPIRATORY TRACT

A midline sagittal section shows the major structures of the nasal cavity, pharynx, and larynx.

detailed, ectodermally derived. The submucosa underlying the epithelium is thin, has seromucous (minor salivary) glands arranged in distinct lobules (fig. 1-3), normally contains a mixed inflammatory cell infiltrate including mature lymphocytes and scattered plasma cells but no lymphoid follicles/aggregates, and has a distinct vascular component consisting of large thick-walled blood vessels. The vascular structures are particularly prominent along the inferior and middle turbinates, resemble erectile tissue owing to the prominent smooth muscle wall, and may be mistaken for a hemangioma (fig. 1-4) (4).

The nasal septum separates the nasal cavities and contains elastic cartilage and lamellar bone. The nasal mucosa is closely apposed to the underlying structures of the nasal septum, with the periosteum and perichondrium attached so closely as to constitute a single membrane, referred to as mucoperiosteum (fig. 1-5). Along the anterior part of the nasal septum the submucosa is rich in thin-walled blood vessels. This location is referred to as Little, or Kiesselbach, area and represents a frequent site of nose

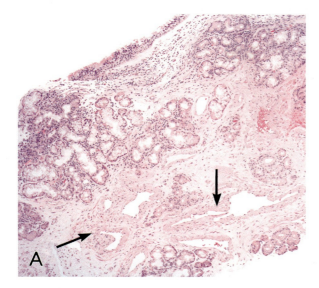
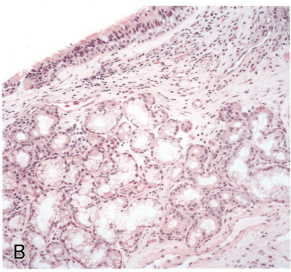
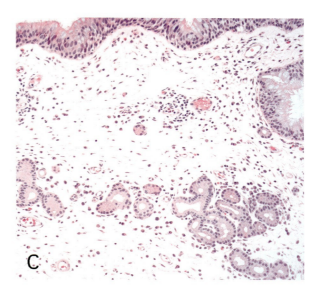

Figure 1-3

HISTOLOGY OF THE SINONASAL TRACT

A: Ciliated respiratory epithelium lines the entire sinonasal tract, including the nasal cavity and paranasal sinuses. It overlies submucosal seromucous glands arranged in lobules with subjacent thick-walled blood vessels (arrows).

B: At higher magnification, the serous and mucous cells are evident.

C: The submucosa contains an admixture of inflammatory cells, including mature lymphocytes and scattered plasma cells.

bleeds (fig. 1-6) (4). The nasal cartilage is of the hyaline type and has a bluish, translucent, homogeneous appearance.

Melanocytes migrating from their origin in the neural crest are present in the normal mucosa of the entire upper aerodigestive tract. In the sinonasal tract, melanocytes are present in the respiratory epithelium as well as in submucosal seromucous glands (5).

The vomeronasal organ of Jacobson (VNO) is a chemosensory structure that develops from the vomeronasal primordia, bilateral epithelial thickenings on the nasal septum (1). Invagination of the primordia gives rise to the tubular VNO between day 37 and 43 (1). The VNO ends blindly posteriorly and reaches its greatest development between 12 and 14 weeks (1). The VNO is consistently present in the form of a bilateral duct-like structure on the nasal septum, superior to the paraseptal cartilage, at all ages (1). Gradual replacement of the receptor cell population with patchy ciliated cells occurs. The human VNO is a true homolog of the VNO in other animals (e.g., mammals, reptiles, amphibians) and is lined by chemosensory epithelium similar to the olfactory epithelium except that the VNO chemoreceptors lack cilia, accounting for their highly developed sense of smell (1,4).

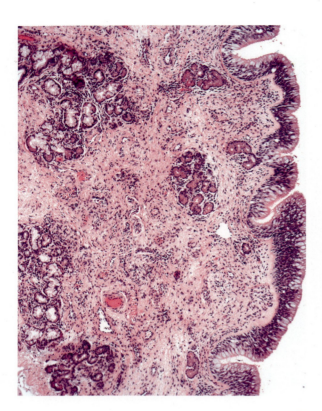 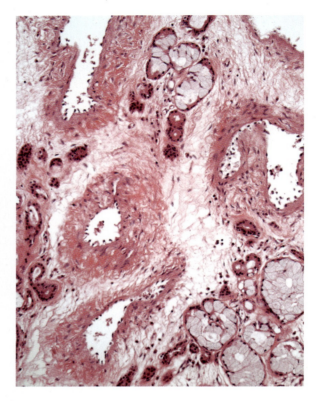

Figure 1-4

HISTOLOGY OF THE SINONASAL TRACT

Left: The nasal turbinates, particularly the inferior and middle turbinates, are normally characterized by the presence of thick-walled vascular structures.

Right: The vascular structures resemble erectile tissue owing to a prominent smooth muscle wall and may be mistaken for a vascular neoplasm.

Figure 1-5

HISTOLOGY OF THE SINONASAL TRACT

The nasal mucosa is closely apposed to the underlying structures of the nasal septum, with the periosteum and perichondrium attached so closely as to constitute a single membrane, referred to as the mucoperiosteum.

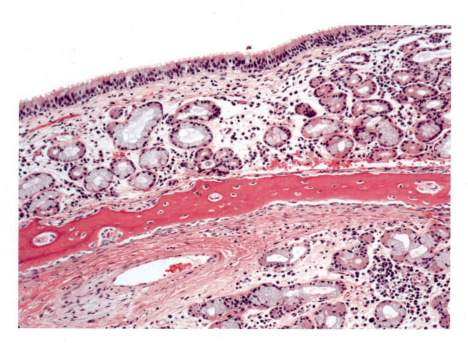

The olfactory mucosa is located in the most superior portion of the nasal cavity, involving the superior portion of the superior turbinate (cribriform plate) and approximately a third of the superior nasal septum (fig. 1-7). The olfactory epithelium consists of bipolar, spindle-shaped olfactory neural (receptor) cells composed of myelinated axons that penetrate the basal lamina to protrude from the mucosal surface and nonmyelinated proximal processes that traverse the cribriform plate, columnar sustentacular or supporting cells, rounded basal cells that lie on basal lamina, and olfactory or Bowman glands in the lamina propria that represent purely serous type glands (fig. 1-8) (3,4). The olfactory epithelial cells are reactive for neuron-specific enolase (NSE) (fig. 1-8).

EMBRYOLOGY, ANATOMY, AND HISTOLOGY OF THE PARANASAL SINUSES

Embryology

The paranasal sinuses (maxillary, ethmoid, sphenoid, and frontal) develop as outgrowths of the walls of the nasal cavities and become air-filled extensions of the nasal cavities (fig. 1-9). Some of the nasal sinuses (the maxillary and portions of the ethmoidal sinuses) develop during late fetal life and others (frontal and sphenoid sinuses) are not present at birth but develop during the early years of life.

Anatomic Borders

Maxillary Sinus. The maxillary sinus represents the largest of the paranasal sinuses and is located in the body of the maxilla (2,3). From above, the maxillary sinus has a triangular

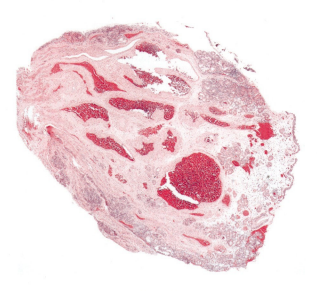

Figure 1-6

HISTOLOGY OF THE SINONASAL TRACT

Along the anterior part of the nasal septum the submucosa is rich in thin-walled blood vessels. This location is referred to as Little or Kiesselbach area and represents a frequent site of nose bleeds.

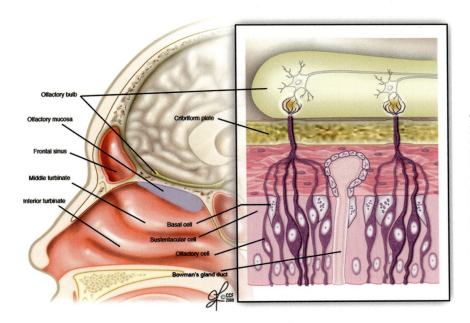

Figure 1-7

NASAL CAVITY

The olfactory mucosa is confined to the most superior portion of the nasal cavity (blue shading). It involves the superior portion of the superior turbinate, the cribriform plate, and the superior approximately one third of the nasal septum. In adults, the distribution becomes patchy, due to multifocal replacement by nonolfactory mucosa. The olfactory cells send processes through the cribriform plate to connect with the olfactory bulb.

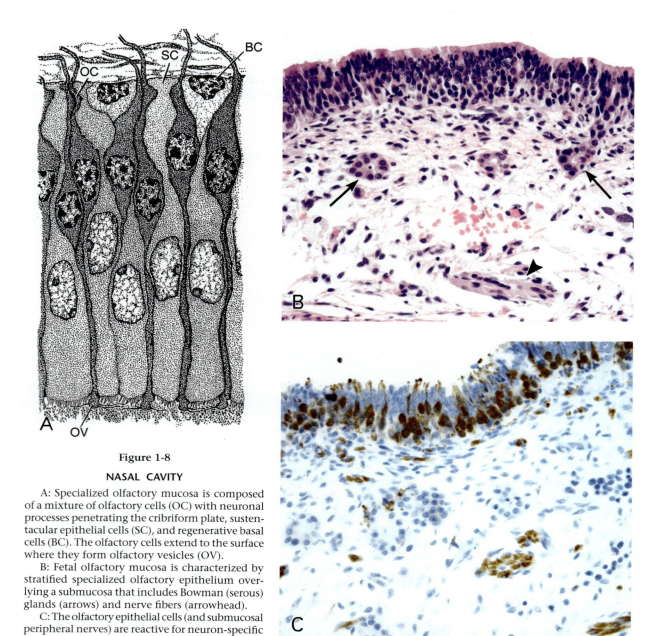

Figure 1-8

NASAL CAVITY

A: Specialized olfactory mucosa is composed of a mixture of olfactory cells (OC) with neuronal processes penetrating the cribriform plate, sustentacular epithelial cells (SC), and regenerative basal cells (BC). The olfactory cells extend to the surface where they form olfactory vesicles (OV).

B: Fetal olfactory mucosa is characterized by stratified specialized olfactory epithelium overlying a submucosa that includes Bowman (serous) glands (arrows) and nerve fibers (arrowhead).

C: The olfactory epithelial cells (and submucosal peripheral nerves) are reactive for neuron-specific enolase (NSE).

shape, with the base formed by the lateral wall of the nasal cavity and the apex projecting into the zygomatic arch. Its borders include: 1) the superior aspect (roof) composed of the orbital surface of the maxilla (floor of the orbit); 2) the inferior aspect (floor), composed of the alveolar and palatine process of the maxilla; 3) the anterolateral aspect, composed of the facial surface of the maxilla; 4) the posterior aspect, composed of the infratemporal surface of the maxilla; and 5) the medial aspect, composed of the lateral wall of the nasal cavity. The maxillary ostium (hiatus semilunaris) is on the highest part of the medial wall of the sinus and does not open directly into the nasal cavity but into the posterior ethmoid infundibulum (uncinate groove), which opens into the middle meatus of the nasal cavity.

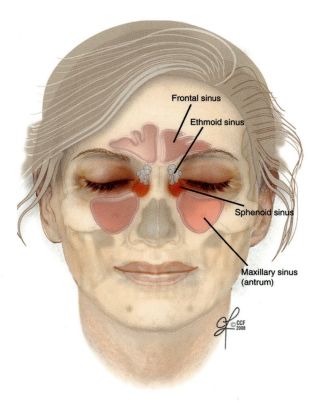

Figure 1-9

PARANASAL SINUSES

The frontal sinuses are most anterior, the maxillary sinuses are beneath the cheek, the ethmoid sinuses occupy the interorbital region, and the sphenoid sinuses are most posterior, just beneath the base of the brain.

Osteomeatal Complex or Unit. This not a discrete anatomic structure but refers to a functional unit of structures that include the maxillary sinus ostium, ethmoid infundibulum, hiatus semilunaris, and frontal recess. It is the common final pathway for drainage of secretions from the maxillary, frontal, anterior, and middle ethmoid sinuses into the middle meatus. Obstruction of the osteomeatal complex plays a pivotal role in the development and persistence of sinusitis. Coronal high resolution computerized tomography (HRCT) provides exquisite detail of these structures.

Ethmoid Sinuses. The ethmoid sinuses are thin-walled cavities in the ethmoidal labyrinth completed by the frontal, maxillary, lacrimal, sphenoidal, and palatine bones. They vary in size and number, usually consisting of 2 to 8 anterior and middle ethmoid cells, and 2 to 8 posterior ethmoid cells (2,3). Based on the relation to the ethmoid infundibulum, the ethmoid cells are grouped into an anterior group, in which the ostia open directly to the ethmoid infundibulum; a middle or bullous group, in which the ostia open on or above the ethmoid infundibulum; and a posterior group, in which the ostia open into the superior meatus.

Frontal Sinuses. The frontal sinuses are roughly pyramidal shaped and located in the vertical part of the frontal bone. These sinuses are frequently asymmetric in size and often contain septa dividing the cavity. The ostia of the frontal sinus opens into the anterior part of the middle meatus. An important anatomic relationship includes the proximity to the anterior cranial fossa and orbit, which are separated from these structures by only a thin plate of bone.

Sphenoid Sinuses. The sphenoid sinuses are contained within the sphenoid bone, situated posterior to the upper part of the nasal cavity. They are related above to the optic chiasm and the hypophysis cerebri, and on each side to the internal carotid artery and cavernous sinus. They open into the sphenoethmoidal recess lying above and behind the superior nasal concha.

Histology

All of the sinuses are lined by ciliated pseudostratified, columnar epithelium, which, together with the nasal cavity, is called the schneiderian membrane. The sinonasal epithelium is ectodermally derived, in contrast with the similar-appearing epithelium lining the nasopharynx, which is of endodermal derivation. Although the epithelium of the paranasal sinuses is the same as that of the nasal cavity, the mucous membranes of the paranasal sinuses are thinner and less vascular than those of the nasal cavity, and have a fibrous layer adjacent to the periosteum (4). Seromucous glands are scattered throughout the paranasal sinus submucosa, particularly in the ostial areas.

CLASSIFICATION

The classification of non-neoplastic lesions of the sinonasal tract is seen in Table 1-1.

DEVELOPMENTAL LESIONS

Heterotopic Central Nervous System (Glial) Tissue

Definition. *Heterotopic central nervous system (glial) tissue* (HCNST) is a midline congenital developmental error composed of altered brain tissue that occurs in or near the bridge of the nose, but without a patent connection to the cranial cavity. It is commonly referred to as *nasal glioma*, but "glioma" is more appropriately used for glial neoplasms. It is also referred to as *glial heterotopia*.

Embryogenesis. HCNST seems to be sporadic, and is only rarely found with other congenital abnormalities (fig. 1-10). Such rare associations may be coincidental and the abnormality is not part of a congenital "syndrome" or a constellation of developmental abnormalities. There is, however, some embryologic association with nasal dermoids and encephaloceles (see below). In early embryogenesis, the prenasal space contains a projection of dura that transiently contacts the overlying ectoderm (6). An abnormal persistence of this contact could produce an effect that would result in some embryonic CNS tissue being abnormally positioned toward the ectodermal area.

Clinical Features. HCNST have been estimated to occur in approximately 1 of 4,000 births. There is no familial association and the gender incidence is roughly equal. The heterotopias usually present within the first year of life, although occurrence in adults has been reported (7). HCNST most commonly occurs in and around the nasal cavity, usually associated with the septum; a midline location with swelling in the nasal bridge area is common (fig. 1-11). The lesion is usually not always midline but may occur more laterally (paramidline), toward or near the inner canthus of the eye. Other sites of involvement include the ethmoid sinus, palate, middle ear, tonsil, and pharyngeal area.

HCNST may be extranasal, intranasal, or mixed. Extranasal lesions make up approximately 60 percent of cases (8). Such lesions present as a subcutaneous blue or red mass along the bridge of the nose; the skin overlying the swelling or mass may be slightly erythematous. This appearance may clinically simulate the appearance of a hemangioma (9), however, the lesion is usually firmer than a hemangioma, as well as an encephalocele (10).

Table 1-1

CLASSIFICATION OF NON-NEOPLASTIC LESIONS OF THE SINONASAL TRACT

Developmental
 Heterotopic central nervous system tissue and encephalocele
 Nasal dermoid sinus and cyst
 Primary ciliary dyskinesia

Noninfectious Inflammatory and Tumor-like
 Sinonasal inflammatory polyps
 Paranasal sinus mucocele
 Sinonasal hamartomas
  Respiratory epithelial adenomatoid hamartoma (REAH)
  Seromucinous hamartoma
  Chondro-osseous and respiratory epithelial (CORE) hamartoma
  Nasal chondromesenchymal hamartoma
 Granulomatosis with polyangiitis (formerly referred as Wegener granulomatosis)
 Myospherulosis
 Extranodal sinus histiocytosis with massive lymphadenopathy (Rosai-Dorfman disease)
 Necrotizing sialometaplasia
 Eosinophilic angiocentric fibroma
 Sarcoidosis
 Rhinophyma
 Relapsing polychondritis

Infectious
 Fungi (noninvasive and invasive fungal sinusitis, others)
 Bacteria (rhinoscleroma, others)
 Protozoa (leishmaniasis, amebiasis)
 Viruses
 Rhinosinusitis

Intranasal lesions represent approximately 30 percent of cases (8) and present with obstruction and/or septal deviation (11,12). Intranasal lesions are clinically confused with nasal polyps. Nasal attachment occurs high within the nasal vault, along the lateral wall of the nasal fossa or middle turbinate. Rare reports of visual loss in adults have been attributed to HCNST (13).

Mixed extranasal and intranasal lesions represent approximately 10 percent of cases. Communication occurs through a defect in the nasal bone. Patients with HCNST have a negative Furstenberg test, which is the absence of swelling or a pulsating lesion following pressure on the ipsilateral jugular vein; typically patients with a positive Furstenberg test have an encephalocele.

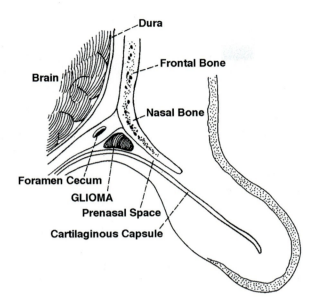

Figure 1-10

HETEROTOPIC GLIAL TISSUE/NASAL GLIOMA

Sagittal section of the nose shows the resultant glioma following closure of the foramen cecum. (Fig. 3 from Katz A, Lewis JS. Nasal gliomas. Arch Otolorynogol 1971;94:353.)

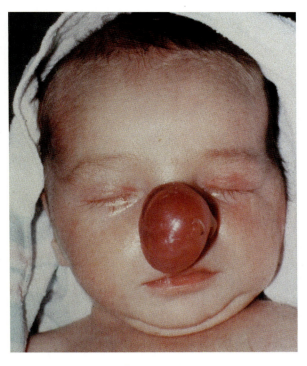

Figure 1-11

HETEROTOPIC NASAL GLIAL TISSUE

Sixty percent of heterotopic glial tissue arises as subcutaneous lesions anterior to the nasal bone.

Although growth is slow and limited, there often is some enlargement of the mass over many months. The size is generally limited to several centimeters in diameter, and the heterotopias do not reach as large a size as do some encephaloceles. Radiographic studies are indicated in order to rule out a bony defect which may identify communication to the cranial cavity, thereby representing an encephalocele.

There are rare reports of a dermal sinus (14) or overlying tuft of hair (15) associated with nasal glial heterotopia. This suggests an embryologic-developmental relationship to nasal dermoids.

Gross Findings. HCNSTs are firm, solid nodules that are 1 to 2 cm in diameter. They are gray to yellow, and are often streaked with white bands.

Microscopic Findings. Histologically, HCNST is composed of astrocytes, including those of the gemistocytic type, and neuroglial fibers associated with fibrous, vascularized connective tissue (fig. 1-12). Cells in the glial tissue may resemble plump fibroblasts (fig. 1-12). Ependymal cells may on rare occasion be identified (7). Usually there are thick fibrous septa within the lesion that can cause the entire tissue to be misjudged as fibrous (fig. 1-12). The fibrous bands tend to circumscribe nodules of glial tissue, and the resulting lobular architecture (albeit subtle on hematoxylin and eosin [H&E]-stained slides) is a frequently found characteristic feature.

The histologic diagnosis is usually uncomplicated, but in contrast to most encephaloceles, the tissue may not be so obviously "brain-like" in appearance, characterized by markedly sclerosed stroma in which the glial cells are fairly inconspicuous (16). Such lesions tend to be found in older patients and can cause problems in diagnosis. The tendency not to show a brain-like appearance is likely due to several factors. First, although rarely there may be a few neurons in the tissue (7,17), but usually there are none. Second, the finely fibrillary quality of the glial matrix may not be obvious. The CNS tissue is substantially different or altered from normal brain tissue and this may result from the development of the abnormal (heterotopic) lesion having been initiated very early and having proceeded extracranially in

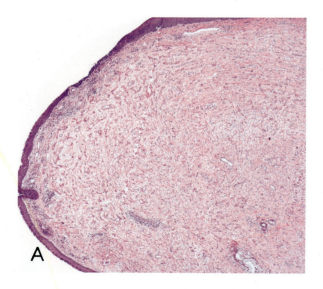
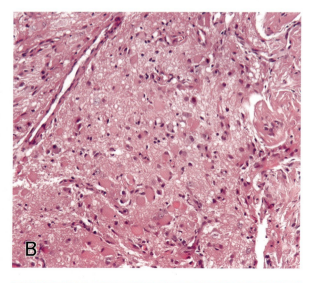

Figure 1-12

HETEROTOPIC NASAL GLIAL TISSUE

A: A polypoid, submucosal, nondescript proliferation is seen.

B: There is a variably cellular proliferation of astrocytes, enlarged (gemistocytic) multinucleated cells, and fibrillary glial processes.

C: In this example, the heterotopic lesion is less apparent given the presence of thick fibrous tissue within the lesion creating the appearance of a fibrous proliferation.

D: Even at higher magnification, the glial nature of the lesion may be difficult to appreciate.

E: The trichrome stain is positive in the fibroconnective tissue (upper left) while absent in the glial proliferation. Diffuse and intense immunoreactivity for glial fibrillary acidic protein (GFAP) confirms the glial nature of the proliferation (right).

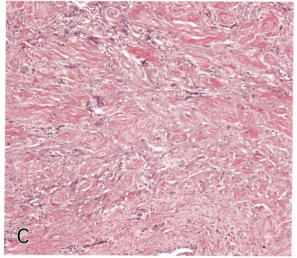
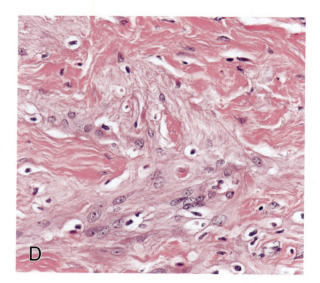
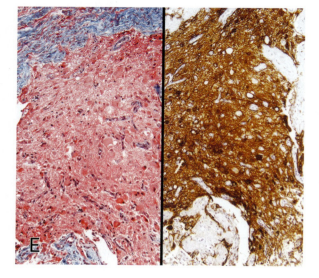

a fibrous microenvironment. If the diagnosis is suspected, however, the difference between the fibrous tissue and the glial tissue can be strikingly highlighted by a trichrome stain (fig. 1-12) and more definitively by immunoreactivity for glial fibrillary acidic protein (GFAP) (fig. 1-12) as well as S-100 protein (7,16).

Differential Diagnosis. Distinction from an encephalocele is important because of the definite communication of the latter with the cerebrospinal fluid (CSF) space. Since some glial HCNSTs have a fibrous stalk projecting to the cranial base and since some encephaloceles have only a meager cranial base defect, a feasible inference is that the heterotopias and encephaloceles may be manifestations of a similar developmental defect (18), with the heterotopias being the more meager or more "arrested" manifestation of the defect. In any event, distinction between the two may be difficult. Although radiographic features and surgical operative findings are the most definitive features of differentiation, the histopathologic features are important for diagnosis. The lobular architecture formed by circumscribing fibrous septa is more characteristic of a heterotopia. The finding of neurons favors an encephalocele but the absence of definite neurons, however, does not exclude an encephalocele. In general, an encephalocele is composed of tissue that is more obviously brain-like than is the case with the heterotopias.

If the glial nature of the tissue is overlooked, an intranasal glial heterotopia may be misinterpreted as an inflammatory polyp, especially if the child is older than an infant (with inflammatory nasal polyps being virtually absent in infants). The tissue of the heterotopia should be less edematous and less inflammatory than is expected in an inflammatory polyp.

Careful scrutiny of the tissue should allow distinction from a neurofibroma. The latter tends to have more spindled and elongated cells than a heterotopia.

Astrocytes within the glial tissue can sometimes be very gemistocytic and occasionally can cause some concern about a malignant lesion (19). Awareness of this phenomenon in this setting obviates the error of a malignant diagnosis.

When the glial nature of the lesion is discerned, the possibility of olfactory neuroblastoma may be considered, particularly since olfactory neuroblastomas are well known to occur mostly in young children. Olfactory neuroblastomas, however, although they certainly occur in pediatric patients, are not a primarily pediatric tumor; occurrence in an infant is not expected. Histologically, an olfactory neuroblastoma is distinctly more cellular than a congenital HCNST.

Treatment and Prognosis. Left untreated, the HCNSTs do not spontaneously regress. There is a small tendency for enlargement (20), perhaps via increased accumulation of reactive fibrous tissue (21), so operative removal is generally indicated. Every reasonable effort should be made to preoperatively judge the likelihood of a CSF communication (i.e., an encephalocele) so that the requirement of repair can be planned. If the lesion is indeed a heterotopia, the prognosis is excellent; these lesions do not produce a deforming hypertelorism (22) and operative removal produces no risk of CNS infection.

Encephaloceles

Definition. *Encephaloceles* are herniations of brain tissue beyond the confines of the cranial cavity. The abnormality is associated with a congenital developmental skull defect or an acquired condition, often related to some injury that results in a skull defect. The condition is called a meningoencephalocele when the meninges are present, but the shortened form of encephalocele is often understood to imply that the meninges are probably also involved in the formation of the lesion.

Encephaloceles are sincipital, occipital, and basal (23,24). A sincipital encephalocele is situated in the anterior part of the skull and is interfrontal (cranial defect lies between the two frontal bones) or frontoethmoidal (nasofrontal, nasoethmoidal, nasoorbital). Occipital encephaloceles are cervico-occipital, low occipital involving the foramen magnum, or high occipital above the intact rim of the foramen magnum. Basal encephaloceles are rare and are categorized by their point of passage through the skull and the area where they extend to: midline basal encephaloceles (transsphenoidal type, sphenoethmoidal type, transethmoidal type) and lateral basal encephaloceles (sphenorbital and sphenomaxillary types) (23).

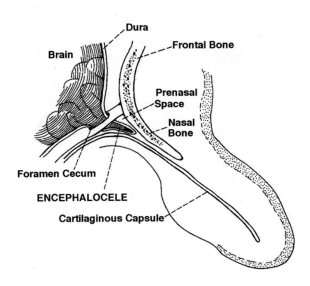

Figure 1-13

ENCEPHALOCELE

A sagittal section of the nose shows a developing encephalocele. (Fig. 2 from Katz A, Lewis JS. Nasal gliomas. Arch Otoloryngol 1971;94:352.)

Embryogenesis. Almost all encephaloceles seem to be sporadic and not related to recognized genetic syndromes (fig. 1-13). Occipital encephaloceles may be associated with other neural tube closure defects such as myelomeningocele; associated anomalies include cleft lip, cleft palate, nasal tip malformation, ocular abnormalities, and craniosynostosis (23,25,26). While occipital encephaloceles may be associated with other neural tube closure defects, anterior (sincipital or nasofrontal and basal) encephaloceles are seldom so associated.

One theory of genesis is a hypothetical failure of anterior neuropore closure. Since anterior encephaloceles are not associated with other neural tube closure defects, however, and there is no dysraphism of the brain underlying such an encephalocele, this seems to be an unlikely explanation. Also, the postembryonic site of anterior neuropore closure is in the area of the sphenoid sinus and this theory would not explain sincipital encephaloceles.

Another theory is a failure of ossification at foci in the anterior skull base. At the outset, this would seem to be a feasible theory, but embryologic-anatomic studies have indicated that the meningeal-neural protrusions that eventuate in an encephalocele are present quite early, and before ossification normally occurs, i.e., the failure of bone formation occurs around the protrusion defect as a secondary effect.

Perhaps the most likely explanation is that after the neural tube fissure closes, there may be connections ("adhesions") between the neural tissue and the overlying cutaneous ectodermal structures. If such a connection persists abnormally, then this could explain both the neural protrusion or herniation and the associated skull defect (the latter being a result of the former). In the sincipital area, this explanation has the appealing added capacity of explaining the formation of the dermoids that occur in the frontonasal area. The traction produced by the neural tube-ectodermal connection (adhesion) could either "pull out" neural tissue, resulting in glial heterotopia or encephalocele, or it could "pull in" cutaneous ectoderm, resulting in a dermoid. This common mechanism of genesis for both the frontonasal neural anomalies and dermoids is supported by a few reports suggesting that in rare instances there is evidence of both lesions in the same patient, i.e, a tuft of hair associated with a glial heterotopia (27) or some neural elements associated with a dermoid (28).

Clinical Features. The prevalence of congenital encephaloceles varies in different parts of the world from about 0.8 to 4.0 per 10,000 live births (25). They are more common in Asia than in the western hemisphere. The ratio of sincipital to occipital lesions also varies geographically. Sincipital encephaloceles are about nine times more frequent than occipital ones in Southeast Asia, but in Europe and North America, occipital lesions are more common. Basal encephaloceles are rare (2 to 10 percent of cases) in all geographic regions. The incidence of acquired sinonasal encephaloceles in adults is difficult to ascertain. Since some of these are postsurgical complications, they are seldom reported or catalogued. Also, many of these lesions are probably misdiagnosed as "heterotopias," with their true nature and genesis unrecognized.

Some acquired encephaloceles are probably related to head trauma other than a surgical cause. The cause of others is not clear. Such lesions conceivably develop from arachnoid granulations projecting into thinner areas of the

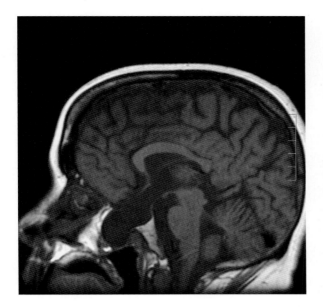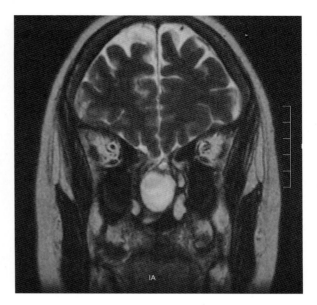

Figure 1-14

SPHENOETHMOIDAL ENCEPHALOCELE

Axial spin echo T1- (left) and coronal FSE T2-weighted (right) images demonstrate a defect in the sphenoid bone. A meningocele containing cerebrospinal fluid (CSF) and meninges extends through the sphenoid sinus into the posterior nasal cavity. (Courtesy of Dr. A. Khorsandi, New York, NY.)

skull base. Slowly, over many years, such projections can eventuate in resorbtive increased thinning ("remodeling") of the bone focally and occasionally cause an acquired encephalocele. Although not congenital, this cause of acquired encephalocele could be thought of as developmental in the broadest sense of the term.

Sincipital congenital encephaloceles usually form a visible midline or paramidline mass in the region of the bridge (root) of the nose and glabella, and are almost always evident at birth. Often these lesions are much larger than the glial heterotopias and are more compressible than the heterotopias. Hypertelorism may often be associated.

Basal encephaloceles do not produce a visible facial mass but rather are masses in the nasal or nasopharyngeal cavities (traversing the sphenoethmoid sinus areas), the posterior orbital region, or the sphenomaxillary fossa. The basal (internal) lesions may not be evident during infancy and may not present until the patient is significantly older, accounting for a "second peak" of encephalocele incidence around the age of 5 to 10 years (29). Likely the lesions slowly enlarge and thus tend to eventually become more symptomatic. Sometimes these lesions are clinically mistaken for an inflammatory nasal polyp, a potentially important error. For both the sincipital and basal lesions, it is important to search radiographically for evidence of a CNS (CSF) connection (fig. 1-14) so that the lesion is known not to be a heterotopia and the proper operative repair can be planned.

Gross Findings. Encephaloceles may be small but often are impressively large masses. The masses are moderately firm and pinkish, and surrounded by a pseudocapsule. They are usually solid, although there may be small cystic areas or collapsed spaces. These latter areas represent either extensions from the ventricular system (meningoencephalocystocele) or areas of degeneration of the brain tissue. The lesions are seldom recognizable as brain tissue grossly.

Microscopic Findings. Because of the nutritional impairment of the herniated brain tissue that constitutes an encephalocele, the tissue has degenerative-reactive alterations (of varying degrees and of variable chronicity). Neurons may disappear and gliosis may be prominent. Changes secondary to congestion or hemorrhage also contribute to the appearance. Even if neurons

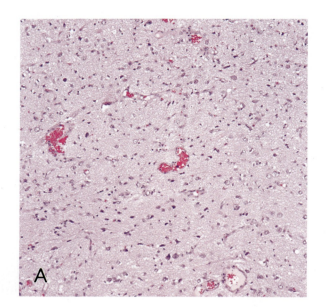
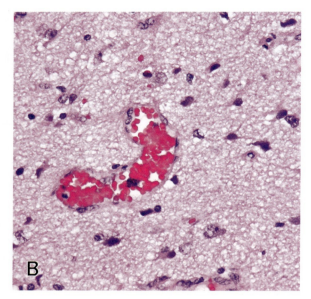
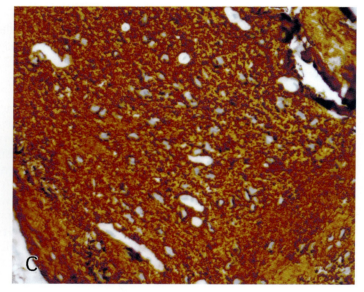

Figure 1-15

NASAL ENCEPHALOCELE

A,B: The encephalocele consists of mature glial tissue, including astrocytes.
C: GFAP staining is diffuse.

are not found, the tissue of encephaloceles usually is more similar to normal brain tissue than the tissue of a congenital heterotopia (fig. 1-15). Diffuse and strong immunoreactivity for GFAP is present (fig. 1-15)

Differential Diagnosis. The histologic distinction from heterotopic CNS tissue is discussed above. From a clinical standpoint, if the lesion presents in an adult patient, it is unlikely to be a congenital heterotopia. The chance of the lesion being a congenital heterotopia that was inapparent for decades and yet significant enough to become symptomatic in the adult is unlikely, although some basal-sinonasal encephaloceles presenting in adults (usually young adults) are actually congenital rather than acquired. Most, however, are acquired. Patients with encephaloceles have a positive Furstenberg test, characterized by swelling or a pulsating lesion following pressure on the ipsilateral jugular vein; typically patients with heterotopic CNS tissue have a negative Furstenberg test.

It is important not to mistake an encephalocele for a common inflammatory nasal polyp. Since the CNS tissue quality of an encephalocele is readily apparent, anything beyond a cursory examination of the tissue should obviate this error.

The histologic appearance may suggest a possible low-grade astrocytoma or other intracranial neoplasm. Clinical considerations should resolve the issue: a low-grade CNS neoplasm arising within the cranial cavity and presenting within the sinonasal tract, without an obvious intracranial origin, does not seem feasible.

Treatment and Prognosis. Congenital sincipital-basal encephaloceles require transcranial resection (30,31). If gross hypertelorism has developed, orbital translocation may be required. The developmental outcome has been normal in approximately 60 percent of cases (25). In adults, acquired encephaloceles may not be very large and the most important part of surgical removal may entail repair of a CNS leak and prevention of infection. The prognosis generally is good.

Nasal Dermoid Sinus and Cyst

Definition. *Nasal dermoid cyst* is a congenital developmental lesion that is virtually identical to dermoid cysts found in other anatomic locations. A congenital developmental origin is usually obvious for these nasal cysts since they usually present in infants or young children. A distinction should be made between nasal dermoids and so-called nasopharyngeal dermoids; the latter are not cysts and are considered to be ectopic accessory auricles (32). *Craniofacial dermoid cyst* is a synonym.

Embryogenesis. Although a few nasal dermoids are found in the lower and lateral regions (e.g., near the ala) of the nose, most are midline structures in the nasal bridge. As such, they are in the same location as glial heterotopias. The development of these two lesions seems related. It is useful to think of both as resulting from the cutaneous-neural connection or synechium in this location (33), with the glial tissue resulting from neural tissue being "pulled out" and the dermoid formed when cutaneous tissue is "pulled in" (although this may not quite literally describe the developmental dynamics).

Clinical Features. There is no gender predilection. Nasal dermoid cysts usually present in infants or young children, but may occur in adults (34). They are usually midline swellings at the root of the nose and make up approximately 10 percent of all dermoids in the cervicofacial region (35). Small lesions or deeply seated cysts may not be apparent until after they become infected and inflamed. A sinus tract with an epidermal opening may be present. Intracranial extension may occur (36–38). Rarely, patients present with a median upper lip fistula (37). Coexistence of a dermal sinus tract, dermoid cyst, and encephalocele has been reported in a patient presenting with nasal cellulitis (40).

Preoperative radiologic evaluation is essential to rule out intracranial extension. Computerized tomography (CT) and magnetic resonance imaging (MRI) are indicated to delineate deep tissue involvement and to exclude possible associated intracranial extension.

Nasal dermoid cysts and sinuses may be associated with or coexist with other congenital developmental malformations such as Gorlin syndrome (41). They may be familial (42).

Gross and Microscopic Findings. The macroscopic and microscopic findings are similar to those of dermoid cysts in more common locations. Grossly, these cysts vary in size from a few millimeters to several centimeters. On cut section, skin and hair are often readily identifiable and the contents of the cyst may include grumous and greasy material. Histologically, the cyst is lined by keratinized squamous epithelium; sebaceous glands, hair follicles, and sweat glands are typically identified. The wall of the cyst is thick with fibrovascular tissue. Respiratory epithelium may be identified. Endodermal and mesodermal elements are not found.

Differential Diagnosis. The histologic appearance usually is diagnostic. Problems can arise, however, if the tissue is mistaken for portions of the normal skin surface or if the features are obscured because of marked alterations secondary to infection. These potential problems should be kept in mind when examining a specimen from this anatomic location.

Treatment and Prognosis. Complete surgical resection is the treatment of choice and is usually curative (43–45). The most important treatment concern is the possibility of the associated existence of a deeply seated cyst or its related sinus tract involving the anterior midline skull base (46). Radiographic examination to judge the deep extent of the lesion is important in planning operative removal. Good cosmetic results and only a low recurrence rate can be expected (35). Lesions with intracranial extension have traditionally been managed with lateral rhinotomy, midface degloving, and external rhinoplasty approaches combined with a frontal craniotomy (38). Alternatively, a subcranial approach has been proposed that offers excellent exposure, minimizes frontal lobe retraction, reduces the likelihood of CSF leak, provides an excellent cosmetic result, and has shown long-term follow-up with no recurrence or negative effect on craniofacial growth (37).

Primary Ciliary Dyskinesia

Definition. *Primary ciliary dyskinesia* (PCD) is a multisystem disease caused by ultrastructural defects of the respiratory cilia and sperm tails. It is characterized by recurrent respiratory tract infections, sinusitis, bronchiectasis, and male subfertility; in about 50 of percent patients it is associated with situs inversus totalis (Kartagener syndrome). Synonyms include *immotile cilia syndrome* and *ciliary dysfunction*.

Pathogenesis. PCD is a heterogenetic disorder, usually inherited as an autosomal recessive trait, but pedigrees showing autosomal dominant or X-linked recessive modes of inheritance have been reported (47). Most cases are congenital and are due to an inborn genetic error, but some are acquired, usually the result of epithelial alterations subsequent to inflammatory disease. The acquired forms of the disorder are referred to as *secondary ciliary dyskinesia*. Ciliopathies are a category of diseases caused by the disruption of the physiologic functions of cilia (48–50).

Ciliary dysfunction results in a broad range of phenotypes, including renal, hepatic, and pancreatic cyst formation; situs abnormalities; retinal degeneration; anoxmia; cerebellar or other brain anomalies; postaxial polydactyly; bronchiectasis; and infertility. The specific clinical features are dictated by the subtype, structure, distribution, and function of affected cilia.

Genetic Mutations. PCD is genetically heterogenous. Currently, biallelic mutations in 31 genes are linked to PCD, allowing a genetic diagnosis in approximately 60 percent of cases (51). Ciliary gene mutations are now known to cause single organ disease, as well as complex syndromes. Different genes are involved in different patients; loss of function mutations in *ARMC4* cause PCD with situs inversus and cilia immotility, associated with a loss of the distal outer (but not inner) dynein arms (52).

Biochemical analysis in *Chlamydomonas* reveals that the C21orf59 ortholog FBB18 is a flagellar matrix protein that accumulates specifically when cilia motility is impaired (53). The *Chlamydomonas* ida6 mutant identifies CCDC65/FAP250 as an essential component of the nexin-dynein regulatory complex. Two genes associated with PCD-causing mutations elucidate two mechanisms critical for cilia motility and polarization: dynein arm assembly for *C21orf59/Kurly* (KUR) (53,54) and assembly of the nexin-dynein regulatory complex for CCDC65 (55). Mutations in *SPAG1* cause PCD with ciliary outer dynein arm and inner dynein arm defects (56).

Exome sequencing has identified loss of function mutations in *CCDC114* as a cause of PCD (57,58). ZMYND10 is a cytoplasmic protein required for inner and outer dynein arm assembly and its variants cause ciliary dysmotility and PCD (59). Loss of function *DYX1C1* mutations, a newly identified dynein axonemal assembly factor (DNAAF4), is found in patients with PCD (60). *RSPH1* mutations appear as a major etiology for a PCD phenotype that includes central complex and radial spoke defects (61). *RSPH3* mutations cause PCD with central complex defects and near absence of radial spokes, showing that *RSPH3* plays a key role in the proper building of radial spokes and central complexes in humans (62). Founder mutations in *RSPH4A* are a common cause of PCD without situs abnormalities in patients of Hispanic (Puerto Rican) descent (63). Mutations in *CCDC39* and *CCDC40* are the major cause of primary ciliary dyskinesia with axonemal disorganization and absent inner dynein arms (64,65).

Ultrastructural analysis (see below) and molecular genetics combined increase the diagnostic yield of PCD. Ciliary biopsy is unreliable as the sole criteria for a definitive diagnosis. Molecular genetic analysis can be used as a complementary test.

Clinical Features. PCD typically presents in the early neonatal period (66). If the diagnosis is considered in older children or adults and a reasonably reliable clinical history is devoid of evidence of prominent and persistent respiratory tract problems dating from early infancy,

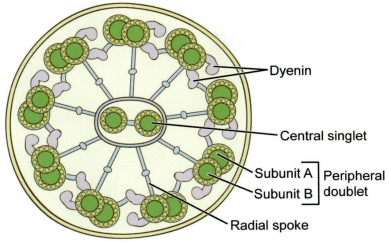

Figure 1-16

NORMAL CILIARY STRUCTURE

Schematic representation of a cross section of a ciliary axoneme (main body of the organellum) detailing the normal ciliary structures including the classic 9 + 2 microtubular pattern. (Courtesy of J. Gregory, Mount Sinai Health System.)

the diagnosis is probably incorrect. Almost all patients have sinusitis and otitis media; associated persistent mucopurulent rhinorrhea is often striking. Chronic bronchitis, recurrent pneumonia, and atelectasis are common. The presence of situs inversus in association with chronic bronchitis, recurrent pneumonia, and atelectasis is virtually pathognomonic for Kartagener syndrome and this clinical scenario generally does not require cilia evaluation for the diagnosis. Approximately 50 percent of patients lack situs inversus and in this setting ultrastructural examination of cilia is required for diagnosis.

Nitric Oxide Measurements. Exhaled and nasal nitric oxide (NO) measurements have been used to detect PCD in children (67). Nasal NO is significantly lower in children with proven PCD compared to those with negative biopsy results and healthy control subjects (68). Nasal NO has been reported to have 91 percent sensitivity and 96 percent specificity for PCD (69), and is thus a useful tool. Collins et al. (70), however, report that the predictive values of nasal NO are good in the referral population but extending screening to more general populations would result in excessive false positives. These authors indicate that although nasal NO remains a useful test, a normal result with a classic clinical history should still indicate a need for further testing.

Ultrastructural Findings. Ultrastructural examination of cilia is considered the "gold standard" for diagnosing PCD. For ultrastructural analysis a nasal cavity biopsy is usually the most easily obtained specimen. The anterior ends of the nasal turbinates are a readily accessible biopsy location, but these areas are where epithelial metaplastic changes are common, and in patients with the chronic rhinitis that occurs in PCD, the presence of squamous metaplasia of the anterior turbinate regions is likely. A biopsy from these areas will in all probability contain no cilia. In such a situation, a specimen is best obtained more toward the posterior part of the nasal cavity.

If lower respiratory tract endoscopy is done as a part of the patient's evaluation, obtaining a tracheal mucosal brushing or biopsy has a much higher chance of producing a specimen with abundant cilia. The difficulties with interpreting ultrastructural studies of clinical specimens increases the importance and applicability of fresh specimen "wet-prep" examinations of ciliary function as a low-cost effective means of excluding PCD (71).

The internal structure of the axoneme of normal cilia has classic 9 + 2 microtubular pattern (fig. 1-16). This includes a pair in the center composed of single microtubules (singlets), a peripheral row of 9 double-barreled (doublets) microtubules composed of subunits A and B, two short diverging arms (dynein arms) that project clockwise from subunit A of each doublet toward the next doublet, and radial spokes that connect subunit A to a central sheath surrounding the central singlets.

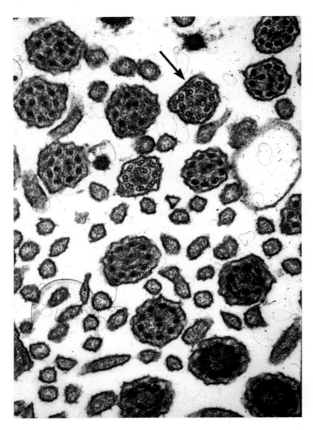 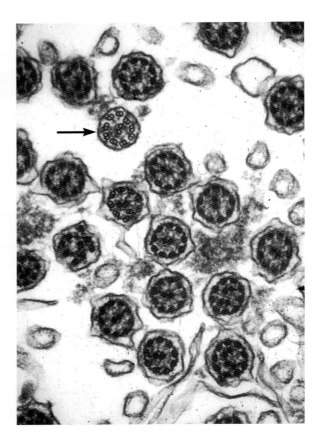

Figure 1-17

PRIMARY CILIARY DYSKINESIA

Electron microscopic evaluation shows absence of dynein arms (arrows), confirming the clinical suspicion of primary ciliary dyskinesia.

The structural abnormality that is most confidently diagnosed by ultrastructural examination is the absence of dynein arms (fig. 1-17). Dynein arms are necessary for the translational movement of ciliary peripheral doublet tubules with respect to one another (via a biochemico-physical "ratcheting-walking" mechanism). The absence of the arms results in a lack of capability for kinetic (i.e., dynamic) movement. In the presence of dynein arms, the diagnosis excludes the condition of "absence of dynein arms." Achieving technical results satisfactory for interpretation remains a significant challenge.

The evaluation of a dynein arm abnormality is problematic. The diagnosis requires that the sample have multiple ciliary cross-sections that have clear structural detail; otherwise, the lack of perception of the arms may be artifactual. Even in the most technically excellent photographic specimens, arms are not apparent on every peripheral tubule doublet because the arms are spaced along the longitudinal axis. If the technical results are mediocre or poor (as most seem to be), it is difficult to clearly see any arms even if the cilia are entirely normal.

These problems make the diagnosis of "partial absence of arms" or "shortened" or "defective" arms extremely difficult and of suspect validity in most instances; this is especially true of "absent inner arms" since the inner arms usually are seen less well than the outer. Having abundant cilia in the specimen is critical because it is often difficult to discern dynein arms, in part due to the fact that: the arms are tiny structures that are focally spaced along the ciliary axonemal tubules and, therefore, the quantity of electron dense material presented by the tiny arm is meager; the arms are tiny so high magnification is required; and combined with the meager density of the arm, the need for high magnification results in only a faint image with consequent visual resolution problems.

If the results strongly suggest a structural defect, it is probably best to obtain another sample from a different anatomic location to see if the same results are obtained. Genetic defects are universal in all of the patient's cilia and are permanent; obtaining samples from different locations or at significantly different times can help increase confidence in the diagnosis (72).

Diagnosis of PCD. Most patients are currently diagnosed with PCD based on the presence of defective ciliary ultrastructure. However, the diagnosis often remains challenging due to several issues. The clinical phenotype and ciliary ultrastructural changes are very variable. Approximately 21 percent of patients with PCD have normal ciliary ultrastructure, further confounding the diagnosis (69). Only 63 percent of pediatric ciliary biopsies are adequate for morphologic evaluation (73). A genetic test for PCD exists but is of limited value because it investigates only a limited number of mutations in only two genes. The genetics of PCD are complicated owing to the complexity of the axonemal structure, which is highly conserved through evolution and composed of multiple proteins. Identifying a PCD-causing gene is challenging due to locus and allelic heterogeneity. And finally, the presence of a limited number of known PCD-causing genes explains only 50 percent of PCD cases; hence, more genes need to be identified.

The diagnosis of PCD lacks a "gold standard" test. European guidelines recommend that PCD be confirmed in a specialist center using appropriate diagnostic testing (74). The symptoms of PCD are nonspecific. The diagnosis is based on a combination of tests including nasal NO level, high-speed video microscopy analysis (HSVMA), genotyping, and transmission electron microscopy (TEM) (69). Recently, a diagnostic predictive tool, referred to as PICADAR, was reported (75). PICADAR applies to patients with persistent wet cough and has seven predictive parameters including full-term gestation, neonatal chest symptoms, neonatal intensive care admittance, chronic rhinitis, ear symptoms, situs inversus, and congenital cardiac defects. PICADAR represents a simple diagnostic clinical prediction tool with good accuracy and validity for selecting patients for further diagnostic testing.

Differential Diagnosis. The diagnosis and differential diagnosis essentially rely on the presence of normal cilia versus abnormal cilia. Diagnosing a ciliary abnormality, with its implication of an incurable genetic defect, should be avoided, as such a diagnosis sentences a patient to an unwarranted pessimistic prognosis that could be of major negative emotional impact. If the results strongly suggest a structural defect, it is probably best to obtain another sample from a different anatomic location to see whether the same results are obtained.

Treatment and Prognosis. The presence of a ciliary abnormality represents a universal and permanent genetic defect in all of the patient's cilia. Early recognition and initiation of both otolaryngologic and pulmonary management may reduce potential long-term morbidities. The mainstays of therapy include, at a minimum, regular airway clearance, routine microbiological surveillance, antibiotic treatment for pulmonary exacerbation, and health vaccinations (76).

NONINFECTIOUS INFLAMMATORY AND TUMOR-LIKE PROCESSES

Sinonasal Inflammatory Polyps

Definition. *Sinonasal inflammatory polyps* are non-neoplastic inflammatory swellings of the sinonasal mucosa.

Clinical Features. There is no gender predilection. Sinonasal inflammatory polyps occur at all ages but are commonly seen in adults over 20 years of age and rarely seen in children less than 5 years of age. The exception to this age restriction occurs in patients with cystic fibrosis, who develop nasal polyps in the first and second decades of life. Most polyps arise from the lateral nasal wall or from the ethmoid recess. Both the nasal cavity and paranasal sinuses may be involved. Polyps may be unilateral or bilateral, single or multiple.

The symptoms include nasal obstruction, rhinorrhea, and headaches. The triad of nasal polyps, asthma, and aspirin intolerance is well recognized, and is referred to as Samter triad (77). Mulberry turbinate is a clinical term that refers to swollen nasal turbinate tissue formed

Non-Neoplastic Diseases of the Head and Neck

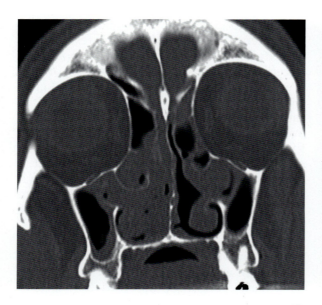 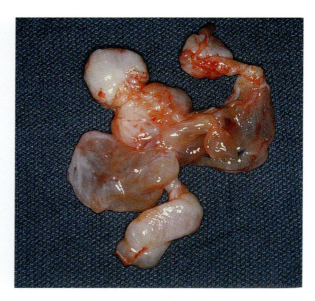

Figure 1-18

SINONASAL INFLAMMATORY POLYPS

Left: Coronal bone window image through the paranasal sinuses demonstrates multiple polypoid-appearing lesions involving the nasal cavity and the maxillary and ethmoid sinuses. (Courtesy of Dr. A. Khorsandi, New York, NY.)

Right: Large multilobular sinonasal inflammatory polyp with smooth and glistening to myxoid, mucoid, and fleshy appearance.

as a result of edema interspersed among the thick vessel walls of the prominent (essentially normal) turbinate vasculature; this appearance may clinically suggest a pathologic process such as a vascular malformation.

The radiologic appearance of sinonasal inflammatory polyps include soft tissue densities, air-fluid levels, mucosal thickening, and opacification of the paranasal sinuses (fig. 1-18). When extensive, inflammatory polyps may expand and even destroy bone.

Pathogenesis. The etiology is linked to multiple factors, including allergy (atopy), infections, cystic fibrosis, diabetes mellitus, and aspirin intolerance (78). Allergy and "atopy" are thought to be the main factors in generating inflammatory polyps (79), with infection, vasomotor instability, and, in rare instances, a condition such as cystic fibrosis, also considered causative. Although marked eosinophilic content probably has some association with allergic causation, quantitative variations in histologic features are poorly correlated with clinical impressions of causation.

The common occurrence of nasal polyps is probably related to the fact that the normal physiologic parameters of lateral nasal cavity mucosa are such that prominent edema forms in the mucosal lamina propria very readily. Thus, it is likely that polyps result from many mild stimuli or causative factors as long as they are chronic. Recently, hemokines, such as regulated on activation normal T-cell expressed and secreted (RANTES), have been implicated in the activation of inflammatory cells within the lamina propria of nasal polyps, possibly representing an important cytokine associated with cystic fibrosis–related polyps (80).

Gross Findings. Sinonasal polyps are soft, fleshy, polypoid lesions with a myxoid or mucoid appearance (fig. 1-18). They vary in size, ranging up to several centimeters in diameter.

Microscopic Findings. Characteristically, the overall low-magnification appearance is that of a polypoid lesion in which the stroma is markedly edematous and noteworthy for the absence of seromucous glands (fig. 1-19). A mixed chronic inflammatory cell infiltrate predominantly composed of eosinophils, plasma cells, and lymphocytes is present (fig. 1-19); neutrophils may predominate in polyps of infectious origin. In addition, the stroma

Nasal Cavity and Paranasal Sinuses

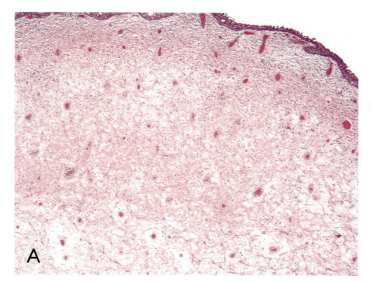
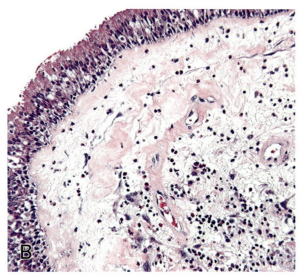
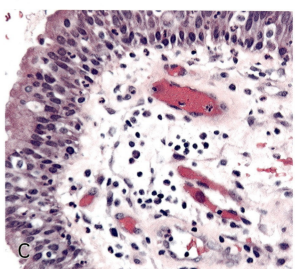

Figure 1-19

SINONASAL INFLAMMATORY POLYP

A: The polypoid lesion has an edematous stroma, the latter lacking seromucous glands.

B: Edematous stroma with mixed chronic inflammatory cells is seen below the intact ciliated respiratory epithelium with a slightly thickened basement membrane.

C: There are mixed inflammatory cells including mature lymphocytes, plasma cells, and eosinophils, and prominent vascularity including capillaries and larger vascular spaces.

contains bland-appearing fibroblasts and small to medium-sized blood vessels.

The stroma may have spaces containing a watery fluid and simulate the appearance of lymphatic spaces (pseudolymphangioma), suggesting a possible diagnosis of lymphangioma (fig. 1-20). However, in contrast to lymphangioma, these spaces lack an endothelial cell lining and do not stain for D2-40 (podoplanin). The surface epithelium of the inflammatory polyp is composed of intact respiratory epithelium that may show squamous metaplasia. Basement membrane thickening with an eosinophilic appearance may be present.

Secondary alterations include surface ulceration, fibrosis, infarction, granulation tissue, deposition of an amyloid-like stroma, osseous and/or cartilaginous metaplasia, glandular hyperplasia, granuloma formation, and atypical stromal cells. Granulomas result from ruptured mucous cysts, cholesterol granulomas, or as a reaction to medicinal intranasal injections (steroids) or inhalants. A prominent vascular component, variably termed angiomatous or angioectatic nasal polyps, may clinically and histologically simulate a malignant tumor.

Although both the gross and histologic appearances of prominent nasal polyps are well

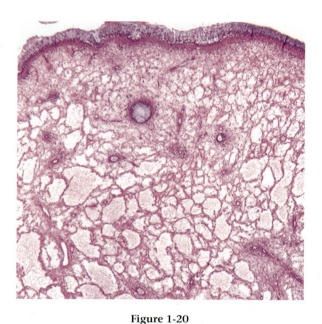

Figure 1-20

SINONASAL INFLAMMATORY POLYP

The stroma has spaces containing watery fluid, simulating the appearance of lymphatic spaces and suggesting a possible diagnosis of lymphangioma (pseudolymphangiomatous polyp). In contrast to lymphangiomas, the spaces in pseudolymphangiomatous inflammatory polyps lack an endothelial cell lining and are negative for D2-40 (podoplanin) (not shown).

known and generally not problematic to diagnose, in some instances, it may be difficult on a histologic basis to decide whether sinonasal tissue should be classified as only manifesting mild nonspecific ("physiologic") edema or labeled as inflammatory polyp(s). The clinical-surgical findings and the gross pathologic quantity of tissue can serve as a guide. It is likely, however, that small amounts of slightly edematous and slightly inflamed sinonasal tissues are "overdiagnosed" as inflammatory polyps by surgical pathologists.

Association with Other Histologic Lesions. Numerous specific sinonasal pathologic conditions, including neoplastic ones, are frequently accompanied by inflammatory polypoid tissues. This may be because inflammatory polyps are common and the association is coincidental. In many instances, however, the apparent polypoid tissues may not be de novo polyps but rather polypoid tissues engendered by the presence of the encountered specific pathologic condition. A case in point is the common (almost "routine") finding of markedly edematous stroma (indistinguishable from that of inflammatory polyps) as an integral part of most sinonasal (Schneiderian) papillomas. The frequency and blatancy of this finding have led some in the past to interpret (inverted type) sinonasal papillomas as an extensive metaplastic change in polyps rather than as an instance of benign neoplasia. In most instances, however, the polypoid stroma does not represent "true" inflammatory polyps but rather it is polypoid edema generated by the formation and presence of the papilloma. Thus, aside from some uncommon conditions such as cystic fibrosis, the apparent association of inflammatory polyps with most other sinonasal pathologic lesions is probably either coincidental or more apparent than real (i.e., a spurious finding of edematous tissue as an integral part of the lesion in question).

Antrochoanal Polyps. This is a clinically distinctive variant of inflammatory polyp that originates within the maxillary sinus (mostly from the medial wall) and extends via a small stalk through the ostium of the sinus into the nasal cavity; most of the growth occurs in the nasal cavity (fig. 1-21). The growth may be prominent, and sometimes this type of polyp extends well into the nasopharynx (fig. 1-21), hangs into the oropharynx, and is observable through the open mouth (fig. 1-21). Roughly 5 percent of surgically treated polyps are of the antrochoanal type (81), but this percentage is significantly increased in children. Nasal polyps are uncommon in children, but a polyp in a child is likely to be the antrochoanal type.

Since the polyp may be a large mass with a small stalk, and since the stalk extends through a small channel, these polyps are particularly subject to secondary changes resulting from chronic or subacute vascular compromise. These changes may range from a simple increase in stromal fibrosis (fig. 1-22) to the more striking alterations described in the next two variants.

Polyps with Atypical Stromal Cells. Some inflammatory sinonasal polyps (particularly the antrochoanal type) develop a striking atypia of some of the stromal cells (fig. 1-23) that can be mistaken for malignancy (82–84). The atypical stromal cells are bizarre-appearing cells with enlarged, pleomorphic and hyperchromatic nuclei, indistinct to prominent nucleoli, and

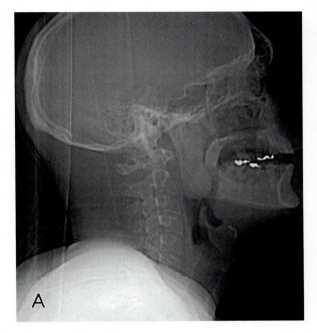
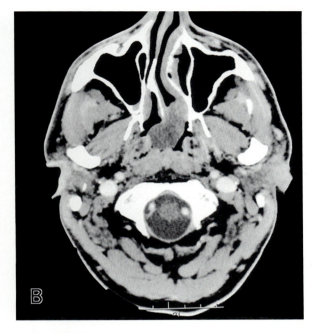
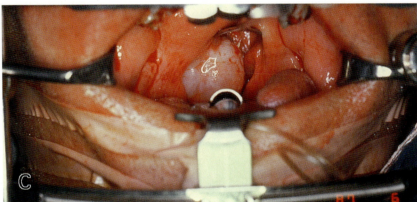

Figure 1-21

ANTROCHOANAL POLYP

A,B: Lateral radiograph (A) and axial soft tissue image (B) of the neck show a nasal polyp protruding into the nasopharyngeal airway. (Courtesy of Dr. A. Khorsandi, New York, NY.)

C: Intraoperative appearance of an antrochoanal polyp appearing as a polypoid smooth-contoured mass extending into the oropharynx and observable through the open mouth.

Figure 1-22

ANTROCHOANAL POLYP

Among a variety of secondary changes that can be seen in association with antrochoanal polyps is the presence of stromal fibrosis.

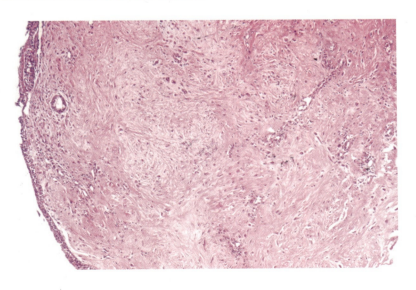

Figure 1-23

SINONASAL POLYP WITH ATYPICAL STROMAL CELLS

A: The atypical stromal cells (arrows) tend to cluster near areas of tissue injury, including near thrombosed vascular spaces.

B,C: The atypical stromal cells are bizarre-appearing, with enlarged, pleomorphic and hyperchromatic nuclei, indistinct to prominent nucleoli, and eosinophilic to basophilic cytoplasm. The atypical cells represent reactive myofibroblasts and typically show immunoreactivity for vimentin, actins (smooth muscle and muscle specific), and desmin but are negative for myoglobin and myogenin as well as epithelial markers (cytokeratins) although they may rarely be keratin positive.

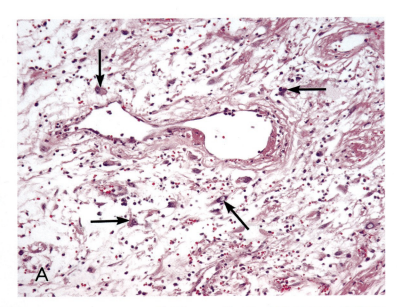

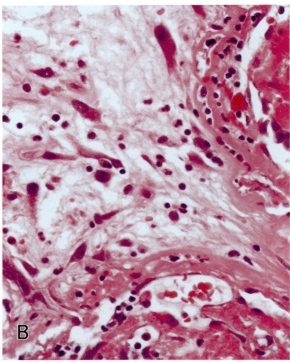

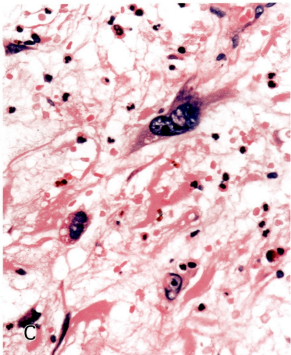

eosinophilic- to basophilic-appearing cytoplasm. These cells tend to cluster near areas of tissue injury (e.g., near thrombosed vascular spaces) (fig. 1-23). In the past, the tissue usually was mistaken for rhabdomyosarcoma, a mistake that was enhanced when the lesion was found in a child, which was frequently the case. Fortunately, the advent of immunohistochemistry has helped to prevent this error since the atypical cells do not stain like rhabdomyoblasts. Immunoreactivity is present for vimentin and actins (smooth muscle and muscle specific), and occasionally for desmin, but is negative for myoglobin and myogenin (MYF-4). The atypical stromal cells may show some keratin reactivity (84) and this has introduced the "new" problem of sometimes suggesting the diagnosis of spindle cell squamous carcinoma (sarcomatoid carcinoma).

The atypical cells may be (at least partly) a response to injury, such as thrombosis or trauma, and represent reactive ("pumped up") myofibroblasts. Such cells usually are widely dispersed or only focally present, and in conjunction with their tendency to cluster near areas of injury, help differentiate the lesion from either sarcoma or sarcomatoid carcinoma, both of which should have at least some areas with more densely distributed atypical cells. Also, although the cells are large and moderately darkly staining, the nuclei, while also large, are round or oval and not irregular in outline. Further, there usually is an ample amount of cytoplasm so that there is no substantive increase in the nuclear to cytoplasmic ratio.

Polyps with Partial Infarction. Occasionally, inflammatory nasal polyps are partially or extensively infarcted, presumably through compromise of the vascular supply at their base (85). The small stalk of antrochoanal polyps explains why this variant is particularly subject to this alteration. When the infarction occurs, the tissues are subject to hemorrhage and this can be extensive (fig. 1-24). The latter is particularly true when the patient has a bleeding diathesis, as is sometimes the case.

Since inflammatory polyps are sometimes quite large and extensive tissue masses (enhanced by the ubiquitous prominent edema), when the hemorrhagic infarction ensues it can eventuate in an even more impressively large or extensive process simulating a neoplastic proliferation. For reasons that are not entirely clear, the hemorrhage and subsequent reactive-organizational changes often result in bone erosion of the lateral nasal cavity-medial maxillary sinus wall, and this bone loss can be extensive (86). Because of the radiographic features of the lesion (which often is strictly unilateral), the clinical concern for a malignant neoplasm can be strong. Of course, extensive necrosis and hemorrhage could obscure a small amount of neoplastic tissue and a diagnosis of nothing more than infarcted polyps must be made carefully. Usually, however, the amount of tissue surgically removed is large (because of the clinical concern for neoplasm), and if this tissue is thoroughly examined, the diagnosis can usually be confidently rendered. The organizational changes in the hemorrhagic tissues usually include extensive neovascularization (fig. 1-24), with or without papillary endothelial hyperplasia (fig. 1-24) (87), and it is important not to mistake this for a vascular neoplasm (see Differential Diagnosis below).

Polyps and Cystic Fibrosis. Cystic fibrosis (CF) tends to promote the formation of nasal polyps and this may occur in young children. Since nasal polyps in young children otherwise are uncommon, their presence may be a sign of CF. It has been claimed that the polyps in a CF patient are histologically a bit different from "ordinary" polyps (88), but the spectrum of variation of the usual polyps is so broad that it is unlikely that such features are reliable in a practical situation.

Minor Variations and Histologic Alterations. Although the stroma of inflammatory polyps normally is markedly edematous, occasionally small patches of nonedematous collagen are scattered in the polyp. For some reason these patches may have inflammatory cells aggregated around the periphery and the appearance can suggest a granuloma. When closely examined, however, these *pseudogranulomas* are seen not to be composed of a core of histiocytes but rather of more fibrous tissue (albeit perhaps somewhat altered by a mild inflammatory cell infiltrate).

A *pseudolymphangioma* can form in a polyp when the edema is so massive that wisps of collagen are spread apart to form a network and the intervening spaces only contain watery fluid. This fluid disappears during processing and the resulting multiple empty spaces can superficially resemble a lymphangioma. Although a few scattered fibrocytic nuclei may remain, close examination reveals an absence of endothelial cells lining the faint septa, and this can prevent a misinterpretation.

The clinical term of *mulberry turbinate* refers to swollen nasal turbinate tissue that has formed because of edema interspersed among the thick vessel walls of the prominent turbinate vasculature. The histologic contrast with the pale edema fluid makes the thick-walled vessels stand out more clearly than normal, and the resulting picture can suggest a vascular malformation, suggested also by the clinical abnormality of an enlarged turbinate. The vascularity, however, is essentially normal.

Non-Neoplastic Diseases of the Head and Neck

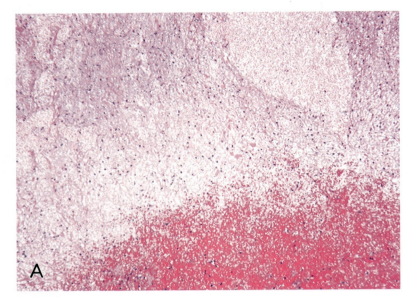

Figure 1-24

INFARCTED INFLAMMATORY POLYP

A: Hemorrhagic change is seen.

B,C: The organizational changes in the hemorrhagic tissues include extensive neovascularization.

C: Papillary endothelial hyperplasia may be present.

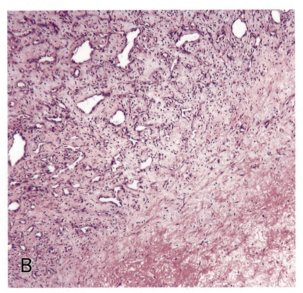
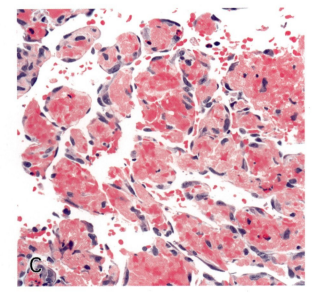

Differential Diagnosis. Almost any nasal neoplasm can be clinically polypoid, and a lesion labeled as a "nasal polyp" at surgery may on occasion result in a major surprise for the surgical pathologist. The surprise may histologically be obvious or subtle. It is the last instance that is potentially problematic because of the proclivity to overlook the correct diagnosis when a nasal inflammatory polyp is expected. The clinical location may provide a clue. For example, inflammatory polyps are not expected to arise from the septum or from the nasopharynx proper and if the lesion is clinically from either of these locations, another diagnosis is suspected. Since some nasal cavity hamartomas (see later in this chapter) arise from the septum and since histologically they can have a stroma similar to that of polyps, this locational information can be useful.

Nasal cavity tissues often manifest some edema without necessarily forming a clinical polyp. Usually, frank polyps are massively edematous and the gross appearance of the tissues suggests the diagnosis. Before making a diagnosis of inflammatory polyps, the clinical or gross pathologic evidence to suggest the presence of a polypoid mass should be considered.

Sinonasal (Schneiderian) papillomas may occur in the background of histologic changes similar to those seen in a sinonasal inflammatory polyp. The endophytic or exophytic surface epithelial proliferation seen in association with sinonasal (Schneiderian) papillomas is absent in sinonasal inflammatory polyps.

Antrochoanal polyps may extend well into the nasopharynx as a mass lesion. Since these polyps have a propensity for occurring in young persons, it is not surprising that occasionally they are mistaken (both clinically and histopathologically) as a (juvenile) nasopharyngeal angiofibroma (NPAF). The clinical knowledge that the origin of the mass is anterior in the nasal cavity (which is not compatible with NPAF), helps avoid a misdiagnosis.

The exuberant organizational vascular proliferation that develops in infarcted polyps can be mistaken for angiosarcoma. The hemorrhage that usually occurs in association with such infarction produces a hematoma with platelets and clotting factors that is an extravascular analogy of an intravascular thrombus; the hematoma can develop "papillary endothelial hyperplasia" (fig. 1-24) identical to that in an organizing thrombus (87). Accordingly, the pathologist's familiarity with the latter helps distinguish organized infarcted polyps from angiosarcoma. Also, compared with the common benign (reactive) vascular proliferations that occur in the sinonasal tract (e.g., lobular capillary hemangioma) (89), actual angiosarcomas are rare.

Altered brain tissue may not be immediately recognized as such, and acquired encephaloceles may be mistaken for inflammatory polyps. Any suggestion on routine light microscopic staining of the possibility of CNS tissue should prompt use of appropriate immunostains (e.g., GFAP) to check this possibility further.

Treatment and Prognosis. Surgical excision includes polypectomy for nasal polyps and medial maxillectomy (Caldwell-Luc procedure) to include removal of the stalk for antrochoanal polyps. Following surgery, recurrence rates are highest in patients with aspirin intolerance and asthma (90). For antrochoanal polyps, if the surgical resection does not include the stalk, then recurrence rates of up to 30 percent occur. The development of functional endoscopic sinus surgery (FESS) has decreased the morbidity of sinonasal surgery and the recurrence of nasal polyposis, including antrochoanal polyps (91), especially when combined with medial maxillectomy; these modalities allow for better visualization of the maxillary sinus walls and, therefore, easier resection of the remnant polyp (92).

Patients with cystic fibrosis and sinonasal disease may respond to medical therapy but surgical resection may be required. Systemic steroid treatment is effective in decreasing polyp size and in controlling mucosal inflammation (93); it may also help prevent recurrence.

Paranasal Sinus Mucocele

Definition. The term "mucocele" has been used for several conditions that are distinctly different from one another etiologically, radiographically, clinically, and histopathologically. A *paranasal sinus mucocele* (PSM) is a distinct clinicopathologic entity that is frequently overdiagnosed (i.e., misdiagnosed) both clinically and pathologically because most physicians are not well versed with its specific features.

PSM is a slow-evolving expansion of a sinus cavity caused by obstruction of the outflow tract (ostium or duct). The lining of the sinus continues to secrete mucus and the continuously accumulating mucus produces the expansion of the sinus cavity. The expansion of the bony walls of the sinus or air cell cavity is the *sine qua non*, the essential elements of PSM.

Pathogenesis. Obstruction of sinus egress is often caused by some type of trauma, and patients often have a history of prior sinonasal surgery which is likely the cause of the obstruction (94,95). This is especially true in the case of frontal sinus or fronto-ethmoid mucoceles (by far the most common location for "true" PSMs). The fronto-nasal duct is long and narrow, and thus can easily be obstructed. In patients without a history of surgery or other trauma, the cause may be inflammatory-reactive sequelae, although often the specific cause is not confidently known.

Clinical Features. There is no gender predilection and PSM occurs in all age groups. With the quantity of mucus that can be generated by the sinonasal mucosa (especially evident if the patient has a cold or allergic condition), it seems likely that a PSM would develop quickly if sinus outflow was completely obstructed. This is not a characteristic of PSM, however. Either

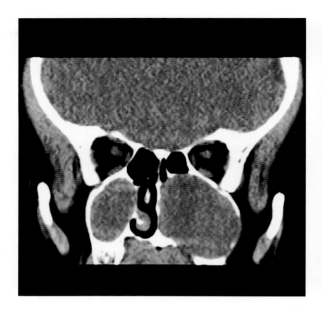 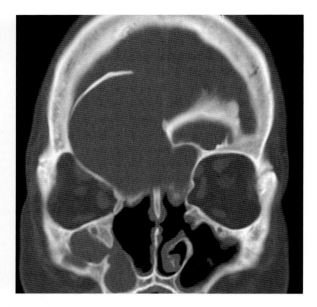

Figure 1-25

SINUS MUCOCELE

Left: Coronal soft tissue window image demonstrates an expansile lesion completely opacifying the left maxillary sinus with associated dehiscence of the lateral and inferior osseous periphery.

Right: Coronal bone window image of the sinus demonstrates complete opacification of an expansile right frontal sinus with dehiscence of the superior sinus wall in the patient who had previous sinus surgery. (Courtesy of Dr. A. Khorsandi, New York, NY.)

obstruction is almost never complete, or there is some resorption of mucus components, attenuation of mucus production, or some other factor that results in the slow expansion of the sinus. Consequently, symptoms and signs are not acute and, aside from eventual marked enlargement of the sinus, generally not severe.

PSMs occur in the frontal and ethmoid sinuses in over 90 percent of cases (96); the maxillary sinus is a less frequent site of occurrence with less than 10 percent of cases occurring in that location (97). Rarely, the sphenoid sinus is involved. Symptoms depend on the site of involvement as well as the direction and extent of expansion, and include pain, facial swelling or deformity, proptosis, enophthalmos, visual disturbances (e.g., diplopia, loss of vision, sudden blindness), optic neuropathy rhinorrhea, and nasal obstruction. Expansion of a mucocele is in the direction of least resistance and extension into the cranial cavity may occur (98). The clinical picture may be mistaken for a neoplasm, rhinorrhea, or nasal obstruction.

With the slow enlargement of the sinus cavity, the bony walls of the cavity manifest the same radiographically, that is, the cavity has a smoothly contoured expanded wall with reactive bony thickening. The lesion often is strikingly rounded and, together with the homogeneous mucoid contents, the radiographic findings are highly characteristic (fig. 1-25).

Gross Findings. Although the gross findings at surgery (large cavity with fairly smooth walls and a large amount of thick mucoid contents) are helpful, the gross features of the pathologic specimen are nonspecific. The mucus is never thickened or inspissated enough to be submitted to pathology; the mucus apparently goes into the surgeon's aspirator or otherwise disappears. The removed tissues are fragmented and there is none of the architecture apparent that is so helpful in the radiographic findings. In this situation, it is best to consider the more informative radiographic findings as a substitute for gross pathology.

Microscopic Findings. Like the gross pathologic features, the histologic findings are usually disappointingly nonspecific. The specimen may contain a moderately large portion of the bony wall of the lesion, and the slightly curved and

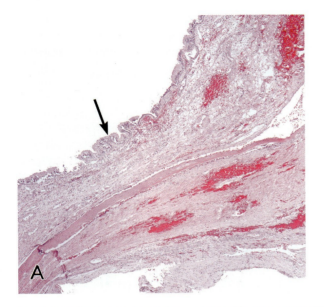
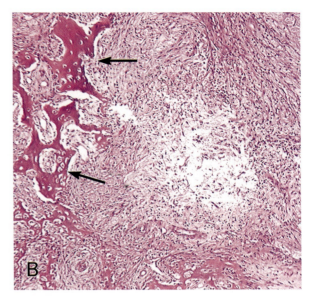
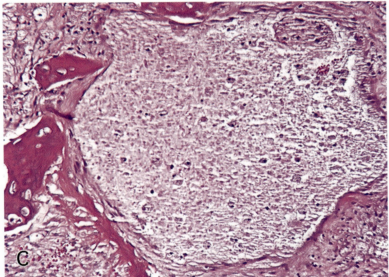

Figure 1-26

PARANASAL SINUS MUCOCELE

A: Like the gross pathologic features, the histologic findings are disappointingly nonspecific and include intact surface epithelium (arrow) closely applied to and following the smooth contour of the bone.

B: Secondary alterations that assist in the histologic diagnosis include reactive new bone formation (arrows).

C: Extravasated mucus is present within soft tissues of the sinus (mucicarmine stain).

smoothly contoured architecture of this bone, together with mucosal surface epithelium being closely applied to and following the smooth contour of the bone, provide histologic support for the diagnosis (fig. 1-26). The bone often manifests a suggestion of reactive new bone formation and this adds to the histologic picture (fig. 1-26). Otherwise, soft tissues and mucosal epithelium often do not show any helpful features.

Occasionally, some of the mucus that had been in the mucocele cavity focally escapes into soft tissues and a mucicarmine stain can highlight this finding (fig. 1-26). It is surprising that the respiratory epithelium lining the mucocele usually shows no metaplastic alterations. If increased pressure inside the cavity is the genesis of the expansile lesion (and this indeed is the working hypothesis), then some chronic alteration of the lining epithelium is expected. The explanation for this negative finding is not completely clear; perhaps the pressure increase, if very minimal, only accomplishes the bony expansion by acting over a very long period of time and the pressure increase is not sufficient to injure the epithelium.

Differential Diagnosis. Relatively nonspecific histologic findings are expected with PSM, and if there are more specific features, an alternative diagnosis may be suspected. Extensive masses of mucoid material with inflammatory cells is not expected with PSM. The probable diagnosis in this case would be allergic fungal sinusitis (see below). The presence of prominent inflammatory polypoid tissue suggests inflammatory polyps. Extensive or densely packed inflammatory cells point toward some inflammatory condition and not PSM.

The importance of considering the radiologist's opinion as to whether the diagnosis of PSM is likely correct or incorrect cannot be overemphasized. For example, there are pseudocysts and retention cysts of the maxillary sinus that sometimes are clinically referred to and pathologically diagnosed as mucoceles, but the radiographic features are completely distinctive.

Treatment and Prognosis. Surgical resection is the treatment of choice (99,100). The prognosis following complete removal is excellent.

Sinonasal Hamartomas

The classification of *sinonasal hamartomas* is listed in Table 1-2. Sinonasal hamartomas are uncommon. Most are of the pure epithelial type (respiratory epithelial adenomatoid hamartoma and seromucinous hamartoma); mesenchymal hamartomas or mixed epithelial-mesenchymal hamartomas occur less commonly. The various features among sinonasal hamartomas are contrasted in Table 1-3. Since cases show the histologic features of both respiratory epithelial adenomatoid hamartoma and seromucinous hamartoma, these lesions may represent a spectrum of the same lesion rather than different lesions.

On the basis of the presence of increased fractional allelic loss (FAL) reported in respiratory epithelial adenomatoid hamartomas, it remains an open issue whether these lesions are non-neoplastic or neoplastic. Our understanding of the nature of these hamartomas is still evolving, and as such, this text classifies these lesions as non-neoplastic, and separates respiratory epithelial adenomatoid hamartoma and seromucinous hamartoma, although any given case may show the histologic features of both.

Table 1-2
CLASSIFICATION OF SINONASAL HAMARTOMAS

Epithelial
Respiratory epithelial adenomatoid hamartoma (REAH)
Seromucinous hamartoma (SH)

Mixed Epithelial and Mesenchymal
Chondro-osseous and respiratory epithelial (CORE) hamartoma

Mesenchymal
Nasal chondromesenchymal hamartoma (NCMH)

Table 1-3
COMPARISON OF SINONASAL HAMARTOMAS

	REAH[a]	SH	CORE	NCMH
Age/Gender	M>F; 3rd to 9th decades, median 6th decade	M>F; 2nd decade to 9th decades	M = F; 2nd to 8th decades	M>F; most occur in newborns within the first 3 months of life but may occur in the 2nd decade, and occasionally in adults
Site(s) of Occurrence	Nasal cavity, in particular posterior nasal septum; involvement of other intranasal sites occurs less often and may be identified along the lateral nasal wall, middle meatus, and inferior turbinate; other sites of involvement include the nasopharynx, ethmoid sinus, and frontal sinus	Posterior nasal septum although may occur in the lateral nasal wall, paranasal sinuses, and nasopharynx	Nasal cavity most common; other sites include nasopharynx, ethmoid sinus, and splenoid sinus	Intranasal mass or facial swelling; may erode into the cranial cavity (through the cribriform plate area)

Table 1-3, continued

	REAH[a]	SH	CORE	NCMH
Histology	Glandular proliferation composed of widely spaced, small to medium-sized glands separated by stromal tissue; glands arise in direct continuity with the surface epithelium, which invaginates downward into the submucosa; glands are round to oval and composed of multilayered ciliated respiratory epithelium often with admixed mucin-secreting (goblet) cells; characteristic finding is the presence of stromal hyalinization with envelopment of glands by a thick, eosinophilic basement membrane; atrophic glands may be lined by a single layer of flattened to cuboidal-appearing epithelium; reactive seromucinous gland proliferation present between glandular proliferations	Dense serous gland proliferation with back-to-back appearance resembles a cribriform pattern of growth; glands are lined by low cuboidal to flat epithelial cells with round to oval nuclei and a variable amount of basophilic to eosinophilic to clear cytoplasm; invagination of the surface respiratory epithelium with at least focal merging with the glandular proliferation; periglandular hyalinization may be present; lack a significant mucinous cell component although focal mucinous change may be found; residual seromucinous glands with retention of their lobular architecture and haphazard growth of glands represent important findings that allow for differentiation from sinonasal low-grade adenocarcinoma	Histologic features of REAH (although adenomatoid components tend to be less prominent) and intimate association with cartilaginous and/or osseous trabeculae	Nodules of cartilage varying in size, shape, and contour; loose spindle cell stroma or abrupt transition to hypocellular fibrous stroma present at the periphery of the cartilaginous nodules; other patterns include a myxoid to spindle cell stroma, fibro-osseous proliferation with cellular stromal component and ossicles or trabeculae of immature (woven) bone; focal osteoclast-like giant cells in the stroma and erythrocyte-filled spaces resembling those of the aneurysmal small bone cyst; mature adipose tissue; proliferating epithelial elements are not a prominent feature
IHC	Cytokeratin positive (AE1/AE3, CAM5.2, CK7); negative for CK20 and CDX2; p63 and CK903 (34βE12) staining of basal (myoepithelial) cells but may be absent; S-100 protein may or may not be positive; low proliferation rate	Seromucinous glands reactive for CK7, CK17, CK19, HMWK; negative for CK14, CK20; p63, calponin, MSA typically negative but in any given case may be positive; S-100 protein staining is limited to the seromucinous glands; collagen type IV and laminin staining present around the glandular proliferation; low proliferation rate	None reported	Cartilaginous nodules and mesenchymal stromal component S-100 protein positive (more intense staining in cartilaginous components); spindle cell stroma vimentin and smooth muscle actin positive; muscle-specific actin (HHF35) may be present
Molecular Findings	Increased fractional allelic loss (as compared to chronic sinusitis but less than that for adenocarcinoma)	Higher mutation rate in comparison to normal seromucinous glands	None reported	12;17 translocation, t(12;17)(q24.1;q21)
Associated Lesions	Sinonasal inflammatory polyps; hyperplasia and/or squamous metaplasia of the surface epithelium unrelated to the adenomatoid proliferation; osseous metaplasia; rare association with inverted type schneiderian papillomas, and solitary fibrous tumor; reported instances of low-grade adenocarcinomas associated with REAHs	Sinonasal inflammatory polyps; REAH	None reported	Pleuropulmonary blastoma

[a]REAH = respiratory epithelial adenomatoid hamartoma; SH = seromucinous hamartoma; CORE = chondro-osseous and respiratory epithelial (CORE) hamartoma; NCMH = nasal chondromesenchymal hamartoma; IHC = immunohistochemistry; HMWK = high molecular weight keratin; MSA = muscle-specific actin.

Respiratory Epithelial Adenomatoid Hamartoma

Definition. *Respiratory epithelial adenomatoid hamartoma* (REAH) is a benign acquired non-neoplastic overgrowth of indigenous glands of the nasal cavity, paranasal sinuses, and nasopharynx arising from the surface epithelium and devoid of ectodermal, neuroectodermal, and mesodermal elements. Synonyms include *glandular hamartoma* and *nasal hamartoma*.

Pathogenesis. These are not congenital lesions and occur virtually only in adults. Consequently, some may object to the classification as hamartoma, since the latter are considered developmental. In the broadest sense, however, development does not cease in childhood and, in any case, apparently non-neoplastic tissue masses can develop from the overgrowth of otherwise normal adult tissues. Most pathologists accept REAH as being within the spectrum of hamartomas.

Considered to be an acquired lesion, the possible stimulus for growth may relate to an underlying chronic inflammatory condition (101). This possibility is supported by occurrence in the setting of inflammatory polyps, raising a possible developmental induction secondary to the inflammatory process. There is no association with any specific etiologic agent such as environmental or occupational exposure, tobacco use or alcohol abuse.

The FAL of 31 percent for REAL falls between an FAL of 1 percent for chronic sinusitis and 64 percent for sinonasal adenocarcinoma (102). Based on the appreciable allelic loss within hamartomas, which is considered unusually high for a non-neoplastic entity, the possibility that REAH is a benign neoplasm rather than a hamartoma has been suggested (102), but remains uncertain.

Clinical Features. REAHs occur in adults of a wide age range, from the third to the ninth decades of life. They form nondestructive nasal cavity masses that become symptomatic because of nasal obstruction. They may be polypoid and may be mistaken for nasal polyps. Often, however, there are features that are not expected with inflammatory polyps. The most frequent site of origin is from the nasal septum, especially from the extreme posterior edge of the septum (101), while inflammatory polyps arise from the lateral portions of the sinonasal tract and hardly ever from the septum. Also, these hamartomas are often firmer than are most inflammatory polyps, and this may lead the clinician to suspect something unusual.

Microscopic Findings. The histopathologic changes are dominated by the presence of a glandular proliferation composed of widely spaced, small to medium-sized glands separated by stromal tissue, including the presence of clusters of seromucinous glands (fig. 1-27). In areas, the glands arise in direct continuity with the surface epithelium, which invaginates downward into the submucosa (fig. 1-27). These histologic findings differentiate REAH from inflammatory polyps. The link with the surface epithelium usually can be seen, but the branching growth can be so marked that most of the proliferation is cross-sectioned and appears as gland-like formations which resemble an adenoma (hence, "adenomatoid"). The epithelium lining the glandular proliferation is identical to the ciliated surface epithelium, and this finding is different from what is seen in a "true" (i.e., neoplastic) adenoma (fig. 1-27).

The glands are round to oval and composed of multilayered ciliated respiratory epithelium, often with admixed mucin-secreting (goblet) cells (fig. 1-28). A characteristic finding is the presence of stromal hyalinization and the envelopment of glands by a thick, eosinophilic basement membrane (fig. 1-28). Some of the glands become quite cystically distended with mucus. Atrophic changes include the presence of an attenuated single layer of flattened to cuboidal epithelium (fig. 1-29). Small reactive-appearing seromucinous glands are seen around the larger glandular proliferation; sometimes, marked proliferation of seromucinous glands with features of a seromucinous hamartoma (see below) are present. The stroma is edematous or fibrous, containing a mixed chronic inflammatory cell infiltrate. Reactive fibrosis in the stroma can cause some of these glands to assume an irregular shape and irregular distribution, suggesting an infiltrative neoplasm, such as an adenocarcinoma.

In addition to the glandular proliferation in REAH, there may be sinonasal inflammatory polyps, epithelial hyperplasia, squamous metaplasia of the surface epithelium, and osseous metaplasia. Rarely, sinonasal (Schneiderian) papillomas and solitary fibrous tumor are

Nasal Cavity and Paranasal Sinuses

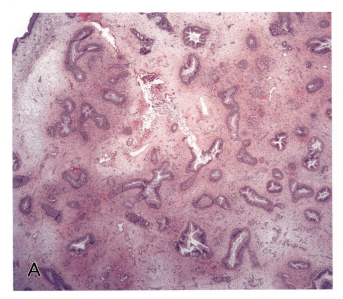
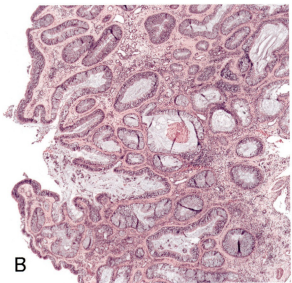
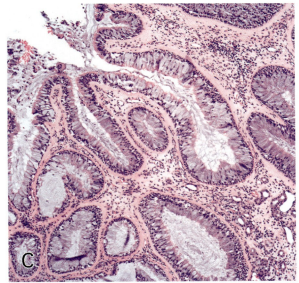

Figure 1-27

RESPIRATORY EPITHELIAL ADENOMATOID HAMARTOMA (REAH)

A: Low magnification shows a prominent glandular proliferation in which the glands have a branched pattern of growth.

B: The glands arise in direct continuity with the surface epithelium (left), and invaginate downward into the submucosa. In addition, residual normal seromucous glands are found between the glandular proliferation.

C: The histologic features of REAH include a glandular proliferation originating from the surface epithelium with invagination into the submucosa, a submucosal glandular proliferation lined by epithelium that is identical to the ciliated surface epithelium, stromal hyalinization enveloping the submucosal glands, glands separated by clusters of seromucous glands (lower right), and edematous to fibrous stroma containing a mixed chronic inflammatory cell infiltrate.

associated with REAHs (101). Reported association of low-grade adenocarcinomas and REAH prompted the consideration that REAH is a precursor lesion for at least a subset of sinonasal low-grade adenocarcinomas (103); however, there is no definitive proof of this.

Immunohistochemical Findings. The glandular proliferation (surface and submucosal) is reactive for cytokeratins, including AE1/AE3, CAM5.2, and CK7 but is negative for CK20 and CDX2. p63 and CK903 (34βE12) stain basal (myoepithelial) cells but in any given case or in areas of any given lesion such staining may be absent (104). The absence of p63-positive myoepithelial/basal cells does not confer a diagnosis of adenocarcinoma, unlike in other organ systems, including the breast and prostate gland, where in conjunction with appropriate light microscopic findings, the absence of myoepithelial/basal cells by immunohistochemical staining with p63, smooth muscle actin, and smooth muscle myosin heavy chain supports a diagnosis of adenocarcinoma. S-100 protein may or may not be reactive. Ki-67 (MIB1) staining is either absent or shows a very low proliferation rate (1 to 2 percent).

Figure 1-28
RESPIRATORY EPITHELIAL ADENOMATOID HAMARTOMA

A: The submucosal glands are separated by fibrous stroma and enveloped by eosinophilic basement membrane-like material (arrows).

B,C: At higher magnification, the glands are round to oval, composed of ciliated respiratory epithelium and enveloped by eosinophilic basement membrane material of variable thickness.

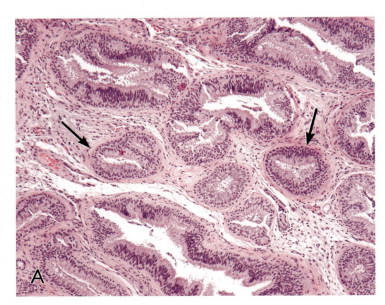
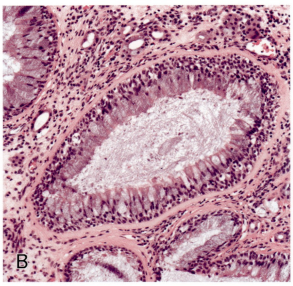
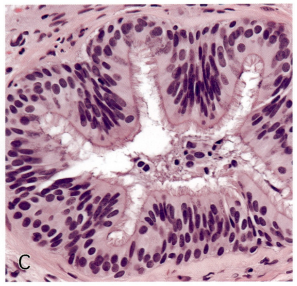

Differential Diagnosis. The most important error to avoid is mistaking REAH for an adenocarcinoma, which has occurred (105). Unless the biopsy is small and the ciliated epithelium atrophically thinned with loss of cilia, the characteristic ciliated respiratory epithelial proliferative component which is the essence of this type of lesion, distinguishes it from adenocarcinoma. Also, although the pattern of some of the small glands can be worrisome, other areas with more clearly normal seromucous glands (with lobularity of appropriate size and shape) and the gradual transition between and similarity among these glands and the atypical ones, contribute to the impression that the atypical glands are likely just reactively altered and not neoplastic.

Distinction from inverted type sinonasal (Schneiderian) papilloma is important, and fortunately is usually not too difficult. Sinonasal papillomas of the inverted type characteristically are composed of a significantly thickened epithelium (squamous compared to normal respiratory epithelium), with associated microcysts, scattered mucocytes, and inflammatory cells. The invaginations of REAH lack these features and are lined by normally thick respiratory epithelium (101).

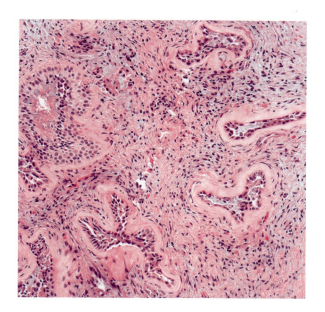 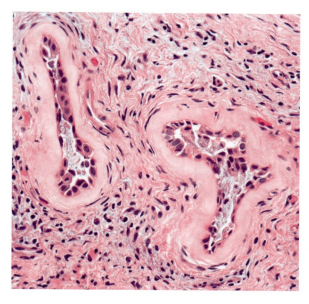

Figure 1-29

ATROPHIC CHANGES IN RESPIRATORY EPITHELIAL ADENOMATOID HAMARTOMA

Left, right: The glands are lined by a flattened to cuboidal layer of epithelium. Stromal hyalinization of increased thickness envelopes the glands.

Inflammatory polyps can have a few respiratory epithelial inclusion cysts without being hamartomatous. The degree of the epithelial proliferation in the hamartomas, however, is usually strikingly beyond what is usual in inflammatory polyps.

Treatment and Prognosis. Although these lesions can form moderately large masses, their growth potential is probably limited (as would be expected with a hamartomatous condition). Conservative (but complete) surgical removal is expected to be curative, with little or no chance of recurrence (101).

Seromucinous Hamartoma

Definition. *Seromucinous hamartoma* (SH) is a benign, acquired, non-neoplastic overgrowth of indigenous glands of the sinonasal tract, and rarely of the nasopharynx, arising from submucosally situated seromucinous glands. Synonyms include *glandular hamartoma* (106) and *microglandular adenosis* (107).

Clinical Features. There is a slight male predilection. SHs occur over a wide age range, from the second to ninth decades of life. SHs most commonly occur as an incidental finding seen in surgical material removed for clinical diagnoses such as chronic sinusitis and sinonasal inflammatory polyps. Symptomatic patients may present with nasal obstruction and epistaxis. The most common site of occurrence is the posterior nasal septum, although the lateral nasal wall, paranasal sinuses, and nasopharynx (108) are also affected. Usually limited in extent, SHs may extend into adjacent sinuses (e.g., maxillary, ethmoid). There are no known etiologic factors although there may be an association with chronic sinusitis, inflammatory polyps, rheumatoid arthritis, and Parkinson disease (108). Radiographically, SHs may appear as polypoid lesions without evidence of aggressive growth such as bone destruction.

Gross Findings. SHs are polypoid to exophytic lesions. They measure 6 mm to 4 cm in greatest dimension.

Microscopic Findings. A characteristic finding is the presence of a submucosal epithelial proliferation of small glands, serous acini, and tubules growing in clusters and lobules, although haphazard arrangements with larger glands and cysts are seen (fig. 1-30). The retention of the lobular architecture and the haphazard growth of glands separated by a variable amount of edematous to fibrous stroma with mixed inflammatory cells (fig. 1-30) represent

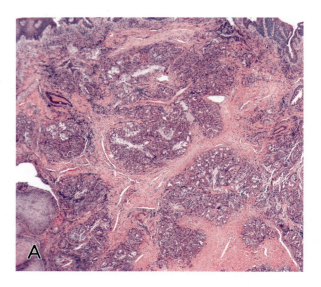
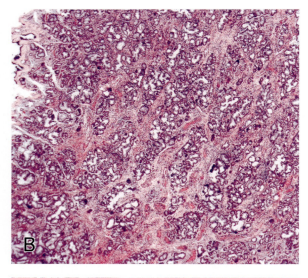
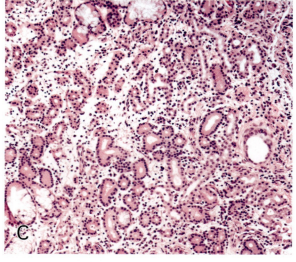
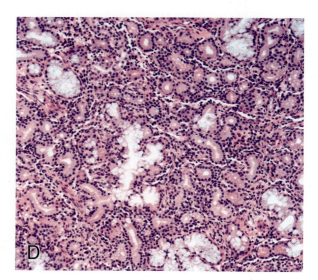
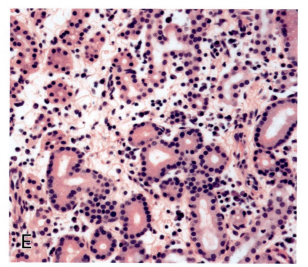

Figure 1-30

SEROMUCINOUS HAMARTOMA

A: This polypoid to exophytic-appearing lesion has a submucosal epithelial proliferation of small glands, serous acini, and tubules growing in clusters and lobules.

B: More diffuse growth of a submucosal seromucinous gland proliferation.

C: The glands separated by edematous stroma with variable admixed inflammatory cells.

D: More densely packed seromucinous glands with little to absent intervening stroma.

E: The glands are lined by low cuboidal to flat epithelial cells, with round to oval nuclei and a variable amount of basophilic to eosinophilic to clear cytoplasm. There is an absence of significant nuclear pleomorphism, increased mitotic activity, and necrosis.

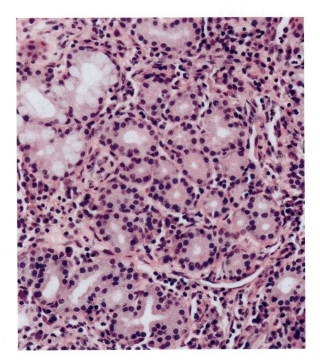 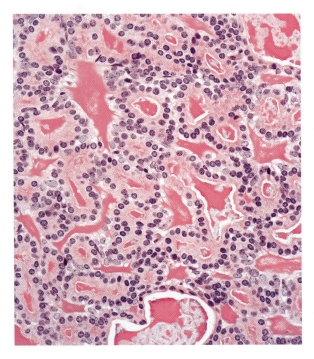

Figure 1-31

SEROMUCINOUS HAMARTOMA

Left: The serous glands are densely packed with a back-to-back appearance that resembles a cribriform pattern of growth. The retention of the lobular architecture and the haphazard growth of glands separated by stromal tissue (see fig. 1-30) represent important findings that allow for differentiation from sinonasal low-grade adenocarcinoma.

Right: Sinonasal low-grade adenocarcinoma, nonintestinal, nonsalivary gland type is characterized by the presence of complex glandular growth with back-to-back (cribriform) glands, without intervening stroma, composed of a single cell type lacking significant nuclear pleomorphism, increased mitotic activity, and necrosis. The immunoprofile of low-grade sinonasal adenocarcinoma overlaps with that of seromucinous hamartoma including an absence of basal/myoepithelial cells, so that differentiation between these two entities is primarily on the basis of histologic features but may be extremely difficult in any one case.

important findings that allow for differentiation from sinonasal low-grade adenocarcinoma. In some cases, the serous glands are densely packed with a back-to-back appearance that may resemble a cribriform pattern of growth and prompt a possible diagnosis of low-grade adenocarcinoma (fig. 1-31).

The glands are lined by low cuboidal to flat epithelial cells with round to oval nuclei and a variable amount of basophilic, eosinophilic, or clear cytoplasm. There is an absence of significant nuclear pleomorphism, increased mitotic activity, and necrosis. The glands are round, oval, angulated, or branching and stellate and contain luminal mucin material. There is generally an absence of a significant mucinous cell component although focal mucinous change may be found.

SHs are covered by benign ciliated respiratory epithelium that may show squamous metaplasia and often have an associated hypocellular edematous, myxoid or fibrous stroma, similar to that seen in sinonasal inflammatory polyps. A mixed chronic inflammatory cell infiltrate composed of mature lymphocytes and plasma cells may be seen, but a significant population of eosinophils is not typically present. In any given case, the histologic changes may be similar to those of respiratory epithelial adenomatoid hamartoma, including invagination of the surface respiratory epithelium with at least focal merging with the glandular proliferation and the presence of periglandular hyalinization (fig. 1-32).

Immunohistochemical Findings. The surface epithelium and the seromucinous glands are

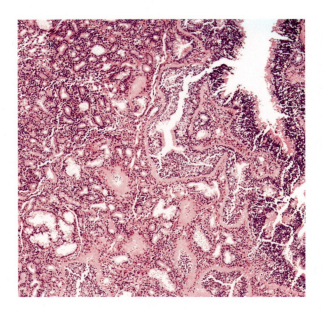 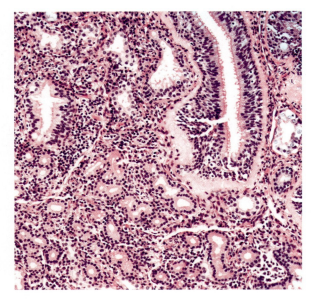

Figure 1-32

SEROMUCINOUS HAMARTOMA

Seromucinous hamartomas have foci showing the histologic features of REAH.
Left: One feature is the invagination of the surface respiratory epithelium (right), with a glandular proliferation enveloped by hyalinized stroma, merging with the seromucinous gland proliferation.
Right: Higher magnification shows ciliated respiratory epithelial-lined glands with periglandular hyalinization merging with a seromucinous gland proliferation.

reactive for cytokeratins, including CK7, CK17, CK19, and high molecular weight cytokeratin (HMWK) but negative for CK14 and CK20. The surface respiratory epithelium shows the presence of p63-positive basal cells. The seromucinous glands are typically negative (109), but may be positive (110). Calponin and muscle-specific actin are usually negative in both the surface respiratory epithelium and the seromucinous glands. The absence of myoepithelial/basal cells by immunohistochemical staining does not confer a diagnosis of adenocarcinoma, unlike in other organ systems, including the breast and prostate gland, where in conjunction with appropriate light microscopic findings, the absence of myoepithelial/basal cells by immunohistochemical staining with p63, smooth muscle actin, and smooth muscle myosin heavy chain supports a diagnosis of adenocarcinoma. S-100 protein staining is limited to the seromucinous glands. Collagen type IV and laminin are present around the glandular proliferation. Ki-67 (MIB1) staining is either absent or shows a very low proliferation rate (1 to 2 percent).

Molecular Genetic Findings. DNA mutation analysis shows a higher mutation rate for SH in comparison to normal seromucinous glands (0.83 percent) (107). This finding is supportive of SH as a benign process, although it is not clear whether such findings support a non-neoplastic or neoplastic lesion.

Differential Diagnosis. The most significant entity in differential diagnosis is sinonasal adenocarcinoma, low-grade, nonintestinal, nonsalivary gland type. This adenocarcinoma is characterized by the presence of complex glandular growth characterized by back-to-back (cribriform) glands without intervening stroma, composed of a single cell type lacking significant nuclear pleomorphism, increased mitotic activity, and necrosis (fig. 1-31). Some cases are characterized by the presence of papillary projections. The immunoprofile of low-grade sinonasal adenocarcinoma overlaps with that of SH, including the absence of basal/myoepithelial cells. The histologic features of SH that differ from adenocarcinoma include retention of a lobular growth pattern and absence of complex

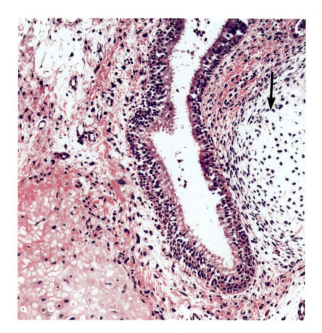 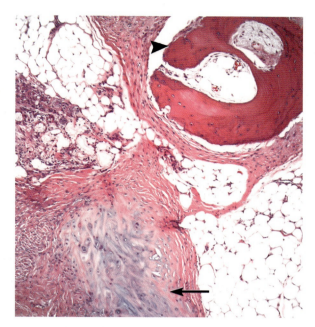

Figure 1-33

CHONDRO-OSSEOUS AND RESPIRATORY EPITHELIAL (CORE) HAMARTOMA

Left: This polypoid proliferation has the histologic features of REAH, including respiratory epithelial-lined glands but is associated with cartilage (arrow) and/or bone (not shown).

Right: This CORE hamartoma has a focus of bone (arrowhead) and "immature-appearing" mesenchyme (arrow). The glandular component, which in CORE hamartomas tends to have reduced prominence, is absent.

back-to-back (cribriform) growth. Nevertheless, in limited tissue samples, or even in adequate sampled material, differentiating low-grade sinonasal adenocarcinoma from SH can be difficult, if not impossible (108). In such circumstances, conservative but complete resection of the lesion, including lesion-free margins is recommended, as such treatment is curative for both SH and low-grade sinonasal adenocarcinoma.

Treatment and Prognosis. Conservative but complete surgical excision is curative. There are no reported recurrences over extended periods of time.

Chondro-osseous and Respiratory Epithelial Hamartomas

Definition. *Chondro-osseous and respiratory epithelial (CORE) hamartomas* are considered to be related to REAHs, but they have the additional feature of chondroid tissue. This tissue may be histologically atypical, and forms a significant histologic difference from the REAH.

Clinical Features. Patients range in age from 11 to 73 years (111). CORE hamartomas present as polypoid lesions most commonly affecting the nasal cavity, but the nasopharynx, ethmoid sinus, and sphenoid sinus may be presenting locations (111).

Microscopic Findings. In addition to the histologic features of REAH, CORE hamartomas have an intimately associated admixture of cartilaginous or osseous trabeculae (fig. 1-33). Also, the respiratory epithelial adenomatoid components tend to be of reduced prominence. A spectrum of chondro-osseous differentiation is present, with some cases manifesting "immature-appearing" mesenchyme in which cartilaginous plates display a zonal phenomenon resembling endochondral ossification in fetal skeletal development, to cases with well-developed bony trabeculae in a myxoid to fibrous stroma.

Differential Diagnosis. It is important not to mistake immature-appearing mesenchyme or cartilage for sarcoma. The presence of the adenomatoid hamartomatous components are helpful in this regard. There is a tendency for immature tissues to occur in younger patients and this may be of some relevance.

Treatment and Prognosis. Conservative but complete resection is curative, although there are rare recurrences.

Nasal Chondromesenchymal Hamartoma

Definition. *Nasal chondromesenchymal hamartoma* (NCMH) is a tumefactive process of the sinonasal tract consisting of an admixture of chondroid and stromal elements with cystic features analogous to chest wall hamartoma. These lesions have some histologic similarities to CORE hamartomas and they may be within the spectrum of that type of lesion. They are distinguished, however, by mostly presenting in the neonatal age group and by a tendency to be larger and more aggressive than the CORE hamartomas (112). Some of these tumors have eroded into the cranial cavity (through the cribriform plate area). Synonyms include *chondroid hamartoma* (113) and *nasal hamartoma* (114).

Clinical Features. This is a rare lesion with less than 30 cases reported in the literature (112,115–117). There is a male predilection. Most lesions occur in newborns within the first 3 months of life but may occur in the second decade of life, and occasionally in adults. The clinical presentation includes respiratory difficulty, an intranasal mass, and facial swelling. Some of these tumors erode into the cranial cavity (through the cribriform plate area), a finding that may clinically simulate the appearance of a meningoencephalocele. NCMH may develop in patients with pleuropulmonary blastoma (PPB), raising the possibility that NCMH is part of the hereditary familial disease complex associated with PPB (117).

Microscopic Findings. Histologically, proliferating epithelial elements are not a prominent feature. The chondromesenchymal elements are fairly cellular and immature, probably reflecting the immature age of the patient. For these reasons, NCMH deserves recognition as a distinct clinicopathologic subgroup of nasal hamartomas.

NCMH is characterized by the presence of nodules of cartilage varying in size, shape, and contour (fig. 1-34). The degree of differentiation varies: some nodules appear similar to the chondromyxomatous nodules of chondromyxoid fibroma and some to nodules of well-differentiated cartilage. A loose spindle cell stroma or abrupt transition to hypocellular fibrous stroma is present at the periphery of the cartilaginous nodules. Additional patterns include a myxoid to spindle cell stroma, fibro-osseous proliferation with a cellular stromal component, and ossicles or trabeculae of immature (woven) bone. Mature adipose tissue may be present and prominent (fig. 1-34).

Immunohistochemical Findings. The cartilaginous nodules and mesenchymal stromal component show S-100 protein staining, which is more intense in the cartilaginous component. The spindle cell stroma shows vimentin and smooth muscle actin reactivity; muscle-specific actin (HHF35) may be present. The presence of actin reactivity supports myofibroblastic differentiation. Epithelial membrane antigen (EMA) reactivity may be present, likely representing nonspecific staining.

Molecular Genetic Findings. A novel 12;17 translocation, t(12;17)(q24.1;q21), has been identified as the sole reported anomaly in a single NCMH patient (11-year-old boy) with a past medical history of PPB (118).

Differential Diagnosis. The differential diagnosis includes REAH, seromucinous hamartoma, and CORE hamartoma. NCMH is distinguished from these hamartomas by presenting in the neonatal age group and by a tendency to be a larger and more aggressive hamartoma.

Treatment and Prognosis. Surgical resection, which may necessitate a combined intranasal and intracranial approach, is the treatment of choice. Malignant transformation in an adult has been reported in one case in which the malignant component was classified by a spindle cell stroma considered to be malignant on the basis of increased nuclear pleomorphism, increased mitotic activity, and increased proliferation index by Ki-67 immunoreactivity (with areas of up to 50 percent reported) (119).

Granulomatosis with Polyangiitis

Definition. *Granulomatosis with polyangiitis* (GPA) is a non-neoplastic, idiopathic, aseptic necrotizing disease with a predilection for the upper/lower respiratory tract and the genitourinary system. It is characterized by granulomatous, necrotizing, and ulcerous inflammatory processes in the respiratory tract (and other internal organs); necrotizing granulomatous vasculitis; and focal glomerulonephritis (120).

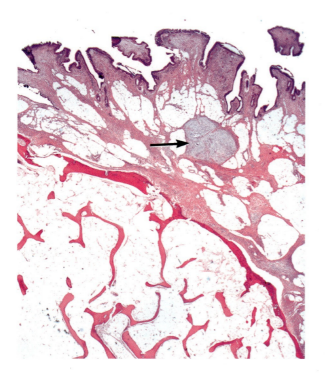
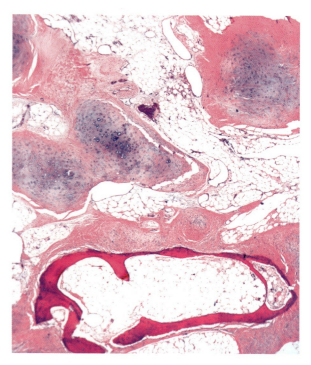

Figure 1-34

CHONDROMESENCHYMAL HAMARTOMA

Left: The polypoid-appearing sinonasal mucosa with submucosal proliferation includes bony trabeculae, mature adipose tissue, and a round cartilaginous nodule (arrow).

Right: Cartilaginous nodules are surrounded by adipose tissue and bone (bottom).

This classic definition calls for involvement of the head and neck region, the lung, and the kidney. Most patients with GPA do not exhibit this classic clinical triad at the time of initial presentation, and the initial biopsy material may originate from lesions of the upper aerodigestive tract (UADT) in the absence of a clinical suspicion of GPA. *Wegener granulomatosis* is a synonym, but a relatively recent recommendation was made to replace Wegener granulomatosis with GPA (121).

Pathogenesis. Despite decades of intensive investigation, the etiology of GPA remains unknown. Although speculative, an infectious etiology (e.g., bacterial) either as the cause or as a cofactor in the disease is suggested on the basis of reported beneficial effects of trimethoprim-sulfamethoxazole therapy on the initial course of the disease. Also, the histologic features of the disease are similar to what might be found in infectious diseases.

Genome-wide analysis of patients with antineutrophil cytoplasmic antibody (ANCA)-associated vasculitides (one of which is GPA) confirms the genetic contribution to the pathogenesis of these conditions (122). A meta-analysis identified 33 genetic variants associated with these vasculitides, supporting a role for alpha-1-antitrypsin, the major histocompatibility complex system, and several distinct inflammatory processes in their pathogenesis. Results indicate that subdivision of ANCA-associated vasculitides based on ANCA serotype has a stronger genetic basis than subdivision based on clinical diagnosis.

Clinical Features. There is a wide patient age range, from early adolescence to old age, although there is a peak incidence in the sixth/seventh decades of life. The sinonasal tract is the most common anatomic area for presenting symptoms, but 80 percent of patients have involvement of other areas. The disease manifests insidiously, often with increasing nasal obstruction that initially is attributed to common nonspecific rhinitis. This is followed

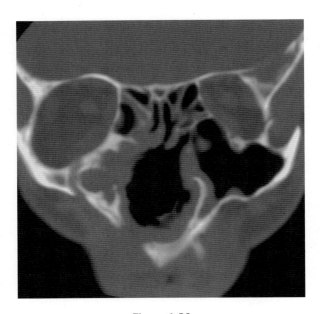

Figure 1-35

GRANULOMATOSIS WITH POLYANGIITIS

Coronal bone window through the sinuses demonstrates extensive erosive osseous changes of the nasal septum, sinus septa, sinus walls, and hard palate, with associated mucosal thickening involving the right maxillary and ethmoid sinuses. (Courtesy of Dr. A. Khorsandi, New York, NY.).

by serosanguinous drainage and crusting of the nasal mucosa. Vague nasal pain may be experienced. Nasal septal perforation and other areas of sinonasal breakdown may ensue, sometimes seemingly accelerated after surgical biopsy or other sinonasal surgical procedures. Patients may develop systemic symptoms and signs out of proportion to the nasal symptoms; these systemic features include increasing malaise, night sweats, migratory arthralgias, and weakness. Ear symptoms are common. Patients with pulmonary and renal involvement may have cough, hemoptysis, and hematuria.

GPA may be systemic or localized. The clinical manifestations vary, such that limited or localized disease may be asymptomatic while with systemic involvement the patient is always sick. The disease may progress from localized to systemic involvement or may remain limited or even regress with treatment. GPA is classified according to the ELK system in which E = ear, nose and throat involvement; L = lung involvement; and K = kidney involvement. Patients with E or EL disease are considered to have the limited form of GPA and patients with renal involvement (i.e., ELK) have systemic GPA (123). The incidence of limited GPA varies from 29 to 58 percent.

Localized UADT GPA tends to affect men more than women, except for laryngeal GPA which is seen predominantly in women. Localized GPA occurs over a wide age range, with the average age of occurrence in the fourth and fifth decades of life. In the UADT, the most common site of occurrence is the sinonasal region, followed by the nasal cavity, maxillary sinus, ethmoid sinus, frontal sinus, and sphenoid sinus. Other sites of involvement include the nasopharynx, larynx (subglottis), oral cavity, ear (external and middle ear including the mastoid), and salivary glands. Symptoms vary according to the site of involvement. Sinonasal tract disease may include sinusitis with or without purulent rhinorrhea, obstruction, pain, epistaxis, anosmia, and headaches. The radiographic features of sinonasal GPA include sinus opacification, bone destruction, ossification of the sinus walls, and soft tissue destruction (fig. 1-35).

Laboratory Findings. Useful laboratory studies in the diagnosis of GPA include elevated erythrocyte sedimentation rate and, in renal disease, elevated serum creatinine and abnormal urinary sediment. More specific (although not pathognomonic) laboratory findings include elevated antineutrophil cytoplasmic antibody (ANCA) and proteinase 3 (PR3). ANCA causes vascular injury that leads to small vessel vasculitis (124). Clinical and experimental evidence supports a pathogenesis that is driven by ANCA-induced activation of neutrophils and monocytes, producing destructive necrotizing vascular and extravascular inflammation (125). Suggestions are made that the pathogenic transformation might be initiated by commensal or pathogenic microbes, legal or illegal drugs, exogenous or endogenous autoantigen complementary peptides, or dysregulated autoantigen expression (125). ANCA has a reported specificity for the diagnosis of GPA of 85 to 98 percent of cases (124,126). ANCA reactivity is seen in the form of cytoplasmic (C-ANCA) versus perinuclear (P-ANCA) staining. GPA is characteristically associated with C-ANCA and only infrequently with P-ANCA, and C-ANCA is of greater specificity than P-ANCA. The sensitivity of the test varies with the extent of disease such that patients with limited GPA have a 50 to 67 percent C-ANCA positivity rate and patients with systemic GPA have a 60 to 100 percent positivity rate. A negative test does not rule out GPA and elevated ANCA levels can be identified in other vasculitides, in inflammatory bowel disease, and in hepatobiliary diseases (127). ANCA titers, however, are not elevated in infections or in lymphomas. ANCA titers follow the disease course: titers revert to normal levels with remission and are elevated with recurrent or persistent disease. A decline in the C-ANCA titer may lag behind clinical evidence of remission by up to 8 weeks.

PR3 is a neutral serine proteinase present in azurophil granules of human polymorphonuclear leukocytes and monocyte lysosomal granules. PR3 serves as the major target antigen of c-ANCA (128–132). ANCA with specificity for PR3 is characteristic for patients with GPA. Patients with GPA have a significantly higher percentage of mPR3-positive neutrophils than healthy controls and patients with other inflammatory diseases. The detection of ANCA directed against PR3 (PR3-ANCA) is highly specific for GPA; ANCA positivity is found only in about 50 percent of the patients with localized GPA, whereas PR3-ANCA positivity is seen in 95 percent of the patients with generalized GPA. In patients with GPA, high expression of PR3 on the surface of nonprimed neutrophils is associated with an rate of relapse. The pathogenesis of vascular injury in GPA is ascribed to ANCA directed mainly against PR3 treatment.

The ANCA-associated vasculites (AAV) include GPA, microscopic polyangiitis (MPA), allergic granulomatous angiitis (AGA), and eosinophilic GPA (Churg-Strauss disease). The major target antigens of AAV are PR3 and myeloperoxidase (MPO), with PR3-ANCA being a marker for GPA and MPO-ANCA related to MPA and AGA. ANCA appears to induce vasculitis by directly activating neutrophils. ANCA specificity is predictive of relapse, with PR3 ANCA-positive patients almost twice as likely to relapse MPO ANCA-positive patients (133).

Gross Findings. GPA of the sinonasal area may result in diffuse ulcerative and crusted lesions with tissue destruction; in advanced cases, septal perforation results in a "saddle nose" deformity. In biopsies of GPA, the gross appearance of the tissue is nonspecific and not helpful.

Microscopic Findings. The histologic features of GPA include the classic triad of: 1) vasculitis, 2) granulomatous inflammation (which may involve vessel walls as well as the supporting tissues), and 3) tissue necrosis (fig. 1-36). Diagnosing GPA from sinonasal biopsies is often a major challenge: often, histologic evidence of vasculitis is not found (134) and the other features usually are not highly specific for the diagnosis. Devaney et al. (134) reviewed 126 head and neck biopsy specimens from 70 patients and reported finding the classic triad of vasculitis, necrosis, and granulomatous inflammation in only 16 percent of the biopsy specimens reviewed; vasculitis and granulomatous inflammation were seen in 21 percent; and vasculitis and necrosis in 23 percent. It is often not possible to unequivocally diagnose GPA on biopsies and a diagnosis of at most "suspicious for GPA" or "cannot exclude GPA" is rendered.

It is to the patient's potential significant benefit, however, not to delay the initiation of treatment longer than is absolutely necessary. To this end, the serologic levels of ANCA and PR3 are critical in trying to establish the diagnosis. Pathologists should note that the characteristic histologic features for GPA are not quite, in a strict sense, those of a granulomatous disease and may not be, in the most basic and fundamental way, solely a vasculitis. While these points are arguable, keeping them in mind can be an aid to learning what to expect when examining a biopsy.

A histologic granuloma is defined as "a localized collection of epithelioid histiocytes, with or without multinucleated giant cells," and which may or may not have "caseation" (histologic degeneration or necrosis). This conjures up the picture of a typical sarcoidal granuloma or a histologic tubercle. This is not the histologic picture of GPA. While the necrotic foci of nasal GPA sometimes manifest a few adjacent histiocytes (and the occasional finding of a few giant cells is important diagnostically), the histiocytes are usually meager and nonspecific. GPA never results in sarcoidal-type granulomas. Rather, scattered, isolated multinucleated giant cells represent the "granulomatous" component of GPA (fig. 1-36). There is no specific localization of the giant cells. In spite of the absence of true granuloma formation, GPA has always been and

Non-Neoplastic Diseases of the Head and Neck

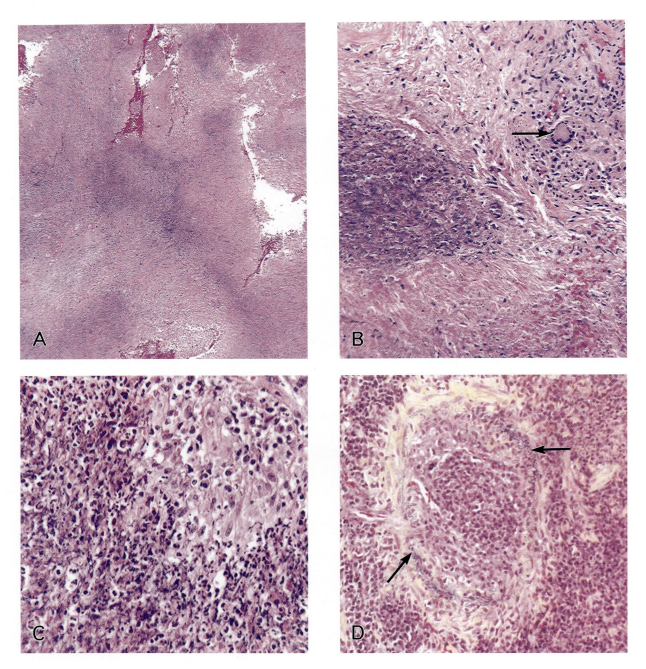

Figure 1-36

GRANULOMATOSIS WITH POLYANGIITIS

A: The disease is best and most basically described as a multifocal necrobiosis characterized by so-called geographic necrosis in the form of patchy foci of degenerated collagen that often has prominent bluish (basophilic) staining.

B: Despite the nomenclature of this disease, well-formed granulomas are not a component of this lesion; rather, scattered multinucleated giant cells (arrow) represent the "granulomatous" component of the lesion.

C: When the patch of necrobiosis is prominent, there is coarse granularity of the degenerated stroma, suggesting a "gritty" or "sandy" texture. In the upper right portion of the figure is an ablated blood vessel surrounded (angiocentric) and "invaded" (angioinvasive) by mixed inflammatory cells, resulting in vascular thrombosis and surrounding ischemic-type necrosis.

D: Elastic stains show disruption of the black staining elastic membranes (arrows) by the angioinvasive benign inflammatory cell infiltrate.

will continue to be considered a granulomatous disease, albeit only in a broad or "loose" concept of granulomatous disease.

GPA is best and most basically described as a multifocal necrobiosis. Nasal GPA most often manifests patchy foci of degenerated collagen that often has a prominent bluish (basophilic) staining pattern (fig. 1-36). When the patch of necrobiosis is prominent, there is a coarse granularity of the degenerated stroma, suggesting a "gritty" texture (fig. 1-36). Some of the larger granules may be from leukocytoclasia, and microabscess formation is another important histologic finding. Similar basophilic granular debris may be found in the base of nonspecific ulcerations unrelated to GPA. As such, if it is found only at the edge of a tissue fragment or in relationship to the surface epithelium, it is not useful. But if the necrobiosis is a patch well within the connective tissue stroma, it is significant. Also, a small questionable focus of incipient necrobiosis is not as helpful as are multiple, well-formed, prominent or large patches of bluish, granular necrobiosis. This latter picture, when it is especially blatant, by itself can be almost diagnostic of sinonasal GPA. While there are other diseases that can manifest patchy necrobiosis, most of those diseases never present in the sinonasal tract. The sole exception is a fungal infection (e.g., mucormycosis, see later) which should always be excluded.

One of the reasons that GPA is usually difficult to confidently diagnose from sinonasal biopsies is the fact that the vasculitis is usually not clearly evident. It is tempting to interpret the patchy necrobiosis as indirect evidence of vasculitis, i.e., as infarctive necrosis "downstream" from affected vessels. Since the nasal tissues are normally quite vascular, it seems unlikely that a subtle and focal vasculitis (i.e., focal enough not to be seen in given sections) would result in prominent patches of necrosis. Also, the histologic character of the bluish necrobiosis does not quite look like what is usually seen with infarction.

The apparent elusiveness of the vasculitis might be explained by a concept that Dr. Wegener himself held: "The primary granulomas form and develop in connective tissue, but without vascular involvement. The vasculitis that accompanies the disease is a secondary feature that presents at a later stage" (120). Feinberg (125), who studied GPA intensively for decades, also considered this idea to be valid. In other words, the pathologic process directly damages fibrous connective tissue, but it also progresses to damage vessel walls. Whether or not this concept is strictly true, the findings in sinonasal biopsies suggest that it is possible and this helps to conceptualize, and therefore understand and remember, the usual findings. Thus, while the findings of definite vasculitis can be of major help in diagnosis, usually it is absent (134) and one can (and should) try to make the diagnosis without requiring demonstrable vasculitis. The finding of prominent "geographic" patches of necrobiosis, occasional multinucleated giant cells, and a few microabscesses may be sufficient to support the diagnosis.

The parenchymal inflammatory infiltrate is predominantly composed of mature lymphocytes, histiocytes, and plasma cells; eosinophils, while generally uncommon, may be numerous on occasion. The intensity and cellular composition of the general nonspecific inflammatory cell infiltrate in the tissues of sinonasal GPA is highly variable from case to case (and to some extent from area to area in an individual case) and is not of significant help in diagnosis. Bacterial superinfection of the diseased mucosa, particularly by *Staphylococcus aureus*, may complicate the clinical picture.

Immunohistochemical Findings. Useful histochemical stains include elastic stains to identify the vasculitis characterized by the disruption of the internal and external elastic membranes by the angioinvasive benign inflammatory cell infiltrate (fig. 1-36). Since GPA is a diagnosis of exclusion, staining for microorganisms should be performed but is invariably negative.

Immunoreactivity is present for both B-cell (CD20) and T-cell (CD3) markers, indicative of a benign (polyclonal) cellular population. Immunohistochemical staining for Epstein-Barr virus (EBV) and in situ hybridization for EBV-encoded RNA (EBER) are negative. IgG4 immunostaining may include increased IgG4-positive cells in sinonasal (or orbital/periorbital) biopsies of GPA (135). This finding could pose a pitfall in the diagnosis of IgG4-related disease. GPA in other organs and controls do not show increased IgG4-positive cells. The biologic or clinical importance of increased IgG4-positive cells in GPA

Table 1-4
CLINICOPATHOLOGIC COMPARISON OF GRANULOMATOSIS WITH POLYANGIITIS, ALLERGIC GRANULOMATOSIS AND VASCULITIS, AND SINONASAL MALIGNANT LYMPHOMAS

	GPA[a]	Allergic Granulomatosis and Vasculitis	Extranodal NK/T-Cell Lymphoma, Nasal Type	DLCBL
Gender/Age	M>F; 4th-5th decades; laryngeal GPA affects F>M	M>F; wide age range (3rd-6th decades)	M>F; 6th decade; most common in Asians; occurs in western population but with less frequency	M>F; 7th decade
Location	Localized UADT GPA most common in nasal cavity > paranasal sinuses; other sites may include nasopharynx, larynx (subglottis), oral cavity, trachea, ear, salivary glands	Multisystem disease including pulmonary, nasal, renal, cutaneous, cardiac, and nervous system involvement	Generally limited to the sinonasal region; extra-sinonasal occurs and represents a higher stage tumor	Nasal cavity and one or more paranasal sinuses
Symptoms	SNT: sinusitis, with or without purulent rhinorrhea, obstruction, pain, epistaxis, anosmia, headaches Larynx: dyspnea, hoarseness, voice changes Oral: ulcerative lesion Ear: hearing loss, pain	Asthma, allergic rhinitis, evidence of eosinophilia in serum and tissue (e.g., eosinophilic pneumonia, eosinophilic gastroenteritis, other), evidence of vasculitis	Destructive process of midfacial region; nasal septal perforation, obstruction, palate destruction, orbital swelling	Nonhealing ulcer, epistaxis, facial swelling, pain cranial nerve manifestations

involving the head and neck region remains uncertain. Similarly, the potential pathogenic relationship between IgG4-related disease and GPA in those cases remains uncertain.

Diagnosis of GPA. The histopathologic diagnosis of GPA is often one of exclusion. Since the histologic findings are often meager, a "negative" biopsy may be of little or no help in excluding GPA. The histomorphologic diagnosis may be limited based on the tissue sampling, therefore, it is imperative that the clinician obtain multiple biopsies, especially in areas from the ulcer bed as well as in areas of more viable-appearing tissue. In any given biopsy, if the histologic features do not support a diagnosis of GPA but the clinical index of suspicion for GPA is high, additional biopsies may be indicated. If the patient has been treated with steroids prior to biopsy, this can suppress the histologic features and make the histologic diagnosis even more difficult and problematic.

Differential Diagnosis. By far, the most important consideration in the differential diagnosis (Table 1-4) is to exclude as well as possible an unusual infection, particularly a fungal infection. Special stains for microorganisms should be performed (e.g., Grocott methenamine silver [GMS], periodic acid–Schiff [PAS]), but cultures of tissue may be important in some cases. Also, a thorough clinical evaluation by a physician specializing in infectious diseases may help to determine how much the general clinical picture suggests GPA versus an infection.

Since NK/T-cell lymphoma, nasal type, is angiocentric, the vessel infiltrate can be mistaken for the vasculitis of GPA. The most important differentiating point is the degree of lymphocytic nuclear atypia. The cytologic characteristics of the lymphoid infiltrate often (but not always) permit distinction between these entities (fig. 1-37). The lymphoid infiltrate in GPA lacks an appreciable degree of cytologic atypia; the presence of nuclear atypia is characteristic of the tumor cells of malignant lymphoma (fig. 1-37). Since there is some degree of subjectivity in the recognition of lymphoid atypia by light microscopic features alone, immunohistochemical or molecular biologic studies are helpful. The NK-cell immunophenotype is cytoplasmic CD3 positive but surface (membranous) CD3 (by flow

	GPA[a]	Allergic Granulomatosis and Vasculitis	Extranodal NK/T-Cell Lymphoma, Nasal Type	DLCBL
Systemic Involvement	ELK classification: E: ear, nose, throat L: lung K: kidney E, EL = limited form GPA ELK = systemic GPA	Typically multisystem involvement although limited forms of disease exist	Majority are localized (stage IE/II/E); may progress to disseminated systemic involvement	Majority are localized (stage IE/II/E); may progress to disseminated systemic involvement
Serology	ANCA and PR3 positive: increased in both primary disease and recurrent disease; C-ANCA more specific than P-ANCA	ANCA and PR3 levels may or may not be present; peripheral eosinophilia; may be associated with antimyeloperoxidase (MPO) ANCA	ANCA and PR3 negative; no specific serologic marker(s)	ANCA and PR3 negative; no specific serologic marker(s)
Histology	Polymorphous (benign) cellular infiltrate; vasculitis; ischemic-type necrosis; isolated multinucleated giant cells (not well-formed granulomas); negative cultures and stains for organisms	Polymorphous (benign) cellular infiltrate, predominantly eosinophils; vasculitis which may be a granulomatous vasculitis (multinucleated giant cells in the wall of involved blood vessels); eosinophilic microabscesses; negative cultures and stains for organisms	Overtly malignant cellular infiltrate but in early phases malignant cells may not be overtly identifiable; angiocentricity and angioinvasion; ischemic-type cells or granulomas; negative cultures and stains for organisms	Diffuse dyscohesive cellular proliferation of medium to large cells with large round to oval vesicular (noncleaved) nuclei, prominent nucleoli, increased mitotic activity, and necrosis
IHC	LCA, B- and T- cell markers, kappa and lambda light chains positive	LCA, B- and T- cell markers positive	CD3 cytoplasmic, CD2, CD56 positive; T-cell markers (CD3, others) positive; cytotoxic granule markers (granzyme B, TIA-1, perforin) positive	LCA and B-cell markers (CD20), CD79) positive; MUM1 positive; p63 may positive (focal to diffuse)
EBV	Negative	Negative	Strong association	No to weak association
Treatment	Cyclophosphamide and prednisone	Systemic corticosteroids	Radiotherapy for localized disease; chemotherapy for disseminated	Radiotherapy and/or chemotherapy
Prognosis	Limited disease associated with a good to excellent prognosis and occasional spontaneous remissions; mortality related to complications of renal and pulmonary involvement	62% 5-year survival; increased morbidity and mortality due to cardiac involvement resulting in CHF or MI	5-year survival for stage I is approximately 50%; local recurrence/relapse and systemic failure common	Dependent on stage; 5-year survival rates vary in the literature from 29 to 80%

[a]GPA = granulomatosis with polyangiitis (formerly referred to as Wegener granulomatosis; also known as Churg-Strauss syndrome as well as eosinophilic granulomatosis and polyangiitis); DLCBL = diffuse large B-cell lymphoma; IHC = immunohistochemistry; EBV = Epstein-Barr virus; ANCA = antineutrophil cytoplasmic antibodies; PR3 = proteinase 3; UADT = upper aerodigestive tract; CHF = congestive heart failure; MI = myocardial infarction; SNT = sinonasal tract; LCA = leukocyte common antigen.

cytometry) negative, CD2 positive, and CD56 positive. Markers of cytotoxic granules are positive, including expression of granzyme B, cytotoxic granule-associated TIA-1, and perforin. EBV is detected in most neoplastic cells in virtually all cases of nasal type NK/T-cell lymphoma by in situ hybridization for EBER (fig. 1-37). In the setting of a sinonasal (midline) destructive disease, the only pathologic entity associated with the presence of EBV is NK/T-cell lymphoma, nasal type. Since EBV-positive cells are typically absent in the nasal cavity mucosa, in inflammatory diseases

Figure 1-37
ANGIOCENTRIC NK/T-CELL LYMPHOMA, NASAL TYPE

A: The angiocentric nature of the cellular infiltrate is evident, with surrounding ischemic type necrosis, similar in appearance to that seen in granulomatosis with polyangiitis (GPA).

B: Usually (but not always) the cytomorphologic characteristics of NK/T-cell lymphoma are those of a malignancy, allowing for distinction between GPA and NK/T-cell lymphoma.

C: The neoplastic cells in angiocentric NK/T-cell lymphoma are positive for Epstein-Barr virus (EBV) and identified by in situ hybridization for EBV-encoded RNA (EBER); the presence of EBV represents a diagnostic feature of NK/T-cell lymphoma, nasal type, differentiating it from other sinonasal midline destructive diseases.

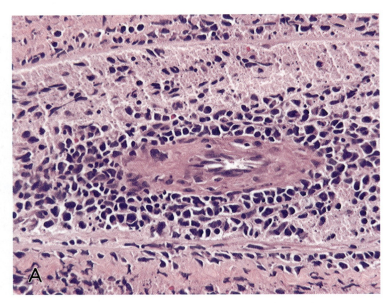

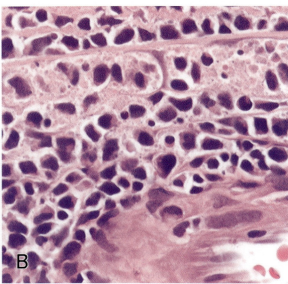

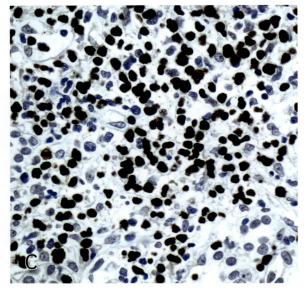

of the sinonasal tract, and in other sinonasal neoplasms, the presence of EBV in conjunction with light microscopy is diagnostic for nasal type NK/T-cell lymphoma even in cases without overtly atypical/malignant-appearing cells. Searching for the microabscesses and scattered giant cells of GPA, which is not expected with malignant lymphoma, is important. C-ANCA and PR3 serologic evaluation is specific for GPA, and is a great help in supporting the diagnosis of GPA and in excluding a diagnosis of a NK/T-cell lymphoma, nasal type, since the latter not associated with elevation of ANCA and PR-3 levels.

Since the inflammatory infiltrate in GPA can include appreciable numbers of eosinophils, the question of allergic granulomatosis and vasculitis (also known as Churg-Strauss granulomatosis) may arise. Churg-Strauss granulomatosis is characterized by asthma, systemic vasculitis, tissue and peripheral eosinophilia, and nasal manifestations; these findings should assist in the differential diagnosis. Further, Churg-Strauss granulomatosis is not expected to clinically present as a sinonasal disorder.

Treatment and Prognosis. Once the diagnosis and extent of disease is determined, most

plasma cells may be present, although this infiltrate may be sparse. Occasional multinucleated giant cells of foreign body type may be seen. Stains for microorganisms are negative.

Differential Diagnosis. Although not common today, in the past in some geographic areas, patients with rhinosinusitis applied or inhaled patent medicines or "homemade" remedies that contained oily substances, particularly oil of Wintergreen. While the histologic reaction may include a more active inflammatory response and a more intense foreign body giant cell reaction, the main help in the differential diagnosis is the history. Not only is the admitted use of an unusual substance important, but the absence of prior surgery is also helpful. In contrast to infectious diseases, especially fungal infections (e.g., rhinosporidiosis, coccidioidomycosis), special stains for microorganisms are negative in myospherulosis.

Treatment and Prognosis. Prevention by the use of nonpetrolatum-based antibiotic substances is most important and indeed, the incidence of this disorder has significantly decreased. In the patient who develops the condition, conservative surgical removal of fibrotic tissue is effective.

Extranodal Sinus Histiocytosis with Massive Lymphadenopathy

Definition. *Extranodal sinus histiocytosis with massive lymphadenopathy* (ESHML) is an idiopathic histiocytic proliferative disorder generally characterized by lymph node-based disease and indolent behavior (143). Extranodal manifestations occur, with the upper respiratory tract among the more common sites of involvement (144). Synonyms include *Rosai-Dorfman disease* and *Destombes-Rosai-Dorfman syndrome*.

Although sinus histiocytosis with massive lymphadenopathy (SHML) is often a nodal-based proliferation occurring as part of a generalized process involving the lymph nodes (145), SHML may involve extranodal sites, independent of the lymph node status. Within the head and neck, there is predilection for the nasal cavity and paranasal sinuses (144).

Clinical Features. Sinonasal tract ESHML is slightly more common in women than in men, and occurs over a wide age range. In descending frequency, extranodal head and neck sites include the sinonasal cavity, orbit/eyelid, salivary gland, oral cavity (palate), lower respiratory tract, nasopharynx and tonsil, middle ear and temporal bone, larynx, and trachea (144).

Symptoms depend on the site of occurrence: in the sinonasal tract, symptoms predominantly relate to nasal obstruction; nonsinonasal tract related symptoms include proptosis, ptosis, decreased visual acuity, pain, stridor, cranial nerve deficits, or a mass lesion. The presentation often includes multiple concurrent sites of involvement and may occur without evidence of lymph node involvement. In general, the diagnosis of ESHML is a pathologic diagnosis and rarely, if ever, suspected by clinical evaluation.

The hematologic and immunologic status is generally intact but there may be polyclonal elevations in serum protein levels and raised erythrocyte sedimentation rates. SHML occurs in association with human immunodeficiency virus (HIV)-infected patients (146,147), Sjögren syndrome (148), amyloidosis (149), and systemic lupus erythematosus (150), and may co-exist with Langerhans cell histiocytosis (151). In the literature, some studies report elevated levels of EBV, as well as human herpesvirus 6 (HHV6), in association with SHML (152,153) while other studies report that SHML cells are not infected by EBV (154) or associated with HHV6 and HHV8 (155). Although some studies implicated SHML as an IgG4-related disease, it is not believed to belong within the spectrum of IgG4-related diseases (156).

Radiographic findings disclose an extensive process. Bone erosion or destruction is common.

Pathogenesis. The cause is unknown. An infectious etiology has been suggested as the cause but an infectious agent has never been isolated. The occurrence in patients with rhinoscleroma suggests a possible etiologic relationship with rhinoscleroma, although this has not been proven (157,158). Other considerations implicated but never substantiated include immunodeficiency, autoimmune disease, or a neoplastic process. The histologic features of SHML have been identified in patients with autoimmune lymphoproliferative syndrome (ALPS), an inherited disorder associated with defects in FAS-mediated apoptosis, suggesting a possible link (159).

Immunophenotypic studies support the interpretation that the SHML cells are part of the mononuclear phagocyte and immunoregulatory effector (M-PIRE) system belonging to the macrophage/histiocytic family (160–162). Stimulation of monocytes/macrophages via macrophage colony-stimulating factor (M-CSF), resulting in immune suppressive macrophages, represents a main mechanism for the pathogenesis of SHML and provides evidence for the monocyte/macrophage but not dendritic cell differentiation of SHML histiocytes. Expression of the chemokine receptors CCR6 and CCR7 in the SHML histiocytes suggests that this may be a general attribute of abnormal histiocytes and may reflect gene activation in a more mature macrophage-derived cell type (163).

Gross Findings. The gross appearance of the lesion varies and includes polypoid, nodular, or exophytic lesions of tan-white or yellow. Tissues are usually removed piecemeal and lesional sizes are not estimable from the pathology specimen.

Microscopic Findings. At low magnification, the histopathologic features include the presence of fibrosis and lymphoid aggregates alternating with pale-appearing areas composed of histiocytes, lymphocytes, and plasma cells within the submucosa. In lymph nodes, the process produces a variegated, patchy appearance because the histiocytes are concentrated in expanded lymph node sinus areas (hence, "sinus histiocytosis"). In the extranodal location of the sinonasal tract, a somewhat similar pattern exists, with lymphoid aggregates composed of mature lymphocytes that may contain histiocytic cells, imparting a mottled appearance to these aggregates (fig. 1-39). True germinal centers are not usually seen. The sheets of histiocytes can have large areas with few lymphocytes adjacent to areas with large patches of lymphocytes (and plasma cells) and few histiocytes. Areas of fibrosis can be prominent and this tissue can outline nodules of the cellular components, adding to the impression of the patchiness of the process. Extension into bone, skeletal muscle, and other soft tissue components occurs.

In addition to the lymphoid aggregates, a polymorphous cellular infiltrate composed of mature lymphocytes, plasma cells, and histiocytes is seen. The histiocytes (so-called SHML cells) appear in clusters or cell nests but may be obscured by the nonhistiocytic cell population (particularly the plasma cells). The histiocytic cells are uniform with mild pleomorphism and are characterized by round to oval, vesicular to hyperchromatic nuclei, with abundant amphophilic to eosinophilic, granular to foamy to clear cytoplasm (fig. 1-39). The nuclei do not demonstrate nuclear lobation, indentation, or longitudinal grooving as seen in Langerhans cell histiocytosis. Nucleoli vary from prominent and eosinophilic to inconspicuous. Mild nuclear pleomorphism and scattered mitoses can be seen. Cell borders are poorly defined but are occasionally delineated by the extracellular deposition of delicate fibrillar material. When some of the histiocytes have cleared or partly foamy cytoplasm, the cytoplasm often has an irregular, "torn" or "ragged" and feathery appearance. While this may be artifact, it is a frequent and characteristic appearance of the histiocytes in this disorder.

As in nodal SHML, a helpful finding in ESHML is the presence of lymphocytes lying in the cytoplasmic field, the so-called emperipolesis, in which the histiocytes ingest (phagocytize) inflammatory cells within their cytoplasm (fig. 1-39). When prominent or definite, this is a particularly characteristic finding although not necessarily pathognomonic (164). The presence of emperipolesis may not be as readily apparent in ESHML as it is in nodal-based disease. The phagocytized cells usually are lymphocytes but plasma cells, erythrocytes, and polymorphonuclear leukocytes are also seen engulfed within the histiocytic cell cytoplasm. The plasma cell component can be prominent and intracytoplasmic eosinophilic globules (Russell bodies) can be seen. Scattered eosinophils may be found and, rarely, they are prominent. Well-formed granulomas or multinucleated giant cells are not a feature.

Immunohistochemical Findings. Special stains for infectious organisms are negative but are required for the differential diagnosis. SHML cells are diffusely S-100 protein positive (fig. 1-39) but are negative for CD1a and langerin. They may also demonstrate immunoreactivity for alpha-1-antichymotrypsin (ACT), CD68 (KP1), lysozyme, and MAC-387. The plasma cells have a polyclonal pattern of proliferation as seen by the cytoplasmic positivity for both kappa and lambda light chains.

Differential Diagnosis. With the prominent S-100-protein–reactive histiocytes, Langerhans

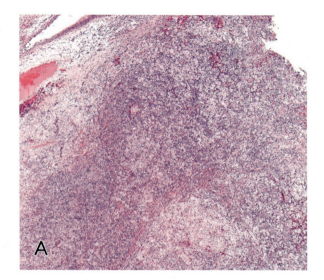
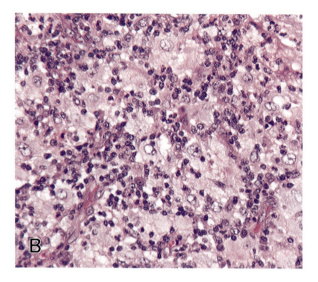
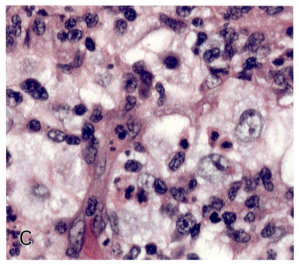

Figure 1-39

EXTRANODAL (SINONASAL) SINUS HISTIOCYTOSIS WITH MASSIVE LYMPHADENOPATHY (SHML) (ROSAI-DORFMAN DISEASE)

A: The sinonasal-based submucosal proliferation shows a variegated, patchy appearance with lymphoid aggregates composed of mature lymphocytes admixed with histiocytic cells that impart a mottled appearance to these aggregates.

B,C: The histiocytes (SHML cells) are characterized by round to oval, vesicular to hyperchromatic nuclei and abundant amphophilic to slightly eosinophilic, granular to slightly foamy to cleared cytoplasm.

D: The presence of emperipolesis, more often seen in nodal-based disease rather than in extranodal sites of involvement, is a helpful diagnostic feature, although emperipolesis can be seen in association with rhinoscleroma.

E: SHML cells are S-100 protein positive (typically diffuse and intense nuclear and cytoplasmic staining) but CD1a and langerin negative (not shown).

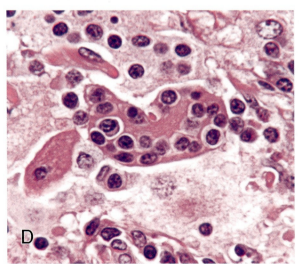
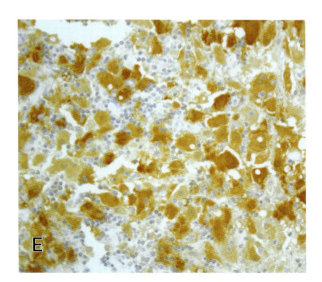

cell histiocytosis (LCH) has to be considered, especially in the extranodal location. The cells of ESHML, however, do not have the CD1a and langerin reactivity expected with LCH. Also, giant cells are not a feature of ESHML but may be found in LCH. The cytoplasm of the cells in LCH does not develop the partly cleared, "ragged" appearance frequently seen with ESHML histiocytes. Although both disorders have some mild nuclear atypia, the clefted appearance of the nuclei in LCH is different from that found in ESHML.

The cleared histiocytes of ESHML can suggest the Mikulicz cells of rhinoscleroma, and the abundant plasma cells add to this impression. Further, emperipolesis may be present in rhinoscleroma (164). Rhinoscleroma is unlikely to have the sheets of histiocytes that are frequent in ESHML. The bacteria in rhinoscleroma *(Klebsiella rhinoscleromatis)* are capricious in their staining properties and may be difficult to demonstrate. With a Warthin-Starry stain, however, the bacteria of rhinoscleroma in the Mikulicz histiocytes are apparent (see later in this chapter).

The heterogenous cell population typical for ESHML as well as the presence of emperipolesis and CD68 and S-100 protein reactivity should allow for differentiation from a hematolymphoid malignancy. While rare, emperipolesis can be seen in association with B-cell lymphomas. SHML on rare occasions has been identified in lymph nodes affected by malignant lymphomas, including non-Hodgkin lymphomas, multiple myeloma, and Hodgkin disease, mixed cellularity type. Transformation of SHML to a high-grade lymphoma has also been reported (165).

Treatment and Prognosis. SHML is considered an indolent, self-limiting disease; severe morbidity and mortality have been attributed to the complications of SHML. There is no ideal treatment for SHML of the head and neck. Treatment protocols should mirror the clinical manifestations and a range of therapeutic modalities are used. In cases of airway compromise, treatment is directed at alleviating the obstruction, which requires surgical intervention. For those patients with extensive or progressive disease, more radical surgical intervention may be required but surgical eradication of disease may prove difficult in cases involving craniofacial bones or the cranial cavity. Radiotherapy and chemotherapy have been utilized, but the efficacy of these agents has not been proven. Extension of disease to vital structures, particularly to the cranial cavity, may result in the death of the patient; however, mortality related to SHML is a rare occurrence (166). Unfavorable prognostic factors include disseminated nodal disease, involvement of multiple extranodal organ systems, and deficiencies in hematologic and immunologic status.

Necrotizing Sialometaplasia

The seromucous glands of the sinonasal tract are similar to the minor salivary glands. They can (albeit seldom) manifest a metaplastic change similar to that of necrotizing sialometaplasia of the oral cavity salivary tissues. The change can be associated with infarcted tissues or otherwise necrotic tissues from sundry causes. As in other locations, sinonasal sialometaplasia can easily be misinterpreted as carcinoma. Usually the metaplasia is a small focus, seldom as extensive as has sometimes been found in the lesions of the palate.

Histologically, the findings are similar to those found in salivary gland locations. The nests of squamous cells within connective tissue can suggest invasive squamous cell carcinoma, but several features prevent this misdiagnosis. The intimate association with glands is important, especially when it appears that the squamous nests are replacing acini through a metaplastic change. This impression is fostered by observing that the squamous nests are about the same size (perhaps slightly larger) as the glands, are rounded, and multiple nests seem to maintain the same lobular architecture and size as the glandular lobule they are transforming. The squamous cells have some reactive atypia, but the cytologic features of malignancy are not present. For a more complete discussion, including illustrations of necrotizing sialometaplasia, see the chapter on salivary glands.

Eosinophilic Angiocentric Fibrosis

Definition. *Eosinophilic angiocentric fibrosis* (EAF) is a rare chronic sclerosing and fibroinflammatory disorder of the upper aerodigestive tract.

Clinical Features. EAF is an uncommon nasal cavity condition that may not be as rare as the dearth of reported cases would suggest.

It is possible that many cases have been diagnosed as nonspecific fibrosis associated with common chronic rhinosinusitis. It has been postulated to represent the mucosal variant of granuloma faciale because of the histologic similarities of early nasal mucosal lesions to those seen in granuloma faciale and the concurrent occurrence of both lesions in approximately 25 percent of cases (167–172).

Women are more often affected; adults have a wide age range. The sites of involvement include the nasal cavity and larynx (subglottis) (170,173–175), orbit, lacrimal gland, and oral cavity (gums). In the nasal cavity, EAF affects the septum more than the lateral wall, is often unilateral but may be bilateral, and rarely extends to the paranasal sinuses (usually maxillary sinus) or orbit. The clinical presentation is that of progressive airway obstruction over several years. Some patients have associated allergies, including allergic rhinitis, chronic urticaria, and sensitivity to penicillin.

The laboratory findings are nonspecific. ANCA levels are not elevated. There are no abnormalities in the erythrocyte sedimentation rate or urinalysis.

Pathogenesis. There is no known etiology. Recent evidence supports including EAF in the spectrum of IgG4-related diseases since some patients with EAF have a serum IgG4 concentration of 1,490 mg/dL (normal, 8 to 140 mg/dL); IgG4-positive plasma cells ranging from 43 to 118 per high-power field; and IgG4 to IgG ratio from 0.68 to 0.97 (176,177).

Microscopic Findings. The main histologic feature is prominent fibrosis; other specific findings can easily be overlooked. Nevertheless, the histologic features described for EAF include an early and late phase, both of which can be seen in any given biopsy. In early lesions, there is an eosinophilic perivascular infiltrate in the lamina propria. Eosinophils surround and extend into capillaries and venules (eosinophilic angiitis); plasma cells and mature lymphocytes may also be present. Thrombosis and "ischemic-" type necrosis are not identified. In late phase lesions, the most characteristic feature is the presence of dense fibrosis with a layered "onion skin-type" perivascular fibrosis (angiocentric fibrosis) (fig. 1-40). The fibrosis is hypocellular, but areas of mixed inflammatory cells remain, including a prominent eosinophilic cell infiltrate (fig. 1-40). Cytologic atypia is not present and there is no evidence of microorganisms, granulomatous inflammation, or giant cells.

Immunohistochemical Findings. Special stains for microorganisms are negative. Immunohistochemical staining shows that the plasma cells are polyclonal and the lymphocytes are predominantly T cells.

Differential Diagnosis. The differential diagnosis includes infectious diseases, granulomatosis with polyangiitis (formerly Wegener granulomatosis), Churg-Strauss disease, fibromatosis, nasal-type NK/T-cell lymphoma, and subglottic stenosis for cases involving the larynx.

Treatment and Prognosis. Excising the area of stenosis may be required in patients with airway obstruction in order to create a patent airway. Corticosteroids and antihistamines are not effective modes of treatment. Disease progression stabilizes over time but typically not prior to the development of airway obstruction.

Sarcoidosis

The sinonasal tract may be involved by *sarcoidosis*, although often the extent may not be enough to cause prominent symptoms. In a patient thought clinically to have sarcoidosis, a nasal mucosal biopsy helps provide support for the diagnosis. In such instances, the granulomas (if found) probably are scattered and scarce. When identified, they are well formed and essentially non-necrotizing, similar in appearance to sarcoid involvement in other anatomic locations. Asteroid bodies and Schaumann bodies may be identified. Occasionally, the involvement of sinonasal tissues may be more intense and this may produce a mass-like lesion. Bone erosion is sometimes present. For a more complete discussion, including illustrations, see the chapter on neck lesions.

Rhinophyma

The clinical appearance (fig. 1-41) of *rhinophyma*, together with the histologic findings of extraprominent sebaceous glands (fig. 1-41), and often chronic inflammation, are well known to pathologists and dermatologists. When a clinicopathologic correlative evaluation is done, the diagnosis of this condition should not be problematic.

Figure 1-40

EOSINOPHILIC ANGIOCENTRIC FIBROSIS

A: The sinonasal mucosa is replaced by prominent dense stromal fibrosis; residual minor salivary glands are present (lower right).

B: The characteristic layered "onion-skin-type" perivascular fibrosis is seen.

C: The mixed inflammatory cell infiltrate includes eosinophils, which may be prominent and may be associated with the small vessel walls, suggesting a small vessel angiitis. It is possible that the areas with inflammatory cells represent an active, "younger" stage of the disorder, with the hypocellular, angiocentric fibrosis being an "older" stage of the process.

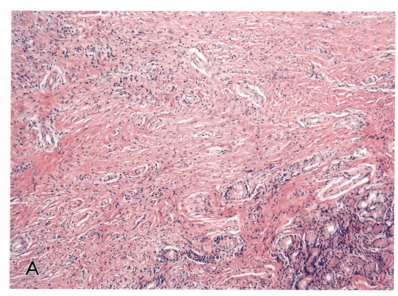

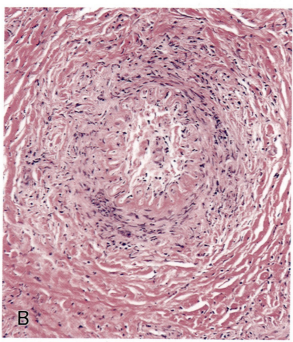

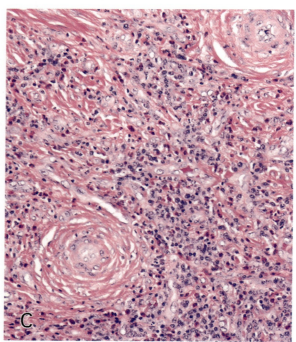

Relapsing Polychondritis

Clinically and histopathologically, the diagnosis of *relapsing polychondritis* (RP) is less problematic when the auricles are affected than when the nasal tissues are solely affected. RP begins as a perichondrial inflammation and since many nonspecific erosions and ulcerations of the nasal septum have inflammation extending to the edges of septal cartilage, the histologic diagnosis of RP in the nose can be especially problematic. Further, the feature often touted in the literature as an aid to diagnosing RP, "loss of basophilia of cartilage," is of limited help. The variations in the basophilic staining qualities of essentially normal cartilage, especially when compounded by variations in laboratory technique, render this feature as potentially more misleading than helpful. For a more complete

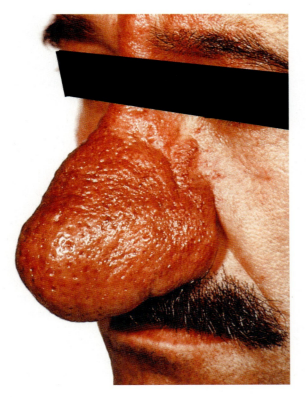 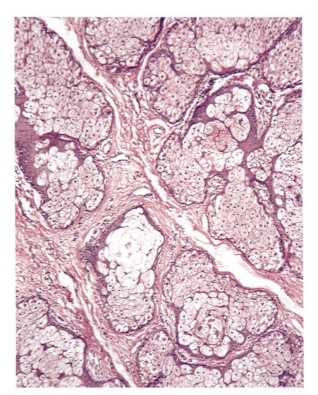

Figure 1-41

RHINOPHYMA

Left: Bulbous-appearing nose.
Right: The histologic findings are those of prominent sebaceous glands.

discussion, including illustrations, see the chapter on the ear.

Pyogenic Granuloma/Lobular Capillary Hemangioma

Definition. *Pyogenic granuloma/lobular capillary hemangiomas* (PG/LCH) are benign polypoid forms of capillary proliferations primarily occurring on skin and mucous membranes. Synonyms include *pregnancy tumor*, *granuloma gravidarum*, and *epulis gravidarum*.

The term pyogenic granuloma is a misnomer in that this lesion is neither an infectious process nor granulomatous. This is a polypoid capillary hemangioma-like growth. Also, the lesion is not purulent, is not likely caused by pyogenic bacteria, and the tissue does not contain granulomas, defined as localized collections of histiocytes. The appellation of "granuloma" for this lesion likely derives from the clinical usage to denote a lesion that is grossly "granulomatous" in the sense of resembling granulation tissue. Nevertheless, this long-used term retains some usefulness

Clinical Features. There is no gender predilection and PG/LCH of the head and neck occurs over a wide age range, most commonly seen in the fourth to fifth decades (178,179). A predilection for males less than 18 years of age has been reported (178), and cases occurring in adolescent girls have also been reported (180) Among head and neck mucosal sites, PG/LCH is most common on the lip, followed by the nose and the oral cavity (oral mucosa more than tongue), but is uncommon in the larynx and trachea (178). In the sinonasal tract, PG/LCH is most often identified in the anterior portion of the nasal septum, referred to as Little area or Kiesselbach triangle; the next most common sinonasal location is the tip of the turbinates.

The most common clinical complaint is epistaxis, followed by painless obstructive symptoms

(179); a minority of patients complain of associated pain (179). PG/LCH appears as a red-brown mass, sometimes with pale areas producing a mottled appearance. Some examples are surprisingly large and extensive. In spite of their vascular nature, surgical removal often does not result in an unusual amount of bleeding.

Many pathologists prefer to diagnose a PG/LCH as a type of capillary hemangioma. This is acceptable, but in general, nasal cavity PPG/LCHs tend to be clinically different from most "true" hemangiomas. The latter are most often deeply seated soft tissue or intraosseous lesions that can be extensive and difficult to treat. PG/LCHs are mostly exophytic lesions that are relatively accessible and therefore more readily treated and cured. Although "true" hemangiomas are uncommon in the sinonasal tract, histologically, they tend to be less cellular than PG/LCHs and often have larger (i.e., cavernous) vascular spaces; they also occur within bone (intraosseous hemangioma). Occasionally a granulation-tissue PG-like reaction can occur as a secondary response to (i.e., be "engrafted upon") another type of lesion, including a benign or a malignant neoplasm. As such, it is important to be reasonably sure that almost all, or at least most, of the clinical lesion has been examined, particularly if there is some reason to suspect that the diagnosis of PG does not explain the clinical findings.

Pathogenesis. The pathogenesis of PG/LCH is controversial. Some consider it to be a reactive hyperplastic process on the basis of its occurrence following trauma, during pregnancy, and during retinoid therapy, while others consider it a neoplasm (i.e., hemangioma) on the basis of its lobular architecture. Some cases are associated with prior trauma (179). PG/LCH may occur in association with pregnancy and in association with oral contraceptive use, suggesting that hormonal factors may be involved. A hormonal role is further supported by the regression of these tumors following parturition. Immunohistochemical evaluation of PC/LCHs, however, failed to identify estrogen or progesterone receptors (180).

The mechanism for the regression of pregnancy-related PG/LCH after parturition remains unclear. Proposed mechanisms for regression include the absence of vascular endothelial growth factor (VEGF) and angiopoietin-2 (ANG-2), causing blood vessels to regress (181).

Whatever the instigation, the lesion appears to be a markedly exuberant overgrowth of reactive vascular tissues.

Gross Findings. The lesions appear as a smooth, lobulated, polypoid red mass. They often have a mottled appearance, especially when sectioned. There are areas that are darker than expected in an inflammatory polyp, and these dark areas probably correlate with regions of congestion, hemorrhage, or necrosis.

Microscopic Findings. These submucosal lesions have characteristic lobular (rather than diffuse) growth clusters composed of central capillaries and smaller ramifying tributaries (fig. 1-42). The lesions are obviously vascular, although edematous stromal tissues comprise a majority of the area of the lesion. The vascular spaces are mostly tiny (capillaries and venules) (fig. 1-42) and often tend to be grouped into moderate-sized, moderately cellular patches surrounded by fairly hypocellular stroma (hence the synonym lobular capillary hemangioma). A larger-caliber central capillary is often present within a patch, and tiny compressed capillaries together with densely packed stromal cells surround the larger central capillary, which may vary in size and shape and may show a staghorn ("hemangiopericytoma-like") appearance. The more cellular regions are composed of cells that, although subtle, give the impression of different cell types (fig. 1-42), e.g., fibrocytes, fibroblasts, myofibroblasts, pericytes, and endothelial cells (within inapparent capillaries, compressed and with lumens obscured).

The endothelial cell lining may be prominent, and may display endothelial tufting and mitoses, but atypical mitoses are not identified. There is no intercommunication of vascular spaces, as may be seen in angiosarcomas, and no true cytologic atypia or atypical mitoses. Mitotic figures can be prominent during the more active growth phases of the lesion. The designation of "active" PG/LCH can be used in conjunction with those tumors showing an increase of mitotic activity, but these "active" lesions carry no additional risk of aggressive behavior or of transformation to an angiosarcoma.

Secondary alterations of inflammation, necrosis, hemorrhage, and vascular organizational proliferations (e.g., papillary endothelial hyperplasia) are common. Similarly, ulceration

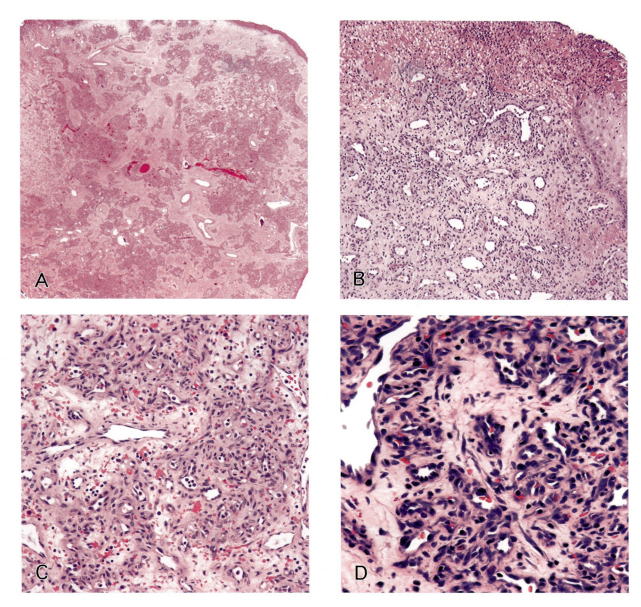

Figure 1-42

NASAL PYOGENIC GRANULOMA/LOBULAR CAPILLARY HEMANGIOMA

A: The submucosal proliferation shows the characteristic lobular growth; ulceration (upper left) and surface epithelial squamous metaplasia (right) are present.

B: The lesion is obviously vascular, composed of capillaries and venules grouped into moderate-sized, moderately cellular (lobular) patches, surrounded by stromal cells surrounding a larger venule and creating a "hemangiopericytic" pattern. Surface ulceration with associated fibrinoid necrosis is present.

C,D: The more cellular regions are composed of an admixture of cell types, creating a granulation tissue-like appearance.

of the surface epithelium with associated fibrinoid necrosis and mixed acute and chronic inflammation are common features. Such changes, however, need not be present, and some large lesions are surprisingly unaltered. Prominently enlarged reactive myofibroblasts, which appear atypical (atypical stromal cells), are not common but can be present.

Immunohistochemical Findings. The lesional cells are reactive for CD31, CD34, and

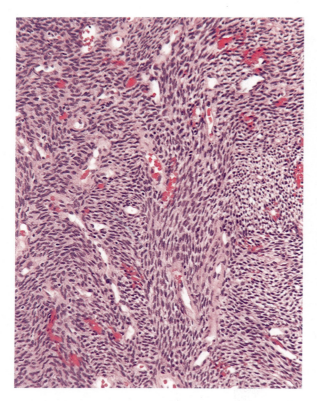 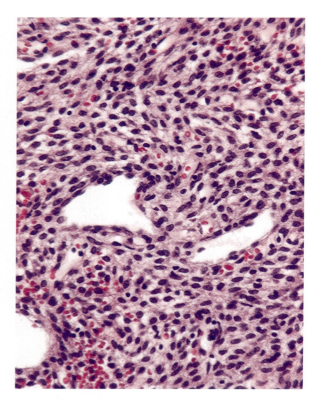

Figure 1-43

SINONASAL GLOMANGIOPERICYTOMA (HEMANGIOPERICYTOMA-LIKE TUMOR)

Left: In contrast to lobular capillary hemangioma (LCH), sinonasal glomangiopericytoma has diffuse (rather than lobular) growth, including a fascicular to storiform pattern. The perivascular hyalinization is a common feature in sinonasal glomangiopericytoma and an uncommon feature in LCH.

Right: In contrast to the mixed cell population of LCH, there is a single cell type seen in sinonasal glomangiopericytoma.

factor VIII-related antigen. No immunoreactivity is present for glucose transporter 1 (GLUT1) and human herpesvirus 8 (HHV-8).

Differential Diagnosis. Occasionally, a few cells have reactive enlargement, a finding that together with the different cell types present can lend a pleomorphic quality to PG/LCH. When mitotic activity is also prominent, a concern for malignancy may arise. All of these features can be a component of PG/LCH, and misdiagnosis as malignancy is unlikely.

The differential diagnosis includes sinonasal glomangiopericytoma (hemangiopericytoma-like tumor) (182). The key to avoiding a misdiagnosis is recognizing the dense cellularity throughout the glomangiopericytoma, with diffuse growth lacking a lobular pattern and composed of one cell type (fig. 1-43). In addition, perivascular hyalinization is often seen with sinonasal glomangiopericytoma, a finding not usually present in PG/LCH. In PG/LCH there often is variable cellularity and patchy lobularity that is uncommon in sinonasal glomangiopericytoma. The neoplastic cells in sinonasal glomangiopericytoma may stain for nuclear β-catenin (183,184), a finding not present in PG/LCH.

PG/LCH may be misdiagnosed as nasopharyngeal angiofibroma (NPAF) (185). NPAF virtually always arises from the anterior upper nasopharynx-extreme posterior upper lateral nasal cavity area, while nasal cavity PG/LCH usually does not involve this specific area, a reliable feature for excluding NPAF. Histologically, the two lesions are very different. NPAF does not have a significant tiny vessel (e.g., capillary) component (except occasionally near the edges of the tumor where granulation tissue can secondarily form

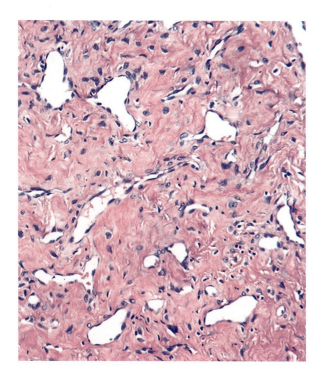

Figure 1-44

NASOPHARYNGEAL ANGIOFIBROMA

The typical histologic appearance includes an admixture of thin-walled, elongated, endothelial-lined blood vessels and surrounding variable cellular fibrous stroma, including stellate-appearing fibroblasts.

as a response to superficial ulceration) and it is not as cellular as PG/LCH. Occasionally, PG/LCH can be hypocellular over large areas, but if so, the stroma usually has an edematous appearance. NPAF tends to have a collagenous stroma without significant edema. NPAF often has moderately large and sometimes stellate stromal cells, but they are sparsely distributed (fig. 1-44). The vascular component of NPAF typically lacks a muscular wall, although many vessels of NPAF have a prominent myoid-collagenous wall and this is generally not a feature of PG/LCH. Immunohistochemical staining of the spindle cells in NPAF includes the presence of (nuclear) β-catenin (185) (and may also include nuclear androgen receptor and testosterone reactivity), not present in PG/LCH.

Treatment and Prognosis. Since PG/LCHs are mostly exophytic and are not expected to be significantly invasive lesions, simple surgical removal usually is sufficient. Recurrences are reported in up to 16 percent of cases (186), but others have reported a significantly lower rate of recurrence (178). In the presence of recurrence, further conservative removal is still appropriate and usually curative.

FUNGAL DISEASES

Fungal Rhinosinusitis

Fungal rhinosinusitis (FRS) comprises a spectrum of disease processes varying in clinical presentation, histologic appearance, and biological significance. It is classified as noninvasive or invasive based on whether fungi have invaded into tissue (Table 1-5) (187). *Noninvasive FRS* includes *allergic fungal rhinosinusitis* (AFRS) and *aspergillus mycetoma* ("*fungus ball*"). *Invasive FRS* includes *acute invasive FRS* and *chronic invasive* and *chronic granulomatous FRS*.

Noninvasive Fungal Rhinosinusitis: Allergic Fungal Rhinosinusitis

Definition. *Allergic fungal rhinosinusitis* (AFRS) is a noninvasive collection of impacted mucus and cellular debris. Similar to allergic bronchopulmonary aspergillosis, the pathologic findings result mainly from a chronic but marked allergic response to the presence of a topical fungal colonization within a sinus cavity rather than a true fungal infection. The allergic response is, nevertheless, a very significant pathologic process and it is engendered by the presence of a fungus in a paranasal sinus; it seems reasonable to consider the process a variant of infectious disease.

First described as a clinicopathologic entity by Katzenstein in 1983 (188), this disorder does not manifest tissue invasion by fungus. The amount of fungal elements present is variable but often is meager. Synonyms include *inspissated mucus, allergic sinonasal aspergillosis, allergic*

Table 1-5

CLASSIFICATION OF FUNGAL RHINOSINUSITIS (FRS)

Noninvasive
 Allergic fungal sinusitis
 Fungus ball
Invasive
 Chronic invasive FRS
 Chronic granulomatous FRS

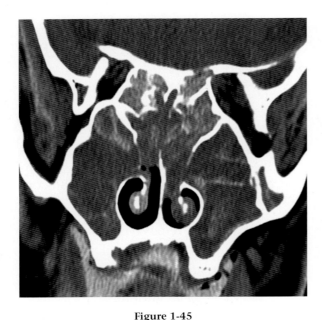

Figure 1-45

ALLERGIC FUNGAL RHINOSINUSITIS

Coronal soft tissue image demonstrates opacified sinuses with contents that are hyperdense to skeletal muscle. There is osseous dehiscence of the sinus septa and along the planum sphenoidale. (Courtesy of Dr. A. Khorsandi, New York, NY.)

fungal sinusitis, eosinophilic fungal rhinosinusitis, eosinophilic mucin rhinosinusitis, and *snotoma*.

Clinical Features. There is no gender predilection. AFRS can present at any age but is most commonly found in children or young adults. In the United States, it tends to be more common in the southwestern part of the country, although increasing incidence has been reported in urban areas in the Midwest and northeastern United States (187). Outside the United States, AFRS is common in India and Middle Eastern countries.

Most patients have a long history of chronic sinusitis, frequently accompanied by headaches and obstructive symptoms. The maxillary and ethmoid sinuses are primarily involved but any sinus may be affected. The clinical presentation includes headaches and airway obstruction. Patients are immunocompetent and commonly present with chronic rhinosinusitis with nasal polyps, inhalant atopy, history of asthma, aspirin insensitivity, blood eosinophilia, and elevated total serum immunoglobulin E (IgE) levels (189).

On radiographic studies, sinus opacification is seen and occasionally, bone erosion is present (fig. 1-45). The sinus CT is always abnormal, showing findings of chronic rhinosinusitis that often include central areas of increased contrast (hyperattenuation). Often the lesion is extensive and, when especially so, the appearance can be alarming, even suggesting a malignant neoplasm. Bone destruction occurs on rare occasion.

Pathogenesis. Originally, AFRS was thought to be almost solely a manifestation of *Aspergillus* species, but other fungi are also causative, particularly dematiaceous fungi such as *Bipolaris, Exserohilum, Curvularia, Drechslera,* and *Alternaria* (190). *Aspergillus* is a member of the Moniliaceae family, Hyphomycetes class, Deuteromycota phylum. *Aspergillus* is abundant in soil and in decaying matter; the mode of transmission is via inhalation. In the United States, most of AFRS cases (over 70 percent) are associated with dematiaceous fungi (187). In India and Middle Eastern countries, the most common fungal organism is *Aspergillus flavus* (187). *Schizophyllum commune,* a basidiomycetous fungus, is a rare cause of AFRS confirmed by sequence analysis (191).

The pathogenesis of AFRS is thought to represent an immunological reaction to fungal antigens and not a fungal infection. AFRS is thought to develop via multiple immunologic pathways that impact host responses (192). Type I hypersensitivity is established by high serum levels of allergen-specific IgE to various fungal antigens and positive Bipolaris skin test results. Type III hypersensitivity is established by an IgG-mediated process defined by the presence of allergen-specific IgG which forms complexes with fungal antigen, inducing an immunologic inflammatory response (192). Recent studies implicate superantigens and non-IgE)-mediated mechanisms in the development of AFRS (193).

Staphylococcus aureus has been implicated as a disease modifier in chronic rhinosinusitis with polyps through superantigen-mediated mechanisms (193). A higher prevalence of *S. aureus* is found in patients with AFRS than in those without, supporting a potential role for *S. aureus* in the pathogenesis.

Gross Findings. The sinus contains thick, rubbery, translucent to brown or greenish-brown material, often in copious quantity.

Microscopic Findings. The characteristic finding in AFRS is an abundant amount of amorphous material with variable patches of degenerated cells, an appearance that may at first suggest necrotic tissue. Closer examination, however, fails to reveal a substrate of necrotic cells and, instead, the material has a slightly "stringy" or laminated visual texture (fig. 1-46). This material is inspissated, gelatinized mucus, and a mucin stain can help delineate it. This material has been called allergic mucin, or more recently eosinophilic mucin, given the debate questioning whether the mucinous material in AFRS is or is not allergic (194–197). When present in huge amounts, allergic (eosinophilic) mucin is highly characteristic (and virtually diagnostic) of AFRS. The diagnosis is confirmed by special stains for fungus. The fungal elements may be frequent enough to be readily identified, but sometimes they are surprisingly scarce.

The patches and laminations of the cellular debris are usually detected as degenerated and distorted inflammatory cells, including many polymorphonuclear cells. Charcot-Leyden crystals may be seen. The inflammatory component is most often composed of eosinophils (fig. 1-46) and neutrophils; scattered plasma cells, lymphocytes, and histiocytes are also seen. Charcot-Leyden crystals, with an elongated and needle-like appearance, may be seen in the eosinophilic infiltrate (fig. 1-46); such crystals are composed of lysophospholipase and stain purple-red with a trichrome stain. Desquamated respiratory epithelial cells can be identified within this amorphous material.

The surgical specimen may or may not include significant mucosal tissues. If it does, these tissues may have prominent chronic inflammation but they are not expected to show evidence of an invasive fungal infection.

Histochemical Findings. Fungal hyphae and spores may be seen by light microscopic evaluation (i.e., hematoxylin and eosin [H&E] stain) but are best identified by histochemical staining including Gomori methenamine silver (GMS) (fig. 1-46) or periodic acid–Schiff (PAS). *Aspergillus* sp. is histologically characterized by thin (2 to 5 µm) hyphae with acute angle (45°) branching and septation. While fungal forms are identifiable by special stains, at times they are scarce; in such circumstances, microbiologic culture for speciation is an important diagnostic tool for their identification. The presence of "allergic mucin" is virtually diagnostic for AFRS even in the absence of fungal identification by special stains. Guo et al. (198) reported that by conventional GMS staining fungi were detected in only 27 percent (9 of 34) of specimens but after predigesting the specimen with trypsin there was dramatic improvement in visualization of fungi to 91 percent (31 of 34).

Immunohistochemical Findings. Antibodies targeting chitinase and *Alternaria* sp. antigens have increased the identification of fungi to as high as 100 percent of cases with allergic (or eosinophilic) mucin, even in cases that were negative for fungal identification by histochemical stains (198). The histologic appearance may suggest an epithelial neoplasm, such as a pleomorphic adenoma, but staining for epithelial markers (e.g., cytokeratins, p63) or myoepithelial markers is negative.

In Situ Hybridization (ISH). ISH as an important adjunct for the diagnosis of fungal diseases: it helps define the genus and species of the fungus seen in surgical resection material (199). Using ISH, approximately 50 percent of patients with AFRS harbor *Aspergillus* or *Penicillium* rRNA in the allergic or eosinophilic mucin (200). ISH for fungal rRNA sequences may provide a means for detecting dematiaceous fungi and prove useful for differentiating dematiaceous fungi from other filamentous fungi in fungal rhinosinusitis (201).

Differential Diagnosis. If the surgical specimen contains mostly tissue and only a small amount of inspissated mucus, the mucus may be nonspecific. The histologic appearance of this mucus may be similar to the mucus of AFRS, except inflammatory cells usually are fewer and fungal elements are absent.

It is important (since the treatment probably will differ) not to mistake a "fungus ball" (fungal mycetoma, see next section) in the sinus for AFRS. A fungal stain shows that the mycetoma is composed of myriads of densely packed fungal elements without the marked amount of mucus that is present with AFRS.

When the inflammatory cells are especially dense, they are often degenerated and have on occasion been mistaken for necrotic tumor cells. Familiarity with the histologic features of AFRS

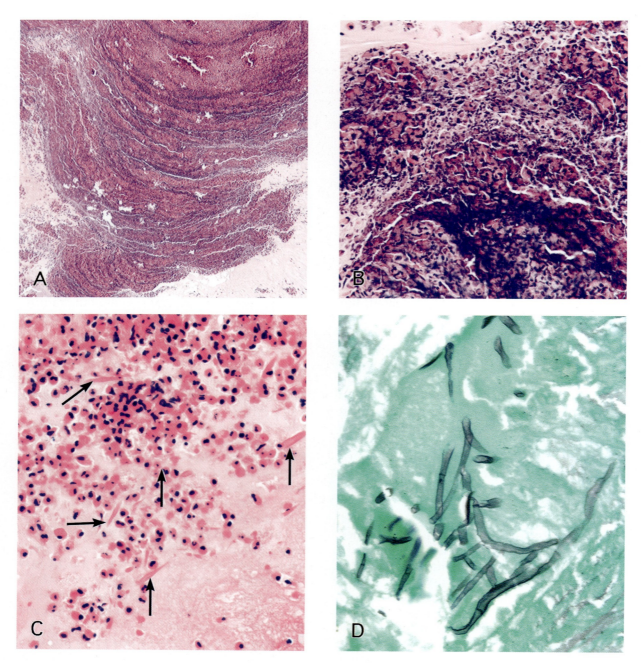

Figure 1-46

ALLERGIC FUNGAL RHINOSINUSITIS

A: Allergic (eosinophilic) mucin is characterized by abundant amorphous material with variable patches of degenerated cells, suggesting necrotic tissue at low-power magnification.

B: At higher magnification, this material is inspissated mucus with associated cellular debris representing degenerated inflammatory cells, including many polymorphonuclear cells and eosinophils.

C: Eosinophils with associated extracellular Charcot-Leyden crystals (arrows).

D: The presence of allergic (eosinophilic) mucin is highly characteristic and virtually diagnostic of allergic fungal rhinosinusitis; as seen in this figure, the Gomori methenamine silver (GMS) stain confirms the presence of fungal forms (hyphae and spores). The fungal elements may be frequent enough to be readily identified, but sometimes they are surprisingly scarce. Even in the absence of fungal elements, the presence of allergic mucin is felt to be diagnostic for allergic fungal sinusitis.

precludes an erroneous interpretation and, if necessary, immunohistochemical staining for epithelial markers will be negative.

Treatment and Prognosis. Treatment includes surgical debridement and evacuation of involved sinus(es). Postoperative steroid therapy is augmented by immunotherapy directed toward the patient's specific allergen sensitivities (192,202). The primary rationale for immunotherapy is to control the allergic diathesis that may be contributing to the patient's chronic sinus inflammation. Systemic antifungal drugs are not indicated since this is not a tissue infection. Local topical antifungal agents to reduce antigen load would be a logical treatment, but the efficacy of such measures has not clearly been determined. Some patients have recurrences, even after clinically adequate initial therapy. Approximately 20 percent of patients may demonstrate paranasal sinus expansion and bone erosion involving surrounding anatomic structures (203). Such patients may have clinical findings involving the orbit and cranial vault.

Fungus Ball

Definition. A *fungus ball* is a noninvasive accumulation of dense fungal hyphae in sinus cavities, most often the maxillary sinus, where a mass is formed. Synonyms include *Aspergillus mycetoma*, *mycetoma*, and *aspergilloma*.

Clinical Features. The clinical presentation is nonspecific, similar to nonspecific chronic sinusitis, except that the symptoms usually are unremitting, and the diagnosis is suspected on imaging studies (204). There are reports that fungal balls tend to predilect middle-aged and elderly women (205,206). The maxillary sinus is the area most often affected; less often, the sphenoid and ethmoid sinuses are involved (205,206). Fungal balls may develop secondary to blockage of the sinonasal orifices as occurs when a neoplasm causes obstruction.

Radiographs demonstrate sinus opacification (fig. 1-47). Calcium oxylate deposition, which can be detected radiographically, commonly accompanies the growth of *Aspergillus*, which is extensive.

Microscopic Findings. Histologically, the fungal hyphae are extramucosal and noninvasive. They are composed of densely packed fungal elements (hyphae) (fig. 1-48). Although

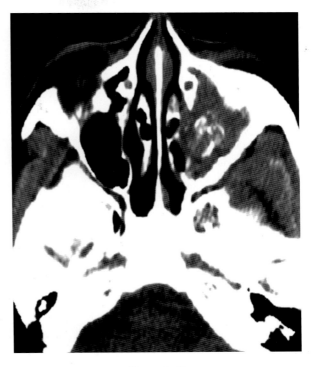

Figure 1-47

FUNGUS BALL (MYCETOMA)

An axial soft tissue window through the sinuses demonstrates a hyperdense, calcified, round lesion involving an opacified left maxillary sinus. (Courtesy of Dr. A. Khorsandi, New York, NY.)

there is associated mucosal dense chronic inflammation, usually there is no tissue invasion by the fungus. Also, there is no granulomatous inflammation. The low magnification features may initially be confused with features of allergic (eosinophilic) mucin seen in allergic fungal rhinosinusitis, however, it becomes evident at higher magnification that the mass is entirely composed of fungal forms. Histochemical staining for fungi (GMS or PAS) makes the fungal form even more apparent (fig. 1-48). Fungal cultures are typically negative (205,206).

Treatment and Prognosis. Surgical removal (functional endoscopic sinus surgery [FESS]) of the mass, consisting of opening the infected sinus cavity at the level of its ostium and removing fungal concretions while sparing the normal mucosa, is the treatment of choice. Increased aeration of the sinus may be all that is necessary to prevent recurrence. Antifungal therapy is not required.

Figure 1-48

FUNGUS BALL (MYCETOMA)

A: At low magnification, the features are suggestive of allergic (eosinophilic) mucin as seen in allergic fungal rhinosinusitis; the fungal hyphae are densely packed and due to distortion may not be recognized immediately as a mass of hyphae.

B: It is evident at higher magnification that the mass is entirely comprised of fungal forms.

C: Fungi are readily apparent by GMS stain. In contrast to invasive fungal sinusitis, the fungal mass does not invade adjacent tissues.

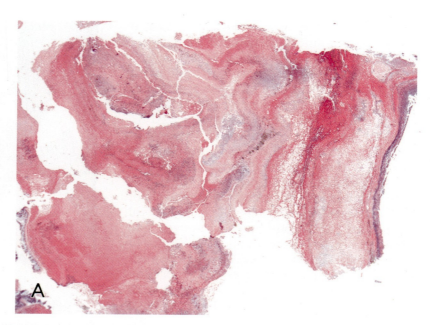

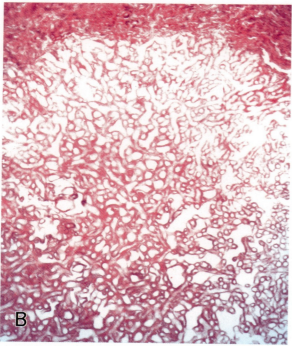

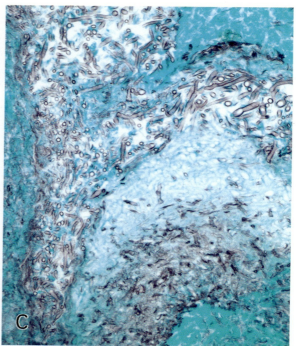

Invasive Fungal Rhinosinusitis: Acute Invasive FRS

Definition. *Acute invasive FRS* is an acute, fulminant fungal infestation of the sinonasal tract characterized by rapid onset and aggressive clinical course, resulting in destruction of the involved sinus(es) within days. The disease course varies (among different patients) from an indolent infection to a fulminant infection. The latter condition is virtually restricted to patients with immune compromise of some type. This is also known as *acute fulminant aspergillus sinusitis*.

Clinical Features. The clinical features of fulminant infection may be more similar to those of mucormycosis than to other forms of sinonasal aspergillosis. Typically, immunocompromised patients are affected, in particular, patients with hematologic malignancies (in particular acute myeloid leukemia and prolonged neutropenia [absolute neutrophil count less than 500/mm^3 for more than 10 days]) (207,208) and diabetics (209). The clinical presentation includes nasal discharge and sinus pain; swelling of the face (maxillary area and periorbital region) may be present (209). With progression of disease, blindness may occur (210).

Patients may require immediate surgical debridement, which in turn may necessitate intraoperative consultation (i.e., frozen section) in order to determine the cause of the fulminant clinical picture (211,212). In this setting, the presence of fungi is histologically evaluated and intraoperative samples sent for microbiologic culture in order to determine the causative fungus.

Pathogenesis. Culture results may be necessary to be sure of the causative fungus. The most common organisms identified include *Aspergillus* sp. and *Rhizopus* sp. but other pathogens, including dematiaceous fungi and *Fusarium* sp. may be identified. Fungal cultures are negative in approximately 30 percent of patients (207,213,214).

Microscopic Findings. Fungal forms are identified throughout the resected tissue; fungi can be seen within mucosal and submucosal tissues, as well as in and around vascular spaces (angioinvasion) (fig. 1-49). Vascular thrombosis may present. Tissue necrosis is evident but an inflammatory response often is very limited. Histochemical stains for fungi (e.g., GMS, PAS) delineate the fungal forms (fig. 1-49).

ISH using specific fungal probes (biotin-labeled oligonucleotide probes targeting *Aspergillus* sp.; *Fusarium* sp.; *Rhizopus* sp.; and a sequence identified in dematiaceous fungi) can effectively identify fungi in (acute) invasive FRS as well as in specimens with negative cultures (215).

Differential Diagnosis. The primary entity in the differential diagnosis is mucormycosis (see below).

Treatment and Prognosis. The treatment for invasive fungal rhinosinusitis is reversing the underlying immunosuppression, initiating of antifungal therapy, and aggressive surgical debridement (216). With early diagnosis and treatment, invasive FRS can be treated and patient survival increased. Disease specific survival and overall survival rates remain low for patients with acute invasive FRS (209). Intracranial involvement and cranial neuropathy at presentation are significantly associated with shortened survival (209).

Chronic Invasive and Chronic Granulomatous FRS

Definition. *Chronic invasive* and *chronic granulomatous FRS* are diseases of immunocompetent patients, usually seen in endemic areas including India, Saudi Arabia, and Sudan (217–219) but are rare in the United States (220). By definition, these forms of chronic rhinosinusitis occur in patients with at least one major and one minor clinical symptom and sign (see below) for more than 12 weeks without complete relief in the intermittent period (217). *Chronic invasive FRS* is a fungal sinonasal infection with fungal tissue invasion but no granulomatous inflammation. *Chronic granulomatous FRS* is a fungal sinonasal infection characterized by granulomatous inflammation, with or without fungal tissue invasion.

Clinical Features. These types of FRS typically occur in adults, with no gender predilection. The major symptoms and signs include facial pain, facial congestion, nasal obstruction, nasal discharge, and hyposmia/anosmia (217). Minor symptoms include headache, fever, fatigue, dental pain, cough, and ear fullness, pressure, or pain (217). Proptosis may be present. Multiple paranasal sinuses may be involved, with or without bone erosion and remodeling; the disease may extend to adjacent areas including brain, cavernous sinus, and orbit.

Pathogenesis. Chronic invasive FRS is most commonly associated with *Aspergillus fumigatus* (221) and occurs in patients with non-neutropenic immunosuppression, uncontrolled diabetes mellitus, or chronic renal failure (222). Chronic granulomatous FRS is almost exclusively associated with *Aspergillus flavus* (217), most likely the result of prolonged exposure to large numbers of fungi. In an epidemiologic study, *Aspergillus* spores were present in large numbers in the air in the wheat-thrashing areas of northern India (i.e., Punjab, Haryana) with significantly higher counts of *A. flavus* during the winter months (217). The fungus may be found in straw roofs, bedding, stored grains, and earthen floors (218).

Microscopic Findings. Chronic invasive FRS is characterized by invasion of the sinonasal

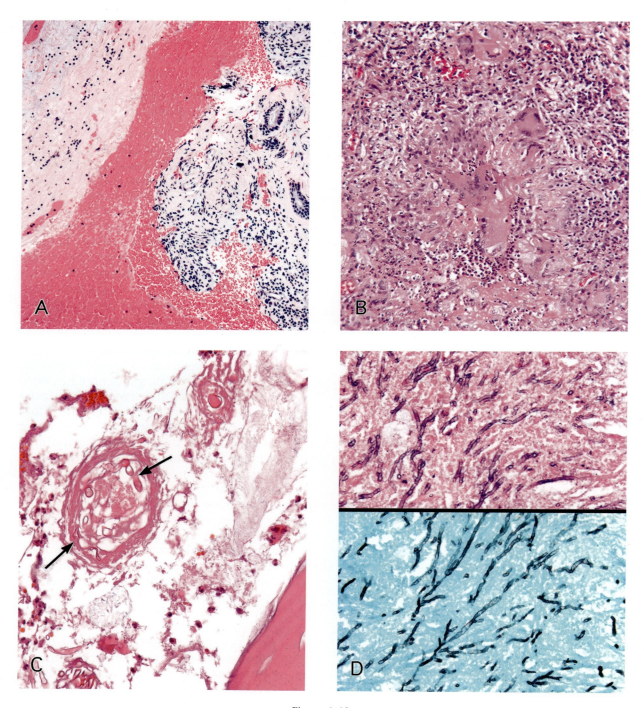

Figure 1-49

INVASIVE FUNGAL RHINOSINUSITIS

A: Submucosal hemorrhage and tissue necrosis (left) of the sinonasal mucosa, with a relative paucity of inflammation. Residual identifiable seromucous glands are seen (right).

B: Granulomatous inflammation and an acute inflammatory cell infiltrate are present.

C: The fungi are in and around the vascular spaces (angioinvasion) (arrows) as well as outside of the vascular spaces (lower right).

D: Histochemical stains for fungi, including periodic acid–Schiff (PAS) (top) and GMS (bottom), delineate the fungal forms.

mucosa by numerous fungal microorganisms (dense accumulation of hyphae), occasional presence of angioinvasion, and associated mixed acute and chronic inflammation. Angioinvasion may be seen but is an uncommon finding. There is an absence of granulomatous inflammation, in contrast to chronic granulomatous FRS.

Chronic granulomatous FRS is characterized by the presence of granulomatous inflammation, including well-formed noncaseating or caseating granulomas and multinucleated giant cells within the submucosa, extensive fibrosis, and the presence of fungal hyphae (fig. 1-50). The fungal forms may be limited in number and only focally identified. A variable mixed inflammatory cell infiltrate is present, including neutrophils and mixed chronic inflammatory cells. Fungal tissue invasion is typically absent as is angioinvasion. GMS and PAS stains assist in delineating the fungal forms.

Treatment and Prognosis. Both chronic invasive FRS and chronic granulomatous FRS are treated by surgical debridement and systemic antifungal therapy. Wide surgical excision of the disease is recommended in order to completely remove the fungal infection (222).

Sinonasal Mucormycosis

Definition. *Sinonasal mucormycosis* is an acute, rapidly evolving fungal infection of the sinonasal region caused by the Zygomycetes class of primitive fungi. Synonyms include *mucormycosis*, *zygomycosis*, and *rhinocerebral* or *rhinorbitocerebral mucormycosis*, terms that may be used because the sinonasal disease often involves adjacent anatomic areas (especially the brain).

Human pathogens in the Zygomycetes class include the orders Mucorales and Entomophthorales. Three fungal genera, designated *Rhizopus*, *Mucor*, and *Absidia*, are included within the order Mucorales, family Mucoraceae. These infections are also sometimes labeled after the higher level class grouping of Zygomycetes, formerly Phycomycetes. Some species in the order Entomophthorales can cause mild infections, but this is not the severe clinicopathologic entity generally implied by mucormycosis.

Clinical Features. The mode of transmission is thought to occur via inhalation. Patients present with the signs of a common cold, with blood-tinged nasal discharge (223). It primarily occurs in adult immunocompromised patients, but rarely in pediatric immunocompromised patients as well (224,225). The typical occurrence is in patients with diabetes mellitus (226), particularly those with the complication of diabetic ketoacidosis, or in immunocompromised patients, including patients with hematologic malignancies (227) and patients following bone marrow transplantation (228,229). Owing to immunosuppression or diabetic acidosis, the body defenses are not sufficient to ward off the invading organism. In the immunocompromised patient, the presentation may include fever, rhinorrhea, facial erythema, and edema (225).

The lesions appear as black necrotic crusts on the nasal mucosa. Nasal septal perforation may follow. Gangrenous change may develop rapidly, and unless aggressive therapeutic intervention ensues, the process may spread to facial skin, eyes and periorbital tissues, and into the central nervous system; spread to distal anatomic sites may occur.

The radiographic findings include evidence of a sinonasal destructive process, including extension into the central nervous system (fig. 1-51) (230). Extension of disease from the nasal cavity and paranasal sinus may include orbital involvement, resulting in extension of the inflammatory process along the infraorbital fissure into the infratemporal fossa and the cavernous sinus. Clinically, orbital involvement may include proptosis, ptosis, ophthalmoplegia, loss of vision, and orbital cellulitis.

Pathogenesis. Although Phycomycetes were originally thought to be the only saprophyte in humans, particularly when found in the oral cavity, nasal passages, or stool, other genera can cause some of the most acutely fatal mycoses known in humans. Of the three genera that cause sinonasal mucormycosis, *Rhizopus* sp. is the most commonly cultured agent. *Mucorales* organisms have large/broad (10 to 20 µm), nonseptated hyphae that branch at haphazard angles. Rare septations may be seen, however, and the presence of septation does not exclude the diagnosis. Partially distorted hyphae are often seen and frequently appear twisted.

Gross Findings. Surgical debridement in order to save the patient's life results in a radical surgical specimen that includes abundant bone.

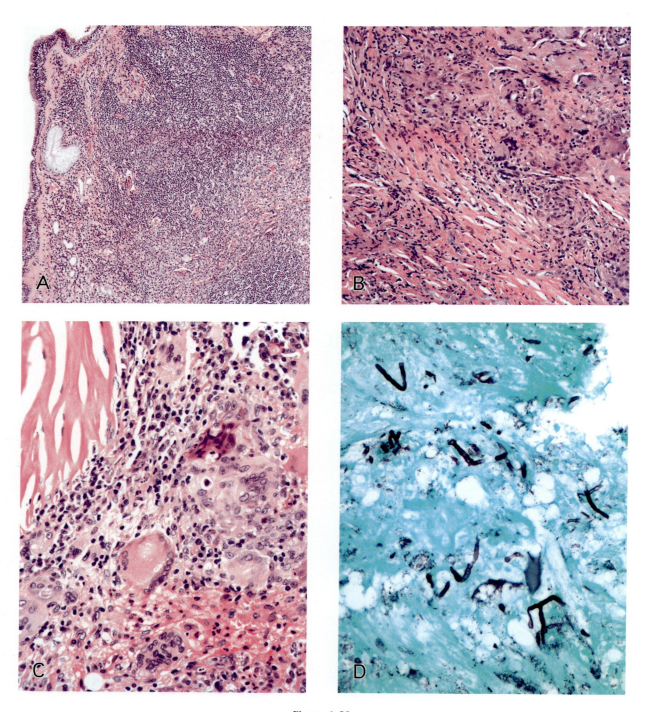

Figure 1-50

CHRONIC GRANULOMATOUS FUNGAL RHINOSINUSITIS

A: The sinonasal mucosa shows a dense submucosal chronic inflammatory cell infiltrate, focal fibrosis, and numerous multinucleated giant cells (bottom).

B,C: At higher magnification, the multinucleated giants cells have associated fibrosis and a mixed chronic inflammation.

D: The GMS stain shows the presence of fungal hyphae and spores. The fungal forms may be limited in number and only focally identified.

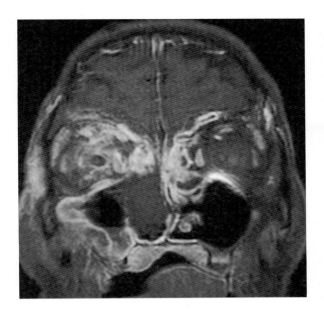 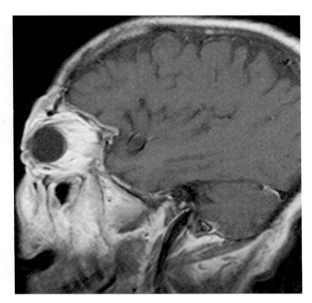

Figure 1-51

SINONASAL MUCORMYCOSIS

This patient had acute myeloid leukemia (AML) and rhinocerebral infection.
Left: Postgadolinium fat suppressed coronal spin echo T1-weighted and postgadolinium sagittal spin echo T1-weighted images demonstrate nasal and ethmoid sinus disease. There is diffuse reticular enhancement of the right retrobulbar fat indicative of orbital cellulites.
Right: The sagittal image also demonstrates inferior frontal dural enhancement.

There are areas of dark discoloration resulting from tissue necrosis.

Microscopic Findings. The soft tissue has prominent areas of infarctive necrosis. The diagnostic finding is the presence of fungal hyphae within the resected tissues. The fungi are angiotropic, with perivascular localization and angioinvasion (fig. 1-52). Invasion through the blood vessel wall and into the lumen may result in complete obstruction, thrombosis, and tissue necrosis ("gritty" type necrosis) in a geographic pattern. Similar findings can be seen in aspergillosis, granulomatosis with polyangiitis (formerly Wegener granulomatosis), and nasal type NK/T-cell lymphoma.

The fungi are large in diameter, generally nonseptate (a rare septum does not exclude the diagnosis), and have hyphae that branch at haphazard angles (fig. 1-52). Some hyphae may be as small as 3 or 4 μm but mostly they are 10 to 15 μm. Partially distorted hyphae are often seen and frequently appear twisted (fig. 1-52). The fungi are usually well seen in H&E-stained slides, without the need for special stains. Nevertheless, PAS and GMS stains assist in the identification of the fungi.

Surrounding tissues have a mixed inflammatory cell infiltrate, hemorrhage, and necrosis. Rarely, foreign body-type multinucleated giant cells are identified, within which fungi may be identified.

Since the seriousness and acuteness of mucormycosis does not allow much time for culturing of the fungus before clinical treatment decisions have to be made, the histologic contribution to these clinical decisions may have to be done without the benefit of culture results. This is seldom a problem because the clinicopathologic features of mucormycosis are very different from those of an indolent fungal infection. In this setting, the histologic evaluation for the presence of fungi by intraoperative consultation (i.e., frozen section) is necessary. Frozen section is a specific and sensitive method to make a quick initial diagnosis of sinonasal mucormycosis (231). In addition to immediate histologic assessment, intraoperative samples should be sent for microbiologic culture in order to be sure of the causative fungus.

Differential Diagnosis. The main consideration is to morphologically distinguish the hyphae of the causative phycomycete from those

Figure 1-52
SINONASAL MUCORMYCOSIS

A: There is ischemic-type necrosis of the sinonasal mucosa. Fungal forms invade the vascular spaces and create a thrombus-like effect and resultant infarctive necrosis.

B: PAS stain delineates the fungi, which are large in diameter, nonseptate, and branch at haphazard angles.

C: The GMS stain shows partially distorted hyphae which appear twisted.

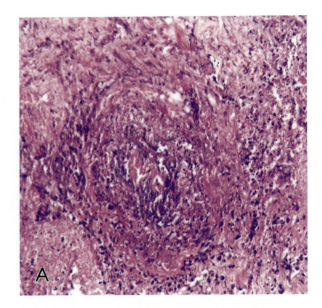
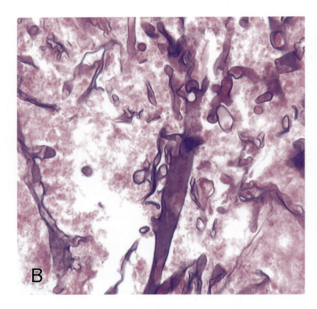
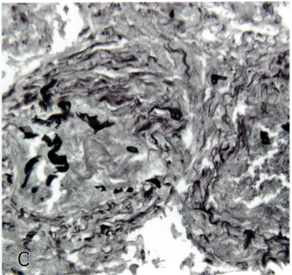

of an *Aspergillus* sp. or an *Aspergillus*-like fungus. The commonly used criteria are the generally smaller, more uniform size of the *Aspergillus* sp. together with a more uniform acute branching of the hyphae. Although a phycomycete may appear to have a rare septation, the presence of multiple definite septa is an important feature of *Aspergillus* and related fungi.

Treatment and Prognosis. Therapy includes surgical removal of necrotic or gangrenous tissue and administration of amphotericin B (232,233). There is increased morbidity and mortality unless prompt therapy is initiated; even with prompt therapy, the prognosis remains guarded. The overall mortality remains high with only half of the patients surviving. Diabetic patients appear to have a better overall survival rate than patients with other comorbidities. Patients who have intracranial involvement, or who do not receive surgery as part of their therapy, have a poor prognosis (227,234).

Rhinosporidiosis

Definition. *Rhinosporidiosis* is a chronic infectious disease of the upper respiratory tract (nasal cavity and nasopharynx) characterized by the

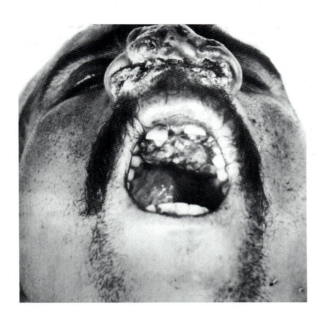

Figure 1-53

RHINOSPORIDIOSIS

There is extensive involvement and destructive growth of the nasal cavity extending into the oral cavity.

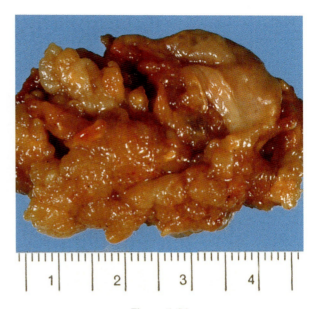

Figure 1-54

SINONASAL RHINOSPORIDIOSIS

A polypoid mass grossly resembles a sinonasal inflammatory polyp.

formation of polypoid masses and caused by the sporulating organism *Rhinosporidium seeberi*.

Clinical Features. Rhinosporidiosis is endemic in India, Sri Lanka, and Brazil, with only sporadic occurrence in the United States. It is more common in men than in women, and affects all ages but is most common in the second to fourth decades of life (235). The infection usually is limited to the upper respiratory mucosa. The most common sites of involvement are the nasal cavity (inferior turbinate along the lateral nasal wall) and the nasopharynx (fig. 1-53) (235,236). Infection may involve the mucosa of the larynx, tracheobronchial tree, esophagus, pharyngeal-oral area, palpebral conjunctiva, and ear (237–239). The most common symptoms include nasal obstruction, epistaxis, and rhinorrhea. The clinical features often are similar to those for usual inflammatory nasal polyps.

Pathogenesis. *R. seeberi* is a fungal organism that does not grow on synthetic media (although it has been propagated in cell culture media). The natural habitat of the organism is not known for certain, but is thought to be a zoonotic organism since it is seen in cattle, horses, and mules. The mode of transmission is thought to occur via water or dust, from which the endospore penetrates the nasal cavity mucosa and matures into sporangium within the submucosal compartment; following maturation, the sporangia burst and endospores are released into the surrounding tissue. The infection is chronic and indolent, and the causative organism does not seem to be contagious.

Gross Findings. While removed tissues may resemble inflammatory polyps, they are more multinodular or papillary in architecture than are polyps (fig. 1-54). The color is a variegated pink to purplish, with a glistening mucoid surface. Sectioning the tissue may reveal whitish microcysts in the submucosal stroma.

Microscopic Findings. The appearance is striking and diagnostic and often does not require special stains. Cystic structures, which are actually sporangia, measuring 100 to 200 µm in diameter, are readily observed within the epithelium but are predominantly submucosal in location (fig. 1-55). These sporangia have varied numbers of sporangiospores (endospores) (fig. 1-55) that are roughly of two size ranges: the smaller spores are about 1 to 2 µm and the larger are 5 to 10 µm in diameter. The larger spores are the more mature form of the endosporulation process. The larger spores tend to congregate toward the center, and the smaller ones are more peripheral, producing a zonated appearance related to spore size.

Smaller cystic structures (without sporangiospores), ranging from 10 to 100 μm, are also seen (fig. 1-55); these are called trophocysts and are considered to result from autoinfection when mature sporangiospores are released from ruptured sporangia. Both the trophocysts and sporangia have a deeply eosinophilic "chitinous" wall, several micrometers thick (fig. 1-55). Occasional collapsed cysts have a half-moon shape.

The mucosal-submucosal tissues surrounding the cysts have a prominent, dense, mixed inflammatory cell infiltrate consisting of lymphocytes, plasma cells, and eosinophils accompanying the microorganisms. Rupture of the cysts induces an acute inflammatory response, however, a granulomatous reaction is not seen. The overlying epithelium may be hyperplastic or demonstrate squamous metaplasia. The microorganisms stain with PAS and mucicarmine stains.

Differential Diagnosis. The cylindrical cell variant of sinonasal (Schneiderian) papilloma tends to have collections of mucus within the epithelium that often attract numerous inflammatory cells, which aggregate within the mucus (fig. 1-56). The mucus cysts might be mistaken for the sporangia (or trophocysts) and the inflammatory cells for the endospores of rhinosporidiosis. A helpful feature is the limitation of the microcysts of the papilloma to an intraepithelial location; with rhinosporidiosis, most of the cystic structures are submucosal.

The rhinosporidial sporangia might be mistaken for those of *Coccidioides immitis*. *R. seeberi*, however, is usually much larger and the wall stains with a mucin stain; *C. immitis* is mucin negative.

Treatment and Prognosis. The only effective treatment is surgical excision. No drug has proven to be effective for this disease. Recurrences, necessitating additional surgical excision, may be seen in 10 percent of cases. Occasionally, the disease spontaneously regresses.

Other Fungi

Other fungal diseases of the sinonasal tract include *sporotrichosis*, *blastomycosis*, *coccidioidomycosis*, *cryptococcosis*, and *histoplasmosis*. Sinonasal infection by these fungal diseases is rare.

Nasal Cavity Sporotrichosis. *Sporotrichum schenckii* is a fungus that is introduced into the extremity through abrasions caused by splinters or thorns (rose bushes). Sporotrichosis is endemic in Rio de Janeiro, Brazil. Cases are associated with human immunodeficiency virus (HIV) infection or acquired immunodeficiency syndrome (AIDS) (240,241). The infection starts as a red papular lesion and then develops into an abscess. This spreads to the regional lymph nodes, resulting in multiple granulomas, which occur along the course of the lymphatics, and ulcerate as the area is ruptured. Subcutaneous inoculation with the ubiquitous fungus *sporothrix schenckii* leads to chronic granulomatous infection that involves skin and subcutaneous tissues. Although rare, *Sporotrichum schenckii* can cause a primary nasal cavity infection, resulting in pansinusitis with nasal discharge, sneezing, and nasal obstruction (242), or invasive sinusitis (241). Because of the rarity of this infection and the fact that the causative organism may be sparse and difficult to find, the correct diagnosis is likely to be missed and other diagnoses entertained.

The histologic findings include microabscesses and a granulomatous reaction (fig. 1-57), which are also features of granulomatosis with polyangiitis (formerly Wegener granulomatosis). The neutrophils are surrounded by multinucleated giant cells, epithelioid cells, and lymphocytes. It is important not to mistake a case of sporotrichosis for granulomatosis with polyangiitis. Sporotrichosis has more pronounced (and larger) microabscess formation and more epithelioid histiocytes than sinonasal granulomatosis with polyangiitis (see previous discussion in this chapter).

Typically there are only a few yeasts visible, which are difficult to see with H&E stains. Special stains (PAS and GMS) are needed for visualization of the organism (fig. 1-57). The Splendore-Hoeppli phenomenon may be present.

Supersaturated potassium iodide is the treatment of choice. Lymphocutaneous disease generally can be treated orally with this drug, while patients with pulmonary or deep infection require amphotericin or ketoconazole.

Sinonasal Blastomycosis, Coccidioidomycosis, Cryptococcosis, and Histoplasmosis. These fungal infections rarely encroach upon the sinonasal tract, and are usually limited to

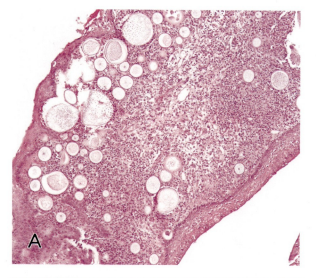
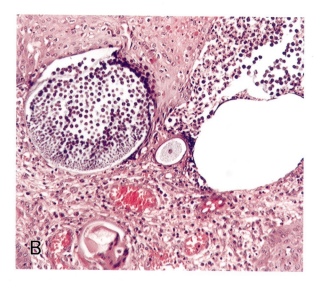
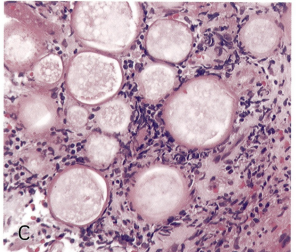
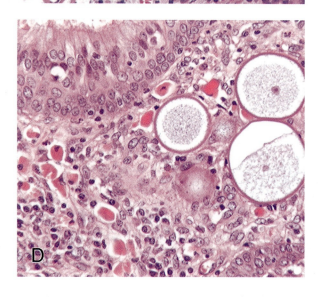
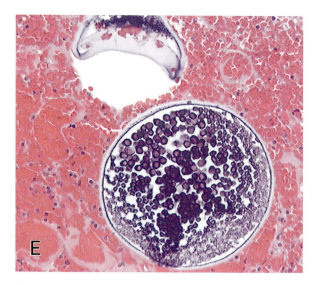

Figure 1-55

SINONASAL RHINOSPORIDIOSIS

A: The polypoid lesion shows variably sized cysts within the submucosa as well as within the surface epithelium.

B: Sporangia contain numerous sporangiospores (endospores).

C: Cystic structures without sporangiospores are referred to as trophocysts and are considered to result from auto-infection via mature sporangiospores being released from ruptured sporangia.

D,E: Both the trophocysts (D) and sporangia (E) have a deeply eosinophilic "chitinous" wall several micrometers thick; one sporangia is collapsed with the a half-moon shape.

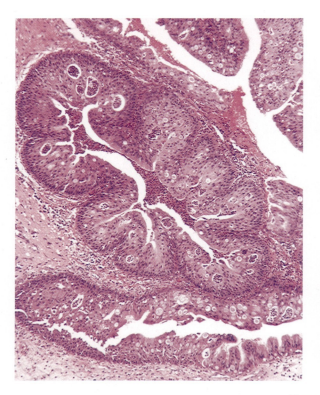 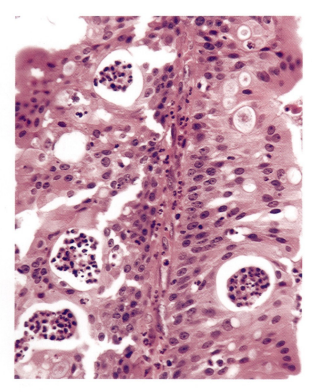

Figure 1-56

SINONASAL PAPILLOMA, CYLINDRICAL CELL TYPE

Left: This benign neoplasm of the sinonasal tract is characterized by an epithelial proliferation of cells with oncocytic-appearing cytoplasm, scattered mucocytes, and (mucus) cysts limited to the epithelial proliferation and not in the submucosa.

Right: At higher magnification, the cysts contain inflammatory cells rather than the endospores of rhinosporidia.

the anterior nasal vestibule area (figs. 1-58–1-61). Usually there is an associated facial skin infection which is more prominent than the nasal cavity involvement and which is an important clue to the diagnosis. Infection of other sites (especially the lungs) is often part of the clinical picture. These fungi may cause pseudoepitheliomatous hyperplasia, which clinically and pathologically may suggest an epithelial neoplasm.

BACTERIAL DISEASES

Bacterial Rhinoscleroma

Definition. *Rhinoscleroma* is a chronic granulomatous infection of the nasal cavity (and occasionally the pharynx or laryngotrachea) caused by *Klebsiella rhinoscleromatis*. Synonyms include *scrofulous lupus* and *scleroma*.

Clinical Features. The disease is endemic in Egypt, parts of Central and South America, North and Central Africa, and Eastern Europe (243–246). This geographic involvement currently is not as clearly apparent as formerly, and sporadic cases can be found in any geographic area but are uncommon in the United States. There is no gender predilection. It can appear in a patient of almost any age, but most commonly is found in young or middle-aged adults (244,245). It has a greater prevalence among persons in lower socioeconomic groups and in persons from rural areas in which poor living conditions and malnutrition foster the growth and spread of the disease.

The infection manifests initially in the nasal cavity and spreads posteriorly to the nasopharynx; other sites of involvement include the paranasal sinuses, orbit, larynx, tracheobronchial tree, and middle ear. Rhinoscleroma has been reported in association with extranodal sinus histiocytosis with massive lymphadenopathy (Rosai-Dorfman

Nasal Cavity and Paranasal Sinuses

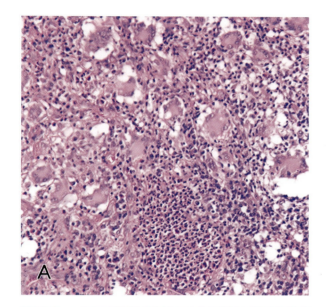

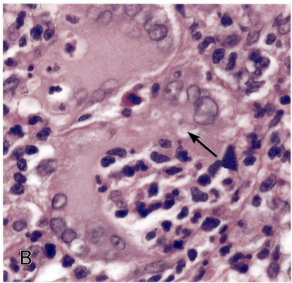

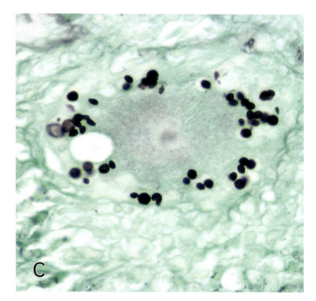

Figure 1-57

NASAL CAVITY SPOROTRICHOSIS

A,B: The histologic features include microabscess formation and granulomatous reaction, including multinucleated giant cells. The microorganism is seen in the giant cells (arrow).

C: The GMS stain highlights the presence of *Sporotrichum schenckii* within the multinucleated giant cells.

disease) (247), HIV-positive patients (243), and patients with a familial history (243).

There are three clinical phases/stages. A rhinitic, exudative, or catarrhal stage is characterized by mucopurulent nasal discharge. The symptoms in the rhinitic stage can resemble those of a prolonged "cold" or chronic low-grade nasal allergy. This stage can continue for many months or even years, and the presence of a granular-appearing nasal mucosa heralds the progression to the next stage. The exudative (florid) stage (fig. 1-62) is marked by mucosal thickening that may result in nasal obstruction. The infected mucosa is pale. The diffuse nodular thickening may result in a mass-like growth composed of firm nodules (consistency of cartilage). The mass may cause nasal expansion and deformity, with some facial mutilation. Bone erosion may contribute to the radiographic findings, suggesting a malignancy. The diagnosis is usually made at this point. The fibrotic or cicatricial stage represents resolution of disease. The resultant "burnt-out" fibrosis causes deformity but nasal discharge abates (dry nose) and without further progression locally. Spread to other areas of the respiratory tract may occur

Non-Neoplastic Diseases of the Head and Neck

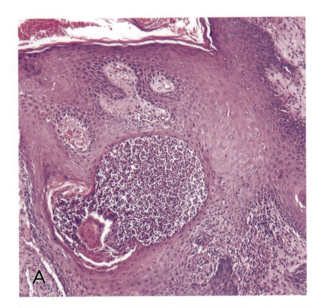

Figure 1-58

SINONASAL BLASTOMYCOSIS

A: The hyperplastic squamous epithelium has an associated microabscess.

B: At higher magnification, multinucleated giant cells are seen in association with the microabcess; the microorganism can be seen in the giant cells (arrow).

C: The PAS stain shows the microorganisms within the giant cells.

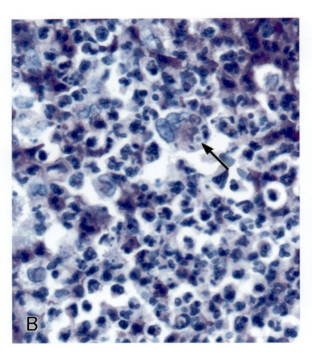

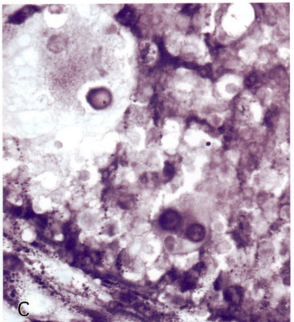

during this phase. This stage generally follows therapy, which is usually instigated during the second stage.

Pathogenesis. *K. rhinoscleromatis* is a Gram-negative diplobacillus of the family Enterobacteriaceae. The organism measures about 2.5 µm, is encapsulated with a slime mucopolysaccharide, and can be cultured on simple media. The infection is not considered contagious (or is only minimally so).

Microscopic Findings. The characteristic histology seen in the florid or proliferative phase consists of a submucosal granulomatous infiltrate composed of macrophages (also referred to as Mikulicz cells), with small nuclei and strikingly clear to foamy cytoplasm (fig. 1-63) intimately associated with an admixture of lymphocytes and numerous plasma cells. The number of plasma cells present may be unusually prominent for a nasal cavity inflammation

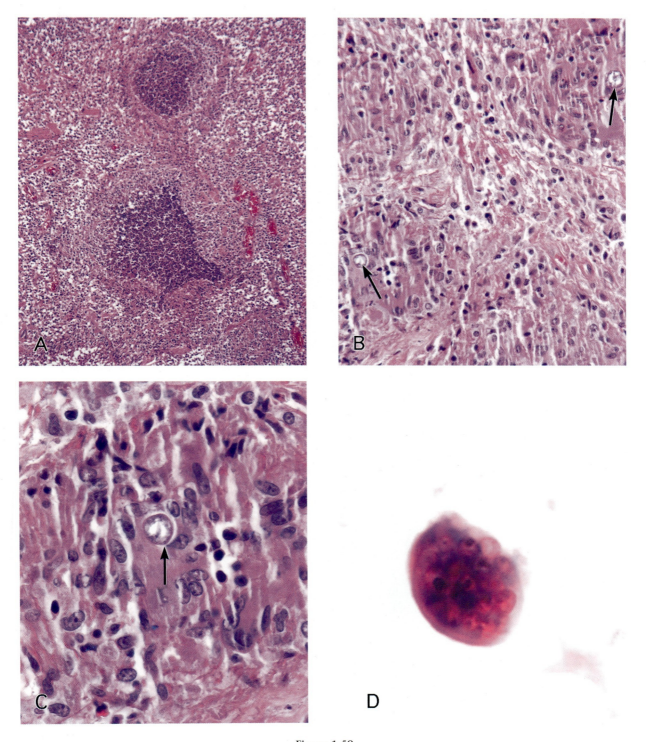

Figure 1-59

SINONASAL COCCIDIODOMYCOSIS

A: Suppurative granulomatous inflammation is present.
B,C: Granulomatous inflammation with identifiable yeast (*C. immitis*) (arrows).
D: Mature sporangium containing sporangiospores (endospores).

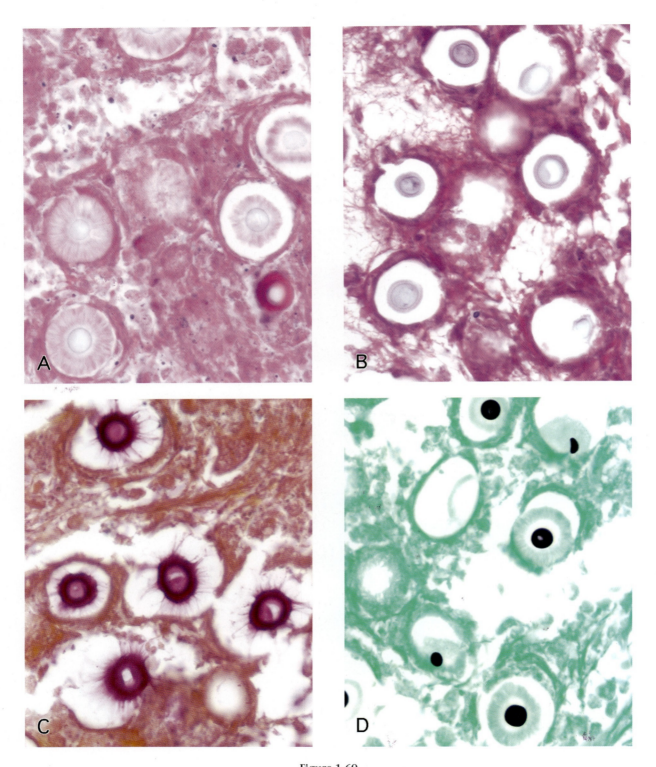

Figure 1-60
SINONASAL CRYPTOCOCCAL INFECTION
A: Hematoxylin and eosin (H&E) stain highlights encapsulated microorganisms.
B–D: Organisms are delineated as well by PAS (B), mucicarmine (C), and GMS (D) stains.

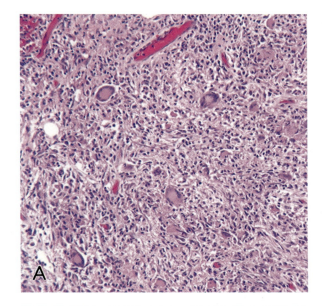

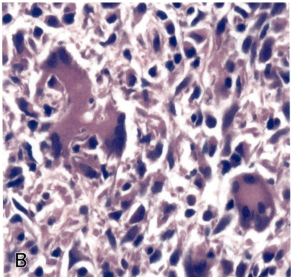

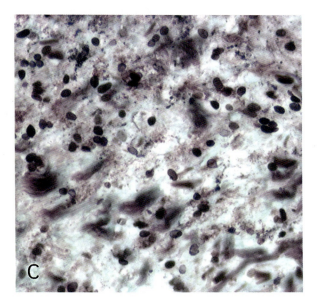

Figure 1-61

SINONASAL HISTOPLASMOSIS

A,B: There is an admixture of histiocytes and multinucleated giant cells.

C: The microorganisms are located within the giant cells, requiring special stains (GMS) for identification.

and this is a clue to the diagnosis given the anatomic location. The plasma cells may contain intracytoplasmic eosinophilic inclusions (globules), referred to as Russell bodies, which represent immunoglobulins.

The macrophages (Mikulicz cells) harbor the bacteria. The presence of some component in the wall of the causative bacterium leads to the histiocytes being expanded by an osmotic hydropic alteration (248). The number of macrophages varies with the stage of the disease; in the proliferative stage, they are plentiful and readily identifiable. The macrophages may be difficult to identify in the fibrotic phase. Emperiopolesis, in which the histiocytes ingest (phagocytize) inflammatory cells within their cytoplasm, is a feature that can be seen in the macrophages in rhinoscleroma (249).

The overlying respiratory epithelium may demonstrate squamous metaplasia or pseudoepitheliomatous hyperplasia. Rarely, ulceration is seen.

Immunohistochemical Findings. The key to confirming the diagnosis is the histologic demonstration of the bacterial rods, mostly in or associated with the macrophages. The best stain is the Warthin-Starry silver impregnation,

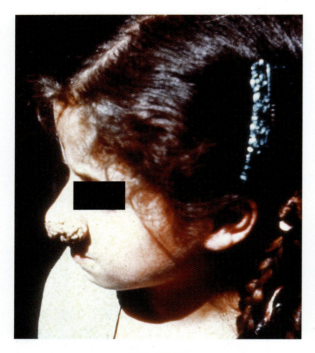

Figure 1-62

NASAL RHINOSCLEROMA

The florid or proliferative stage is characterized by an intranasal mass with expansion and deformity as well as nasal obstruction.

which make the bacteria apparent (fig. 1-63). The bacteria are sometimes visualized with Giemsa, GMS, or Brown and Hopps stains, but for unclear reasons the staining is surprisingly capricious and "falsely negative" with these stains. The macrophages are CD68 positive immunohistochemically but negative for S-100 protein, CD1a, and langerin.

Differential Diagnosis. Clinically, midline destructive diseases such as granulomatosis with polyangiitis or malignant lymphoma may be considered, but rhinoscleroma is not as destructive as it is proliferative. The presence of a submucosal macrophage proliferation with admixed lymphocytes and plasma cells may suggest a possible diagnosis of extranodal sinus histiocytosis with massive lymphadenopathy (Rosai-Dorfman disease), especially in the presence of emperipolesis. Differentiation can be accomplished by either identifying the causative microorganism in rhinoscleroma by Warthin-Starry staining or by immunohistochemistry; the macrophages (histiocytes) in rhinoscleroma are CD68 positive and S-100 protein negative while the histiocytes in extranodal sinus histiocytosis with massive lymphadenopathy are CD68 positive and S-100 protein positive.

Included in the differential diagnosis are other infections such as leprosy, yaws, mucocutaneous leishmaniasis, paracoccidioidomycosis (South American blastomycosis), rhinosporidiosis, syphilis, and tuberculosis. The lepra cells in leprosy (see below), especially histologically, mimic the macrophages of rhinoscleroma. Otherwise, the demonstration of the bacterial rods of *K. rhinoscleromatis* is the key to confident diagnosis. In this situation, the most important point leading to diagnosis is to consider rhinoscleroma so that appropriate stains are done. The disease is uncommon enough in some countries, such as the United States, that the diagnosis may not be considered in the differential diagnosis. Some cases have been misinterpreted as a pseudotumorous inflammation such as plasma cell granuloma (250).

Treatment and Prognosis. The treatment of choice is long-term antibiotic therapy (tetracycline, streptomycin, thiophenicol, ciprofloxacin) followed by surgical debridement. Surgical resection may be necessary to correct functional and aesthetic disorders (246) or when airway obstruction may be life threatening. The prognosis is good following initiation of antibiotic therapy, although recurrence/relapse occur, which may necessitate additional biopsies (243). Recurrence rates of up to 25 percent within 10 years of diagnosis have been reported (244,245). Owing to the potential for recurrence/relapse, long-term follow-up is advised (248).

Sinonasal Botryomycosis

Sinonasal botryomycosis is a chronic bacterial infection analogous to a fungus ball except that the mass of microorganisms is composed of bacteria, usually *Pseudomonas* sp. It usually is a cutaneous (skin and subcutaneous tissue) lesion and uncommonly is mucosal based (251). The term botryomycosis is used to describe a lesion resembling mulberry, or a "bunch of grapes," (Greek botryos), which was initially believed to be caused by a true fungus. *Bacteria ball* is a synonym.

Botryomycosis primarily occurs as a skin-related lesion; it rarely affects viscera (e.g., lung, liver, kidney, bowel, brain, orbit, spleen, lymph

Nasal Cavity and Paranasal Sinuses

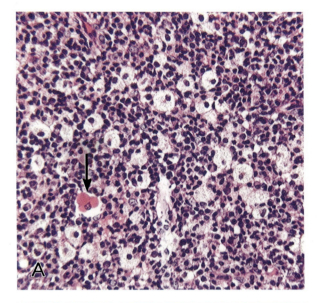

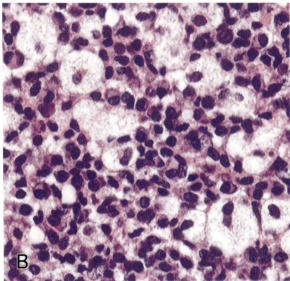

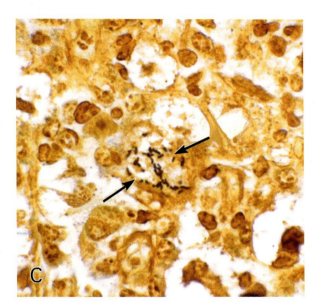

Figure 1-63

SINONASAL RHINOSCLEROMA

A,B: The characteristic histologic features include the presence of Mikulicz cells, which are histiocytes with small nuclei with strikingly clear expanded cytoplasm associated with a prominent mature plasma cell infiltrate. A Russell body (A, arrow) is characterized by a plasma cell with intracytoplasmic eosinophilic inclusion globules indicative of immunoglobulins.

C: The causative bacteria are present within the histiocytes (arrows), requiring special stains (Warthin-Starry) for their identification.

nodes, tonsil, sinonasal tract). It tends to be a localized lesion that may clinically simulate an aggressive neoplasm. It occurs in healthy individuals, patients with chronic disease, and immunocompromised patients (e.g., with cystic fibrosis, diabetes mellitus, chronic granulomatous disease, AIDS) (251). Patients with sinonasal disease may present with persistent headache and bulging eyes. Radiographic evidence of an expansile paranasal sinus lesion with bony erosion may be present (251).

The histologic findings include the presence of amorphous, acellular material, with deposition of proteinaceous material and inorganic compounds (fig. 1-64). Separate, rounded eosinophilic grains or granules, associated with a neutrophilic infiltrate, are seen. The grains or granules contain the causative bacterial organisms (fig. 1-64). Club-like or radiating projections form along the periphery of the acellular material, referred to as the Splendore-Hoeppli phenomenon, which is an antigen-antibody reaction seen in association with other organisms including actinomyces, fungi, bacteria, helminthes, mycetoma, phycomycosis, as well as in association with the presence of silk sutures.

Figure 1-64

SINONASAL BOTRYOMYCOSIS

A: The amorphous, acellular material contains proteinaceous material and inorganic compounds.

B: At higher magnification, separate, rounded eosinophilic grains or granules associated with a neutrophilic infiltrate are seen; the grains or granules contain the causative bacterial organisms (i.e., *Pseudomonas aeruginosa*).

C: Filamentous Gram-negative bacilli morphologically compatible with *P. aeruginosa* are present (Gram stain) but may be difficult to identify.

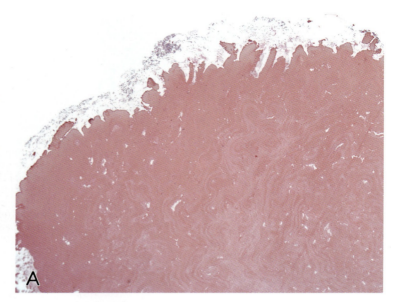
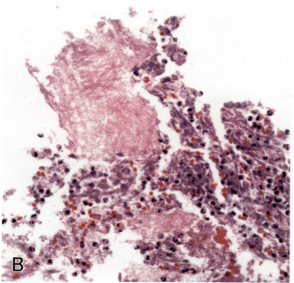
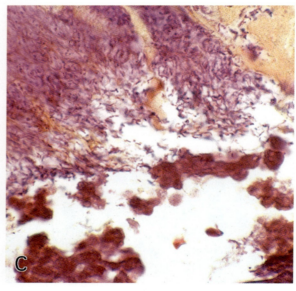

The microscopic features of surgically removed material may be perplexing to the pathologist because the amorphous and variegated appearance of the material is likely to be difficult to recognize as aggregated bacteria. This may be due to the secondary deposition of proteinaceous material and inorganic compounds that largely obscure the bacteria. Histochemical stains for bacteria (e.g., Gram and Brown and Hopps) delineate the filamentous Gram-negative *P. aeruginosa*. The bacteria may not be readily identifiable, and if the diagnosis is not considered or if the pathologist is not familiar with the entity, the diagnosis may be overlooked. Microbiologic cultures confirm a *Pseudomonas* infection.

Surgical evacuation is curative. Botryomycotic lesions are generally resistant to antimicrobial therapy because of associated fibrosis and the compactness of the granules characteristic of botryomycotic lesions. Therapeutic drugs may not reach the microorganisms.

Miscellaneous Sinonasal Bacterial Infections

Although *leprosy* is not expected to present clinically solely as a nasal infection, nasal involvement is very common in patients with this infection. Indeed, nasal infection may be important in the transmission of the disease.

Other mycobacterial infections also present, rarely, in the sinonasal tract, but in immunocompromised individuals (e.g., those with AIDS) such infections are more frequent, especially with atypical mycobacteria. In this setting, the host's inflammatory response may be histologically surprisingly nonspecific and without "tubercular" granulomatous features; a "high index of suspicion" may be required to perform the acid-fast staining, but once this is done the diagnosis is obvious because of the large number of organisms.

In patients with a clinical "midline destructive" condition in the nasal cavity (with the clinical suspicion centered mainly around granulomatosis with polyangiitis or angiocentric NK/T-cell lymphoma), the possible destructive effects of *tertiary syphilis* should be considered. Also, the presence of sinonasal mucosa-based plasma cell-rich inflammatory infiltrate could conceivably represent secondary syphilis. The histology of such lesions may suggest plasma cell endarteritis. In either of these situations, the diagnosis will not likely be syphilis, but it is easy to have a serologic test performed, including nontreponemal (nonspecific) antibody tests and treponemal (specific) antibody tests (tests that tend to be most reactive in the secondary stage of disease). The diagnosis of syphilis is easy to overlook in contemporary times.

PROTOZOAL DISEASES

Mucocutaneous Leishmaniasis

Leishmaniasis is a protozoal infection caused by different species of *Leishmania*; the parasite is transmitted by the bite of an infected female phlebotomine sandfly. A clinical history, especially including travel to an endemic area, may be necessary to suspect the possibility of this infection. The disease is prevalent throughout the world.

There are three forms of disease: cutaneous, mucocutaneous, and visceral. *Cutaneous leishmaniasis (oriental or tropical sore)* is caused by *Leishmania tropica* (in Asia and Africa) and *Leishmania mexicana* (in Central and South America). It is endemic in the Middle East, around the eastern Mediterranean, in North Africa, and in parts of Asia. Acute lesions are usually single papules

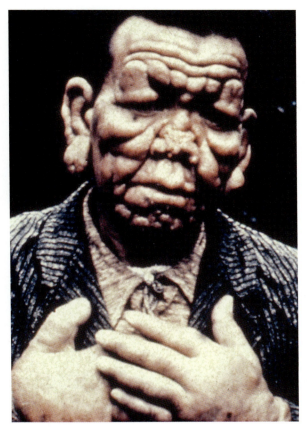

Figure 1-65

MUCOCUTANEOUS LEISHMANIASIS

Leishmania braziliensis with extensive cutaneous involvement as well as mucosal involvement of the sinonasal tract.

that may become nodules that ulcerate, heal, and leave a scar. Chronic lesions (persisting for 1 to 2 years) are single or occasionally multiple, raised nonulcerated plaques. The recidivous (lupoid) form includes erythematous papules, often circinate, near scars of previously healed lesions. The disseminated form (primary diffuse cutaneous leishmaniasis) develops in anergic individuals as widespread nodules and macules without ulceration or visceral involvement (some authorities consider diffuse cutaneous leishmaniasis to represent a fourth form of disease). The tardive form is the development of a lesion at the site of recent cutaneous surgery, with the likely source of infection occurring over five decades previously.

Mucocutaneous leishmaniasis (fig. 1-65) is caused by *Leishmania braziliensis*. It is endemic to Central and South America or in travelers to those areas.

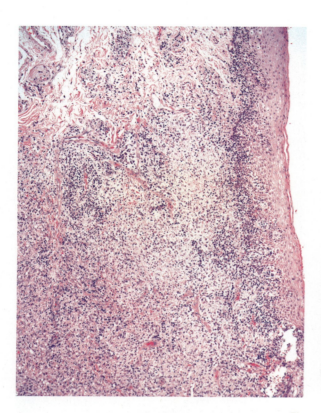 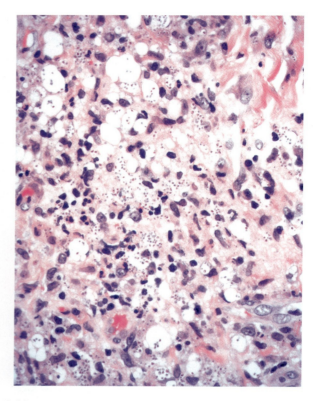

Figure 1-66

MUCOCUTANEOUS LEISHMANIASIS

Left: Diffuse anergic leishmaniasis is characterized by a dermal inflammatory cell infiltrate composed of histiocytes, with associated lymphocytes and plasma cells, and absence of granulomatous inflammation.

Right: The microorganisms *L. braziliensis*, referred to as amastigotes, are readily seen within the histiocytes by H&E staining, appearing as small, ovoid to round structures with a thin cell membrane and absence of a capsule, a differentiating feature from *Histoplasma capsulatum*.

The initial lesions resemble those of the cutaneous form. The rare disseminated anergic form may occur in immunocompromised individuals (252). The development of destructive ulcerative lesions of the mucous membranes is referred to as *espundia*. The upper aerodigestive tract sites of involvement include the sinonasal tract, nasopharynx, and oral cavity (tongue) (253).

Visceral leishmaniasis (synonyms include *Kala-azar, dumdum fever,* and *black fever*) is an acute or chronic infection caused by *Leishmania donovani*; it is widely distributed, but occurs predominantly in South America, Africa, the Mediterranean basin (Italy, Greece), and Asia. Multiple organs are affected and may result in fever, hepatosplenomegaly, weight loss, anemia, and thrombocytopenia. The visceral form is a leading cause of death from tropical parasitic infections, second only to malaria (254).

Leishmaniasis usually starts as a cutaneous lesion at any of a number of sites. Sinonasal mucocutaneous infection represents secondary spread from cutaneous infection (fig. 1-66). The histologic features of mucocutaneous infection include surface ulceration with a marked lymphoplasmacytic cell infiltrate and granulation tissue. Pseudoepitheliomatous hyperplasia of the surface epithelium may be present. In the immune competent patient, the inflammatory response may be vaguely granulomatous, with some epithelioid histiocytes and scattered giant cells, as well as necrosis (necrotizing granuloma). In this setting, the number of microorganisms present may be sparse.

In diffuse anergic leishmaniasis, there is no granulomatous inflammation but numerous large histiocytes with associated lymphocytes and plasma cells. In this setting, numerous microorganisms are present (fig. 1-66). The microorganisms, referred to as amastigotes, are found within histiocytes and can be seen by H&E stain but often require oil immersion for identification. They tend to be localized at the periphery of the macrophages (so-called marque sign), and are small, ovoid to round and measure 1.5 to 3.0 μm in diameter. They have a thin cell membrane, large nucleus, and a rod-shaped kinetoplast. The nucleus and kinetoplast are accentuated by the Giemsa stain. The absence of a capsule assists in differentiating *Leishmania* from *Histoplasma capsulatum*. Molecular biologic techniques (polymerase chain reaction) assist in detecting the presence of microorganisms (252,255,256).

Various drugs, including antifungal ketoconazole, as well as miltefosine, pentamidine, and metronidazole are effective in the treatment of leishmaniasis (252). The most promising drug is an anticancer compound, miltefosine, which belongs to the alkylphosphocholines (252). Its limitations include that it cannot be given during pregnancy, results in severe gastrointestinal side effects, and is costly. Other drugs such as paromomycin, allopurinol, and sitamaquine result in variable cure rates. Most of these compounds, however, are not as efficient as amphotericin B (257–259).

Amebiasis

The nasal cavity is the portal of entry for acute and fatal cerebral infections due to *Naegleria fowleri* (260) and the more chronic granulomatous amebic encephalitis due to *Acanthamoeba* sp. (or *B. mandrillaris*) (261). Since the clinical manifestations are the result of the encephalitis, and this is the location of most infections, a diagnosis from a nasal cavity surgical specimen is not expected (262,263). Such has occurred, however, on rare occasions and such a finding should be considered.

VIRAL DISEASES

Upper respiratory tract viral infections are probably the most common type of human infection, but in the field of surgical pathology, sinonasal viral infections hardly come into diagnostic consideration. It is true that human papillomavirus (HPV) and EBV genomes play a role in important neoplastic conditions, but these are not discussed here.

RHINOSINUSITIS

Definition. *Rhinosinusitis* is a nonspecific or specific inflammation of the sinonasal tract that may be isolated to the nasal cavity (rhinitis), isolated to the paranasal sinuses (sinusitis), or involve both nasal cavity and paranasal sinuses (rhinosinusitis).

Clinical Features. The causes of rhinosinusitis are numerous (Table 1-6) and include allergies (most common), infections, aspirin intolerance or aspirin-exacerbated respiratory disease (AERD), nonallergic rhinosinusitis with eosinophilia (NARES), idiopathic conditions, occupational or environmental exposure, systemic diseases (e.g., asthma, cystic fibrosis), structural or mechanical causes (e.g., deviated nasal septum, neoplasms), immotile cilia syndrome, medications, and pregnancy (264–273). Medication-induced rhinosinusitis is referred to as *rhinosinusitis medicamentosa* and may be caused by topical or systemic medications such as propranolol, oral contraceptives, reserpine, and nasal sprays. Pregnancy-related rhinosinusitis is thought to result from the combined effects on the nasal mucosa of pregnancy-related hormones, increased blood volume, and airway resistance (271,274,275).

Radiologic Findings. Often, the diagnosis of rhinosinusitis is straightforward and does not require radiographic imaging or tissue sampling (276). There are, however, exceptions in which

Table 1-6
CAUSES OF RHINOSINUSITIS

Allergic (most common)
Infectious
Aspirin intolerance or aspirin-exacerbated respiratory disease (AERD)
Nonallergic rhinosinusitis with eosinophilia (NARES)
Idiopathic
Occupational or environmental exposure
Systemic diseases
Structural or mechanical causes
Medication induced
Pregnancy

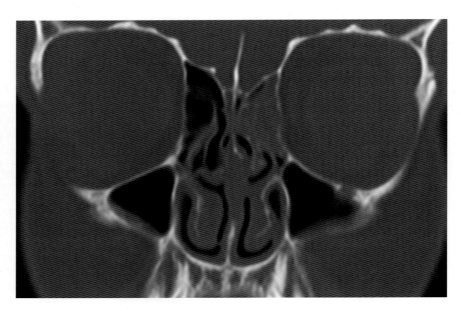

Figure 1-67

CHRONIC RHINOSINUSITIS

Coronal bone window image demonstrates thickening of the mucosal surfaces of the floor and lateral walls of each inferior meatus in a patient with inflammatory change involving the ethmoid sinuses. (Courtesy of Dr. A. Khorsandi, New York, NY.)

both radiographic imaging and biopsies are required in order to establish the diagnosis and to exclude other possible diseases that cause or are associated with rhinosinusitis.

Radiologic air-fluid levels represent the best diagnostic clue to acute rhinosinusitis, characterized by bubbly appearing secretions within a sinus with mucosal thickening. It is most common in the ethmoid and maxillary sinuses, creating a "foam on water" appearance. The sinus lumen size remains normal, without expansion or reduction in volume, but sinus reduction in volume can be seen with chronic rhinosinusitis. This is not considered accurate for assessing extent of inflammation.

In chronic rhinosinusitis, the radiologic findings include mucosal thickening or soft tissue opacification of a nonexpanded sinus, with thickening and sclerosis of sinus bony walls (fig. 1-67) (277). It is most common in this ethmoid sinus followed by maxillary, frontal, and sphenoid sinuses. The sinus lumen size remains normal or is decreased in volume.

Computerized tomography (CT) findings in acute rhinosinusitis include peripheral soft tissue mucosal thickening within a sinus, with inflammatory tissue obstructing the drainage pathways of the osteomedial complex (277). Contrast enhancement shows inflamed mucosa but not central secretions.

Magnetic resonance imaging (MRI) is not frequently performed for rhinosinusitis but is used to evaluate for orbital and intracranial complications. MRI findings can be used to differentiate fungal from other inflammatory diseases and to differentiate inflammatory lesions from neoplasms.

CT findings in chronic sinusitis include mucosal thickening or opacification of the sinus without sinus expansion. There is variable density (isodense to hyperdense) of secretions depending on content (protein, water, fungi). CT is better at detecting luminal sinus disease than endoscopic evaluation but there is a lack of correlation between symptomatology and imaging findings.

Microscopic Findings. The histologic changes of nonspecific chronic sinusitis include a submucosal mixed inflammatory cell infiltrate, including mature lymphocytes with a variable admixture of plasma cells, eosinophils, histiocytes, and neutrophils, and submucosal edema. Other findings include surface epithelial squamous metaplasia, which is often (but not uniformly) present, minimal fibrosis, and a vascular proliferation. In longstanding or recurrent/persistent disease, inflammatory epithelial hyperplasia may be present, clinically referred to as *hyperplastic papillary sinusitis*. Histologically, the changes include a papillary appearance to the surface mucosa, which is lined by a single layer of columnar cells and goblet cells, and abundant inflammatory cells in the lamina propria (fig. 1-68).

Nasal Cavity and Paranasal Sinuses

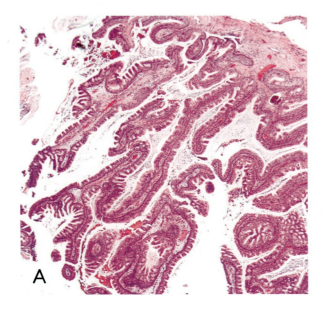

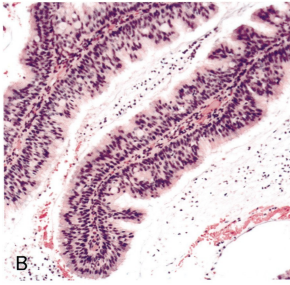
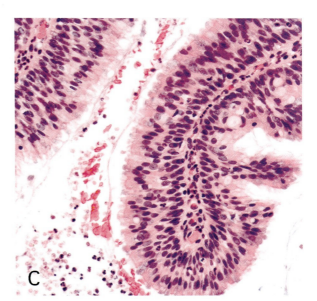

Figure 1-68

PAPILLARY SINUSITIS

A secondary alteration that occurs in longstanding cases of chronic sinusitis is a prominent papillary architecture composed of ciliated pseudostratified columnar epithelial cells with intermixed goblet cells. This appearance is clinically referred to hyperplastic papillary sinusitis and should not be mistaken for either a sinonasal papilloma or low-grade (papillary) adenocarcinoma.

Differential Diagnosis. The differential diagnosis includes a more specific cause of sinusitis (e.g., specific infectious etiology) and sinonasal inflammatory polyp. In the presence of papillary epithelial hyperplasia, the differential diagnosis includes sinonasal (Schneiderian) papilloma and less often sinonasal adenocarcinoma.

Treatment and Prognosis. Rhinosinusitis is a spectrum of diseases and defining its various subtypes alters management to include medical treatment (e.g., steroids, antibiotics) and surgery (e.g., functional endoscopic sinus surgery [FESS]). Management often involves a combination of systemic and topical therapies, with surgery reserved for patients who fail medical therapy. FESS is among the most common surgeries performed for sinonasal disease refractory to maximal medical therapy.

Over the past decades, the average life expectancy for patients with cystic fibrosis has increased; with increasing survival and improved pulmonary management, otolaryngologists are now seeing increasing numbers of cystic fibrosis patients with chronic rhinosinusitis (278). For adult and pediatric cystic fibrosis patients with sinusitis, FESS yields clinical improvement measured primarily by sinonasal symptoms and endoscopic findings. In general, sinusitis is not life threatening, but depending on cause, may result in ongoing and persistent morbidity.

Allergic Rhinosinusitis

In adults, allergies are the most common cause of rhinosinusitis; in children, allergies are second to viral upper respiratory infection (279,280). There is no gender predilection and allergic rhinosinusitis occurs over a wide age range. Allergic rhinosinusitis is caused by exposure to an allergen in a sensitized patient. It is mediated via a type I IgE immune reaction. Among the more common allergens are pollens, animal dander, dust mites, and mold. Allergic rhinosinusitis may predispose patients to recurrent or chronic sinusitis. Allergic rhinosinusitis may be familial (280).

In a sensitized patient, exposure results in an allergic reaction that produces nasal congestion with rhinorrhea, sneezing, and itching. In noninfected patients, the nasal secretions appear clear; in infected patients, the nasal secretions appear purulent. The reaction begins within minutes of exposure, peaking about 15 minutes later. The endoscopic appearance of the sinonasal mucosa is pale to bluish; inflammatory polyps may or may not be identified.

Generally, the gold standard for allergy testing is skin testing, representing a reaction between antigen and sensitized mast cells in the skin that results in a wheal and flare skin response. Occasionally, skin testing may be negative in allergic rhinosinusitis patients due to local (nasal) synthesis of IgE, with the local (nasal) tissue being more sensitive than the distant (cutaneous) site (281).

The histopathologic findings of allergic rhinosinusitis include submucosal edema with a mixed inflammatory cell reaction dominated by the presence of eosinophils. Squamous metaplasia of the surface epithelium may be present. Neutrophils can be identified, especially in the presence of secondary bacterial infection.

The treatment for allergic rhinosinusitis includes antihistamines, nasal cromolyn preparations (stabilizes mast cells against degranulation and release of inflammatory mediators), topical corticosteroids, and immunotherapy for documented IgE-mediated allergies.

Infectious Rhinosinusitis

Infectious rhinosinusitis is caused by a variety of microorganisms, the most common of which are viruses and bacteria. There is no gender predilection and it occurs over a wide age range.

Viral Rhinosinusitis

Viral rhinosinusitis results in the common cold. Symptoms include nasal congestion and a watery nasal discharge. Among the more common viruses implicated in causing disease are rhinoviruses, influenza and parainfluenza viruses, adenoviruses, and respiratory syncytial virus. In the setting of viral rhinosinusitis, secondary infection by bacteria may occur and is manifested by a mucopurulent discharge. Viral rhinosinusitis usually follows a self-limiting disease course.

Bacterial Sinusitis

The more common bacteria implicated in causing *bacterial sinusitis* include *Streptococcus pneumoniae*, *Haemophilus influenzae*, and α-hemolytic streptococci. Bacterial sinusitis is associated with pain that is usualy localized over the infected site; headaches are uncommon. Bacterial sinusitis may be acute, subacute, or chronic. *Acute bacterial sinusitis* is worsening symptoms of longer than 7 days but less than 3 weeks; in *subacute bacterial sinusitis* symptoms last 3 weeks to 3 months; in *chronic bacterial sinusitis* symptoms last more than 3 months. Patients with resistant or refractory chronic sinusitis have an increased incidence of *S. aureus*, anaerobic bacteria, and Gram-negative organisms. *Pseudomonas aeruginosa* is a commonly cultured organism in patients who have received multiple courses of antibiotics over extended periods of time; the culturing of *Pseudomonas* suggests an immune deficiency condition. Appropriate antibiotic therapy is curative.

Atrophic Rhinosinusitis

Atrophic rhinosinusitis is also referred to as *ozena* (stench) and occasionally *rhinitis sicca*. It is more common in women and tends to begin in childhood, often in the second decade of life at the onset of puberty. Atrophic rhinosinusitis is characterized by atrophy of the nasal mucosa, crust formation, and foul smelling odor from the nasal cavity. Symptoms also include nasal obstruction, headaches, anosmia, epistaxis, and halitosis. It is caused by a variety of factors including chronic bacterial infection, nutritional (e.g., vitamin A, iron) deficiencies, chronic exposure to irritants, prior radiation or surgery, end stage of chronic infections, hypoestrogenemia, and autoimmune disease (282,283).

Biopsies show squamous metaplasia of the mucosal surface epithelium, submucosal edema with nonspecific chronic inflammation, fibrosis, atrophic and decreased numbers of seromucous glands, and vascular dilatation. The histologic findings are nonspecific. The clinical impression of the atrophic appearance of the nasal cavity tissues (e.g., turbinates) is important in the diagnosis; excluding evidence of other possible diseases is necessary.

Medical therapy (e.g., antibiotics, nutritional supplements [vitamin A, iron, estrogen) and surgery have been used to treat atrophic rhinosinusitis (284). There is no known cure; over time, the active disease may spontaneously arrest, with the disappearance of the nasal crusting and foul odor.

Aspirin Intolerance or Aspirin-Exacerbated Respiratory Disease

Aspirin intolerance or *aspirin-exacerbated respiratory disease* (AERD), is also referred to as *Samter triad* or *syndrome,* includes aspirin (or nonsteroidal anti-inflammatory drug) hypersensitivity, sinonasal polyps, and asthma (285,286). Approximately 7 percent of asthmatics are aspirin sensitive but the prevalence doubles in severe asthmatics (287). Unlike allergic asthma, this disease tends to develop in adulthood, occurs in patients without an atopic history, and displays a slightly higher prevalence in females (288).

Within hours of ingestion of aspirin or nonsteroidal anti-inflammatory medications, patients experience bronchoconstriction and rhinorrhea. Symptoms also include nausea, vomiting, and diarrhea with gastrointestinal cramping. The symptoms are believed to be induced by pharmacologic interference in the metabolism of arachidonic acid rather than an allergic response (289). Hallmark features include eosinophilia, expression of Th2 cytokines, and elevated levels of cysteinyl leukotrienes (CysLTs) (290–292). A prominent role for interferon (IFN)-γ in the maturation of eosinophil progenitors in AERD has been recently proposed (293). Nonallergic rhinosinusitis with eosinophilia syndrome (NARES) or eosinophilic chronic rhinosinusitis syndrome (ECRS) may be a precursor to the aspirin intolerance syndrome (294,295).

The polyps associated with aspirin intolerance usually are bilateral. The polyps are histologically similar to sinonasal inflammatory polyps (previously discussed in this chapter) not occurring in aspirin intolerant patients. Patients with nasal polyps have more severe symptoms with less improvement after operative intervention and a significantly higher need for revision surgery.

Treatment includes avoidance of instigating medications, symptomatic relief, and polypectomy. Leukotriene modifiers and aspirin desensitization are also used (288). FESS may improve sinonasal and asthma symptom severity and frequency, and quality of life (296).

Nonallergic Rhinosinusitis with Eosinophilia Syndrome and Eosinophilic Chronic Rhinosinusitis Syndrome

Nonallergic rhinosinusitis with eosinophilia syndrome (NARES) and *eosinophilic chronic rhinosinusitis syndrome* (ECRS) are forms of rhinosinusitis characterized by sneezing, pruritus, profuse watery rhinorrhea, and lacrimation in association with eosinophilia of 20 percent or greater and a negative dermal skin test (265,297). Symptoms occur in an "on again, off again" manner. The eosinophilia is frequently, but not exclusively, caused by IgE-mediated hypersensitivity and is dominated by the associated cytokine milieu of Th2 inflammation (265,297). NARES and ECRS encompass a wide variety of etiologies (265,297) and recent evidence suggests that they may be precursors to aspirin intolerance (294,295). The treatment includes avoidance of instigating medications, symptomatic relief, and polypectomy.

REFERENCES

Embryology, Anatomy, and Histology

1. Moore KL, Persaud TV. Development of nasal cavities. In: Moore ML, Persaud TVN, ed. The developing human: clinically oriented embryology, 7th ed. Philadelphia: Saunders, Elsevier, 2003: 227-230.
2. Hollinshead WH. The nose and paranasal sinuses. In: Hollinshead WH, ed. Anatomy for surgeons, vol. 1, 3rd ed. Philadelphia: Harper and Row; 1982:223-267.
3. Standring S. Nose, nasal cavity and paranasal sinuses. In: Standring S, ed. Gray's anatomy. The anatomical basis of clinical practice, 40th ed. Edinburgh: Elsevier Churchill Livingstone; 2008:547-559.
4. Pantanowitz L, Balogh K. Mouth, nose, and paranasal sinuses. In: Mills SE, ed. Histology for pathologists, 4th ed. Philadelphia: Lippincott Williams & Wilkins; 2012:433-459.
5. Zak FG, Lawson W. The presence of melanocytes in the nasal cavity. Ann Otol Rhinol Laryngol 1974;83:515-519.

Heterotopic Glial Tissue

6. Hoshaw TC, Walike JW. Dermoid cysts of the nose. Arch Otolaryngol 1971;93:487-491.
7. Penner CR, Thompson L. Nasal glial heterotopia: a clinicopathologic and immunophenotypic analysis of 10 cases with a review of the literature. Ann Diagn Pathol 2003;7:354-359.
8. Kapadia SB, Popek EJ, Barnes L. Pediatric otorhinolaryngic pathology: diagnosis of selected lesions. Pathol Annu 1994;29(Pt 1):159-209.
9. Skolnick EM, Campbell JM, Meyers RM. Dermoid cysts of the nose. Laryngoscope 1971;81:1632-1637.
10. Bradley PJ, Singh SD. Nasal glioma. J Laryngol Otol 1985;99:247-252.
11. Adil E, Huntley C, Choudhary A, Carr M. Congenital nasal obstruction: clinical and radiologic review. Eur J Pediatr 2012;171:641-650.
12. Gnagi SH, Schraff SA. Nasal obstruction in newborns. Pediatr Clin North Am 2013;60:903-922.
13. Majithia A, Liyanage SH, Hewitt R, Grant WE. Adult nasal glioma presenting with visual loss. J Laryngol Otol 2010;124:1309-1313.
14. Whitaker SR, Sprinkle PM, Chou SM. Nasal glioma. Arch Otolaryngol 1981;107:550-554.
15. Ziter FM, Bramwit DN. Nasal encephaloceles and gliomas. Brit J Radiol 1970;43:136-138.
16. Theaker JM, Fletcher CD. Heterotopic glial nodules: a light microscopic and immunohistochemical study. Histopathology 1991;18:255–260.
17. Mirra SS, Pearl GS, Hoffman JC, Campbell WG Jr. Nasal 'glioma' with prominent neuronal component: report of a case. Arch Pathol 1981; 105:540-541.
18. Hughes GB, Sharpino G, Hunt W, Tucker HM. Management of the congenital midline nasal mass: a review. Head Neck Surg 1980;2:222-233.
19. Black BK, Smith DE. Nasal glioma: two cases with recurrence. AMA Arch Neurol Psychiatry 1950; 64:614-630.
20. Walker EA Jr, Resler DR. Nasal gliomas. Laryngoscope 1963;73:93-107.
21. Yeoh GP, Bale PM, de Silva M. Nasal cerebral heterotopia: the so-called nasal glioma or sequestered encephalocele and its variants. Pediatr Pathol 1989;9:531-549.
22. Dawson RL, Muir IF. The fronto-nasal glioma. Brit J Plast Surg 1955;8:136-143.

Encephaloceles

23. Naidich TP, Blaser SI, Bauer BS, Armstrong DC, McLone DG, Zimmerman RA. Embryology and congenital lesions of the midface. In: Som PM, Curtin HD, eds. Head and neck imaging, 4th ed. St. Louis: Mosby. 2003:3-86.
24. Suwanwela C, Suwanwela N. A morphological classification of sincipital encephalomeningoceles. J Neurosurg 1972;36:201-211.
25. Macfarlane R, Rutka JT, Armstrong D, Phillips J, Posnick J. Encephaloceles of the anterior cranial fossa. Pediatr Neurosurg 1995;23:148-158.
26. Naidich TP, Altman NR, Braffman BH, McLone DG, Zimmerman RA. Cephaloceles and related malformations. AJNR 1992;13:655-690.
27. Ziter FMH Jr, Bramwit DN. Nasal encephaloceles and gliomas. Brit J Radiol 1970;43:136-138.
28. Hughes GB, Sharpino G, Hunt W, Tucker HM. Management of the congenital midline nasal mass: a review. Head Neck Surg 1980; 2:222-233.
29. Blumenfeld R, Skolnik EM. Intranasal encephaloceles. Arch Otolaryngol 1965;82:527-531.
30. Ogiwara H, Morota N. Surgical treatment of transsphenoidal encephaloceles: transpalatal versus combined transpalatal and transcranial approach. J Neurosurg Pediatr 2013;11:505-510.
31. Tirumandas M, Sharma A, Gbenimacho I, et al. Nasal encephaloceles: a review of etiology, pathophysiology, clinical presentations, diagnosis, treatment, and complications. Childs Nerv Syst 2013;29:739-744.

Nasal Dermoid Cyst

32. Heffner DK, Thompson LDR, Schall D, Anderson V. Pharyngeal dermoids ("hairy polyps") as accessory auricles. Ann Otol Rhinol Laryngol 1996;105:819-824.

33. Hoshaw TC, Walike JW. Dermoid cysts of the nose. Arch Otolaryngol 1971;93:487-491.
34. Vaghela HM, Bradley PJ. Nasal dermoid sinus cysts in adults. J Laryngol Otol 2004;118:955-962.
35. Denoyelle F, Ducroz V, Roger G, Garabedian EN. Nasal dermoid sinus cysts in children. Laryngoscope 1997;107:795-800.
36. Cheng ML, Chang SD, Pang D, Adler JR. Intracranial nasal dermoid sinus cyst associated with colloid cyst of the third ventricle. Case report and new concepts. Pediatr Neurosurg 1999;31:201-206.
37. Kellman RM, Goyal P, Rodziewicz GS. The transglabellar subcranial approach for nasal dermoids with intracranial extension. Laryngoscope 2004;114:1368-1372.
38. Meher R, Singh I, Aggarwal S. Nasal dermoid with intracranial extension. J Postgrad Med 2005;51:39-40.
39. Locke R, Kubba H. A case of a nasal dermoid presenting as a median upper lip sinus. Int J Oral Maxillofac Surg 2011;40:985-987.
40. Karandikar M, Yellon RF, Murdoch G, Greene S. Coexistence of dermal sinus tract, dermoid cyst, and encephalocele in a patient presenting with nasal cellulitis. J Neurosurg Pediatr 2013;11:91-94.
41. Pivnick EK, Walter AW, Lawrence MD, Smith ME. Gorlin syndrome associated with midline nasal dermoid cyst. J Med Genet 1996;33:704-706.
42. Anderson PJ, Dobson C, Berry RB. Nasal dermoid cysts in siblings. Int J Pediatr Otorhinolaryngol 1998;44:155-159.
43. Blake WE, Chow CW, Holmes AD, Meara JG. Nasal dermoid sinus cysts: a retrospective review and discussion of investigation and management. Ann Plast Surg 2006;57:535-540.
44. Holzmann D, Huisman TA, Holzmann P, Stoeckli SJ. Surgical approaches for nasal dermal sinus cysts. Rhinology 2007;45:31-35.
45. Winterton RI, Wilks DJ, Chumas PD, Russell JL, Liddington MI. Surgical correction of midline nasal dermoid sinus cysts. J Craniofac Surg 2010; 21:295-300.
46. Sessions R. Nasal dermal sinuses—new concepts and explanations. Laryngoscope 1982;92(Pt 2; suppl 29):1-28.

Primary Ciliary Dyskinesia

47. Horani A, Ferkol TW, Dutcher SK, Brody SL. Genetics and biology of primary ciliary dyskinesia. Paediatr Respir Rev 2016;18:18-24.
48. Hildebrandt F, Benzing T, Katsanis N. Ciliopathies. N Engl J Med 2011;364:1533-1543.
49. Ferkol TW, Leigh MW. Ciliopathies: the central role of cilia in a spectrum of pediatric disorders. J Pediatr 2012;160:366-371.
50. Ware SM, Aygun MG, Hildebrandt F. Spectrum of clinical diseases caused by disorders of primary cilia. Proc Am Thorac Soc 2011;8:444-450.
51. Werner C, Onnebrink JG, Omran H. Diagnosis and management of primary ciliary dyskinesia. Cilia 2015;4:2.
52. Onoufriadis A, Paff T, Antony D, et al. Splice-site mutations in the axonemal outer dynein arm docking complex gene CCDC114 cause primary ciliary dyskinesia. Am J Hum Genet 2013;92:88-98.
53. Austin-Tse C, Halbritter J, Zariwala MA, et al. Zebrafish Ciliopathy screen plus human mutational analysis identifies C21orf59 and CCDC65 defects as causing primary ciliary dyskinesia. Am J Hum Genet 2013;93:672-686.
54. Jaffe KM, Grimes DT, Schottenfeld-Roames J, et al. c21orf59/kurly Controls both cilia motility and polarization. Cell Rep 2016;14:1841-1849.
55. Horani A, Brody SL, Ferkol TW, et al. CCDC65 mutation causes primary ciliary dyskinesia with normal ultrastructure and hyperkinetic cilia. PLoS One 2013;8:e72299.
56. Knowles MR, Ostrowski LE, Loges NT, et al. Mutations in SPAG1 cause primary ciliary dyskinesia associated with defective outer and inner dynein arms. Am J Hum Genet 2013;93:711-720.
57. Onoufriadis A, Shoemark A, Munye MM, et al. Combined exome and whole-genome sequencing identifies mutations in ARMC4 as a cause of primary ciliary dyskinesia with defects in the outer dynein arm. J Med Genet 2014;51:61-67.
58. Wu DH, Singaraja RR. Loss-of-function mutations in CCDC114 cause primary ciliary dyskinesia. Clin Genet 2013;83:526-527.
59. Moore DJ, Onoufriadis A, Shoemark A, et al. Mutations in ZMYND10, a gene essential for proper axonemal assembly of inner and outer dynein arms in humans and flies, cause primary ciliary dyskinesia. Am J Hum Genet 2013;93:346-356.
60. Tarkar A, Loges NT, Slagle CE, et al. DYX1C1 is required for axonemal dynein assembly and ciliary motility. Nat Genet 2013;45:995-1003.
61. Kott E, Legendre M, Copin B, et al. Loss-of-function mutations in RSPH1 cause primary ciliary dyskinesia with central-complex and radial-spoke defects. Am J Hum Genet 2013;93:561-570.
62. Jeanson L, Copin B, Papon JF, et al. RSPH3 mutations cause primary ciliary dyskinesia with central-complex defects and a near absence of radial spokes. Am J Hum Genet 2015;97:153-162.
63. Daniels ML, Leigh MW, Davis SD, et al. Founder mutation in RSPH4A identified in patients of Hispanic descent with primary ciliary dyskinesia. Hum Mutat 2013;34:1352-1356.
64. Antony D, Becker-Heck A, Zariwala MA, et al. Mutations in CCDC39 and CCDC40 are the major cause of primary ciliary dyskinesia with axonemal disorganization and absent inner dynein arms. Hum Mutat 2013;34:462-472.

65. Blanchon S, Legendre M, Copin B, et al. Delineation of CCDC39/CCDC40 mutation spectrum and associated phenotypes in primary ciliary dyskinesia. J Med Genet 2012;49:410-416.
66. Schidlow DV. Primary ciliary dyskineasia (the immotile cilia syndrome). Ann Allergy 1994;73:457-469.
67. Leigh MW, Hazucha MJ, Chawla KK, et al. Standardizing nasal nitric oxide measurement as a test for primary ciliary dyskinesia. Ann Am Thorac Soc 2013;10:574-781.
68. Collins SA, Gove K, Walker W, Lucas JS. Nasal nitric oxide screening for primary ciliary dyskinesia: systemic review and meta-analysis. Eur Respir J 2014;44:1589-1599.
69. Jackson CL, Behan L, Collins SA, et al. Accuracy of diagnostic testing in primary ciliary dyskinesia. Eur Respir J 2016;47:837-848.
70. Collins SA, Behan L, Harris A, Gove K, Lucas JS. The dangers of widespread nitric oxide screening for primary ciliary dyskinesia. Thorax 2016; 71:560-561.
71. Bent JP 3rd, Smith RJ. Intraoperative diagnosis of primary ciliary dyskinesia. Otolaryngol Head Neck Surg 1997;116:64-67.
72. Mierau GW, Agostini R, Beals TF, et al. The role of electron microscopy in evaluating ciliary dysfunction: report of a workshop. Ultrastruct Pathol 1992;16:245-254.
73. Simoneau T, Zandieh SO, Rao DR, et al. Impact of cilia ultrastructural examination on the diagnosis of primary ciliary dyskinesia. Pediatr Dev Pathol 2013;16:321-326.
74. Barbato A, Frischer T, Kuehni CE, et al. Primary ciliary dyskinesia: a consensus statement on diagnostic and treatment approaches in children. Eur Respir J 2009;34:1264–1276.
75. Behan L, Dimitrov BD, Kuehni CE, et al. PICADAR: a diagnostic predictive tool for primary ciliary dyskinesia. Eur Respir J 2016;47:1103-1112.
76. Polineni D, Davis SD, Dell SD. Treatment recommendations in primary ciliary dyskinesia. Paediatr Respir Rev 2016;18:39-45.

Inflammatory Polyps

77. Pfaar O, Klimek L. Aspirin desensitization in aspirin intolerance: update on current standards and recent improvements. Curr Opin Allergy Clin Immunol 2006;6:161-166.
78. Moloney JR. Nasal polyps, nasal polypectomy, asthma and aspirin sensitivity: their association in 445 cases of nasal polyps. J Laryngol Otol 1977;91:837-846.
79. Settipane GA, Chafee FH. Nasal polyps in asthma and rhinitis. A review of 6,037 patients. J Allergy Clin Immunol 1977;59:17–21.
80. Scapa VI, Ramakrishnan VR, Mudd PA, Kingdom TT. Upregulation of RANTES in nasal polyps from patients with cystic fibrosis. Int Forum Allergy Rhinol 2011;1:157-160.
81. Ryan RE Jr, Neel HB 3rd. Antral-choanal polyps. J Otolaryngol 1979;8:344-346.
82. Compagno J, Hyams VJ, Lepore ML. Nasal polyposis with stromal atypia. Review of follow-up study of 14 cases. Arch Pathol Lab Med 1976;100:224-226.
83. Kindblom LG, Angervall L. Nasal polyps with atypical stromal cells: a pseudosarcomatous lesion. A light and electron microscopic and immunohistochemical investigation with implications on the type and nature of the mesenchymal cells. Acta Pathol Microbiol Immunol Scand Sect A 1984;92:65-72.
84. Nakayama M, Wenig BM, Heffner DK. Atypical stromal cells in inflammatory nasal polyps: Immunohistochemical and ultrastructural analysis in defining histogenesis. Laryngoscope 1995; 105:127-134.
85. Sheahan P, Crotty PL, Hamilton S, Colreavy M, McShane D. Infarcted angiomatous nasal polyps. Eur Arch Otorhinolaryngol 2005;262:225-230.
86. Winestock DP, Bartlett PC, Sondheimer FK. Benign nasal polyps causing bone destruction in the nasal cavity and paranasal sinuses. Laryngoscope 1978;88:675-679.
87. Safneck JR, Alguacil-Garcia A, Dort JC. Intranasal papillary endothelial hyperplasia. Otolaryngol Head Neck Surg 1995;113:766-770.
88. Oppenheimer EH, Rosenstein BJ. Differential pathology of nasal polyps in cystic fibrosis and atopy. Lab Invest 1979;40:445-449.
89. Yfantis HG, Drachenberg CB, Gray W, Papadimitriou JC. Angiectatic nasal polyps that clinically simulate a malignant process: report of 2 cases and review of the literature. Arch Pathol Lab Med 2000;124:406-410.
90. Brescia G, Marioni G, Franchella S, et al. Post-operative steroid treatment for eosinophilic-type sinonasal polyposis. Acta Otolaryngol 2015;135:1200-1204.
91. Choudhury N, Hariri A, Saleh H. Endoscopic management of antrochoanal polyps: a single UK centre's experience. Eur Arch Otorhinolaryngol 2015;272:2305-2311.
92. Kelles M, Toplu Y, Yildirim I, Okur E. Antrochoanal polyp: clinical presentation and retrospective comparison of endoscopic sinus surgery and endoscopic sinus surgery plus mini-Caldwell surgical procedures. J Craniofac Surg 2014;25:1779-1781.
93. Berkiten G, Salturk Z, Topaloglu I. Efficacy of systemic steroid treatment in sinonasal polyposis. J Craniofac Surg 2013;24:e305-308.

Paranasal Sinus Mucocele

94. Evans C. Aetiology and treatment of fronto-ethmoidal mucocele. J Laryngol Otol 1981;95:361-375.

95. Koudstaal MJ, van der Wal KG, Bijvoet HW, Vincent AJ, Poublon RM. Post-trauma mucocele formation in the frontal sinus; a rationale of follow-up. Int J Oral Maxillofac Surg 2004;33:751-754.
96. Weber AL. Inflammatory diseases of the paranasal sinuses and mucoceles. Otolaryngol Clin North Am 1988;21:421-437.
97. Thio D, Phelps PD, Bath AP. Maxillary sinus mucocele presenting as a late complication of a maxillary advancement procedure. J Laryngol Otol 2003;117:402-403.
98. Close LG, O'Conner WE. Sphenoethmoidal mucoceles with intracranial extension. Otolaryngol Head Neck Surg 1983;91:350-357.
99. Har-El G. Endoscopic management of 108 sinus mucoceles. Laryngoscope 2001;111:2131-2134.
100. Serrano E, Klossek JM, Percodani J, Yardeni E, Dufour X. Surgical management of paranasal sinus mucoceles: a long-term study of 60 cases. Otolaryngol Head Neck Surg 2004;131:133-140.

Respiratory Epithelial Adenomatoid Hamartoma

101. Wenig BM, Heffner DK. Respiratory epitheial adenomatoid hamartomas of the sinonasal tract and nasopharynx: a clinicopathologic study of 31 cases. Ann Otol Rhinol Laryngol 1995;104:639-645.
102. Ozolek JA, Barnes EL, Hunt JL. Basal/myoepithelial cells in chronic sinusitis, respiratory epithelial adenomatoid hamartoma, inverted papilloma, and intestinal-type and nonintestinal-type sinonasal adenocarcinoma: an immunohistochemical study. Arch Pathol Lab Med 2007;131:530-537.
103. Jo VY, Mills SE, Cathro HP, Carlson DL, Stelow EB. Low-grade sinonasal adenocarcinomas: the association with and distinction from respiratory epithelial adenomatoid hamartomas and other glandular lesions. Am J Surg Pathol 2009;33:401-408.
104. Ozolek JA, Hunt JL. Tumor suppressor gene alterations in respiratory epithelial adenomatoid hamartoma (REAH). Comparison to sinonasal adenocarcinoma and inflamed sinus mucosa. Am J Surg Pathol 2006;30:1576-1580.
105. Graeme-Cook F, Pilch BZ. Hamartomas of the nose and nasopharynx. Head Neck 1992; 14:321–327.

Seromucinous Hamartoma

106. Baillie EE, Batsakis JG. Glandular (seromucinous) hamartoma of the nasopharynx. Oral Surg Oral Med Oral Pathol 1974;38:760-762.
107. Ambrosini-Spaltro A, Morandi L, Spagnolo DV, et al. Nasal seromucinous hamartoma (microglandular adenosis of the nose): a morphological and molecular study of five cases. Virchows Arch 2010;457:727-734.
108. Khan RA, Chernock RD, Lewis JS Jr. Seromucinous hamartoma of the nasal cavity: a report of two cases and review of the literature. Head Neck Pathol 2011;5:241-247.
109. Weinreb I, Gnepp DR, Laver NM, et al. Seromucinous hamartomas: a clinicopathological study of a sinonasal glandular lesion lacking myoepithelial cells. Histopathology 2009;54:205-213.
110. Fleming KE, Perez-Ordoñez B, Nasser JG, Psooy B, Bullock MJ. Sinonasal seromucinous hamartoma: a review of the literature and a case report with focal myoepithelial cells. Head Neck Pathol 2012;6:395-399.

Chondro-osseous and Respiratory Epithelial Hamartomas

111. Adair CF, Thompson LD, Wenig BM, Heffner DK. Chondro-osseous and respiratory epithelial hamartomas of the sinonasal tract and nasopharynx. Mod Pathol 1996;9:100A.

Nasal Chondromesenchymal Hamartoma

112. McDermott MB, Ponder TB, Dehner LP. Nasal chondromesenchymal hamartoma: an upper respiratory tract analogue of the chest wall mesenchymal hamartoma Am J Surg Pathol 1998;22:425-433.
113. Kim DW, Low W, Billman G, Wickersham J, Kearns D. Chondroid hamartoma presenting as a neonatal nasal mass. Int. J Pediatr Otorhinolaryngol 199;47:253-259.
114. Terris MH, Billman GF, Pransky SM. Nasal hamartoma: case report and review of the literature. Int. J. Pediatr Otorhinolaryngol 1993;28:83-88.
115. Johnson C, Nagaraj U, Esguerra J, Wasdahl D, Wurzbach D. Nasal chondromesenchymal hamartoma: radiographic and histopathologic analysis of a rare pediatric tumor. Pediatr Radiol 2007;37:101-104.
116. Ozolek JA, Carrau R, Barnes EL, Hunt JL. Nasal chondromesenchymal hamartoma in older children and adults. Series and immunohistochemical analysis. Arch Pathol Lab Med 2005;129:1444-1450.
117. Priest JR, Williams GM, Mize WA, Dehner LP, McDermott MB. Nasal chondromesenchymal hamartoma in children with pleuropulmonary blastoma—a report from the International Pleuropulmonary Blastoma Registry registry. Int J Pediatr Otorhinolaryngol 2010;74:1240-1244.
118. Behery RE, Bedrnicek J, Lazenby A, et al. Translocation t(12;17)(q24.1;q21) as the sole anomaly in a nasal chondromesenchymal hamartoma arising in a patient with pleuropulmonary blastoma. Pediatr Dev Pathol 2012;15:249-253.

119. Li Y, Yang QX, Tian XT, Li B, Li Z. Malignant transformation of nasal chondromesenchymal hamartoma in adult: a case report and review of the literature. Histol Histopathol 2013;28:337-344.

Granulomatosis with Polyangiitis

120. Wegener F. Wegener's granulomatosis. Thoughts and observations of a pathologist. Eur Arch Otorhinolaryngol 1990;247:133-142.
121. Jennette JC, Falk RJ. Nosology of primary vasculitis. Curr Opin Rheumatol 2007;19:10-16.
122. DeRemee RA, McDonald TJ, Harrison EG, Coles DT. Wegener's granulomatosis. Anatomic correlates, a proposed classification. Mayo Clin Proc 1976;51:777–781.
123. Falk RJ, Terrell RS, Charles LA, Jennette JC. Anti-neutrophil cytoplasmic autoantibodies induce neutrophils to degranulate and produce oxygen radicals in vitro. Proc Natl Acad Sci USA 1990;87:4115-4119.
124. Jennette JC, Falk RJ. Pathogenesis antineutrophil cytoplasmic autoantibody-mediated disease. Nar Rev Rheumatol 2014;10:463-473.
125. Fienberg R, Mark EJ, Goodman M, McCluskey RT, Niles JL. Correlation of antineutrophil cytoplasmic antibodies with the extrarenal histopathology of Wegener's (pathergic) granulomatosis and related forms of vasculitis. Hum Pathol 1993;24:160-168.
126. Hardarson S, Labrecque DR, Mitros FA, Neil GA, Goeken JA. Antineutrophil cytoplasmic antibody in inflammatory bowel and hepatobiliary diseases. High prevalence in ulcerative colitis, primary sclerosing cholangitis, and autoimmune hepatitis. Am J Clin Pathol 1993;99:277-281.
127. Brockmann H, Schwarting A, Kriegsmann J, et al. Proteinase-3 as the major autoantigen of c-ANCA is strongly expressed in lung tissue of patients with Wegener's granulomatosis. Arthritis Res 2002;4:220-225.
128. Schreiber A, Busjahn A, Luft FC, Kettritz R. Membrane expression of proteinase 3 is genetically determined. J Am Soc Nephrol 2003;14:68-75.
129. van Rossum AP, Rarok AA, Huitema MG, Fassina G, Limburg PC, Kallenberg CG. Constitutive membrane expression of proteinase 3 (PR3) and neutrophil activation by anti-PR3 antibodies. J Leukoc Biol 2004;76:1162-1170.
130. von Vietinghoff S, Schreiber A, Otto B, Choi M, Göbel U, Kettrritz R. Membrane proteinase 3 and Wegener's granulomatosis. Clin Nephrol 2005;64:453-459.
131. Winek J, Mueller A, Csernok E, Gross WL, Lamprecht P. Frequency of proteinase 3 (PR3)-specific autoreactive T cells determined by cytokine flow cytometry in Wegener's granulomatosis. J Autoimmuno 2004;22:79-85.
132. Lionaki S, Blyth ER, Hogan SL, et al. Classification of antineutrophil cytoplasmic autoantibody vasculitides: the role of antineutrophil cytoplasmicautoantibody specificity for myeloperoxidase or proteinase 3 in disease recognition and prognosis. Arthritis Rheum 2012;64:3452-3462.
133. Rahmattulla C, Mooyaart AL, van Hooven D, et al. Genetic variants in ANCA-associated vasculitis: a meta-analysis. Ann Rheum Dis 2016;75: 1687-1692.
134. Devaney KO, Travis WD, Hoffman G, Leavitt R, Lebovics R, Fauci AS. Interpretation of head and neck biopsies in Wegener's granulomatosis. A pathologic study of 126 biopsies in 70 patients. Am J Surg Pathol 1990;14:555-564.
135. Chang SY, Keogh KA, Lewis JE, et al. IgG4-positive plasma cells in granulomatosis with polyangiitis (Wegener's): a clinicopathologic and immunohistochemical study on 43 granulomatosis with polyangiitis and 20 control cases. Hum Pathol 2013;44:2432-2437.
136. Pagnoux C, Guillevin L. Treatment of granulomatosis with polyangiitis (Wegener's). Expert Rev Clin Immunol 2015;11:339-348.
137. Zand L, Specks U, Sethi S, Fervenza FC. Treatment of ANCA-associated vasculitis: new therapies and a look at old entities. Adv Chronic Kidney Dis 2014;21:182-193.
138. Guillevin L, Pagnoux C, Karras A, et al. Rituximab versus azathioprine for maintenance in ANCA-associated vasculitis. N Engl J Med 2014; 371:1771-1780.
139. Smith RM. Update on the treatment of ANCA associated vasculitis. Presse Med 2015;44(Pt 2): e241-249.

Myospherulosis

140. Coulier B, Desgain O, Gielen I. Sinonasal myospherulosis and paraffin retention cysts suggested by CT: report of a case. Head Neck Pathol 2012;6:270-274.
141. Wheeler TM, Sessions RB, McGavran MH. Myospherulosis: a preventable iatrogenic nasal and paranasal entity. Arch Otolaryngol 1980;106: 272-274.
142. Rosai J. The nature of myospherulosis of the upper respiratory tract. Am J Clin Pathol 1978;69; 475-481.

Extranodal Sinus Histiocytosis with Massive Lymphadenopathy

143. Rosai J, Dorfman RF. Sinus histiocytosis with massive lymphadenopathy: a newly recognized benign clinicopathologic entity. Arch Pathol 1969;87:63–70.

144. Wenig BM, Abbondanzo SL, Childers EL, Kapadia SB, Heffner DR. Extranodal sinus histiocytosis with massive lymphadenopathy (Rosai-Dorfman disease) of the head and neck. Hum Pathol 1993;24:483-492.
145. Rosai J, Dorfman RF. Sinus histiocytosis with massive lymphadenopathy: a pseudolymphomatous benign disorder. Analysis of 34 cases. Cancer 1972;30:1174–1188.
146. Delacretaz F, Meuge-Moraw C, Anwar D, Borisch B, Chave JP. Sinus histiocytosis with massive lymphadenopathy (Rosai-Dorfman disease) in an HIV-positive patient. Virchows Arch A Pathol Anat Histopathol 1991;419:251-254.
147. Perry BP, Gregg CM, Myers S, Lilly S, Mann KP, Prieto V. Rosai-Dorfman disease (extranodal sinus histiocytosis) in a patient with HIV. Ear Nose Throat J 1998;77:855-858.
148. Drosos AA, Georgiadis AN, Metafratzi ZM, Voulgari PV, Efremidis SC, Bai M. Sinus histiocytosis with massive lymphadenopathy (Rosai-Dorfman disease) in a patient with primary Sjogren's syndrome. Scand J Rheumatol 2004;33:119-122.
149. Rocken C, Wieker K, Grote HJ, Muller G, Franke A, Roessner A. Rosai-Dorfman disease and generalized AA amyloidosis: a case report. Hum Pathol 2000;31:621-624.
150. Kaur PP, Birbe RC, DeHoratius RJ. Rosai-Dorfman disease in a patient with systemic lupus erythematosus. J Rheumatol 2005;32:951-953.
151. Wang KH, Cheng CJ, Hu CH, Lee WR. Coexistence of localized Langerhans cell histiocytosis and cutaneous Rosai-Dorfman disease. Br J Dermatol 2002;147:770-774.
152. Levine PH, Jahan N, Murari P, Manak M, Jaffe ES. Detection of human herpesvirus 6 in tissues involved by sinus histiocytosis with massive lymphadenopathy (Rosai-Dorfman disease). J Infect Dis 1992;166:291-295.
153. Luppi M, Barozzi P, Garber R, et al. Expression of human herpesvirus-6 antigens in benign and malignant lymphoproliferative diseases. Am J Pathol 1998;153:815-823.
154. Tsang WY, Yip TT, Chan JK. The Rosai-Dorfman disease histiocytes are not infected by Epstein-Barr virus. Histopathology 1994;25:88-90.
155. Ortonne N, Fillet AM, Kosuge H, Bagot M, Frances C, Wechsler J. Cutaneous Destombes-Rosai-Dorfman disease: absence of detection of HHV-6 and HHV-8 in skin. J Cutan Pathol 2002;29:113-118.
156. Liu L, Perry AM, Cao W, et al. Relationship between Rosai-Dorfman disease and IgG4-related disease: study of 32 cases. Am J Clin Pathol 2013;140:395-402.
157. Kasper HU, Hegenbarth V, Buhtz P. Rhinoscleroma associated with Rosai-Dorfman reaction of regional lymph nodes. Pathol Int 2004;54:101-104.
158. Kumari JO. Coexistence of rhinoscleroma with Rosai-Dorfman disease: is rhinoscleroma a cause of this disease? J Laryngol Otol 2012;126:630-632.
159. Maric I, Pittaluga S, Dale JK, et al. Histologic features of sinus histiocytosis with massive lymphadenopathy in patients with autoimmune lymphoproliferative syndrome. Am J Surg Pathol 2005;29:903-911.
160. Eisen RN, Buckley PJ, Rosai J. Immunophenotypic characterization of sinus histiocytosis with massive lymphadenopathy (Rosai–Dorfman disease). Semin Diagn Pathol 1990;7:74–82.
161. Foucar K, Foucar E. The mononuclear phagocyte and immunoregulatory effector (M-PIRE) system: evolving concepts. Semin Diagn Pathol 1990;7:4–18.
162. Paulli M, Rosso R, Kindl S, et al. Immunophenotypic characterization of the cell infiltrate in five cases of sinus histiocytosis with massive lymphadenopathy (Rosai–Dorfman disease). Hum Pathol 1992;23:647–654.
163. Fleming MD, Pinkus JL, Fournier MV, et al. Coincident expression of the chemokine receptors CCR6 and CCR7 by pathologic Langerhans cells in Langerhans cell histiocytosis. Blood 2003;101:2473-2475.
164. Chou TC, Tsai KB, Lee CH. Emperipolesis is not pathognomonic for Rosai-Dorfman disease: rhinoscleroma mimicking Rosai-Dorfman disease, a clinical series. J Am Acad Dermatol 2013;69:1066-1067.
165. Moore JC, Zhao X, Nelson EL. Concomitant sinus histiocytosis with massive lymphadenopathy (Rosai-Dorfman Disease) and diffuse large B-cell lymphoma: a case report. J Med Case Rep 2008;2:70.
166. Foucar E, Rosai J, Dorfman RF. Sinus histiocytosis with massive lymphadenopathy: an analysis of 14 deaths occurring in a patient registry. Cancer 1984;54:1834-1840.

Eosinophilic Angiocentric Fibrosis

167. Burns BV, Roberts PF, De Carpentier J, Zarod AP. Eosinophilic angiocentric fibrosis affecting the nasal cavity. A mucosal variant of the skin lesion granuloma faciale. J Laryngol Otol 2001;115:223-226.
168. Chinelli PA, Kawashita MY, Sotto MN, Nico M. Granuloma faciale associated with sinonasal tract eosinophilic angiocentric fibrosis. Acta Derm Venereol 2004;84:486-487.
169. Narayan J, Douglas-Jones AG. Eosinophilic angiocentric fibrosis and granuloma faciale: analysis of cellular infiltrate and review of literature. Ann Otol Rhinol Laryngol 2005;114:35-42.

170. Nogueira A, Lisboa C, Duarte AF, et al. Granuloma faciale with subglottic eosinophilic angiocentric fibrosis: case report and review of the literature. Cutis 2011;88:77-82.
171. Roberts PF, McCann BG. Eosinophilic angiocentric fibrosis of the upper respiratory tract: a mucosal variant of granuloma faciale? A report of three cases. Histopathology 1985;9:1217-1225.
172. Yung A, Wachsmuth R, Ramnath R, Merchant W, Myatt AE, Sheehan-Dare R. Eosinophilic angiocentric fibrosis—a rare mucosal variant of granuloma faciale which may present to the dermatologist. Br J Dermatol 2005;152:574-576.
173. Altemani AM, Pilch BZ, Sakano E, Altemani JM. Eosinophilic angiocentric fibrosis of the nasal cavity. Mod Pathol 1997;10:391-393.
174. Jain R, Robblee JV, O'Sullivan-Mejia E, et al. Sinonasal eosinophilic angiocentric fibrosis: a report of four cases and review of literature. Head Neck Pathol 2008;2:309-315.
175. Thompson LD, Heffner DK. Sinonasal tract eosinophilic angiocentric fibrosis. A report of three cases. Am J Clin Pathol 2001;115:243-248.
176. Deshpande V, Khosroshahi A, Nielsen GP, Hamilos DL, Stone JH. Eosinophilic angiocentric fibrosis is a form of IgG4-related systemic disease. Am J Surg Pathol 2011;35:701-706.
177. Ferry JA, Deshpande V. IgG4-related disease in the head and neck. Semin Diagn Pathol 2012;29:235-244.

Pyogenic Granuloma/Lobular Capillary Hemangioma

178. Mills SE, Cooper PH, Fechner RE. Lobular capillary hemangioma: the underlying lesion of pyogenic granuloma. A study of 73 cases from the oral and nasal mucous membranes. Am J Surg Pathol 1980;4:471–479.
179. Smith SC, Patel RM, Lucas DR, McHugh JB. Sinonasal lobular capillary hemangioma: a clinicopathologic study of 34 cases characterizing potential for local recurrence. Head Neck Pathol 2013;7:129-134.
180. Nichols GE, Gaffey MJ, Mills SE, Weiss LM. Lobular capillary hemangioma. An immunohistochemical study including steroid hormone receptor status. Am J Clin Pathol 1992;97:770–775.
181. Yuan K, Lin MT. The roles of vascular endothelial growth factor and angiopoietin-2 in the regression of pregnancy pyogenic granuloma. Oral Dis 2004;10:179-185.
182. Thompson LD, Miettinen M, Wenig BM. Sinonasal-type hemangiopericytoma: a clinicopathologic and immunophenotypic analysis of 104 cases showing perivascular myoid differentiation. Am J Surg Pathol 2003;27:737-749.
183. Agaimy A, Haller F. CTTNB1 (β-catenin)-altered neoplasia: A review focusing on soft tissue neoplasms and parenchyma lesions of uncertain histogenesis. Adv Anat Pathol 2016;23:1-12.
184. Lasota J, Felisiak-Golabek A, Aly FZ, Wang ZF, Thompson LD, Miettinen M. Nuclear expression and gain-of-function β-catenin mutation) in glomangiopericytoma (sinonasal-type hemangiopericytoma): insight into pathogenesis and a diagnostic marker. Mod Pathol 2015;28:715-720.
185. Heffner DK. Problems in pediatric otorhinolaryngic pathology, II. Vascular tumors and lesions of the sinonasal tract and nasopharynx. Int J Pediatr Otorhinolaryngol 1983;5:125-138.
186. Bhaskar SN, Jacoway JR. Pyogenic granulomas—clinical features, incidence, histology, and result of treatment: report of 242 cases. J Oral Surg 1966;24:391-398.

Allergic Fungal Rhinosinusitis

187. Montone KT. Pathology of fungal rhinosinusitis: a review. Head Neck Pathol 2016;10:40-46.
188. Katzenstein AL, Sale SR, Greenberger PA. Pathologic findings in allergic Aspergillus sinusitis: a newly recognized form of sinusitis. Am J Surg Pathol 1983;7:439-443.
189. Cody DT 2nd, Neel HB 3rd, Ferreiro JA, Roberts GD. Allergic fungal sinusitis: the Mayo Clinic experience. Laryngoscope 1994;104:1074-1079.
190. Friedman GC, Hartwick RW, Ro JY, Saleh GY, Tarrand JJ, Ayala AG. Allergic fungal sinusitis. Report of three cases associated with dematiaceous fungi. Am J Clin Pathol 1992;96:368-372.
191. Won EJ, Shin JH, Lim SC, Shin MG, Suh SP, Ryang DW. Molecular identification of Schizophyllum commune as a cause of allergic fungal sinusitis. Ann Lab Med 2012;32:375-379.
192. Doellman MS, Dion GR, Weitzel EK, Reyes EG. Immunotherapy in allergic fungal sinusitis: The controversy continues. A recent review of literature. Allergy Rhinol (Providence) 2013;4:e32-35.
193. Clark DW, Wenaas A, Luong A, Citardi MJ, Fakhri S. Staphylococcus aureus prevalence in allergic fungal rhinosinusitis vs other subsets of chronic rhinosinusitis with nasal polyps. Int Forum Allergy Rhinol 2013;3:89-93.
194. Chakrabarti A, Das A, Panda NK. Controversies surrounding the categorization of fungal sinusitis. Med Mycol. 2009;47(suppl 1):S299-308.
195. Chakrabarti A, Denning DW, Ferguson BJ, et al. Fungal rhinosinusitis: a categorization and definitional scheme addressing current controversies. Laryngoscope 2009;119:1809-1818.
196. Montone KT. Role of fungi in the pathophysiology of chronic rhinosinusitis: an update. Curr Allergy Asthma Rep 2013;13:224-228.

197. Montone KT. The molecular genetics of inflammatory, autoimmune, and infectious diseases of the sinonasal tract: a review. Arch Pathol Lab Med 2014;138:745-753.
198. Guo C, Ghaderoshi S, Kephart GM, et al. Improving the detection of fungi in eosinophilic mucin: seeing what we could not see before. Otolaryngol Head Neck Surg 2012;147:943-949.
199. Montone KT, Guarner J. In situ hybridization for rRNA sequence sin anatomic pathology specimens, applications for fungal pathogen detection: a review. Adv Anat Pathol 2013;20:168-174.
200. Perez-Jaffe LA, Lanza DC, Loevner LA, Kennedy DW, Montone KT. In situ hybridization for Aspergillus and Penicillium in allergic fungal sinusitis: a rapid means of speciating fungal pathogens in tissues. Laryngoscope 1997;107:233.
201. Montone KT, LiVolsi VA, Lanza DC, et al. Rapid In-situ hybridization for dematiaceous fungi using a broad-spectrum oligonucleotide DNA probe. Diagn Mol Pathol 2011;20:180-183.
202. Hall AG, deShazo RD. Immunotherapy for allergic fungal sinusitis. Curr Opin Allergy Clin Immunol 2012;12:629-634.
203. Reitzen SD, Lebowitz RA, Jacobs JB. Allergic fungal sinusitis with extensive bone erosion of the clivus presenting with diplopia. J Laryngol Otol 2009;123:817-819.

Fungus Ball

204. Grosjean P, Weber R. Fungus balls of the paranasal sinuses: a review. Eur Arch Otorhinolaryngol 2007;264:461-470.
205. Dufour X, Kauffman-Lacroix C, Ferrie JC, Goujon JM, Rodier MH, Klossek JM. Paranasal sinus fungal ball epidemiology, clinical features, and diagnosis. A retrospective analysis of 175 cases from a single center in France 1989–2002. Med Mycol 2006;44:61–67.
206. Nicolai P, Lombardi D, Tomenzoli D, et al. Fungus ball of the paranasal sinuses: experience in 160 patients treated with endoscopic surgery. Laryngoscope 2009;119:2275–2279.

Invasive Fungal Rhinosinusitis

207. Campo M, Lewis RE, Kontoyiannis DP. Invasive fusariosis in patients with hematologic malignancies at a cancer center: 1998–2009. J Infect 2010;60:331–337.
208. Chen CY, Sheng WH, Cheng A, et al. Invasive fungal sinusitis in patients with hematological malignancy: 15 years experience in a single university hospital in Taiwan. BMC Infect Dis 2011;11:250.
209. Monroe MM, McLean M, Sautter N, et al. Invasive fungal rhinosinusitis: a 15-year experience with 29 patients. Laryngoscope 2013;123:1583-1587.
210. Mauriello JA Jr, Yepez N, Mostafavi R, et al. Invasive rhinosino-orbital aspergillosis with precipitous visual loss. Can J Ophthalmol 1995;30:124-130.
211. Ghadiali MT, Deckard NA, Farooq U, Astor F, Robinson P, Casiano RR. Frozen-section biopsy analysis for acute invasive fungal rhinosinusitis. Otolaryngol Head Neck Surg 2007;136:714-719.
212. Taxy JB, El-Zayaty S, Langerman A. Acute fungal sinusitis: natural history and the role of frozen section. Am J Clin Pathol 2009;132:86–93.
213. Derber C, Elam K, Bearman G. Invasive sinonasal disease due to dematiaceous fungi in immunocompromised individuals: case report and review of the literature. Int J Infect Dis 2010:14(Suppl 3):e329–332.
214. Montone KT, LiVolsi VA, Feldman MD, et al. Fungal rhinosinusitis: a report of 400 patients at a single university medical center. Int J Otolaryngol 2012;2012:684835.
215. Montone KT, LiVolsi VA, Lanza DC, et al. In situ hybridization for specific fungal organisms in acute invasive fungal rhinosinusitis. Am J Clin Pathol 2011;135:190-199.
216. Duggal P, Wise SK. Chapter 8: Invasive fungal rhinosinusitis. Am J Rhinol Allergy 2013;27(Suppl 1):S28-30.

Chronic Invasive and Chronic Granulomatous FRS

217. Chakrabarti A, Rudramurthy SM, Panda N, Das A, Singh A. Epidemiology of chronic fungal rhinosinusitis in rural India. Mycoses 2015;58:294-302.
218. Currens J, Hutcheson PS, Slavin RG, Citardi MJ. Primary paranasal Aspergillus granuloma: case report and review of the literature. Am J Rhinol 2002;16:165-168.
219. Veress B, Malik OA, El Tayeb AA, el-Daoud S, Mahgoub ES, el-Hassan AM. Furthrer observations on the primary paranasal Aspergillus granuloma in the Sudan. A morphological study of 46 cases. Am J Trop Med Hyg 1973;22:765-772.
220. Busaba NY, Colden DG, Faquin WC, Salman SD. Chronic invasive fungal sinusitis: a report of two atypical cases. Ear Nose Throat J 2002;81:462-466.
221. Montone KT. Pathology of fungal rhinosinusitis: a review. Head Neck Pathol 2016;10:40-46.
222. Pagella F, De Bernardi F, Dalla Gasperina D, et al. Invasive fungal rhinosinusitis in adult patients: our experience in diagnosis and management. J Craniomaxillofac Surg 2016;44:512-550.

Sinonasal Mucormycosis

223. Ferguson BJ. Mucormycosis of the nose and paranasal sinuses. Otolaryngol Clin North Am 2000;33:349-365.

224. Ganesan P, Swaroop C, Ahuja A, Thulkar S, Bakhshi S. Early onset sinonasal mucormycosis during induction therapy of acute lymphoblastic leukemia: good outcome without surgical intervention. J Pediatr Hematol Oncol 2009;31:152-153.
225. Rassi SJ, Melkane AE, Rizk HG, Dahoui HA. Sinonasal mucormycosis in immunocompromised pediatric patients. J Pediatr Hematol Oncol 2009;31:907-910.
226. Parfrey NA. Improved diagnosis and prognosis of mucormycosis. A clinicopathologic study of 33 cases. Medicine (Baltimore) 1986;65:113-123.
227. Ketenci I, Unlü Y, Kaya H, et al. Rhinocerebral mucormycosis. J Laryngol Otol 2011;125:e3.
228. Gaziev D, Baronciani D, Galimberti M, et al. Mucormycosis after bone marrow transplantation: report of four cases in thalassemia and review of the literature. Bone Marrow Transplant 1996;17:409-414.
229. Morrison VA, McGlave PB. Mucormycosis in the BMT population. Bone Marrow Transplant 1993;11:383-388.
230. Press GA, Weindling SM, Hesselink JR, Ochi JW, Harris JP. Rhinocerebral mucormycosis: MR manifestations. J Comput Assist Tomogr 1988;12:744-749.
231. Hofman V, Castillo L, Betis F, Guevara N, Gari-Toussaint M, Hofman P. Usefulness of frozen section in rhinocerebral mucormycosis diagnosis and management. Pathology 2003;35:212-216.
232. Alobid I, Bernal M, Calvo C, Vilaseca I, Berenguer J, Alos L. Treatment of rhinocerebral mucormycosis by combination of endoscopic sinus debridement and amphotericin B. Am J Rhinol 2001;15:327-331.
233. Raj P, Vella EJ, Bickerton RC. Successful treatment of rhinocerebral mucormycosis by a combination of aggressive surgical debridement and the use of systemic liposomal amphotericin B and local therapy with nebulized amphotericin—a case report. J Laryngol Otol 1998;112:367-370.
234. Munir N, Jones NS. Rhinocerebral mucormycosis with orbital and intracranial extension: a case report and review of optimum management. J Laryngol Otol 2007;121:192-195.

Rhinosporidiosis

235. Makannavar JH, Chavan SS. Rhinosporidiosis—a clinicopathological study of 34 cases. Indian J Pathol Microbiol 2001;44:17-21.
236. Satyanarayana C. Rhinosporidiosis with a record of 225 cases. Acta Otolaryngol 1960;51:348-356.
237. Arora R, Gupta R, Dinda AK. Rhinosporidiosis of trachea: a clinical cause for concern. J Laryngol Otol 2008;122:e13.
238. Madana J, Yolmo D, Gopalakrishnan S, Saxena SK. Laryngotracheal rhinosporidiosis. Ear Nose Throat J 2013;92:E27-30.
239. Madana J, Yolmo D, Gopalakrishnan S, Saxena SK. Rhinosporidiosis of the upper airways and trachea. J Laryngol Otol 2010;124:1139-1141.

Nasal Sporotrichosis

240. Freitas DF, de Siqueira Hoagland B, do Valle AC, et al. Sporotrchiosis in HIV-infected patients: report of 21 cases of endemic sporotrchosis in Rio de Janeiro, Brazil. Med Mycol 2012;50:170-178.
241. Morgan M, Reves R. Invasive sinusitis due to Sporothrix schenckii in a patient with AIDS. Clin Infect Dis 1996;23:1319-1320.
242. Kumar R, Kaushal V, Chopra H, et al. Pansinusitis due to Sporothrix schenckii. Mycoses 2005;48:85-88.

Rhinoscleroma

243. de Pontual L, Ovetchkine P, Rodriguez D, et al. Rhinoscleroma: a French national retrospective study of epidemiological and clinical features. Clin Infect Dis 2008;47:1396-1402.
244. Gaafar HA, Gaafar AH, Nour YA. Rhinoscleroma: an updated experience through the last 10 years. Acta Otolaryngol 2011;131:440-446.
245. Mukara BK, Munyarugamba P, Dazert S, Löhler J. Rhinoscleroma: a case series report and review of the literature. Eur Arch Otorhinolaryngol 2014;271:1851-1856.
246. N'gattia KV, Kacouchia N, Koffi-N'guessan L, et al. Retrospective study of the rhinoscleroma about 14 cases in ENT departments of university hospitals (Côte d'Ivoire). Eur Ann Otorhinolaryngol Head Neck Dis 2011;128:7-10.
247. Kumari JO. Coexistence of rhinoscleroma with Rosai-Dorfman disease: is rhinoscleroma a cause of this disease? J Laryngol Otol 2012;126:630-632.
248. Shum TK, Whitaker CW, Meyer PR. Clinical update of rhinoscleroma. Laryngoscope 1982;92:1149-1153.
249. Chou TC, Tsai KB, Lee CH. Emperipolesis is not pathognomonic for Rosai-Dorfman disease: rhinoscleroma mimicking Rosai-Dorfman disease, a clinical series. J Am Acad Dermatol 2013;69:1066-1067.
250. Heffner DK. Plasma cell granuloma in the nasal cavity. Cancer 1991;68:2490.

Botryomycosis

251. Wenig BM, Smirniotopoulos JG, Heffner DK. Botryomycosis ("bacteria ball") of the sinonasal tract caused by Pseudomonas aeruginosa. Arch Pathol Lab Med 1996;120:1123-1128.

Mucocutaneous Leishmaniasis

252. Handler MZ, Patel PA, Kapila R, Al-Qubati Y, Schwartz RA. Cutaneous and mucocutaneous leishmaniasis: differential diagnosis, diagnosis, histopathology. J Am Acad Dermatol 2015;73: 911-926.
253. Daneshbod Y, Oryan A, Davarmanesh M, et al. Clinical, histopathologic, and cytologic diagnosis of mucosal leishmaniasis and literature review. Arch Pathol Lab Med 2011;135:478-482.
254. Handler MZ, Patel PA, Kapila R, et al. Cutaneous and mucocutaneous leishmaniasis: clinical perspectives. J Am Acad Dermatol 2015;73:897-908.
255. Andrade RV, Massone C, Lucena MN, et al. The use of polymerase chain reaction to confirm diagnosis in skin biopsies consistent with American tegumentary leishmaniasis at histopathology: a study of 90 cases. An Bras Dermatol 2011;86:892-896.
256. Weirather JL, Jeronimo SM, Gautam S, et al. Serial quantitative PCR assay for detection, species discrimination, and quantification of Leishmania spp. in human samples. J Clin Microbiol 2011;49:3892-3904.
257. McGwire BS, Satoskar AR. Leishmaniasis: clinical syndromes and treatment. QJM 2014;107:7-14.
258. Rama M, Kumar NV, Balaji S. A comprehensive review of patented antleishmanial agents. Pharm Pat Anal 2015;4:37-56.
259. Sundar S, Chakravarty J. Leishmaniasis: an update of current pharmacotherapy. Expert Opin Pharmacother 2013;14:53-63.

Amebiasis

260. Cope JR, Ratard RC, Hill VR, et al. The first association of primary amebic meningoencephalitis death with culturable Naegleria fowleri in tap water from a US treated public drinking water system. Clin Infect Dis 2015;60:e36-42.
261. Siripanth C. Amphizoic amoebae: pathogenic free-livinh protozoa; review of the literature and review of cases in Thailand. J Med Assoc Thai 2005;88:701-707.
262. Dickson JM, Zetler PJ, Walker B, Javer AR. Acanthamoeba rhinosinusitis. J Otolaryngol Head Neck Surg 2009;38:E87-90.
263. Siripanth C, Punpoowong B, Riganti M. Early detection and identification of amphizoic amoebae from nasal exudates of a symptomatic case. J Med Assoc Thai 2005;88:545-549.

Rhinosinusitis

264. deShazo RD, Kemp SF. Rhinosinusitis. South Med J 2003;96:1055-1060.
265. Ferguson BJ. Categorization of eosinophilic chronic rhinosinusitis. Curr Opin Otolaryngol Head Neck Surg 2004;12:237-242.
266. Gysin C, Alothman GA, Papsin BC. Sinonasal disease in cystic fibrosis: clinical characteristics, diagnosis, and management. Pediatr Pulmonol 2000;30:481-489.
267. Jani AL, Hamilos DL. Current thinking on the relationship between rhinosinusitis and asthma. J Asthma 2005;42:1-7.
268. Kennedy DW. Pathogenesis of chronic rhinosinusitis. Ann Otol Rhinol Laryngol Suppl 2004;193:6-9.
269. Meltzer EO, Szwarcberg J, Pill MW. Allergic rhinitis, asthma, and rhinosinusitis: diseases of the integrated airway. J Manag Care Pharm 2004;10:310-317.
270. Morwood K, Gillis D, Smith W, Kette F. Aspirin-sensitive asthma. Intern Med J 2005;35:240-246.
271. Schatz M, Zeiger RS. Diagnosis and management of rhinitis during pregnancy. Allergy Proc 1988;9:545-554.
272. Smart BA, Slavin RG. Rhinosinusitis and pediatric asthma. Immunol Allergy Clin North Am 2005;25:67-82.
273. Wang X, Kim J, McWilliams R, Cutting GR. Increased prevalence of chronic rhinosinusitis in carriers of a cystic fibrosis mutation. Arch Otolaryngol Head Neck Surg 2005;131:237-240.
274. Ellegard EK. The etiology and management of pregnancy rhinitis. Am J Respir Med 2003;2:469-475.
275. Lekas MD. Rhinitis during pregnancy and rhinitis medicamentosa. Otolaryngol Head Neck Surg 1992;107(Pt 2):845-848.
276. Lanza DC. Diagnosis of chronic rhinosinusitis. Ann Otol Rhinol Laryngol Suppl 2004;193:10-14.
277. Batra PS. Radiologic imaging in rhinosinusitis. Cleve Clin J Med 2004;71:886-888.
278. Mainz JG, Gerber A, Arnold C, Baumann J, Baumann I, Koitschev A. [Rhinosinusitis in cystic fibrosis.] HNO 2015;63:809-820. [German]
279. Engler DB, Grant JA. Allergic rhinitis: a practical approach. Hosp Pract 1991;26:105-112.
280. Naclerio RM. Allergic rhinitis. N Engl J Med 1991;325:860-869.
281. Shatkin JS, Delsupehe KG, Thisted RA, Corey JP. Mucosal allergy in the absence of systemic allergy in nasal polyposisand rhinitis: a meta analysis. Otolaryngol Head Neck Surg 1994;111:553-556.
282. Dutt SN, Kameswaran M. The aetiology and management of atrophic rhinitis. J Laryngol Otol 2005;119:843-852.
283. Shehata MA. Atrophic rhinitis. Am J Otolaryngol 1996;17:81-86.

284. Sinha SN, Sardana DS, Rajvanshi VS. A nine years' review of 273 cases of atrophic rhinitis and its management. J Laryngol Otol 1977;91:591-600.
285. Samter M, Beers RF Jr. Intolerance to aspirin. Clinical studies and consideration of its pathogenesis. Ann Intern Med 1968;68:975-983.
286. Zeitz HJ. Bronchial asthma, nasal polyps, and aspirin sensitivity: Samter's syndrome. Clin Chest Med 1988;9:567-576.
287. Rajan JP, Wineinger NE, Stevenson DD, White AA. Prevalence of aspirinexacerbated respiratory disease among asthmatic patients: a meta-analysis of the literature. J Allergy Clin Immunol 2015;135(3):676.e1-681.e1.
288. Steinke JW, Wilson JM. Aspirin-exacerbated respiratory disease: pathophysiological insights and clinical advances. J Asthma Allergy 2016;9:37-43.
289. Probst L, Stoney P, Jeney E, Hawke M. Nasal polyps, bronchial asthma and aspirin sensitivity. J Otolaryngol 1992;20:60-65.
290. Bachert C, Wagenmann M, Hauser U, Rudack C. IL-5 synthesis is upregulated in human nasal polyp tissue. J Allergy Clin Immunol 1997;99(Pt 1):837-842.
291. Payne SC, Early SB, Huyett P, Han JK, Borish L, Steinke JW. Evidence for distinct histologic profile of nasal polyps with and without eosinophilia. Laryngoscope 2011;121:2262-2267.
292. Sampson AP, Cowburn AS, Sladek K, et al. Profound overexpression of leukotriene C4 synthase in bronchial biopsies from aspirin-intolerant asthmatic patients. Int Arch Allergy Immunol 1997;113:355-357.
293. Steinke JW, Liu L, Huyett P, Negri J, Payne SC, Borish L. Prominent role of interferon-γ in aspirin-exacerbated respiratory disease. J Allergy Clin Immunol 2013;132:856.e3-865.e3.
294. Mascia K, Borish L, Patrie J, Hunt J, Phillips CD, Steinke JW. Chronic hyperplastic eosiniphilic sinusistis as a predictor of aspirin-exacerbated respiratory disease. Ann Allergy Asthma Immunol 2005;94:652-657.
295. Moneret-Vautrin DA, Hsieh V, Wayoff M, et al. Nonallergic rhinitis with eosinophilia syndrome a precursor of the triad: nasal polyposis, intrinsic asthma, and intolerance to aspirin. Ann Allergy 1990;64:513-518.
296. Adelman J, McLean C, Shaigany K, Krouse JH. The role of surgery in management of Samter's triad: A systematic review. Otolaryngol Head Neck Surg 2016;155:220-237.
297. Sok JC, Ferguson BJ. Differential diagnosis of eosinophilic chronic rhinosinusitis. Curr Allergy Asthma Rep 2006;6:203-214.

2 ORAL CAVITY AND JAW

By Drs. Esther L. B. Childers and Mary S. Richardson

EMBRYOLOGY, ANATOMY, AND HISTOLOGY

Embryology

The primitive oral cavity, or stomodeum, partly develops from the surface ectoderm and partly from the endoderm of the cranial end of the foregut (the future site of the pharynx) (1). Initially, the oropharyngeal membrane separates these structures, but at the end of the 4th week of gestation the oropharyngeal membrane disappears, allowing for direct communication of the mouth with the pharynx.

The majority of the epithelium of the oral cavity (lips, gums, palate) is of ectodermal origin. The epithelium of the tongue varies in its development. The anterior two thirds, or oral tongue, is of ectodermal origin, developing from the tuberculum impar and is of 1st branchial arch (mandibular arch) derivation. The posterior, or pharyngeal, portion of the tongue is of endodermal origin, developing from the hypobranchial eminence and is of 3rd branchial arch derivation.

The muscles of mastication (temporalis, masseter, and medial and lateral pterygoids) are derived from the 1st branchial arch. The mandible is formed from the mandibular prominence of the 1st branchial arch. The maxilla, zygomatic bone, and squamous part of the temporal bone derive from the maxillary prominence of the 1st branchial arch.

Anatomy

The anatomic borders of the oral cavity (2,3) include: anterior, the vermilion border of the lips; posterior is a line drawn from the junction of the hard and soft palate to the circumvallate papillae of the tongue; superior, the hard palate until its junction with the soft palate; inferior, the anterior two thirds of the tongue to the line of the circumvallate papillae; and lateral, the buccal mucosa of the cheeks. Many structures are located within the anatomic confines of the oral cavity (fig. 2-1).

Lips. The mucosal lip begins at the junction of the vermilion border with the skin and includes only the vermilion surface or that portion of the lip that comes in contact with the opposing lip. The vermilion border is the junction between the skin and the oral mucosa.

Buccal Mucosa. This includes all the membranes lining the inner surface of the cheeks and lips from the line of contact of the opposing lips to the line of attachment of mucosa of the alveolar ridge (upper and lower) and pterygomandibular raphe.

Alveolar Ridges (Lower and Upper). The mucosa of the lower alveolar ridge overlies the alveolar process of the mandible, which extends from the line of attachment of mucosa in the buccal gutter to the line of free mucosa of the floor of the mouth; posteriorly, it extends to the ascending ramus of the mandible.

The mucosa of the upper alveolar ridge overlies the alveolar process of the maxilla, which extends from the line of attachment of mucosa in the upper gingival buccal gutter to the junction of the hard palate; the posterior margin is the upper end of the pterygopalatine arch.

Retromolar Trigone or Retromolar Gingiva. Attached mucosa overlies the ascending ramus of the mandible from the level of the posterior surface of the last molar tooth to the apex superiorly, adjacent to the tuberosity of the maxilla.

Floor of Mouth. This semilunar or horseshoe-shaped area is situated beneath the movable tongue, between the upper alveolar ridge and the mucous membrane covering the palatine process of the maxillary palatine bones. The floor of the mouth extends from the inner surface of the superior alveolar ridge to the posterior edge of the palatine bone, It consists of the mucous membrane of the oral cavity to the superior surface of the mylohyoid muscle as it unites in the midline from the symphysis

103

of the mandible to the area of the third molar. A fold of tissue, lingual frenulum, extends from the inferior surface of the tongue near the base. A portion of the submandibular gland and the sublingual gland are contained within the contents of the floor of the mouth. The ducts from the sublingual gland and the submandibular gland open into the floor of the mouth at the sublingual papilla (caruncle). Also contained within the floor of the mouth is the sublingual branch of the lingual artery.

Tongue. This is a highly muscular organ of deglutition, taste, and speech. It is attached by muscles to the hyoid bone, mandible, styloid process, soft palate, and pharyngeal wall. The anterior two thirds are the oral tongue and the posterior one third is the pharyngeal or postsulcal part.

The anterior two thirds of the tongue (oral tongue) is the freely mobile portion of the tongue extending anteriorly from the line of circumvallate papillae to the undersurface of the tongue at the junction of the floor of the mouth. It is covered by numerous papillae, some of which bear taste buds. The anterior tongue is composed of four areas: tip, lateral borders, dorsum, and undersurface (nonvillous ventral surface).

The dorsal tongue (fig. 2-1) represents the superior surface related to the hard and soft palates. It is located in floor of the oral cavity. Generally convex in all directions at rest, it is divided by a v-shaped sulcus terminalis into anterior (oral or presulcal) part which faces upward and a posterior (pharyngeal or postsulcal) part which faces posteriorly. The ventral surface of the tongue represents the undersurface (nonvillous ventral surface). It is visible when the tip of the tongue is turned upwards.

The pharyngeal (postsulcal) part of the tongue is the posterior third. Its base is posterior to the palatoglossal arches and it forms the anterior wall of the oropharynx. The mucosa reflects laterally onto the palatine tonsils and the pharyngeal wall, and posteriorly onto the epiglottis by glossoepiglottic folds, surrounding two depressions or valleculae. This portion of the tongue is devoid of papillae. Underlying lymphoid nodules, embedded in the submucosa, are collectively referred to as the lingual tonsil.

Hard Palate. This semilunar area is between the upper alveolar ridge and the mucous membrane covering the palatine process of the maxillary palatine bones. It extends from the inner surface of the superior alveolar ridge to the posterior edge of the palatine bone.

Gingivae (Gums). The mucosal membrane is directly adjacent to an erupted tooth; it is divided into marginal, attached, and interdental areas. The palatal gingiva is contiguous with the palatal mucosa.

Gnathic (Jaw) Bones. These include maxilla and mandible. The maxilla is the largest facial bone, other than the mandible. Jointly both bones form the whole of the upper jaw. Each maxillary bone forms the greater part of the floor and lateral wall of the nasal cavity, floor of the orbit, contributes to the infratemporal and pterygopalatine fossae, and bounds the inferior orbital and pterygomaxillary fissures. Each maxilla has a body and four processes: zygomatic, frontal, alveolar, and palatine.

The mandible is the largest and strongest bone of the face, wholly forming the lower jaw. It consists of a horizontally curved body that is convex forwards and two broad rami that ascend posteriorly. The body of the mandible supports the mandibular teeth within the alveolar process.

The rami bear coronoid and condylar processes. Each condyle articulates with the adjacent temporal bone at the temporomandibular joint, which is a synovial joint between the articular fossa (referred to as glenoid or mandibular fossa), the temporal bone above, and the mandibular condyle. Its articular surface lined by fibrocartilage rather than hyaline cartilage.

Teeth. The teeth are composed of enamel, dentin, and pulp. The enamel is a hard, inert, acellular substance. Dentin is immediately beneath the enamel, and is a less mineralized and more porous structure than enamel. Within the dentin is a chamber for the dental pulp, which is composed of nerve, vascular, and connective tissues. Teeth are supported in the jaw by cementum, periodontal ligament, and alveolar bone.

Normally, there are a total of 32 teeth. The American Dental Association system includes numbering each tooth by one number from #1 to #32 starting from right maxillary third molar moving clockwise

Periodontal Ligament. This ligament supports the teeth, generates the force for tooth eruption, and provides sensory information about tooth position and forces to facilitate

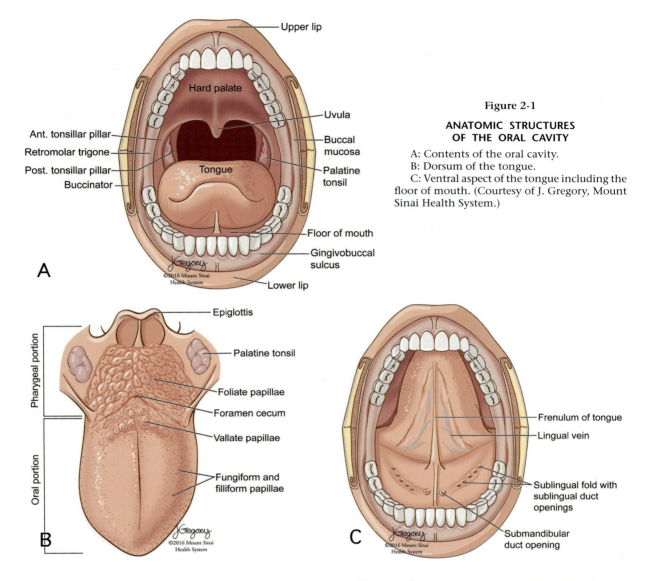

Figure 2-1

ANATOMIC STRUCTURES OF THE ORAL CAVITY

A: Contents of the oral cavity.
B: Dorsum of the tongue.
C: Ventral aspect of the tongue including the floor of mouth. (Courtesy of J. Gregory, Mount Sinai Health System.)

reflex jaw activity. The dense fibrous connective tissue, 0.2 mm wide, contains cells associated with the development and maintenance of alveolar bone (osteoblasts and osteoclasts) and cementum (cementoblasts and odontoclasts). The ligament contains a network of epithelial cells (epithelial cell rests of Malassez) which are the embryologic remnants of an epithelial root sheath; this network has no evident function but may give rise to dental cysts.

Histology

The epithelial surface of the oral cavity mucosa, including the inner surface of the lips, is covered by stratified squamous epithelium and, unlike the skin, under normal conditions keratinization is not present (4). The histology of the epithelial surfaces of the oral cavity mucosa are detailed in Table 2-1.

Lip. The cutaneous portion of the lip is covered by keratinizing squamous epithelium and includes the presence of cutaneous adnexae, including sweat glands, sebaceous glands, and hair follicles; it is richly supplied with sensory nerves (4). The squamous epithelium of the vermilion border is thin, and is densely innervated, but lacking sweat or sebaceous glands. The mucosal surface of the lip is covered by thicker stratified squamous epithelium and contains underlying minor salivary glands and ducts.

Table 2-1

ORAL MUCOSA: HISTOLOGIC FEATURES

Site	Histology
Buccal and labial mucosa (contiguous structures)	Thick nonkeratinizing stratified squamous epithelium with broad, tapered rete ridges
Dorsal tongue	Moderate to thick keratinized squamous epithelium with parakeratosis
Floor of mouth and ventral tongue (contiguous structures and histology similar to soft palate)	Thin nonkeratinizing stratified squamous epithelium with short or poorly formed rete ridges; serous minor salivary glands identified in anterior ventral tongue (glands of Blandin-Nunn) and posterior ventral tongue (von Ebner glands)
Gingiva, attached (histology similar to hard palate)	Thin layer of orthokeratin with thin granular layer of nonkeratinizing stratified squamous epithelium with poorly formed rete ridges; rete ridges tend to be more tapered and slender as compared to hard palate; may contain odontogenic epithelial rests (rests of Serres)
Gingiva, nonattached	Nonkeratinized epithelium
Hard palate (histology similar to attached gingiva)	Thin layer of orthokeratin with thin granular layer of nonkeratinizing stratified squamous epithelium with poorly formed rete ridges; dense lamina propria; submucosal minor salivary glands present
Soft palate	Thin nonkeratinizing stratified squamous epithelium with short or poorly formed rete ridges

Tongue. The epithelium of the tongue is stratified squamous epithelium. A submucous layer is present only on the ventral surface; underneath the mucosa are interlacing bundles of striated muscle (4). The dorsal aspect of the tongue, in particular the anterior portion, is characterized by the presence of numerous mucosal projections forming papillae; these papillae are absent on the ventral surface. The taste buds are pale, oval bodies within the epithelium of the papillae along the dorsal and lateral aspects of the tongue. Minor salivary glands, purely serous type, are identified within the muscular tissue.

Taste Buds. Taste buds tend to be numerous within circumvallate papillae and less numerous in fungiform and foliate papillae as well as elsewhere along dorsal and lateral aspects of tongue (4). The taste buds are intraepithelial sensory receptors appearing as barrel-shaped, lighter staining structures oriented at a right angle to the surface (fig. 2-2). They are composed of three types of spindle cells with elongated nuclei: gustatory or taste cells, supporting or sustentacular cells, and basal cells. The taste buds are immunoreactive for cytokeratins (CAM5.2, CK18) as well as for neuron-specific enolase (fig. 2-2), S-100 protein, and synaptophysin.

Minor Salivary Glands. The minor salivary glands are seen throughout the oral cavity. They appear as scattered, unencapsulated small lobules within the oral cavity mucosa and submucosa. Normally, minor salivary glands are present within muscle; the intramuscular location is associated with the tongue and lips. The minor salivary glands in the tongue are located in the anterior ventral portion (referred to as Blandin or Nuhn glands) and are of pure mucous type; in the region of the circumvallate papillae on the posterior and lateral portion (referred to von Ebner glands) and consist of pure serous type (fig. 2-2); and in the remainder of the oral cavity, where mixed seromucous and mucous glands predominate.

The minor salivary glands are present in the retromolar mandibular ridge. The anterior hard palate and gingiva, however, are typically devoid of minor salivary glands. See chapter 6, Salivary Glands, for a more complete discussion.

Juxtaoral Organ of Chievitz. The juxtaoral organ of Chievitz is a well-delineated, normal microscopic structure of uncertain function normally situated at the angle of the mandible, bilaterally, near the buccotemporal space (4). Recent evidence supports a possible neurosecretory or neuroreceptor function (5). The juxtaoral organ of Chievitz appears as multilobulated, round to elongated nests of squamoid epithelial cells embedded in a fibrous stroma rich in small peripheral nerves (fig. 2-3). The more central cells

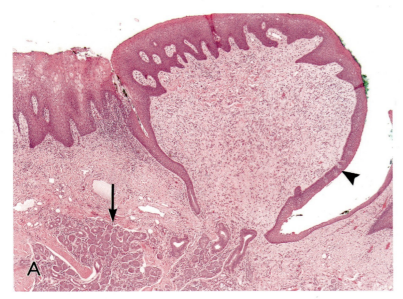

Figure 2-2

CIRCUMVALLATE PAPILLAE

A: Clusters of intraepithelial taste buds (arrowhead), stained lighter than the surrounding epithelium, are seen along the lateral wall of the papilla. Within the submucosa are numerous nerve fibers as well as minor salivary glands composed of serous glands (von Ebner glands) and ducts (arrow).

B: At higher magnification, the intraepithelial taste buds (arrows) appear as barrel-shaped structures composed of cells with elongated nuclei, mostly situated in the basal portion of the buds.

C: The taste buds are immunoreactive for neuron-specific enolase (as well as for synaptophysin and S-100 protein [not shown]) and are in direct contact with nerve fibers in the submucosa that are also reactive for neuron-specific enolase.

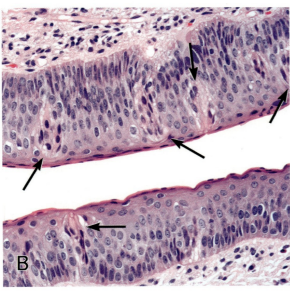
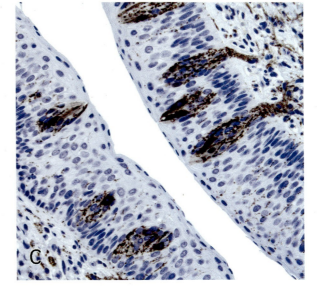

are nonkeratinizing, with identifiable intercellular bridges composed of uniform, bland-appearing nuclei, eosinophilic to clear cytoplasm, and inconspicuous nucleoli. The more peripheral cells are basaloid, with nuclear palisading. Occasionally, duct-like lumens are identified. A delineated/prominent basement membrane is present around the squamoid cell nests. In contrast to squamous cells, the cells of the juxtaoral organ of Chievitz have an absence of keratinization and keratohyaline granules. Melanin pigment may be identified (5). Immunoreactivity may be present for cytokeratin and S-100 protein.

The juxtaoral organ of Chievitz is usually an incidental finding identified during intraoperative consultation (i.e., at frozen section) or in permanent sections in tissue excised for other reasons. In the presence of its normal histology, which includes squamoid cells and normal intimate association with small peripheral nerves (branches of the buccal nerve), diagnostic confusion may arise with an invasive squamous cell carcinoma with neurotropism.

Nonepithelial Intraepithelial Cells. Nonepithelial cells that can be found in the oral mucosa include melanocytes, Langerhans

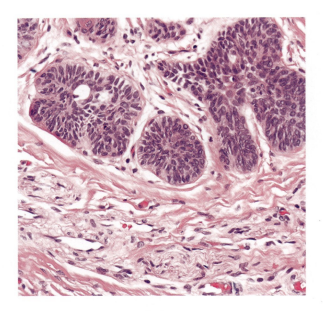

Figure 2-3

JUXTAORAL ORGAN OF CHIEVITZ

Epithelial nests and islands are adjacent to neurovascular structures.

cells, and Merkel cells. Melanocytes are located in the basal layer. They are most common in gingiva but also present in lips, palate, and buccal mucosa. Melanocytes are identified by light microscopy and are further delineated by immunoreactivity for S-100 protein and melanocytic-related markers (e.g., HMB45, melan A, SOX10, MITF1, tyrosinase).

Langerhans (dendritic) cells are mostly located in suprabasal epithelial layers. They play a role in immune response. Their dendritic nature cannot be recognized by routine staining but requires immunohistochemical staining for S-100 protein (best for seeing dendritic processes) and CD1a.

Merkel cells are located in the basal layer, individually or in clusters, and are neuroendocrine cells. Merkel cells are not recognized by routine staining but require immunohistochemical staining for neuroendocrine markers (e.g., synaptophysin, chromogranin), S-100 protein, neuron-specific enolase, and cytokeratins (AE1/AE3, CAM5.2, CK20).

CLASSIFICATION

The non-neoplastic lesions of the oral cavity are delineated in Table 2-2.

DEVELOPMENTAL LESIONS

Heterotopias (Choristomas) and Hamartomas

Heterotopia, also referred to as *choristoma*, *ectopia*, and *aberrant rest*, is a non-neoplastic developmental anomaly of essentially normal tissue; the tissue elements, however, are foreign to the anatomic location. *Hamartoma* is a non-neoplastic developmental anomaly caused by excessive growth of normal cells or tissue indigenous to its site of occurrence.

Fordyce Granules

Definition. *Fordyce granules* are collections of sebaceous glands in the oral cavity. Since sebaceous glands are not a normal histologic component of the oral cavity mucosa, Fordyce granules represent a heterotopic lesion. Synonyms include *Fordyce disease*, *Fordyce condition*, and *ectopic sebaceous glands*.

Clinical Features. Sebaceous glands are present within the oral cavity in 70 to 95 percent of the adult population but they seldom coalesce to form a mass lesion (6–8). While any mucosal site of the oral cavity may be affected, Fordyce granules most commonly occur on the buccal mucosa, upper lip, retromolar region, and tonsillar areas. Fordyce granules are usually asymptomatic, raised, yellow or white papules, with a symmetric distribution, measuring 1 to 3 mm in greatest dimension. Uncommonly, coalescence of smaller papules into a large cauliflower-like lesion may occur.

Microscopic Findings. Because the clinical appearance of Fordyce granules is often diagnostic, these lesions are usually not biopsied. Most often, the histologic diagnosis of Fordyce granules is an incidental finding in biopsies of the oral mucosa for other reasons. Histologically, the typical sebaceous glands are composed of cells with abundant foamy cytoplasm (fig. 2-4); the sebaceous glands are present in one or more lobules and are found within the submucosa immediately beneath an intact squamous epithelium. The latter may be raised owing to the sebaceous gland lesion. In contrast to cutaneous sebaceous glands, those of Fordyce granules are not associated with hair follicles. The adjacent stroma is unremarkable except for the possible presence of an inflammatory cell reaction.

Table 2-2
CLASSIFICATION OF NON-NEOPLASTIC LESIONS OF THE ORAL CAVITY AND JAW

Developmental Lesions
- Heterotopias and hamartomas
- Ectopic thyroid tissue (lingual thyroid)
- Oral choristoma
- Exostoses

Nonodontogenic Cysts
- Mucoceles (mucus extravasation phenomenon, mucus retention cyst, ranula)
- Oral lymphoepithelial cyst
- Nasopalatine duct cyst
- Others

Infectious Diseases
- Fungal
- Viral
- Bacterial
- Others

Epithelial Inflammatory or Tumor-Like Processes
- Verruca vulgaris
- Condyloma acuminatum
- Focal epithelial hyperplasia
- Oral hairy leukoplakia
- Verruciform xanthoma
- Inflammatory papillary hyperplasia
- Pseudoepitheliomatous hyperplasia

Mesenchymal Lesions
- Peripheral ossifying fibroma
- Peripheral odontogenic fibroma
- Fibroma giant cell fibroma
- Giant cell granuloma
- Fibromatoses
- Vascular lesions (pyogenic granuloma)
- Benign fibro-osseous lesions

Pigmented Lesions
- Amalgam tattoo
- Melanotic macule
- Black hairy tongue

Odontogenic Cysts
- Developmental (dentigerous, others)
- Inflammatory (periapical, residual, others)
- Odontogenic keratocyst

Selected Autoimmune, Allergic, Systemic, and Cutaneous-Type Diseases
- Granulomatosis with polyangiitis (formerly referred to as Wegener granulomatosis)
- Aphthous stomatitis
- Lichen planus
- Others

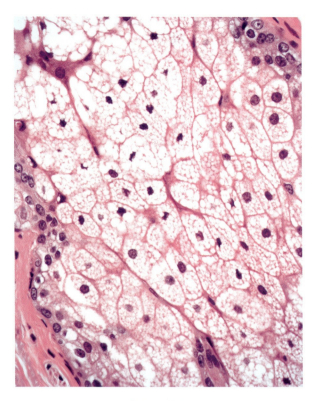

Figure 2-4

FORDYCE GRANULES

Fordyce granules are characterized by submucosal lobules of sebaceous cells with abundant, foamy appearing cytoplasm. In contrast to cutaneous sebaceous glands, those of Fordyce granules are not associated with hair follicles.

Differential Diagnosis. The coalescence of sebaceous glands into a larger mass may suggest sebaceous gland hyperplasia or sebaceous adenoma. Perhaps the differentiation of heterotopia versus hyperplasia versus neoplasia is academic since the treatments for all are similar. Some authors advocate that a clinically distinct lesion requiring a biopsy for diagnosis and composed of no fewer than 15 normal sebaceous lobules should be diagnosed as sebaceous gland hyperplasia (9).

Treatment and Prognosis. Fordyce granules require no treatment. Antibiotic therapy may be required for those lesions that become inflamed or infected. Intraoral sebaceous carcinoma, presumably originating from Fordyce granules, is a rare occurrence (10,11). It is associated with infiltrative growth and may identified by the presence of pagetoid spread of sebaceous cells within the surface epithelium.

Ectopic Thyroid Tissue and Lingual Thyroid

Definition. *Ectopic thyroid tissue* is the presence of thyroid tissue in abnormal locations.

Excluding thyroid tissue seen in association with thyroglossal duct cysts, the presence of ectopic thyroid tissue is rare and is almost exclusively seen in a suprahyoid location (12). The most common ectopic focus for thyroid tissue is the base of the tongue and is referred to as *lingual thyroid*; however, ectopic thyroid may be seen in any location, from the tongue to the suprasternal notch. Synonyms include *ectopic lingual thyroid* and *heterotopic thyroid tissue*.

Embryology. The thyroid gland originates as a diverticulum from the floor of the pharynx during the 4th week of gestation (1). The pharyngeal attachment of the thyroid gland is the foramen cecum, located on the dorsal surface of the tongue, immediately posterior to the circumvallate papillae from where the gland descends into the neck. In its descent the thyroglossal duct courses anterior to the hyoid bone, then loops around the anterioinferior border of the hyoid to lie on its posterior surface prior to descending into its anatomically normal place in the neck (1). Involution of the thyroglossal duct occurs by the 6th or 7th week of gestation. Failure of the duct to involute, however, may result in ectopic thyroid tissue, including cysts, sinuses, or fistulas, anywhere along its path of descent into the neck.

Clinical Features. Lingual thyroid affects women more than men. It most often is diagnosed in adolescence but may occur over a wide age range, from birth to the seventh decade of life. Lingual thyroid most frequently is identified along the midline of the base of the tongue between the foramen cecum and the epiglottis; rarely, the body of the tongue is affected.

Most patients who are symptomatic are women; contributing factors are thought to be related to puberty, pregnancy, and menopause. The most common symptom is dysphagia (13–16). Lingual thyroids may grow large, resulting in dyspnea, orthopnea, and severe respiratory distress. Other symptoms include bleeding, voice changes, a foreign body sensation, snoring, and sleep apnea (17). In greater than 75 percent of patients, cervical thyroid tissue is absent (total migration failure) and the lingual thyroid represents the only thyroid tissue present. In the absence of a normally situated thyroid gland, the surgical removal of the lingual thyroid results in hypothyroidism.

The appropriate preoperative clinical work-up for lingual thyroid includes scintigraphy with technetium or radioiodine studies in order to determine whether normally placed thyroid tissue is present or absent, whether there are other ectopic foci of thyroid tissue (thyroid follicles may be found in the hyoid region), and to evaluate the functional activity of the lingual thyroid tissue. Approximately 70 percent of patients with symptomatic lingual thyroid are hypothyroid and 10 percent suffer from cretinism; hyperthyroidism is a rare finding (18). Incisional biopsies must be performed with caution as this may cause sloughing of the gland, infection, necrosis, or hemorrhage.

Tc-99m pertechnetate scanning is an efficient diagnostic tool that yields high-quality images in this clinical setting. Computerized tomography (CT) shows a mass at the base of the tongue with a greater density than the tongue (19). Magnetic resonance imaging (MRI) shows a well-defined mass of low-intermediate T2 signal in the midline base of the tongue, without an invasive tendency or a cervical thyroid gland in the normal site.

Gross Findings. Lingual thyroid tissue generally is submucosal. It varies in appearance from a smooth, to a lobulated, to a nodular mass, with a red color and soft to firm consistency. It ranges in size from 2 to 3 cm. The overlying mucosa may be intact or ulcerated.

Microscopic Findings. The thyroid tissue is submucosal and unencapsulated (fig. 2-5), and may be nodular and hypercellular. The thyroid follicular epithelial cells are normal in appearance, composed of bland-appearing nuclei lacking features that might be diagnostic for papillary thyroid carcinoma (fig. 2-5). The thyroid tissue may extend into skeletal muscle; the latter finding is not an indication of malignancy.

Although unnecessary, immunohistochemical staining shows the thyroid cells to be reactive for thyroglobulin, thyroid transcription factor 1 (TTF1), PAX8, and CD56. C cells are not present in lingual thyroid tissue and the cells are nonreactive for calcitonin, and neuroendocrine markers (e.g., synaptophysin, chromogranin).

Pathologic alterations of the thyroid tissue may include adenomatoid nodules, lymphocytic thyroiditis, and neoplasia. The development of a thyroid neoplasm in lingual thyroid tissue

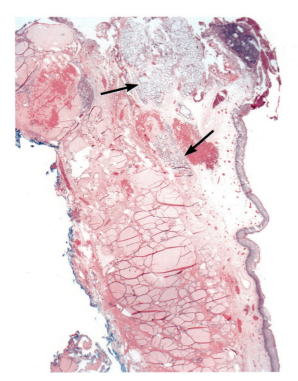 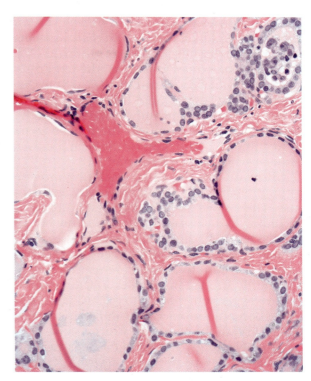

Figure 2-5

LINGUAL THYROID

Left: The thyroid tissue is submucosal and unencapsulated, and in areas lies adjacent to lingual mucous glands (arrows).
Right: The thyroid colloid-filled follicles are lined by attenuated to more cellular areas consisting of uniform-appearing cells with round to oval nuclei and coarse nuclear chromatin. Features that might be diagnostic for papillary thyroid carcinoma are lacking.

is rare; among the types of carcinoma that may develop, the most common is papillary thyroid carcinoma, most often classic type; less often, histologic variants (e.g., follicular variant); and much less frequently follicular carcinoma (20–22). Medullary thyroid carcinoma, owing to different embryologic development, does not occur in association with lingual thyroid or in other cases of thyroid gland ectopia.

Differential Diagnosis. The histologic identification of thyroid tissue is not problematic. In the rare instance of papillary thyroid carcinoma, evaluation for metastasis to the tongue base from a papillary thyroid carcinoma originating from a primary cervical-situated thyroid gland is indicated.

Treatment and Prognosis. Attempts to shrink the mass have included thyroid hormones and radioactive iodine[131] to destroy the lingual thyroid tissue, however, the latter also destroys all other thyroid tissue and may also cause sloughing of the gland and hemorrhage. Surgical excision (intraorally or via pharyngotomy) is used for symptomatic patients (e.g., with dysphagia, dysphonia, dyspnea), patients with uncontrollable hyperthyroidism, or in the presence of hemorrhage. In those individuals with absent cervical thyroid tissue or other ectopic thyroid sites, autotransplantation of thyroid tissue into the neck muscles can be done. The prognosis is good. Malignant transformation with metastasis to cervical lymph nodes and to the lung has been reported (limited to men who are older than 35 years of age) but is rare (20–22).

Oral Choristoma

Definition. An *oral choristoma* is a growth of tissue not normal for the anatomic site within the oral region. The histologic tissue type is usually included in the designation of the choristoma: *cartilaginous choristoma, osseous choristoma, gastric choristoma,* and *glial choristoma* have all been described in the oral region (23–27). Previously known as "osteoma," the term osseous choristoma was coined in 1971 (28) to distinguish these lesions from the skeletal growth of benign bone. Some authors have noted the behavior of these lesions in the tongue to be more tumor-like and propose the term "osseous tumor-like lesion of the tongue" (23).

Clinical Features. Chou et al. (29) provide a comprehensive review of oral cavity choristomas. The lesions are probably best considered according to the tissue type and location, but all soft tissue lesions are nodular, firm masses, with normal overlying mucosa. The age range at diagnosis is newborn to 73 years. Females are more commonly affected than males. The duration of lesions ranges from months to years. Glial choristomas occur in the oral cavity and do not have a connection to the central nervous system.

Gross Findings. The gross findings vary according to the type of tissue present.

Microscopic Findings. Most lesions occur in the tongue, and the most common tissue type is osseous or chondroid (fig. 2-6). More unusual combinations of location and tissue type have been reported, such as gingival choristoma of cartilage and gingival salivary gland choristoma (29). Glial choristoma of the tongue, and gastrointestinal cyst or choristoma of the tongue and of the submandibular region have been reported as well. Although sebaceous glands in the buccal and labial mucosa are generally considered a normal variant, mass lesions of sebaceous glands on the dorsal tongue have been called sebaceous choristoma (30). Intraoral hair follicle has been included in this group of lesions by some authors, although others dispute the classification (29).

Treatment and Prognosis. The treatment consists of simple surgical excision.

Tori and Exostoses

Definition. These are benign, non-neoplastic, slowly growing bony growths or protuberances. They include *torus palatinus* and *torus mandibularis.* Less commonly, they are termed *buccal exostoses* and *palatal exostoses.*

Clinical Features. Torus palatinus is a common exostosis that occurs in the midline of the

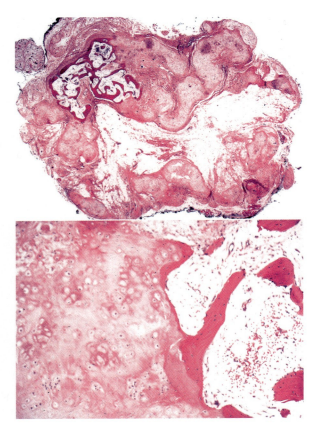

Figure 2-6

ORAL CHORISTOMAS

This diverse group of lesions most commonly occurs in association with the tongue and histologically most often is composed of an admixture of mature bone and cartilage.

hard palate (31). It is more common in women than in men, and primarily occurs in early adulthood (before the fourth decade of life). These tori are usually small (less than 2 cm), are asymptomatic, and do not appear on routine dental radiographs; occasionally, they are large and symptomatic, and appear as a radiopacity.

The torus mandibularis is a common exostosis that develops along the lingual aspect of the mandible, most often in the premolar region (fig. 2-7) (31). These tori are slightly more common in men than in women, and have a peak incidence in early adulthood. They may be single or multiple, and approximately 80 percent are bilateral (21).

Oral cavity exostoses most often occur on the buccal surface of the maxilla, in the molar region. A less common site of occurrence is the

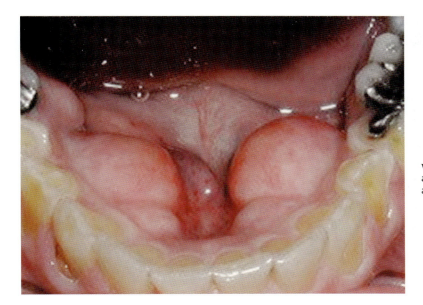

Figure 2-7

TORUS MANDIBULARIS

Bilateral lobular bony protuberances with overlying intact mucosa are located along the lingual aspect of the mandibular alveolar ridge.

labial aspect of the alveolar processes in the anterior segment of the jaw (32). They appear as nodular protuberances or excrescences covered by a thin mucosa.

Pathogenesis. The etiology of the tori is likely a combination of factors, including environmental (e.g., stress) and genetic factors (33).

Microscopic Findings. Histologically, there is a nodular mass of dense, compact bone or a cortex of compact bone, with a central area of cancellous bone. Fatty bone marrow may be present.

Differential Diagnosis. Generally, the clinical and radiographic features of tori and exostoses allow for ready identification. The differential diagnosis may include osteomas, a benign fibroosseous lesion (e.g., ossifying fibroma), and, less often, early osteosarcoma.

Treatment and Prognosis. The treatment includes surgical resection for those patients who require a denture, whose lesion ulcerates repeatedly, or who have interference with oral function. These lesions are not known to undergo malignant transformation.

ORAL CAVITY CYSTS

Oral cavity cysts include epithelial and odontogenic cysts. Some common oral cavity nonodontogenic cysts are described below. Epidermoid cysts, dermoid cysts, and branchial cleft cysts may occur in the oral cavity but are more frequent elsewhere in the head and neck (see chapters on the Neck and Ear and Temporal Bone).

Oral Lymphoepithelial Cyst

Definition. *Oral lymphoepithelial cyst* is a squamous epithelial-lined cystic cavity; a benign lymphoid infiltrate is associated with the cyst wall. It is analogous to lymphoepithelial cysts that occur in other anatomic locations such as salivary gland lymphoepithelial cyst, cervical lymphoepithelial cyst, and pancreatic lymphoepithelial cyst. It is also termed *benign lymphoepithelial cyst*.

Clinical Features. Buchner et al. (34) reported the clinicopathologic features of 38 cases of oral lymphoepithelial cyst. The floor of the mouth was the most common location, followed by the ventral tongue, posterolateral tongue, soft palate, and palatine pillar and buccal vestibules. Oral lymphoepithelial cyst also arises in areas of the oral tonsils and oral lymphoid tissue of Waldeyer ring. In the above study, patients had a wide age range, but the mean age was 38 years; the cyst was more common in males.

The clinical presentation is usually a submucosal nodular mass that is freely mobile and has a slightly yellow color (fig. 2-8). The overlying mucosa is normal or slightly telangiectatic. The diameter of the lesions range from 0.1 to 1.0 cm.

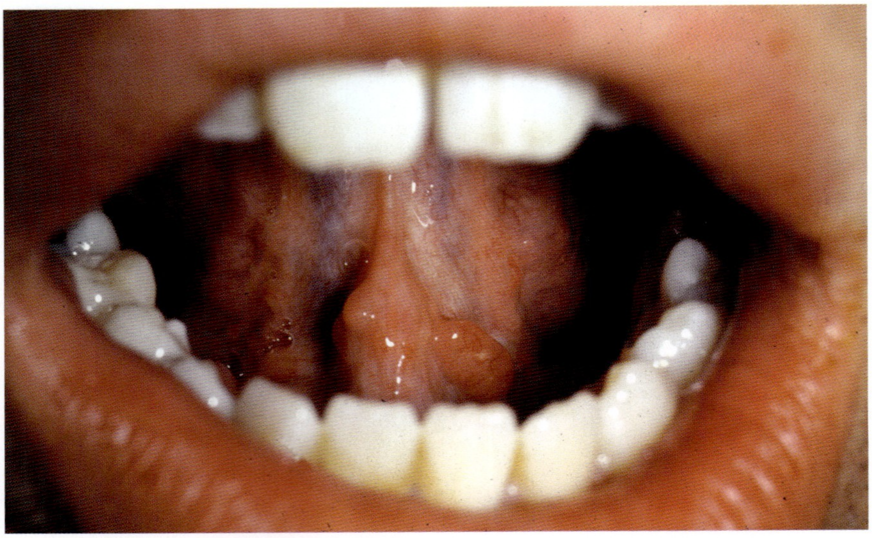

Figure 2-8

LYMPHOEPITHELIAL CYST

Located along the floor of mouth, it appears as a circumscribed submucosal yellowish nodule. On palpation, the nodule was freely mobile and soft.

Oral lymphoepithelial cyst is thought to result from the entrapment of epithelium during embryogenesis or from dilated crypt epithelium (35,36). The source of the epithelium may vary, depending on the location of the cyst. An association with Epstein-Barr virus (EBV) or human immunodeficiency virus (HIV) has not been established. Cytomegalovirus and *Mycobacterium* infection were reported in a HIV-infected patient with acquired immunodeficiency syndrome (AIDS) but were probably not the causative agents of the lymphoepithelial cyst in the parotid gland.

Microscopic Findings. Oral lymphoepithelial cysts are well-circumscribed, benign cysts lined by stratified or simple squamous epithelium, and may transition between the two, but remain unilocular and do not form complex loculations. There may be focal exocytosis of the lymphocytes into the squamous lining (fig. 2-9). The lumen may be filled with keratin or mucoid material sparsely interspersed with polymorphonuclear leukocytes and histiocytes, or it may be empty. Occasional bacterial colonization may be seen in the cystic space. The lumen may be dilated or collapsed. Some cysts are connected to the surface. The cyst wall contains prominent, benign lymphoid follicular hyperplasia. The lymphoid follicles are usually easily identified and may cause bulges into the luminal surface (fig. 2-9), but in some cases the lymphoid proliferation does not form germinal centers.

Differential Diagnosis. It is critical to distinguish the benign epithelial and lymphoid components from malignant counterparts. Squamous cell carcinoma may invoke a profound lymphoid response and should not be confused with lymphoepithelial cyst. Similarly, the atypical lymphoid proliferation of an extranodal marginal zone B-cell lymphoma may exhibit epitheliotropism and form lymphoepithelial complexes, but should not be mistaken for lymphoepithelial cysts.

Treatment and Prognosis. Complete surgical excision is adequate therapy.

Nasopalatine Duct Cyst

Definition. *Nasopalatine duct cyst* is a nonodontogenic oral cavity cyst thought to arise from remnants of the nasopalatine cyst, an embryologic structure connecting the oral and nasal cavities in the area of the incisive canal. It is also known as *median anterior maxillary cyst*.

Clinical Features. Nasopalatine duct cyst is the most common nonodontogenic oral cavity cyst, representing slightly over 70 percent of nonodontogenic cysts and occurring in approximately 1 percent of the population (37–40). Nasopalatine duct cysts occur in two forms: the intraosseous incisive canal cyst and the soft tissue cyst of the palatine papilla; of the two, the incisive canal cyst is more common.

Nasopalatine duct cyst occurs more often in males, and can be seen in all age ranges but is most common in fourth to sixth decades of life.

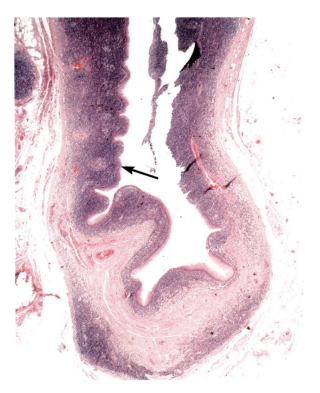 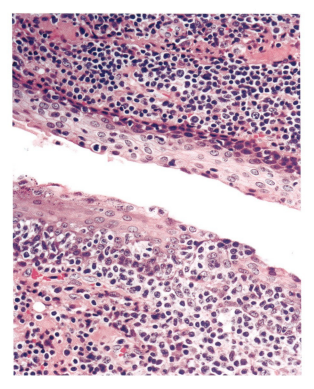

Figure 2-9

LYMPHOEPITHELIAL CYST

Left: Low-power view of excised cyst from the patient in figure 2-8 shows a unilocular epithelial-lined cystic proliferation with a mural benign lymphocytic cell infiltrate that includes lymphoid follicles; these cause bulging of the luminal surface (arrow).

Right: The cyst is lined by stratified squamous epithelium (left) but may also include permeation of the lymphocytes into the squamous epithelium (bottom).

Many patients are asymptomatic, with cysts identified on routine radiographic studies. Those with symptoms have swelling of the anterior palate (i.e., incisive canal), pain, and drainage.

Radiographically, nasopalatine duct cysts are well-circumscribed radiolucencies, most often round to oval, with a sclerotic border identified in or near the midline of the anterior maxilla between and apical to the roots of the maxillary incisor teeth (fig. 2-10) (41). Overlap of the nasal spine may give a "heart-shaped" appearance to the radiograph.

Microscopic Findings. Nasopalatine duct cyst has an epithelial lining that consists of a combination of stratified squamous epithelium (most common), pseudostratified columnar epithelium, and simple cuboidal or columnar epithelium, the latter with or without goblet cells and cilia (fig. 2-11). The cyst wall may include mucous glands (seen in about a third of cases), medium-sized nerves, and muscular arteries and veins. The presence of these structures is due to origin of this cyst from within the incisive canal; finding these structures is diagnostically useful. A mixed chronic inflammatory cell reaction, sometime, including acute inflammatory cells, may be present and varies from mild to marked.

Differential Diagnosis. The differential diagnosis includes other oral cysts, odontogenic and nonodontogenic. The clinical-radiologic-pathologic features of nasopalatine duct cyst allow for diagnosis and differentiation from other oral cysts.

Treatment and Prognosis. The treatment for the symptomatic or large nasopalatine duct cysts is surgical resection. Enucleation is the treatment of choice (39). Recurrences are rare. A squamous cell carcinoma probably originating from a nasopalatine cyst has been reported but is extremely rare (42).

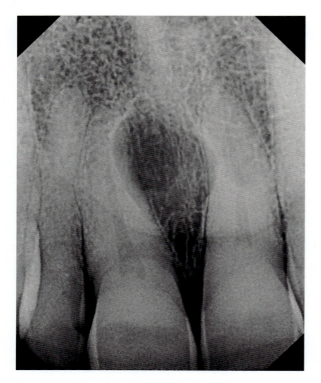

Figure 2-10

NASOPALATINE DUCT CYST

Radiographic imaging shows a well-circumscribed radiolucent lesion between and apical to the roots of the vital maxillary central incisors.

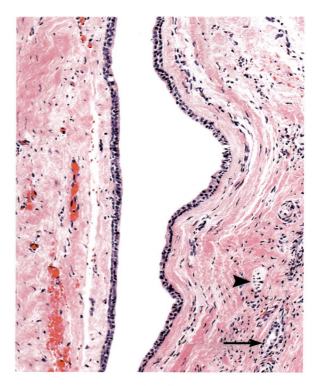

Figure 2-11

NASOPALATINE DUCT CYST

The excised cystic lesion seen in figure 2-10 is lined by pseudostratified columnar epithelium overlying fibroconnective tissue that includes a gland (arrow), small peripheral nerves (arrowhead), and small blood vessels.

INFECTIOUS DISEASES OF THE ORAL CAVITY

Infections of the oral cavity are common and organisms include fungus, virus, bacteria, and protozoa. The breadth of infections diseases of the oral cavity is extensive and this section only focuses on the more common seen by the surgical pathologist.

Fungal Disease: Candidiasis

Definition. *Candidiasis* is an infection caused by the yeast-like fungal microorganisms, *Candida albicans*. Synonyms include *oral thrush*, *moniliasis*, and *candidosis*.

Clinical Features. Candidiasis is the most common oral fungal infection in humans. Clinical forms are varied and include pseudomembranous candidiasis (also known as "thrush"), erythematous candidiasis, mucocutaneous candidiasis, and chronic hyperplastic candidiasis (also referred to as candidal leukoplakia) (43–46). Oral candidiasis often occurs in immune compromised or debilitated patient (43,47), however, oral candidiasis also occurs in immune competent (healthy) patients. Factors that impact on the development of oral candidiasis include the immune status of the patient, the strain of *Candida*, and the status of the oral mucosa environment.

Pseudomembranous Candidiasis (PC) or Thrush. PC is characterized by the presence of white plaques that adhere to the mucosa and give the appearance of cottage cheese (46). Common sites of occurrence include the buccal mucosa, dorsal tongue, and palate. Patients may experience a burning sensation or have a foul taste in their mouths. The plaques may be removed, exposing an underlying erythematous-appearing mucosa.

Erythematous Candidiasis (EC). EC has varying clinical presentations. Early or acute atrophic candidiasis typically follows a course of broad spectrum antibiotics. This *Candida* infection results in the diffuse loss of the filiform papillae of the dorsal tongue, appearing as patchy, denuded foci (48). Patients complain of a burning sensation.

Median rhomboid glossitis (also referred to as *central papillary atrophy of the tongue*) is a feature of chronic EC and was initially erroneously considered to be a developmental defect of the tongue (49–52). The lesions are typically asymptomatic, resulting in filiform papillae of the posterior tongue appearing as well-demarcated, erythematous zones seen in the midline, posterior dorsal tongue. When these lesions are associated with candidiasis of other oral mucosal sites, it is termed *chronic multifocal candidiasis*. Other sites of involvement include the junction of the hard and soft palate, and the angles of the mouth (*angular cheilitis* or *perlèche*). Occurrence under a denture is referred to as *denture stomatosis*.

Chronic Hyperplastic Candidiasis (CHC). CHC is a mucosal white patch that cannot be rubbed off, and is the result of *Candida* infection; this process is also referred to as *candidal leukoplakia* (53). The process of candidal infection producing a leukoplakic lesion is not universally accepted, as opposed to the process of candidal infestation occurring as a secondary process in a pre-existing leukoplakic lesion. The clinical appearance is that of nondescript leukoplakia typically involving the (anterior) buccal mucosa; some lesions are mixed red and white, referred to as *erythroleukoplakia*. The latter, in contrast to a purely leukoplakic lesion, is more apt to harbor underlying significant dysplasia or carcinoma.

Mucocutaneous Candidiasis. This rare acquired or inherited (autosomal recessive) immunologic disorder results in candida infection that is predicated on the extent of the immunologic disorder. The immunologic dysfunction generally manifests in the first few years of life; the intraoral candidal infection manifests as thick, white plaques that do not rub off.

Microscopic Findings. There are several members of the *Candida* genus, but the most common cause of upper aerodigestive tract mucosal candidiasis is *C. albicans*. *C. albicans* is a dimorphic fungus that includes a yeast form and a hyphal form. The hyphal form is considered responsible for tissue invasion and a diagnosis of candidiasis is based on finding hyphae or pseudohyphae. Hyphae vary in length, are branched, and may be apparent by hematoxylin and eosin (H&E) staining (fig. 2-12). However, microorganisms may be difficult to identify by conventional staining and in suspected cases, special stains, including periodic acid-Schiff (PAS) or Gomori methenamine silver (GMS) may be required for definitive identification (fig. 2-12).

In oral mucosal candidiasis, the microorganisms typically are found in the thickened parakeratin layer and in the superficial spinous layer. In conjunction with the fungal infestation, there usually is an associated neutrophilic infiltrate that may or may not coalesce to form microabscesses. The neutrophilic cell infiltrate is not a pathognomonic finding but its presence in the superficial areas should prompt consideration of an infectious etiology, specifically fungal infection. In conjunction with the fungal infection and acute inflammatory cell reaction, additional findings include hyperkeratosis, parakeratosis, orthokeratosis, irregular epithelial hyperplasia with elongated rete ridges, and a submucosal nonspecific chronic inflammatory cell reaction. Reactive basal zone epithelial atypia may be present. Less commonly, fungi are present within the deeper epithelial layers; this is more common in patients with a significant immunocompromised condition.

Differential Diagnosis. In general, a diagnosis of oral mucosal candidiasis is established on clinical grounds. Biopsy of a given lesion may be required for those lesions that are unresponsive to antifungal therapy or in the setting of chronic hyperplastic candidiasis in which the differential diagnosis may include exclusion of significant epithelial dysplasia (i.e., moderate or severe) or carcinoma.

Treatment. Relative to the mucosal candidal infection, irrespective of the clinical setting, antifungal therapy is usually curative of the fungal infection (54).

Other Fungi

Other fungal infections that may occur in the oral cavity (and other upper aerodigestive tract mucosa) include histoplasmosis, cryptococcosis, mucormycosis, blastomycosis, and aspergillosis (see the chapter on the sinonasal tract for images of these infections). More often

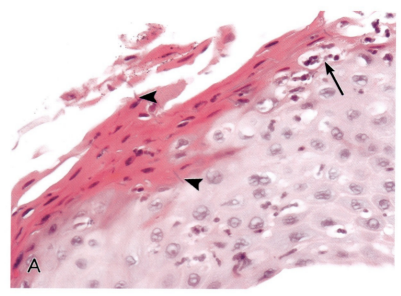

Figure 2-12

CANDIDIASIS

A: Squamous epithelium with a focal neutrophilic cell infiltrate (arrow) shows the presence of fungal hyphae (arrowheads) in the thickened parakeratin layer and in the superficial spinous layer lying perpendicular to the epithelial surface.

B,C: Special stains, including Grocott methenamine silver (GMS) and periodic acid–Schiff (PAS) more clearly delineate the fungal spores and hyphae.

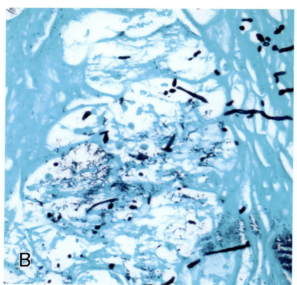

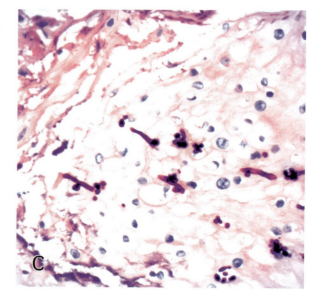

these fungi infect nonoral mucosal sites or the skin. Mucosal infestation by these fungi may be associated with (florid) pseudoepitheliomatous hyperplasia of the surface epithelium.

Viruses

Viral infection of head and neck sites occurs in nonimmunocompromised patients and in patients whose immune system creates an opportunity for fungal infection. Human papillomavirus (HPV) is associated with non-neoplastic and neoplastic lesions of the oral cavity and other sites of the upper aerodigestive tract. The clinical and pathologic findings of specific HPV-associated non-neoplastic diseases are discussed later in this chapter. Viral diseases of the oral cavity and upper aerodigestive tract often occur in immunocompromised patients. Among these immunocompromised disease states are cancer patients, HIV-infected patients, and patients with AIDS. Among the more common viruses that infect head and neck sites in these clinical settings are cytomegalovirus (CMV) and herpes virus (simplex and zoster).

Human Papillomavirus

General Features. HPV represents a large group of small double-stranded circular DNA viruses. It is strongly epitheliotropic. HPV is a sexually and nonsexually transmitted disease (55). It is associated with both non-neoplastic and neoplastic lesions. Non-neoplastic diseases associated with HPV include verrucae (verruca vulgaris or common wart and condyloma acuminatum) and Heck disease, also known as focal epithelial hyperplasia.

Epithelial neoplasms associated with HPV are benign and malignant (55). Benign neoplasms (typically with low-risk HPV 6/11) include papillomas, including sinonasal (Schneiderian) papillomas and other mucosal (squamous) papillomas of various upper aerodigestive tract sites (oral cavity, oropharynx, and larynx). Malignant neoplasms associated with HPV (typically high-risk HPV 16/18) include oropharyngeal (nonkeratinizing) carcinoma, papillary squamous cell carcinoma, and basaloid squamous cell carcinoma (56). For these carcinomas there is evidence for a causal role of HPV in their development (57).

The cells of malignant neoplastic tumors associated with HPV contain HPV DNA and HPV RNA. The role of HPV in neoplastic proliferations may stem from its function as a promoter in the multistep process of carcinogenesis in squamous cells of the upper aerodigestive tract. Two viral oncoproteins of high-risk HPVs, E6 and E7, promote tumor progression by inactivation of p53 and retinoblastoma tumor suppressor gene products, respectively (58). These viral oncoproteins are capable of disrupting the cell-cycle regulatory pathways in the genetic progression to squamous cell carcinoma. In this regard, HPV may play a role in the development of verrucous carcinoma, although a causal association between HPV and verrucous carcinoma has not been established.

Microscopic Findings. Histologically, a feature associated with HPV infection is the presence in epithelial cells of koilocytosis, characterized by cells with condensed, pyknotic or hyperchromatic ("raisin-shaped") nuclei with perinuclear clear areas referred to as halos (fig. 2-13). Binucleated and multinucleated cells may be present.

Immunohistochemical markers are available for the identification of HPV, including a poly-

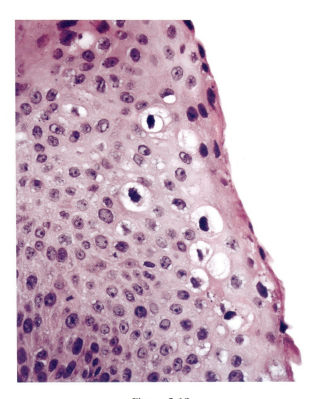

Figure 2-13

HUMAN PAPILLOMAVIRUS (HPV) INFECTION

Histologically, a feature associated with HPV infection is the presence of intraepithelial koilocytosis, characterized by cells with condensed pyknotic ("raisin-shaped") nuclei with perinuclear clear areas ("halos").

clonal marker, as well as more directed markers for specific HPV subtypes. Detection of HPV by in situ hybridization using labeled probes to detect HPV RNA and DNA, as well as in situ polymerase chain reaction (PCR), have increased the detection of HPV. HPV 16 is strongly associated with tonsillar carcinomas, and integration of the virus has been shown to be tightly coupled to the neoplastic process (58–61).

Treatment and Prognosis. There are no specific treatment protocols for HPV of the upper aerodigestive tract. There is no definitive correlation to malignant progression/transformation of a benign lesion/neoplasm in the presence of HPV. Therapy is directed at the underlying or associated pathologic process; however, recent evidence of HPV 16 integration in association with tonsillar carcinoma may represent a meaningful finding for risk assessment, early cancer detection, and disease surveillance.

Epstein-Barr Virus

Epstein-Barr virus (EBV) is an enveloped icosahedral herpesvirus with double-stranded linear DNA. Non-neoplastic diseases associated with EBV include (but are not limited to) infectious mononucleosis (discussed in chapter 3) and oral hairy leukoplakia (see later in this chapter).

Cytomegalovirus

Cytomegalovirus (CMV). CMV is the most common opportunistic pathogen recognized at autopsy in AIDS patients (62–64). Additional clinical settings for CMV infection of the head and neck include immune-compromised patients following stem cell or solid organ transplantation (65). In general, CMV infection involving the head and neck is not common.

CMV appears as a single or as multiple, oval, tan-white, ulcerated lesions with a hyperemic rim, with or without an associated exudate. Histologic findings include mucosal ulceration, necrosis, and cytomegaly (63,64). Characteristic intranuclear or intracytoplasmic inclusions are identified usually in mesenchymal rather than epithelial cells (see chapter 3 for illustrations).

Immunohistochemical stains (anti-CMV reactivity) assist in the detection/diagnosis of CMV infection. DNA sequencing analysis by PCR confirms and identifies CMV (66).

The differential diagnosis primarily includes other viral inclusion diseases such as herpes virus infection. Immunohistochemical stains allow discrimination among these viral inclusion diseases.

Given the occurrence of CMV in the head and neck in association with immune-compromised diseases/states, treatment is usually with systemic antiviral agents that may include ganciclovir, or its prodrug valganciclovir, foscarnet, and cidofovir (62,67,68). Overall, prognosis is dependent on the underlying disease state and the ability to control the local/systemic infection.

Herpes Virus

Two distinct subtypes of herpes simplex virus (HSV) are identified: type 1, referred to as the "oral" type and type 2, referred to as the "genital" type. The virus type, however, is not a reliable indicator of the anatomic site affected, especially with changing sexual habits. Because of its tendency to infect cells of ectodermal origin (skin or mucous membranes) HSV is a frequent cause of mucocutaneous disease in the HIV-positive patient (69). Head and neck manifestations are those of an ulcerated lesion with involvement of intraoral, nasal cavity, lip, external ear, pharynx, and tonsil; in addition, enlargement and tenderness of cervical and submental lymph nodes may be seen. Infection of the pharynx may appear as vesicular lesions which bleed easily and may be covered with a black crust or as shallow tonsillar ulcers covered with gray exudates.

Herpes zoster occurs as *varicella (chicken pox)* or as *dermatomal zoster (shingles)*; the latter, while not specific for HIV infection, appears to be related to HIV infection and may represent an early marker of the immunosuppression associated with HIV infection. Herpes zoster can localize to any dermatome, is neurotropic, and can cause unremitting pain. Head and neck manifestations include involvement of the 8th cranial nerve or geniculate ganglion producing severe ear pain, hearing loss, vertigo, and facial nerve paralysis (Ramsay Hunt syndrome).

Herpes infection may appear as a single lesion or multiple, oval, tan-white, ulcerated lesions with a hyperemic rim with or without associated exudates. There is intraepidermal vesicle formation marked by acantholysis and balloon degeneration of epithelial cells. Intranuclear inclusions may be identified within the degenerating epithelial cells. In herpes zoster virus infection, the intranuclear inclusions are indistinguishable from those of herpes simplex. Multinucleated giant cells may be numerous (see chapter 3 for illustrations).

Herpetic lesions are identified by positive anti-HSV immunoreactivity. DNA sequencing analysis by PCR confirms and identifies HSV (66).

The differential diagnosis primarily includes other viral inclusion diseases such as CMV. Immunohistochemical stains allow for discriminating among these viral inclusion diseases. The treatment for herpetic infection includes antiviral chemotherapy including acyclovir, ganciclovir, and foscarnet.

Bacteria and Spirochetes

Bacterial infections of the oral cavity are common but generally represent a clinical diagnosis rather than a surgical disease. Immunocompromised patients infected by opportunistic microorganisms, however, may require tissue sampling for diagnostic purposes. HIV-infected/AIDS patients may experience an increased incidence of gonorrhea and syphilis.

Gonorrhea

Definition. *Gonorrhea* is a localized and systemic disease caused by *Neisseria gonorrhea*, a pyogenic Gram-negative diplococcus.

Clinical Features. Otolaryngic manifestations include gonococcal pharyngitis, which generally is asymptomatic but may present with sore throat, tonsillar hypertrophy, and cervical adenopathy (70–73). The organism infects mucosal and glandular structures.

Microscopic Findings. This uncommon mucosal disease process has no specific light microscopic features that require special stains for diagnosis. Gram stain smears from the pharynx are unreliable due to the presence of other organisms, so that samples must be cultured on appropriate media (chocolate agar) for identification. DNA amplification testing for the identification of oropharyngeal *N. gonorrhea* offers greater sensitivity than standard cultures (74).

Differential Diagnosis. The differential diagnosis includes nonspecific inflammatory reactions.

Treatment and Prognosis. The treatment of choice for gonorrhea remains penicillin. Penicillin G or procaine is administered parenterally. For those persons allergic to penicillin, either tetracycline or erythromycin are effective alternatives. For penicillinase-producing strains, spectinomycin hydrochloride, cefoxitin sodium, or ampicillin are used.

Syphilis

Definition. *Syphilis* is a systemic venereal disease caused by *Treponemal pallidum*, a member of the family Spirochaetaceae that includes *T. pertenue* (yaws) and *T. carateum* (pinta).

Clinical Features. The clinical stages of syphilis are primary, secondary, tertiary, and congenital, any of which can affect virtually every site in the head and neck and cause an array of clinical manifestations. Tonsillar involvement manifests as a painless solitary chancre, which appears at the site of inoculation in the primary stage; chancres may clinically mimic a neoplasm. Pharyngotonsillitis is a presenting symptom in secondary syphilis and mucosal involvement produces "mucous patches," which are highly contagious (71,73,75). Other head and neck symptoms in the secondary stage may include rhinitis, laryngitis, pharyngitis, cranial nerve deficits, sensorineural deafness, labyrinthitis, and glossitis. Skin lesions and lymphadenopathy are seen in 90 percent of the patients in the secondary or disseminated stage.

Tertiary stage syphilis typically involves the central nervous system (neurosyphilis) and aorta (cardiovascular syphilis); however, localized, nonprogressive lesions may develop in mucosal otolaryngic sites. These are termed *benign tertiary syphilis* or *gummas*; the gummatous reaction represents a pronounced immunologic reaction of the host.

Congenital syphilis develops via transplacental infection and primarily occurs with mucocutaneous and osseous manifestations, including in decreasing percentage, frontal bossing, short maxilla, high palatal arch, saddle nose, mulberry molars and Hutchinson incisors, sternoclavicular thickening, interstitial keratitis, rhagades, and 8th nerve deafness (76–79).

Laboratory evaluation includes two types of serologic tests for syphilis, the nontreponemal (nonspecific) antibody tests and the treponemal (specific) antibody tests. These tests are most reactive in the secondary stage of disease.

Microscopic Findings. An inflammatory infiltrate can be seen that is predominantly composed of plasma cells with scattered histiocytes, lymphocytes, and polymorphonuclear leukocytes. This infiltrate has a tendency to involve small blood vessels, which display endothelial cell proliferation (plasma cell endarteritis); concentric layers are produced that markedly narrow the lumen of the vessel, resulting in obliterative endarteritis (80). The obliterative endarteritis coupled with the inflammatory infiltrate produced by the spirochetes represent the histologic hallmarks of the disease (see chapter 3 for illustrations).

Organisms can be demonstrated in the chancre by the Warthin-Starry stain and appear as elongated, thin rod-like structures. A variety of techniques, including darkfield examination of smears and immunocytochemistry are used to detect organisms

Differential Diagnosis. The differential diagnosis includes nonspecific inflammatory reactions.

Treatment and Prognosis. The treatment of choice for syphilis remains penicillin. Penicillin G is administered parenterally. For those persons allergic to penicillin, either tetracycline or erythromycin are effective alternatives. For penicillinase-producing strains, spectinomycin hydrochloride, cefoxitin sodium, or ampicillin are used.

EPITHELIAL INFLAMMATORY OR TUMOR-LIKE PROCESSES: REACTIVE EPITHELIAL AND EPITHELIAL-RELATED PROLIFERATIONS

Verruca Vulgaris

Definition. *Verruca vulgaris* (VV) is a benign epithelial proliferation due to HPV. It is also termed (common) *wart*.

Clinical Features. VV is more common in men than women, and occurs over a wide age range, but is most common in the third and fourth decades of life; it also occurs in children. The most common sites of occurrence are the lips, palate, and tongue, but any oral mucosal site can be affected. VV presents as a circumscribed, exophytic, white lesion with a firm consistency and a papillary appearance (fig. 2-14). VV is most often a single lesion but multiple lesions may occur. VV is caused by HPV, types 2 and 4, and less often, by types 6 and 16 (81,82).

Pathogenesis. The route of infection is by autoinoculation from a cutaneous lesion (83). Since the advent of highly active antiretroviral therapy (HAART), the incidence of oral VV has increased (84), although the reasons for this occurrence remain uncertain. In contrast to immune-based susceptibility to oropharyngeal candidiasis in HIV-positive persons, susceptibility to oral VV (and oral hairy leukoplakia) may be more associated with factors other than mucosal immune function.

Microscopic Findings. The histology of oral mucosal VV is the same as that of more common cutaneous VV, and is characterized by a papillomatous epithelial proliferation with prominent hyperkeratosis, including thickened external orthokeratosis, and elongated rete ridges (fig. 2-14). A characteristic feature is the orientation of the rete ridges along the periphery angulating angulation toward the center of the lesion. The epithelium is cytologically bland, has a prominent granular layer, and koilocytes are present in the more superficial aspect (fig. 2-14). The koilocytes are cells with condensed, pyknotic or hyperchromatic ("raisin-shaped") nuclei and perinuclear clear areas referred to as halos. A mixed chronic inflammatory cell infiltrate may be present in the subjacent stroma.

Differential Diagnosis. The differential diagnosis includes a (squamous) papilloma, which also may be associated with HPV. From a histologic standpoint, however, papillomas typically lack surface keratinization, a prominent granular cell layer, koilocytes, and angulation of the rete ridges at the periphery toward the center of the lesion.

Treatment and Prognosis. Removal of the lesion is the treatment of choice and can be performed by surgery, cryosurgery, or electrosurgery. Recurrences are rare but any cutaneous lesion may lead to additional autoinoculation and therefore all lesions should be treated simultaneously. Spontaneous regression/disappearance within 1 to 2 years may occur, especially in children.

Condyloma Acuminatum

Condyloma acuminatum (CA) is a benign papillomatous epithelial proliferation caused by HPV and thought to be sexually transmitted. The term condyloma acuminatum is derived from the Greek words *kondylos* (knob or knuckle) and *acumen* (point). Synonyms include *venereal wart* and *venereal condyloma*.

Oral Mucosal Condyloma Acuminatum

Clinical Features. Since CA is a sexually transmitted disease it usually develops in areas of sexual contact such as the anogenital region. Oral mucosal CA has no gender predilection and can be seen in all ages but tends to be most common in teenagers and young adults. The most common oral mucosal sites of occurrence include the tongue, lip, lingual frenum, and soft palate/uvula (83,85–88).

CA is often asymptomatic and appears as a red-pink, broad-based sessile mass with a papillary, cauliflower-like, mulberry appearance. It may be solitary or multiple, and tends to be larger than papillomas, usually measuring 1.0 to 1.5 cm but may reach up to 3.0 cm.

Pathogenesis. HPV types 6 and 11 are found in oral CA (87,89,90) and HPV types 16 and 18 are present in a minority of cases (91,92). The condyloma is very contagious. Primary sexual

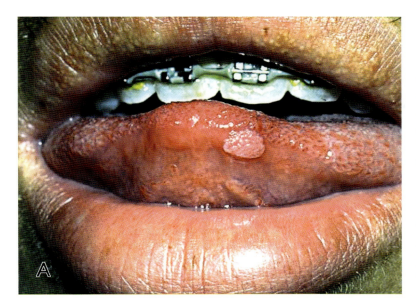

Figure 2-14

VERRUCA VULGARIS

A. Oral (lingual) verruca appears as a circumscribed, exophytic, white lesion with a papillary appearance.

B: At low magnification, the lesion is characterized by a verrucoid to papillomatous epithelial proliferation with prominent hyperkeratosis, including thickened external orthokeratosis and elongated rete ridges. A characteristic feature is the orientation of the rete ridges along the periphery angulating toward the center of the lesion (arrow).

C: The epithelium is cytologically bland and shows cells with hypergranulosis as well as scattered koilocytes, the latter including cells with condensed, pyknotic or hyperchromatic ("raisin-shaped") nuclei with perinuclear clear areas (arrows).

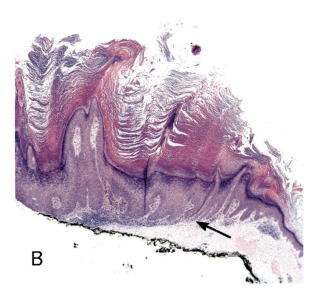

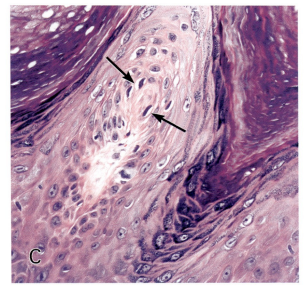

transmission following direct contact is the principal mode of transmission; less often, transmission occurs via hematogenous spread, autoinoculation from anogenital lesions, or perinatal transmission from mother to infant (92,93).

Microscopic Findings. Histologically, there are broad papillary epithelial fronds (mammillated epidermal hyperplasia), with prominent acanthosis, parakeratin crypt formation, and koilocytosis characterized by raisinoid nuclei with perinuclear halos (fig. 2-15). The rete ridges in their depth are bulbous in appearance. Numerous mitotic figures can be seen. The subjacent stroma shows dilated capillaries and a variable mixed chronic inflammatory cell reaction, including mature lymphocytes and plasma cells.

Special Studies. Although unnecessary for the diagnosis, the presence of HPV can be detected by immunohistochemical, electron microscopic, and molecular diagnostic (in situ hybridization and PCR) studies.

Differential Diagnosis. The differential diagnosis includes (squamous) papilloma and verruca vulgaris (VV). The presence of marked acanthosis, parakeratin crypt formation, numerous koilocytes, and a sessile appearance assist

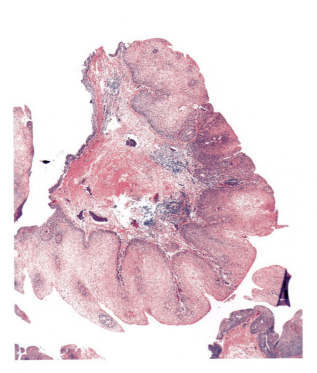 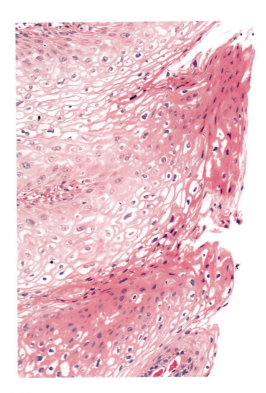

Figure 2-15

CONDYLOMA ACUMINATUM

Left: Broad papillary epithelial fronds (mammillated epidermal hyperplasia) with bulbous-appearing rete ridges are present.
Right: Koilocytosis is characterized by raisinoid-appearing nuclei with perinuclear halos.

in differentiating CA from a papilloma. CA and VV have overlapping histologic features. Differences include the presence of marked hyperorthokeratinization and angulated rete pegs along the periphery toward the center of the lesion in VV, while CA shows more extensive acanthosis as well as the more consistent presence of stromal dilated capillaries and a superficial mixed chronic inflammatory cell infiltrate.

Treatment and Prognosis. Removal of the lesion is the treatment of choice and can be performed by surgery, cryosurgery, or electrocautery. Recurrences are common. Spontaneous regression/disappearance may occur.

Unlike uterine cervical HPV-associated lesions where the HPV association is considered precancerous, the same precancerous nature is not felt to be true in the oral mucosa (88).

Focal Epithelial Hyperplasia

Definition. *Focal epithelial hyperplasia* (FEH) is an HPV-induced benign oral mucosal epithelial proliferation. It is also known as *Heck disease* (94).

Clinical Features. FEH shows no gender predilection and while initially identified in children, it affects all age groups. FEH was originally found in indigenous groups of North, Central, and South America, as well as lower socioeconomic groups in Guatemala (95). This lesion is a flat nodule. It is limited to the oral cavity and is most commonly found (in descending order) on the lower lip, buccal mucosa, tongue, and upper lip (96–99). HPV types 13 and 32 are found in association with FEH; other involved subtypes are HPV-6 and 11, and rarely, high-risk HPV (HPV16) (100–102). FEH represents an oral manifestation of AIDS (103).

Microscopic Findings. The histologic appearance of FEH includes the presence of irregular epithelial hyperplasia with hyperkeratosis, parakeratosis, and acanthosis (fig. 2-16). The rete ridges are widened and may be fused or appear confluent; elongation of the rete ridges

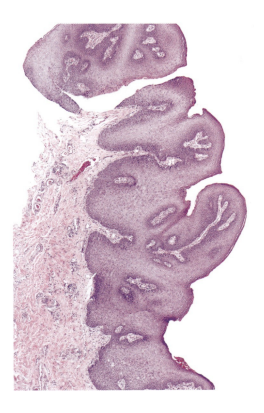 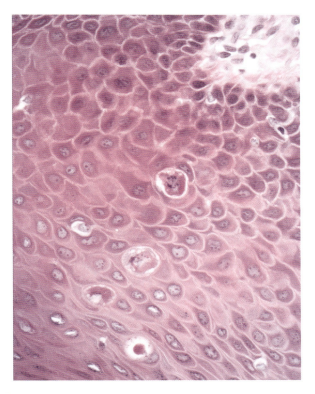

Figure 2-16

FOCAL EPITHELIAL HYPERPLASIA (HECK DISEASE)

Left: Irregular epithelial hyperplasia with hyperkeratosis, parakeratosis, and acanthosis; the lesion has an endophytic growth pattern with widened and fused rete ridges.

Right: A characteristic feature is the presence of mitosoid cells, characterized by collapsed nuclei that take on the appearance of a mitotic figure.

is not usually seen. The thickened epithelial proliferation extends in an exophytic rather than endophytic manner; the latter causes in the rete pegs in the lesion to be at the same level or depth as the adjacent nonlesional epithelial rete pegs. Koilocytes and ballooning cells are seen in cells of the superficial keratinocytes. In addition, mitosoid cells, cells with collapsed nuclei taking on the appearance of a mitotic figure, are seen (fig. 2-16).

Special Studies. Ultrastructural analysis shows virus-like particles in the nuclei and cytoplasm of cells within the spinous layer.

Differential Diagnosis. The differential diagnosis includes a variety of epithelial proliferations including squamous papilloma, verruca vulgaris, condyloma acuminatum, pseudoepitheliomatous hyperplasia, and proliferative verrucoid leukoplakia. The absence of prominent surface projections, absence of endophytic growth, and presence of mitosoid cells assist in differentiating FEH from these other lesions.

Treatment and Prognosis. The lesions of FEH undergo spontaneous regression, usually within months, but may take up to a year or more. As such, there is no specific treatment required. Transformation to carcinoma does not occur.

Oral Hairy Leukoplakia

Definition. *Oral hairy leukoplakia* (OHL) is an EBV-induced verruciform hyperkeratotic lesion of the lateral tongue in AIDS/HIV-infected patients.

Clinical Features. OHL is a lesion that is highly, but not universally, associated with HIV infection, potentially representing an oral mucosal marker for this virus (104–106). OHL has a tendency to affect HIV-infected men more often than HIV-infected women. It is the most common EBV-related lesion in patients with AIDS.

The lesion does not cause symptoms unless secondarily infected (e.g., by *Candida albicans*) and varies in appearance from a well-demarcated, flat, white plaque to a well-demarcated, raised, white lesion with vertical striations or corrugations (107). The lesions typically localize to the lateral tongue but occasionally involve the ventral or dorsal tongue and infrequently other oral sites such as the buccal mucosa (107).

Pathogenesis. Due to its association with AIDS, OHL was initially thought to be caused by a variety of microorganisms, including HIV, EBV, HPV, and HSV. The cause of OHL is EBV (108–110). OHL also occurs in non-HIV-positive but immunocompromised patients, such as renal transplant patients on immunosuppressive therapy (111,112), and in patients on high-dose corticosteroid treatment (113–116).

Microscopic Findings. The histology of OHL includes the presence of irregular epithelial hyperplasia with filiform or hair-like keratin projections, associated parakeratosis and acanthosis, and koilocytosis of superficial epithelial cells lying beneath the parakeratotic layer. Balloon degeneration of edema may be seen within the deeper epithelial layer (fig. 2-17). Koilocytes (fig. 2-17) and cells with Cowdry inclusions (ground-glass appearance and intranuclear inclusions) may be seen in superficial epithelial cells lying beneath the parakeratotic layer. A nonspecific mild chronic inflammatory cell reaction may be seen within the submucosa. Concomitant fungal (*C. albicans*) microorganisms may be present within the superficial keratin layer. The epithelial proliferation lacks dysplasia. In situ hybridization for EBV provides a definitive diagnosis (fig. 2-17).

Differential Diagnosis. The differential diagnosis of OHL includes other oral leukoplakic lesions, hairy tongue, and verrucous carcinoma. Hairy tongue is a benign condition characterized by hyperkeratosis and enlargement of filiform papillae. In contrast to OHL, hairy tongue is a poorly demarcated lesion with diffuse involvement of the dorsum of the tongue. Verrucous carcinoma includes the presence of tiered keratosis and elongated bulbous rete pegs, features not seen in OHL.

Treatment and Prognosis. OHL is a self-limiting disease and in most cases requires no treatment. For diagnostic and differential diagnostic purposes, an incisional biopsy may be performed. OHL has no malignant potential. Morbidity and mortality are associated with HIV- or AIDS-associated opportunistic infections (117). Appropriate antibiotic or antiviral therapy may be required.

Verruciform Xanthoma

Definition. *Verruciform xanthoma* is a non-neoplastic reactive or inflammatory process representing a morphologic rather distinct clinicopathologic entity. It is characterized by epithelial hyperplasia and associated xanthomatous cells (i.e., lipid-laden histiocytes), primarily occurring in the oral mucosa and associated with a variety of diseases. Verruciform means "warty" and xanthos means yellow.

Clinical Features. Verruciform xanthoma is a rare lesion. In a recent review of the literature, males (55.5 percent) were found to be affected slightly more than females (44.5 percent), with a mean age of 44.9 years (118). Verruciform xanthoma primarily affects the oral cavity, and while it may occur in any intraoral site, the gingiva and alveolar mucosa are the most common locations. Verruciform xanthoma uncommonly occurs in other upper aerodigestive tract mucosal sites, including the larynx (epiglottic and glottic areas) and tonsillar region (119).

Given its name, verruciform xanthoma appears as a warty or papillary, yellow to yellow-white lesion that is well-demarcated. It usually measures less than 2 cm in greatest dimension. Verruciform xanthoma may have a reddish color owing to the presence of surface keratinization. It is typically a slow-growing, painless growth; most lesions are solitary, but may be multifocal. It occurs in association with lichen planus, odontogenic keratocyst, warty dyskeratoma (120), lipid storage disease (119), and in immunocompromised patients (121–123).

Pathogenesis. The exact cause of the lesion is unknown. Although HPV has been found in the lesional tissue, most studies indicate that degenerating keratinocytes probably lead to the accumulation of foamy histiocytes without evidence to support an HPV-associated lesion (124). There is no known association with lipid storage diseases nor do patients with verruciform xanthoma have abnormal lipid profiles.

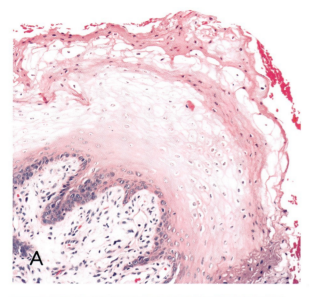
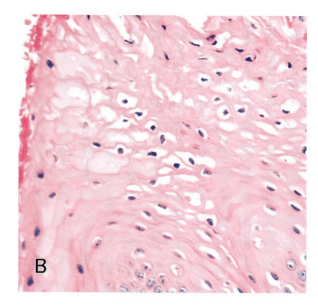
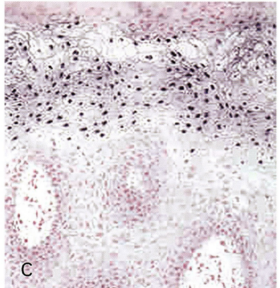

Figure 2-17

ORAL HAIRY LEUKOPLAKIA

A: The oral mucosa shows irregular epithelial hyperplasia with a dense corrugated parakeratotic layer immediately above a band of epithelial cells with pale clear cytoplasm (ballooned cells).
B: Cells with perinuclear halos (koilocytes) are identified.
C: In situ hybridization for Epstein-Barr virus encoded RNA shows positive nuclear staining within the superficial layer and a band of clear cells.

Microscopic Findings. The surface mucosa shows papillary to verrucoid projections with a hyperkeratotic and uniformly acanthotic epithelium (fig. 2-18). Parakeratotic plugs of a bright orange to eosinophilic hue are present between the papillary projections. Accumulations of xanthoma cells or foamy macrophages within the papillary projections of the lamina propria are the characteristic feature of this lesion. The xanthoma cells are limited to the papillae between the elongated rete ridges. The number of macrophages may range from dense to few.

Special Studies. Special stains show that the xanthoma cells contain lipid and have intracytoplasmic diastase-resistant, periodic acid–Schiff (PAS)-positive material. Immunohistochemical staining shows the xanthoma cells to have a monocyte/macrophage phenotype as evidenced by reactivity for CD68 (KP1) and absence of S-100 protein and CD1a (118,124,125).

Differential Diagnosis. The clinical features of verruciform xanthoma may be similar to those of condyloma acuminatum, verruca vulgaris, squamous papilloma, and even a carcinoma

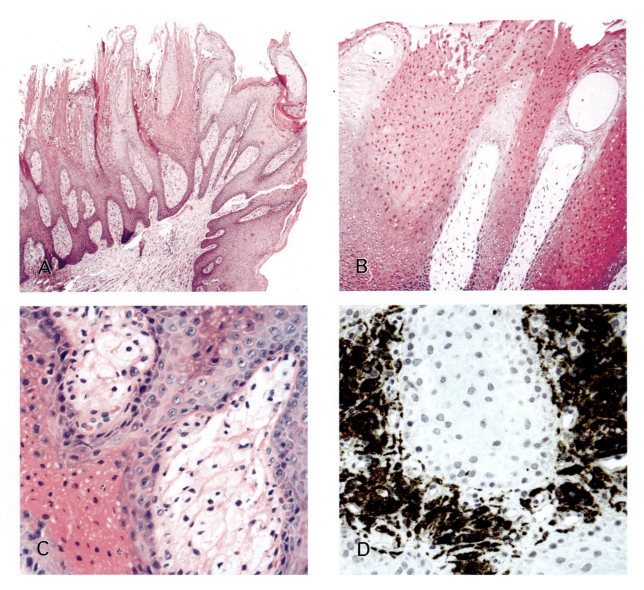

Figure 2-18

VERRUCIFORM XANTHOMA

A: The surface mucosa shows verrucous and papillary projections with a hyperkeratotic and uniformly acanthotic epithelium. Parakeratotic plugs with a bright orange to eosinophilic hue are present between the papillary projections.

B: Accumulation of xanthoma cells (foamy macrophages) within the papillary projections of the lamina propria is a characteristic feature of this lesion.

C: At higher magnification, the xanthoma cells have foamy or clear cytoplasm and are limited to the papillae between the elongated rete ridges.

D: The xanthoma cells are strongly immunoreactive for CD68 (KP1), a histiocytic cell marker.

(verrucous carcinoma, squamous cell carcinoma), but the histologic findings allow for easy differentiation. Other lesions may have associated xanthomatous cells or histiocytes, including fibrous histiocytoma, granular cell tumor, and Langerhans cell histiocytosis. The finding of xanthoma cells within the lamina propria is distinctive for verruciform xanthoma. Aside from the histologic findings, immunohistochemical staining should separate these lesions.

Oral Cavity and Jaw

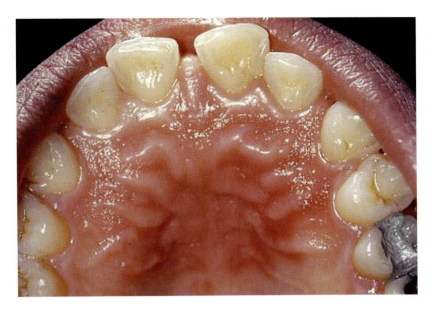

Figure 2-19

INFLAMMATORY PAPILLARY HYPERPLASIA OF THE PALATE
Papillary appearing red lesions.

Treatment and Prognosis. Surgical excision is usually adequate treatment, in cases where verruciform xanthoma is the sole lesion. However, since verruciform xanthoma often occurs in conjunction with other lesions, surgical excision should be complete and microscopic examination thorough. While verruciform xanthoma is not a precancerous lesion, it may be associated with synchronous dysplasia and carcinoma (122,126) or metachronous squamous cell carcinoma (120,127).

Inflammatory Papillary Hyperplasia

Definition. *Inflammatory papillary hyperplasia* (IPH) is a benign, reactive oral epithelial hyperplasia, often associated with an intraoral inflammatory process (e.g., stomatitis).

Clinical Features. IPH is a common oral lesion. The lesions are more common in men than women, and typically occur in the third to fifth decades of life (128). IPH may occur in any intraoral site but is most often found on the palate. IPH is painless, appearing as multiple warty or papillary, red lesions (fig. 2-19).

Pathogenesis. The development of IPH has been linked to patients who have stomatitis as a result of ill-fitting dentures or dental prostheses, especially in those who retain their prosthesis while sleeping and who exhibit poor oral hygiene (129).

Microscopic Findings. IPH appears as a papillary epithelial hyperplasia with hyperkeratosis, parakeratosis, and an absence of epithelial dysplasia (fig. 2-20). Edematous change and a mixed chronic inflammatory cell reaction can be seen in the submucosa. Secondary reactive or degenerative changes of the seromucous glands, including squamous metaplasia (sialometaplasia), fibrosis, atrophy, mucin pool formation, and mixed inflammation may be present in areas overlying the minor salivary glands. Despite these findings, the lobular configuration of the seromucous glands is retained.

Differential Diagnosis. The differential diagnosis includes carcinoma (squamous cell carcinoma, mucoepidermoid carcinoma), however, the overall histologic features of IPH should be recognizable as benign and readily distinguished from a carcinoma.

Treatment and Prognosis. Surgical resection is considered the treatment of choice (128). In those patients with ill-fitting dentures or who exhibit poor oral hygiene, replacement of the prosthesis with a better fitting one and education in proper oral hygiene are indicated. Lesions will not regress simply by the removal of the ill-fitting prosthesis. If present, a fungal infection should be treated with antifungal therapy. IPH is not considered to be a premalignant lesion.

Pseudoepitheliomatous Hyperplasia

Definition. *Pseudoepitheliomatous hyperplasia* (PEH) is an exuberant reactive or reparative overgrowth of squamous epithelium displaying

Figure 2-20
INFLAMMATORY PAPILLARY HYPERPLASIA OF THE PALATE

A–C: Papillary epithelial hyperplasia with associated hyperkeratosis, parakeratosis, and an absence of epithelial dysplasia. Secondary changes that may be present (although not shown here) include sialometaplasia, submucosal fibrosis, and mixed chronic inflammation.

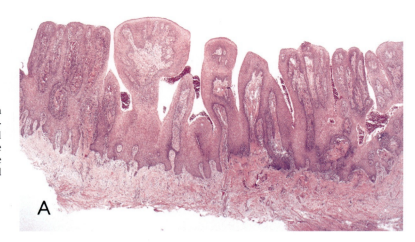
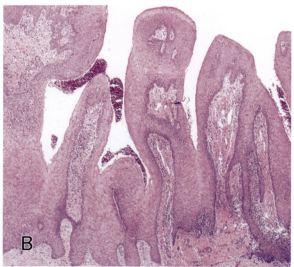
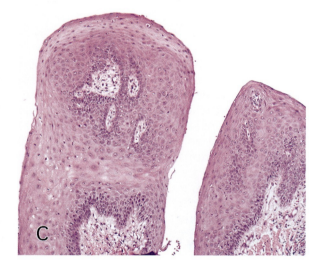

no cytologic evidence of malignancy. It may be mistaken (clinically and histologically) for an invasive squamous carcinoma.

Clinical Features. PEH is not a distinct clinicopathologic entity; rather it represents a morphologic entity (130,131). As such, there is a wide spectrum in demographics and the clinical presentation associated with PEH. PEH may occur as an isolated process, or more often, is the morphologic process associated with or induced by other diseases or lesions. The latter includes trauma, chronic denture irritation, infection (e.g., due to *Candida*, blastomycosis, others) and neoplasms (132,133). Classically, PEH is associated with an underlying granular cell tumor (fig. 2-21).

Microscopic Findings. Histologically, PEH is characterized by a florid epithelial proliferation, with or without associated hyperkeratosis. There is acanthosis with elongation and downward extension of the rete ridges. The rete ridges typically have a rounded or smooth-edged appearance (fig. 2-21). In most examples of PEH, there is limited to absent epithelial dysplasia; however, in some cases and perhaps in PEH associated with a granular cell tumor, the epithelial dysplasia is severe. Further, nests of squamous epithelium may take on a more angulated appearance and simulate an invasive growth pattern (fig. 2-21) (134,135), approaching or even reaching the morphologic level of squamous cell carcinoma (see below). Granular cells are thought to be of neural (Schwann cell) origin and are immunoreactive for S-100 protein, SOX10, and neuron-specific enolase (fig. 2-21).

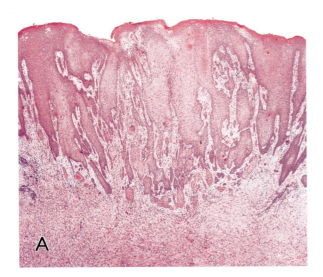
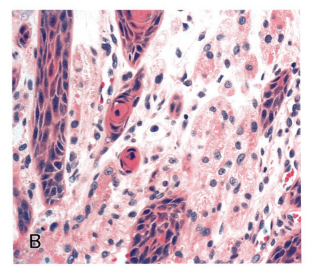
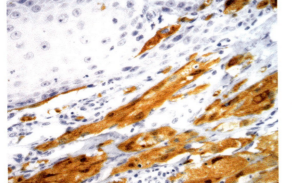
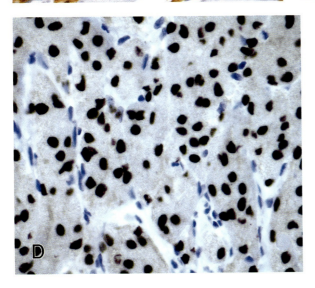
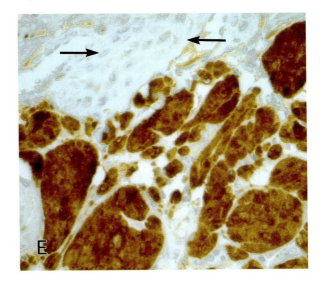

Figure 2-21

PSEUDOEPITHELIOMATOUS HYPERPLASIA (PEH) ASSOCIATED WITH A GRANULAR CELL TUMOR

A: The prominent surface epithelial proliferation includes nests of squamous epithelium with an irregular growth pattern, suggesting infiltration. Lying deep to the PEH is the granular cell tumor, appearing as a diffuse cellular proliferation.

B: At higher magnification, the granular cells have abundant eosinophilic granular cytoplasm; the squamous nests are irregular, with cytologic atypia, raising a possible diagnosis of squamous cell carcinoma (see E).

C,D: The granular cells are diffusely immunoreactive for S-100 protein (nuclear and cytoplasmic) (C) and SOX10 (nuclear) (D).

E: S-100 protein staining is diffusely and strongly reactive in the granular cell tumor but the squamous epithelial nests are negative (between the arrows). In those examples of PEH associated with granular cell tumor in which the squamous cell nests suggest a possible diagnosis of squamous cell carcinoma, the absence of extension of the squamous nests below the granular cell tumor, as seen by light microscopy or S-100 protein staining, assists in the diagnosis.

Differential Diagnosis. In the majority of cases differentiating PEH from a carcinoma is not problematic given the presence of a bland epithelial proliferation with rounded rete ridges and absence of dysplasia (136). However, as noted, sometimes differentiating PEH from squamous cell carcinoma is problematic. In the presence of a granular cell tumor, the associated PEH should not extend below the deepest part of the granular cell tumor. In this case, the squamous proliferation is not considered malignant. However, if the epithelial proliferation does extend below the deepest part of the granular cell tumor, as determined by light microscopy or by S-100 protein staining, or there is definitive evidence (i.e., histologic confirmation) of metastasis (e.g., to cervical lymph node, other sites) of squamous cell carcinoma then, presuming there is no previous history or concurrent presence of another primary mucosal squamous cell carcinoma, a diagnosis of squamous cell carcinoma can be made in association with a granular cell tumor.

PEH may be induced by a fungal infection of the mucosa. If an infectious etiology is suspected, then special stains for microorganisms, in particular for fungi (e.g., Gomori methenamine silver, PAS, mucicarmine) may be required for the diagnosis. The microorganisms should be located within the deeper aspects of the epithelium and not limited to the superficial thickened parakeratin layer and in the superficial spinous layer as seen in fungal colonization.

Although not usually verrucoid, PEH may have associated hyperkeratosis with a verrucoid or papillary appearance, which may need differentiation from proliferative verrucoid leukoplakia (PVL). PVL is considered a premalignant lesion rather than a non-neoplastic reactive process (see below).

Treatment and Prognosis. There is no specific treatment for PEH. If it occurs in association with or induced by another disease, then therapy should be oriented to treating the other process. The latter may include antifungal therapy or surgery for a granular cell tumor.

Proliferative Verrucous Leukoplakia

Definition. *Proliferative verrucous leukoplakia* (PVL) is an aggressive, irreversible form of oral leukoplakia, with a tendency to recur, often with multifocal oral involvement, and to undergo malignant transformation to either verrucous carcinoma or conventional squamous cell carcinoma. It is also known as *verrucous hyperplasia*.

The diagnosis of PVL is determined clinicopathologically and usually is rendered in retrospect. In the early stages, PVL is virtually impossible to diagnose due to the innocuous appearance of the lesion, and the clinical and pathologic features that overlap with those of other types of leukoplakic lesions (137). A recent proposal for a diagnosis of PVL required: involvement of more than two oral cavity subsites, total added size of leukoplakic areas of at least 3 cm, a well-documented period of at least 5 years of disease evolution characterized by spreading and one or more recurrences in a previously treated area (138).

Clinical Features. PVL is an uncommon lesion. It is more common in women than men (4 to 1) and is most common in women over 60 years of age, with mean age in eighth decade of life. PVL typically occurs in the setting of a long history (decades) of oral leukoplakia. The most common site of occurrence is on the buccal mucosa or oral tongue but it may also involve the gingiva, alveolar mucosa, floor of mouth, palate, and lip.

There are no known risk factors associated with PVL including tobacco and alcohol use or abuse (137,139,140). HPV has been reported in PVL but its etiologic significance remains unproven (141,142).

Gross Findings. The lesion is a flat, thickened keratosis with the histologic appearance of a non-dysplastic keratosis. With progression of disease, the lesions become multiple, multifocal, and confluent, with an exophytic or warty (verrucoid) appearance (fig. 2-22); it is in the latter clinical form that squamous cancer (verrucous carcinoma or conventional squamous cell carcinoma) is seen.

Microscopic Findings. PVL is composed of hyperplastic squamous epithelium with regularly spaced, verrucous epithelial projections and associated hyperkeratosis. The lesions are sharply defined, with the hyperplastic epithelium remaining superficial (without submucosal invasion) and not extending deeper than that of the adjacent epithelium (fig. 2-23). Such features contrast to the downward growth into the underlying submucosal compartment by the bulbous

Oral Cavity and Jaw

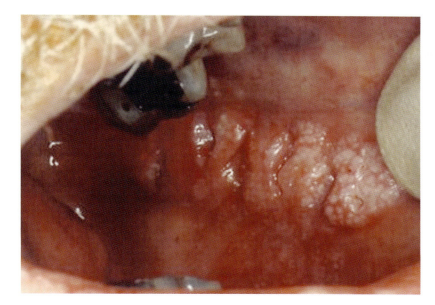

Figure 2-22

PROLIFERATIVE VERRUCOUS HYPERPLASIA

Multiple, confluent, exophytic and warty (verrucoid) lesions are seen on the buccal mucosa.

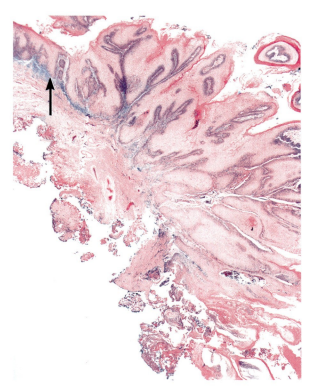 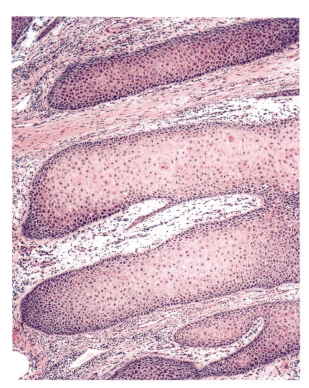

Figure 2-23

PROLIFERATIVE VERRUCOUS HYPERPLASIA

Left: The verrucoid squamous epithelial proliferation has prominent hyperkeratosis ("church-spire" keratosis), markedly elongated rete ridges, and absence of dysplasia. The verrucous epithelial proliferation remains superficial (without submucosal invasion) and does not extend deeper than the adjacent normal epithelium (arrow).

Right: At higher magnification, the epithelial cells lack dysplastic changes. The histologic diagnosis of proliferative verrucous hyperplasia is problematic and typically requires clinicopathologic correlation. It usually is made retrospectively following persistent, recurrent and progressive leukoplakic intraoral lesions.

Table 2-3

DIFFERENTIAL DIAGNOSIS OF PROLIFERATIVE VERRUCOID LEUKOPLAKIA (PVL)

	PVL	COL[a]	VC
Gender	F>M (4:1)	M>F (2:1)	M>F
Age	> 60; mean 8th decade	younger ages	elderly
Most common sites	oral cavity, tongue	anywhere in oral cavity	buccal mucosa, larynx
Risk factor(s)	unknown	tobacco, others	tobacco
Presence of dysplasia	rare	low (5-15%)	no
Progression to malignancy	high[b]	low (1-2%)	yes

[a]COL = conventional oral leukoplakia; VC = verrucous carcinoma.
[b]To verrucous carcinoma or conventional squamous cell carcinoma.

rete ridges in verrucous carcinoma. A lichenoid inflammatory infiltrate is uncommon.

In any given lesion, a combination of verrucous hyperplasia, verrucous carcinoma, and conventional well-differentiated squamous cell carcinoma may be identified. In order to exclude the presence of submucosal invasion, complete excision of the lesion, allowing for histologic examination of the entire lesion, is appropriate. Adequate sampling is imperative, otherwise, there will be diagnostic and differential diagnostic problems on incisional biopsy material.

Differential Diagnosis. The differential diagnosis includes reactive (nonspecific) verrucoid hyperplasia and verrucous hyperkeratosis, oral leukoplakia, and verrucous carcinoma (Table 2-3).

Treatment and Prognosis. Surgical management is the treatment of choice. Surgical resection, however, is generally unsuccessful owing to inherent geographic spread and the progressive nature of PVL. Disease-free survival rates following surgery are low due to recurrence and multifocal involvement. Nonsurgical treatments include radiotherapy, topical agents, cryotherapy, and phototherapy; none are effective in controlling disease.

The therapeutic goal may be one of control rather than cure, maintaining surveillance to detect invasive cancer early and treated by wide excision. Radiotherapy should be reserved for invasive carcinoma with aggressive features. Early recurrence is common, usually accompanied by greater extension and an increase of epithelial changes including dysplasia. Malignant transformation to verrucous carcinoma or conventional squamous cell carcinoma is almost always the outcome (140,143).

Since PVL is associated with verrucous carcinoma in a high percentage of cases, some authors believe that PVL should be considered a premalignant condition or an early biologic form of verrucous carcinoma and treated accordingly. Such a consideration would obviate the confusion, both clinically and pathologically, that surrounds the use of the term verrucous hyperplasia in describing these oral cavity lesions.

The prognosis associated with PVL is considered poor. In one study of 30 patients followed from 1 to 20 years, 43 percent (13 of 30) died of or with their disease (persistent or recurrent), 43 percent (14 of 30) were alive with disease, and 10 percent were alive without disease (144).

MESENCHYMAL LESIONS

Peripheral Ossifying Fibroma

Definition. *Peripheral ossifying fibroma* is a reactive (non-neoplastic) lesion found exclusively as a gingival proliferation of fibrous stroma, with calcified product, presumably arising from the periodontal ligament. The clinical and pathologic features are those of a distinct entity and not just the soft tissue counterpart of ossifying fibroma. Synonyms include *ossifying fibroid epulis*, *peripheral fibroma with calcification*, and *calcifying fibroblastic granuloma*.

Clinical Features. Peripheral ossifying fibroma is a common gingival growth that is more common in women than men; they usually occur in the second decade of life (145–147). The clinical features are not usually sufficient to suggest peripheral ossifying fibroma over other gingival nodules such as peripheral odontogenic fibroma,

fibroma, or pyogenic granuloma, all presenting as firm, nontender gingival swellings.

Peripheral ossifying fibroma is unique to the gingival mucosa, with the majority of cases occurring anterior to the molar region and equally affecting the mandible and maxilla. The lesion presents as a firm, smooth, sessile to pedunculated, dome-shaped nodule of the gingiva (fig. 2-24), measuring up to 1 cm in greatest dimension. It may expand the interdental papilla on the lingual, palatal, or facial aspect. Mucosal ulceration may occur. Peripheral ossifying fibroma occurs only on the gingiva and does not involve the underlying bone.

Periapical radiographs may show slight cupping of the crestal bone, or rarely, the lesional calcifications are of sufficient size and density to be seen (fig. 2-24).

Microscopic Findings. Peripheral ossifying fibroma is an unencapsulated cellular lesion composed of connective tissue and plump-appearing fibroblasts with large, round to oval, vesicular nuclei and mineralized material. The latter includes interlacing trabeculae of bone or osteoid, calcification, or spherules of cementum (fig. 2-25). The lesion is often ulcerated on the surface. This ulceration may be on the portion of the lesion that is adjacent to the tooth, the crevicular epithelium. The portion of the lesion that is exposed to masticatory trauma may also be ulcerated. The ulcerated surface is often associated with superficial bacterial colonization and with acute and chronic inflammatory cells that may permeate deep into the lesion. Mitotic figures are rarely seen, and if present, are typically found in areas of inflammation.

The submucosa includes a variably cellular fibrous stroma composed of spindle-shaped to ovoid cells with indistinct cytoplasmic membranes (fig. 2-26). The fibrous stroma may exhibit increased cellularity in areas of calcified product, but the spindle-shaped cells are bland, with an absence of significant nuclear pleomorphism (fig. 2-26). Droplet calcification may predominate, resulting in a product that closely resembles cementum (fig. 2-27) while the calcified matrix may closely resemble woven bone (fig. 2-27). Dystrophic calcifications, irregular mineralized areas with jagged edges, and basophilic staining may also be seen. The calcified product of the cellular stroma is sparse or plentiful (fig. 2-28).

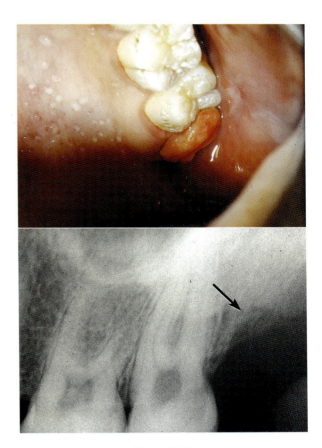

Figure 2-24

PERIPHERAL OSSIFYING FIBROMA

Top: A smooth surfaced, dome-shaped nodule is on distal aspect of the second molar tooth.

Bottom: The imaging findings of the lesion shows slight saucerization or cupping (arrow) of the bone distal to the second molar tooth.

Stroma and product may be a small portion of the biopsy specimen. Multinucleated giant cells are occasionally associated with the bony and calcified portions of the lesion. Small, scattered islands of odontogenic epithelium that resemble remnants of the dental lamina may be seen, but should not comprise a significant portion of the lesion and should not be closely associated with the calcifications. The lesion does not penetrate periosteum or supporting bone.

Differential Diagnosis. The osseous component of peripheral ossifying fibroma may be confused with a fibroosseous process. The cellular stroma and the matrix-producing cells may mimic soft tissue extension of an osteosarcoma, particularly if overlying ulceration incites

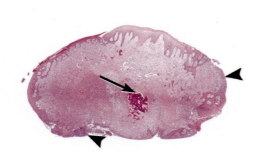
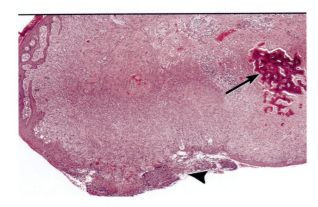

Figure 2-25
PERIPHERAL OSSIFYING FIBROMA
Top, bottom: Polypoid fragment of squamous mucosa with focal surface ulceration (arrowheads) and submucosal benign bony trabeculae (arrows) set in a variably cellular fibrous stroma.

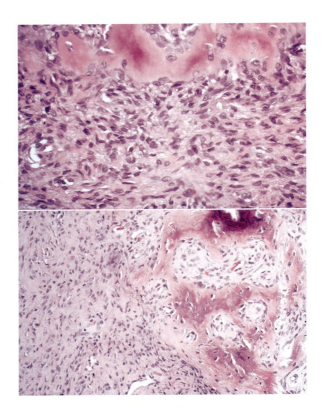

Figure 2-26
PERIPHERAL OSSIFYING FIBROMA
The stroma is composed of small, bland spindle cells with indistinct cell membranes lacking significant nuclear pleomorphism. The calcified product is present as droplets (top) or trabeculae (bottom).

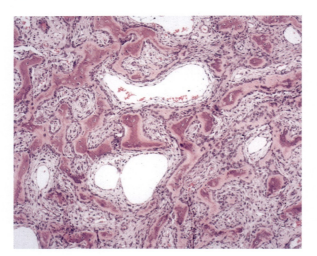
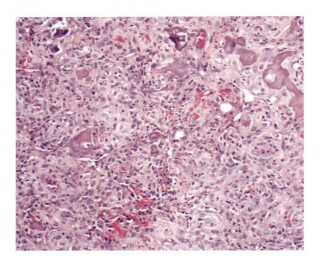

Figure 2-27
PERIPHERAL OSSIFYING FIBROMA
The calcified product may be rimmed by osteoblasts and form trabeculations (left) or appear as droplet type formations (right).

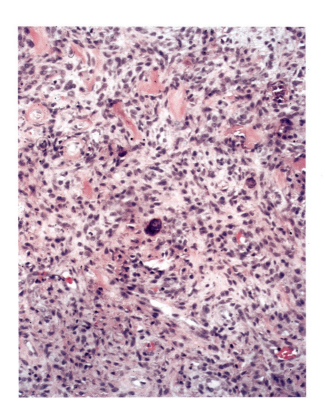 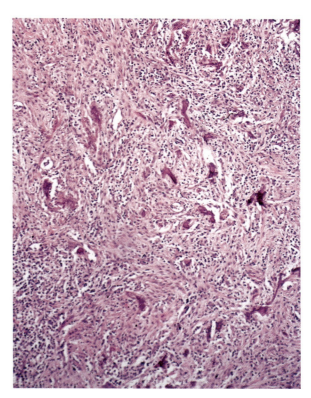

Figure 2-28

PERIPHERAL OSSIFYING FIBROMA

Calcified product is interspersed within the stroma, but may be sparse (left) or abundant (right). The calcified product varies from osteoid-like material to droplet cementum-like product to bone-like.

Table 2-4

DIFFERENTIAL DIAGNOSIS OF COMMON GINGIVAL NODULES

	Fibroma	Peripheral Giant Cell Fibroma	Peripheral Giant Cell Granuloma	Peripheral Ossifying Fibroma	Peripheral Odontogenic Fibroma	Pyogenic Granuloma
Architecture	Nodular	Nodular	Nodular	Nodular	Nodular	Nodular
Vascularity	–[a]	–	++	–	–	++
Calcification	–	–	–	++	+/–	–
Giant cells	–	++	++	–	–	–
Attenuated epithelial surface	+	–	–	–	–	–
Elongated rete ridges	–	+	–	–	–	–

[a]– = not present or inconspicuous; ++ = present in notable proportion; +/– = occasional finding.

occasional mitotic figures. The calcified product in a fibrous stroma may focally resemble fibrous dysplasia, but clinical and radiographic confirmation that the lesion is supraperiosteal proves useful in making this distinction.

Occasional lesions contain varying amounts of odontogenic epithelial rests, leading to consideration of peripheral odontogenic fibroma (Table 2-4). If the lesion is ulcerated, the overlying granulation tissue may mimic pyogenic granuloma.

Rarely, giant cells are associated with the osseous material in peripheral ossifying fibroma, and could be mistaken for a giant cell granuloma. However, the vascular stroma of peripheral giant cell granuloma is lacking.

Treatment and Prognosis. Conservative but complete surgical excision is the treatment of choice and may necessitate excision of the periodontal ligament and periosteum (145, 148). Excision should be followed by clinical examination for local irritation, such as calculus formation, and removal as clinically indicated. Tooth extraction is not usually required. Up to 20 percent of cases recur (145).

Peripheral Odontogenic Fibroma

Definition. *Peripheral odontogenic fibroma* is a rare extraosseous nodule composed of rests and strands of benign odontogenic epithelium in an inactive fibrous stroma. It is found exclusively on the gingiva. The World Health Organization classifies the peripheral odontogenic fibroma as an extraosseous lesion representing the soft tissue counterpart of the central (intraosseous) odontogenic fibroma (149–151). Although related in histologic appearance to the central or intraosseous odontogenic fibroma, the two lesions are distinct. This lesion is also termed *odontogenic epithelial hamartoma* and *peripheral fibroameloblastic fibroma*.

Clinical Features. The age range for patients with peripheral odontogenic fibroma is broad, with few cases in children and the elderly and a peak occurrence in the third decade (149). There is no gender predilection. The clinical features are not usually sufficient to suggest a diagnosis of peripheral odontogenic fibroma as opposed to other gingival nodules such as peripheral ossifying fibroma, fibroma, or pyogenic granuloma; all these lesions present as firm, nontender gingival swellings. The posterior mandible is the most common location for this lesion (151). Nodules range from 1 to 3 cm in greatest diameter. The teeth may be mildly displaced, and calcifications may be seen on radiographs (152).

Microscopic Findings. Peripheral odontogenic fibroma is a nodular growth of the attached gingiva with a fibrous stroma and nests or strands of benign odontogenic epithelium (fig. 2-29). The epithelial cells are low cuboidal to polygonal, with prominent cell membranes, eosinophilic cytoplasm, and nuclei with homogenous nucleoplasm and inconspicuous nucleoli. The epithelial component may be prominent or scarce, and displays reverse polarization but lacks a stellate reticulum (fig. 2-29). There is some overlap with peripheral ossifying fibroma, as some calcified product may be present. The calcified matrix resembles dentin and is directly associated with the odontogenic epithelium. The connective tissue background varies from dense to myxoid. The stroma usually demonstrates increased cellularity in areas of epithelium or calcification, and may show focal hyalinization adjacent to the odontogenic epithelial rests. The fibroblasts are often small, ovoid cells that may be closely packed.

The lesion is not encapsulated, but is usually circumscribed below the lamina propria. The lesion may be ulcerated on the crevicular or oral surface and a concomitant inflammatory cell infiltrate may be seen throughout. Mitoses are rare, and if seen, are confined to areas of inflammation or ulceration.

Differential Diagnosis. There are other peripheral lesions composed of odontogenic epithelium in a fibrous stroma. The distinction between peripheral calcifying epithelial odontogenic tumor, peripheral ameloblastoma, and peripheral ossifying fibroma depends on the quality and quantity of each histologic component. Although there may be some histologic overlap between peripheral ossifying fibroma and peripheral odontogenic fibroma, these two lesions are histologically distinct (Table 2-4). The calcifications in peripheral ossifying fibroma range from small foci of osteoid to vital woven boney trabeculae and are not associated with islands of odontogenic epithelium. In contrast, the calcified material in peripheral odontogenic fibroma, if present at all, more closely resembles dentin or cementum and is associated with the odontogenic epithelium, but is a minor component of the lesion.

Peripheral ameloblastoma is characterized by odontogenic epithelium, with peripheral reverse polarization of the nuclei away from the basement membrane and areas resembling stellate reticulum, in a nonactive fibrous stroma (fig. 2-30). The stroma in peripheral odontogenic fibroma is more often cellular, with small ovoid spindle cells and varying amounts of ground substance.

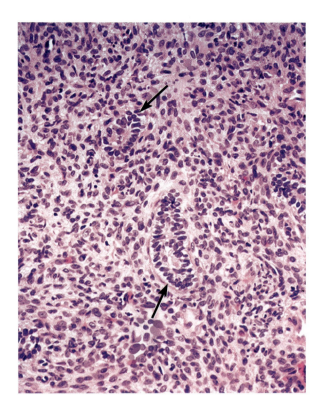 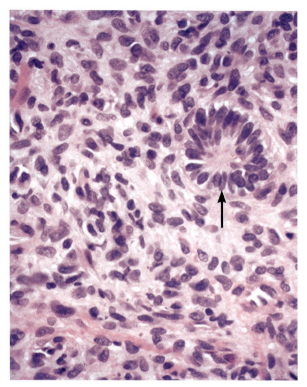

Figure 2-29

PERIPHERAL ODONTOGENIC FIBROMA

Left, right: The densely cellular stroma with small islands of odontogenic epithelium (arrows) resembles ameloblastoma, including the presence of reverse polarization of the nuclei away from the basement membrane. The stellate reticulum that is typically seen in ameloblastoma is absent, however. The stroma includes cells with ovoid to elongated nuclei that, despite the increased cellularity, are bland, without significant nuclear pleomorphism or increased mitotic activity.

Peripheral calcifying epithelial odontogenic tumor is also characterized by the combination of odontogenic epithelium in a fibrous stroma. The polygonal-shaped epithelial cells often exhibit nuclear pleomorphism and the stroma is typically hyalinized and contains small concentric calcifications. The amyloid areas of stroma seen in calcifying epithelial odontogenic tumor often stain with Congo red and demonstrate apple green birefringence when viewed under polarized light.

Treatment and Prognosis. Simple excision is adequate therapy. Recurrence is variably reported in the literature, which may be due to the limited follow-up of the reported cases, but has been reported to be as high as 40 percent (152). Residual lesion is probably responsible for some persistent cases and complete, assured excision is recommended.

Irritation Fibroma

Definition. *Fibroma* is considered the most common soft tissue lesion of the oral cavity to be diagnosed by biopsy, and is considered to be reactive in origin rather than neoplastic (153). Synonyms include *traumatic fibroma*, *focal fibrous hyperplasia*, *fibrous nodule*, *fibrous epulis*, and *fibroepithelial polyp*.

Clinical Features. There is a female predilection and most fibromas are found in adults between 20 and 59 years of age. They are less common in children (153,154).

The lesions are firm, nontender gingival swellings, an appearance similar to other gingival nodules such as peripheral ossifying fibroma, peripheral odontogenic fibroma, or pyogenic granuloma. Fibromas are slow-growing lesions, appearing as well-demarcated nodules with either a sessile or pedunculated base and a

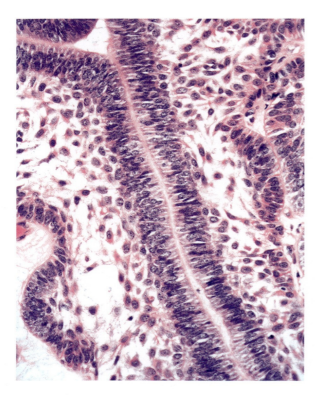 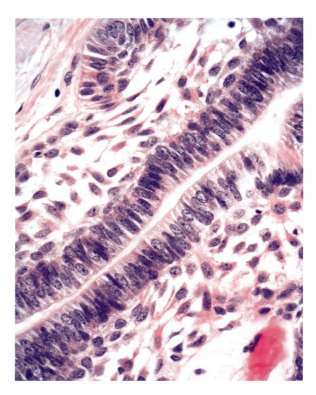

Figure 2-30

PERIPHERAL AMELOBLASTOMA

Features include odontogenic epithelium with reverse polarization of the nuclei away from the basement membrane and areas resembling stellate reticulum. The presence of areas of stellate reticulum contrasts with the odontogenic nests in the peripheral odontogenic fibroma.

smooth domed-shaped elevation (fig. 2-31). The most common location for fibroma is the buccal mucosa, followed by the gingiva, lips, and tongue (151).

The duration of the lesion varies considerably, but may range up to 17 months. A case of bilateral lesions of the hard palate has been reported (151). Periapical radiographs show no evidence of osseous pathology.

The major cause of irritation fibroma is mechanical irriitation secondary to trauma/injury from dentures, lip or cheek biting, or sharp edges of teeth or fillings. Some fibromas, however, have occurred in the absence of a history of trauma or injury, raising the possibility that these lesions are true neoplasms.

Epulis fissuratum is a unique variant of denture-related fibroma typically occurring in the mucosal vestibule and sulcus adjacent to the alveolar ridge, areas where the edge of an ill-fitting denture may traumatize adjacent tissue (155).

The mass represents a redundant fold of tissue running parallel to the edge of the denture. The *retrocuspid papule* is another fibrous oral mass occurring as an asymptomatic, firm papule on the lingual aspect of the mandibular cuspid, either on the gingiva or on the adjacent oral mucosa (156).

Gross Findings. The lesion is a firm nodule of fibrous tissue with a smooth mucosal surface. It is usually received in one piece. The diameter of the lesion ranges from less than 0.5 to 2.0 cm, but is usually from 0.5 to 1.0 cm (156). Upon sectioning, a homogeneous, solid interior is seen. Hemorrhage, cystic space, calcification, or mucus are not appreciable. The biopsy specimen is usually excisional, with a small rim of normal tissue.

Microscopic Findings. Fibroma is a bland, nodular proliferation of fibrous connective tissue surfaced by attenuated stratified squamous epithelium. The perimeter of the lesion is not encapsulated, and blends imperceptibly into

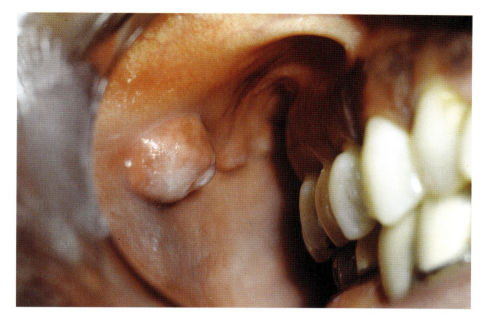

Figure 2-31

IRRITATION FIBROMA

This is a smooth, sessile nodule of the buccal mucosa approximately 0.75 cm in diameter.

Figure 2-32

IRRITATION FIBROMA

The polypoid lesion has intact surface squamous epithelium and submucosal fibrosis that blends imperceptibly into the adjacent connective tissue.

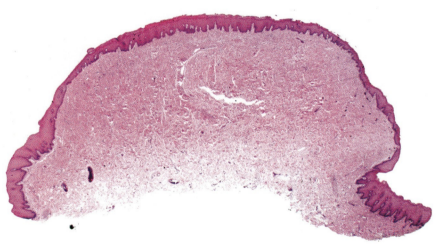

the surrounding connective tissue (fig. 2-32). The fibrous tissue ranges from dense and coarse (fibroma durum) (fig. 2-33) to delicate and fibrillar (fibroma molle) (fig. 2-33), and the proportion of ground substance varies from sparse to abundant. Collagen may be in interlacing, haphazard, or parallel bundles. The nuclei of the fibroblasts are inconspicuous, cigar-shaped, and evenly distributed throughout the lesion. The cytoplasmic borders are not prominent and chromatin is evenly distributed. Mitoses are not seen. There may be mild inflammation present, accompanied by edema, and the surface of the lesion may be ulcerated but is usually normal or attenuated mucosa. Vascularity is limited and the lesion may be avascular.

Epulis fissuratum is histologically similar to an irritation fibroma except that there is often a denser chronic inflammatory cell reaction and a greater tendency for the surface epithelium to be ulcerated. The retrocuspid papule is histologically similar to the giant cell fibroma (see below) except that in occasional cases rests of odontogenic epithelium are identified (156).

Special Studies. Histochemical and immunohistochemical stains have been used in an attempt to better define the characteristics of the collagen and fibrous components of the lesion.

Non-Neoplastic Diseases of the Head and Neck

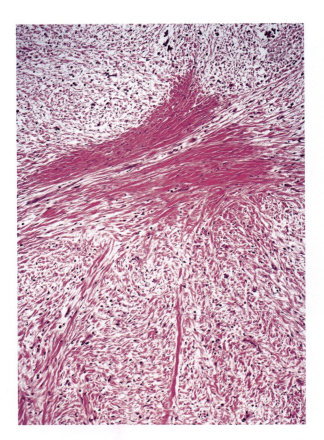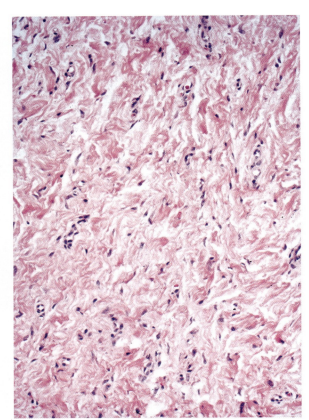

Figure 2-33

IRRITATION FIBROMA

The collagen ranges from coarse bundles (fibroma durum) (left) to delicate fibrils (fibroma molle) (right).

The connective tissue component is a mixture of glycoproteins and fibers, but the pattern of staining does not differentiate between lesions.

Differential Diagnosis. The diagnosis is not often challenging for this lesion. If the surface is ulcerated or the gingival crevice is inflamed, granulation tissue may cause consideration of pyogenic granuloma (lobular capillary hemangioma). Superficial candidiasis may confound the diagnosis (fig. 2-34). The presence of stellate giant cells, multinucleated giant cells, bone or osteoid, or odontogenic epithelium argues against classification as fibroma. The presence of dense fibrous/collagenized and avascular stroma may suggests keloid; the latter rarely, if ever, occurs in the mouth.

Treatment and Prognosis. Surgical excision of the lesion, in conjunction with removal of any apparent source of chronic irritation, is adequate treatment. Recurrence of fibroma is uncommon.

Giant Cell Fibroma

Definition. *Giant cell fibroma* is a benign submucosal fibrous tumor of the oral cavity characterized by large mononuclear and multinucleated giant cells.

Clinical Features. Giant cell fibroma predilects to young people, with the peak occurrence in the second decade, although a broad age range has been reported (151,157–159). There is no significant gender predilection. The most common location is the gingiva, followed by the tongue, palate, buccal mucosa, and lips (158). Periapical radiographs show no evidence of an osseous pathology. Unlike the irritation fibroma, giant cell fibroma does not appear to be associated with chronic irritation (151).

Gross Findings. Giant cell fibroma is a nodular mass usually measuring less than 1.0 cm in greatest dimension, and often less than 0.5 cm.

Oral Cavity and Jaw

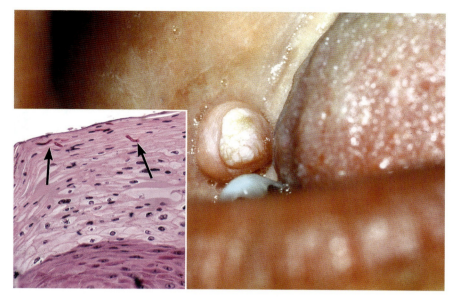

Figure 2-34

FIBROUS NODULE

Thick, white mucosa lies over the nodule. Inset: PAS stain highlights the presence of fungal forms in the superficial aspects of the surface epithelium (arrows).

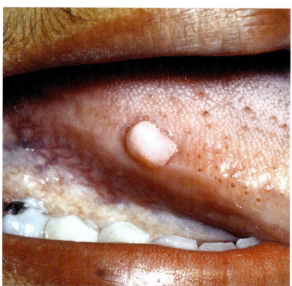

Figure 2-35

GIANT CELL FIBROMA OF TONGUE

The fibroma is a papillary, sessile nodule on the lateral border of the tongue measuring approximately 0.5 cm in diameter.

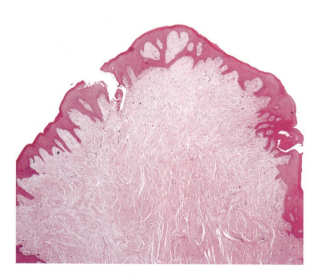

Figure 2-36

GIANT CELL FIBROMA OF TONGUE

The nodular lesion is characterized by a submucosal fibrous proliferation; the surface squamous epithelium includes elongated ("spiky") rete ridges.

The nodule may have a pedunculated or sessile base. The mucosal surface is often papillary and pink, in contrast to the other gingival nodules that are usually covered by smooth surface mucosa (fig. 2-35).

Microscopic Findings. Giant cell fibroma is a bosselated nodule composed of dense submucosal fibroconnective tissue. The stratified squamous surface epithelium may appear papillary and often has prominent elongated and downwardly extending ("spiky") rete ridges (figs. 2-36, 2-37). The fibroblasts/giant cells are identified within the submucosa/connective tissue, as well as between elongated rete ridges.

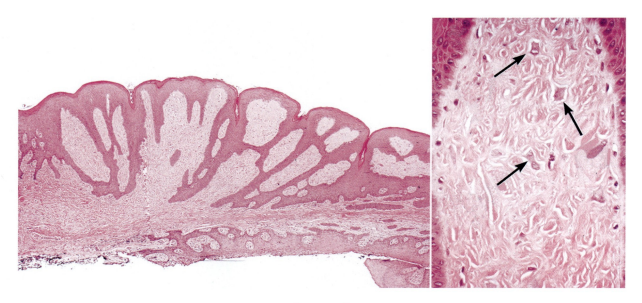

Figure 2-37

GIANT CELL FIBROMA OF GINGIVA

Left: The polypoid or nodular lesion has dense submucosal fibrous connective tissue. The overlying surface squamous epithelium has a bosselated appearance, with elongated and downwardly extending rete ridges.

Right: At higher magnification, stellate-shaped fibroblasts, some with more than one nucleus (arrows), are present within the submucosal dense fibrous connective tissue.

They are stellate in shape and composed of one or multiple round to oval nuclei, vesicular chromatin, prominent nucleoli, and finely granular cytoplasm; there is a low nuclear to cytoplasmic ratio (fig. 2-37). The fibroblasts may be few (fig. 2-37) or numerous (fig. 2-38). Separation artifact is sometimes noted around the stellate fibroblasts (fig. 2-39). Foci of melanin granules may be seen but mitoses are absent. Variable vascularity and chronic inflammation, including mast cells, are present. The fibroblasts may show smooth muscle actin immunoreactivity, supporting a myofibroblastic differentiation.

Differential Diagnosis. The identification of stellate mononuclear and multinuclear fibroblasts in the lamina propria distinguish giant cell fibroma from conventional fibroma. The giant cells of giant cell fibroma are not the "osteoclastic" type giant cells seen in peripheral giant cell fibroma, and the stroma is not as vascular in giant cell fibroma as it is in giant cell granuloma.

Treatment and Prognosis. Simple surgical excision is the treatment of choice. Recurrence is uncommon.

GIANT CELL LESIONS

Giant cell lesions are localized intraosseous and extraosseous proliferations characterized by the presence of a variable admixture of osteoclast-like giant cells, hemorrhage, and fibrous tissue. Since there is no histologic evidence to support a repair phenomenon, the designation "reparative" has been discarded. *Giant cell granuloma* shares many features with aneurysmal bone cyst and in many regards these lesions may be indistinguishable. Those lesions predominantly confined to intraosseous sites (e.g., jaws) are referred to as *central giant cell granulomas*; controversy exists as to whether these lesions represent true neoplasms or reactive processes. Those lesions primarily involving soft tissues (e.g., sinonasal or oral mucosa) are termed *peripheral giant cell granulomas*, which is felt to represent a non-neoplastic reactive process likely occurring secondary to trauma or local irritation (160).

Central and Peripheral Giant Cell Granulomas

Clinical Features. *Central giant cell granulomas* are more common in women than in men, and occur in patients under 30 years of age

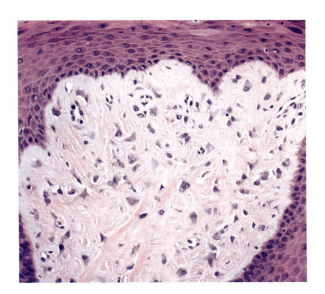 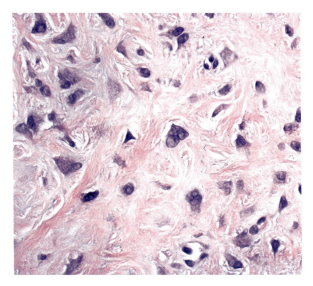

Figure 2-38

GIANT CELL FIBROMA OF GINGIVA

Left: There are numerous and readily identifiable submucosal giant cells.
Right: The giant cells are stellate in shape and composed of one or multiple round to oval nuclei, vesicular chromatin, prominent nucleoli, and finely granular cytoplasm. The nuclear to cytoplasmic ratio is low.

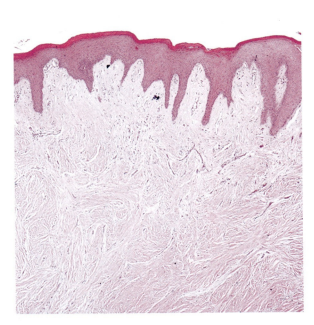 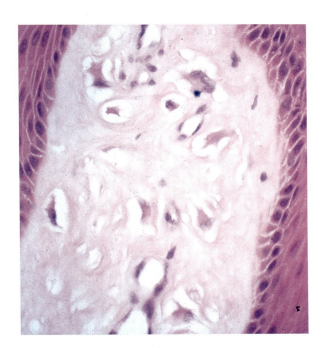

Figure 2-39

GIANT CELL FIBROMA OF GINGIVA

Left: The sessile nodule is characterized by dense submucosal fibrosis and bosselated surface epithelium, with elongated and downwardly extending ("spiky") rete ridges.
Right: Stellate fibroblasts, some multinucleated, are located between the rete ridges. The clear zone around the nuclei represents artifactual separation.

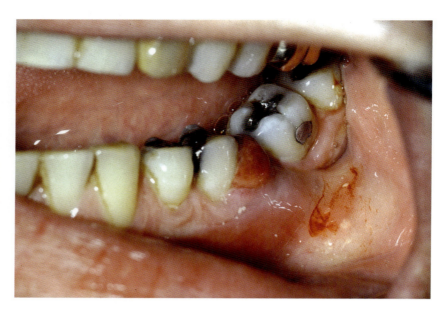

Figure 2-40

PERIPHERAL GIANT CELL GRANULOMA

The gingival nodule fills the interdental space. Radiograph imaging (not shown) was characterized by the presence of saucerization of the bone but without a central (intraosseous) component.

(161). The gnathic bones are the most common sites of occurrence; the mandible is more often involved than the maxilla (161). Rare occurrences in other areas include paranasal sinuses and temporal bone. The clinical presentation is usually that of a painless mass or swelling at the affected site. The radiographic appearance includes a demarcated, multiloculated, or "soap bubble"-appearing intraosseous lesion with expansion and thinning of the cortical plates; the teeth may be displaced (162).

Peripheral giant cell granuloma predilects to women. It may occur over a wide age range, from 3 to 85 years, but tends to occur in patients under 30 years of age (160). The lesion most often occurs in the oral mucosa (gingiva, alveolar mucosa) overlying the mandible and maxilla (tooth-bearing areas); sinonasal tract or nasopharyngeal involvement is uncommon. Peripheral giant cell granuloma is characteristically a painless firm nodule, pedunculated or sessile, mucosal-based, red to blue, well circumscribed, and superficial to the periosteum (fig. 2-40). The surface or the crevicular mucosa may be ulcerated. For both central and peripheral lesions, laboratory values, including serum calcium and serum phosphorus, are within normal limits.

The radiographic appearance of peripheral giant cell granuloma includes a superficial (not intraosseous) location with saucer-like erosion of subjacent bone, and expansion and thinning of the cortical plates. Radiographs should always be reviewed to determine that there is no intrabony involvement, but a slight cupping of the crestal bone may be observed. Multiple lesions in the mandible, particularly if symmetric and bilateral, may suggest a diagnosis of cherubism.

Microscopic Findings. Central and peripheral giant cell granulomas are histologically identical. Peripheral giant cell granulomas are submucosal lesions lying under intact, uninvolved surface epithelium (fig. 2-41). The surface mucosa may be ulcerated or hyperplastic. The surface epithelium is separated from subjacent giant cell granuloma by a zone of uninvolved fibroconnective tissue.

The histologic findings include a submucosal unencapsulated cellular stroma that includes variable numbers of multinucleated giant cells, oval to spindle-shaped fibroblasts, fibrous stroma, and increased vascularity (fig. 2-41). The giant cells tend to aggregate in and around foci of hemorrhage and may be observed within the lumen of vessels (fig. 2-42); the latter may show a prominent endothelial cell proliferation. Less often, giant cells are diffusely distributed in the fibroblastic stroma. Copious foci of hemorrhage, including fresh hemorrhage and hemosiderin deposition, as well as hemosiderin-laden macrophages are characteristically identified (fig. 2-42). Mitotic figures may be seen in association with the fibroblasts but not the giant cells.

The number of nuclei in the multinucleated giant cells ranges from few to many (fig. 2-42).

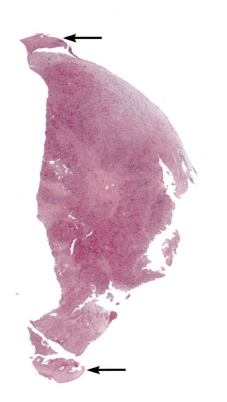 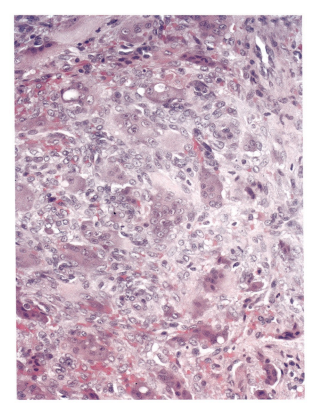

Figure 2-41

PERIPHERAL (MUCOSAL) GIANT CELL GRANULOMA

Left: The gingival mucosal lesion shows dense cellularity; residual squamous epithelium is present (arrows) but most of the surface is ulcerated.

Right: The submucosal proliferation includes numerous multinucleated giant cells.

The nuclei are round to oval, with vesicular chromatin and vary in size from small to large. Small to prominent eosinophilic nucleoli are present. The cytoplasm is granular and eosinophilic to basophilic.

The stroma is cellular with ovoid to spindle-shaped nuclei and indistinct cell membranes. Fibrous tissue is usually present in varying degree (fig. 2-42). The stroma is usually quite vascular and extravasated red blood cells and hemosiderin deposits, either in tissue or within histiocytes, are common (fig. 2-42). Emperipolesis may be identified. An associated chronic inflammatory cell infiltrate, which may include mast cells (feature not typically seen in central lesions), can be identified. Hemosiderin-laden macrophages are typically seen along periphery of the lesion. Calcified product has been reported in peripheral giant cell granuloma (163), but if the osteoid, bone, or cementum is a significant constituent of the lesion, consideration should be given to classification as peripheral ossifying fibroma.

As previously noted, the histology of central giant cell granuloma is identical to that of peripheral giant cell granuloma, but in contrast, the lesion is located within bone (fig. 2-43).

Differential Diagnosis. The differential diagnosis of peripheral giant cell granuloma hinges on clinical and radiographic correlation, since the lesion must be confirmed to be superficial to the periosteum or it could represent soft tissue extension of a central giant cell granuloma. Occasional lesions have minor amounts of osteoid production or odontogenic epithelial rests, but should not be mistaken for peripheral ossifying fibroma or peripheral odontogenic fibroma (Table 2-4).

For central and peripheral lesions, the differential diagnosis includes giant cell tumor,

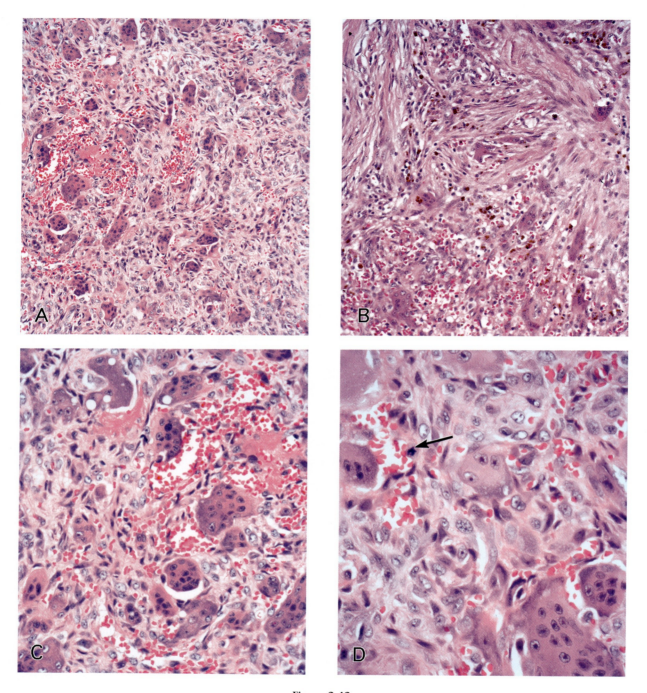

Figure 2-42

PERIPHERAL (MUCOSAL) GIANT CELL GRANULOMA

A: A submucosal proliferation is composed of numerous multinucleated giant cells associated with spindle-shaped fibroblasts; the giant cells tend to aggregate in and around foci of hemorrhage.

B: Multinucleated giant cells and spindle-shaped fibroblasts are associated with fresh hemorrhage and hemosiderin deposition.

C: The number of the nuclei in the giant cells varies from cells with few nuclei to others with many nuclei. The nuclei are round to oval with vesicular chromatin; prominent nucleoli and abundant cytoplasm are present.

D: Mitotic figures (arrow) are seen in the fibroblasts but not the giant cells.

brown tumor of hyperparathyroidism, and aneurysmal bone cyst. Giant cell tumor of bone (osteoclastoma) is a benign but potentially aggressive osteolytic neoplasm of bone composed of stromal mononuclear cells and osteoclast-like giant cells. Histologically, giant cell tumors are characterized by the presence of abundant multinucleated giant cells and stromal mononuclear cells. In contrast to giant cell granulomas, the multinucleated giant cells in a giant cell tumor are diffusely and evenly distributed, are large, and have numerous nuclei (10 to 100) (fig. 2-44). The nuclei are round to oval and tend to cluster in the center of the giant cells. The giant cells may be associated with, or cause, bony destruction. The mononuclear cell stromal component is composed of plump, ovoid or spindle-shaped nuclei, which are similar in appearance to those seen in the giant cells. Mitoses are seen in the stromal mononuclear cells (fig. 2-44) but atypical mitoses are not present. The presence of atypical mitoses is an indicator of malignancy. Additional findings include the presence of foam cells, osteoid, and rarely, chondroid. The presence of chondroid material should engender consideration of another lesion. Cystic degeneration may occasionally occur. The multinucleated giant cells express strong CD68 (KP1) staining (monocytic/histiocytic lineage) and vimentin staining; smooth muscle actin is negative. The mononuclear stromal cells exhibit an osteoblast phenotype, expressing alkaline phosphatase and the receptor activator for nuclear factor kappa B ligand (RANKL), a factor that is essential for osteoclast formation (164,165). They also express osteoprotegrin, an inhibitor of osteoclastogenesis, and TRAIL, a receptor that binds osteoprotegerin (166,167).

Given the histologic similarity of peripheral giant cell granuloma to brown tumor of hyperparathyroidism, the diagnosis includes laboratory evaluation of parathyroid gland function. Abnormalities in parathyroid gland function are not found in central and peripheral giant cell lesions.

Aneurysmal bone cyst (ABC) is a benign non-neoplastic osseous lesion characterized by the presence of numerous blood-filled cavities lacking an endothelial lining. ABC may occur as a de novo process, unrelated to and unassociated with an underlying pre-existing bone lesion, or occurs in association with an underlying

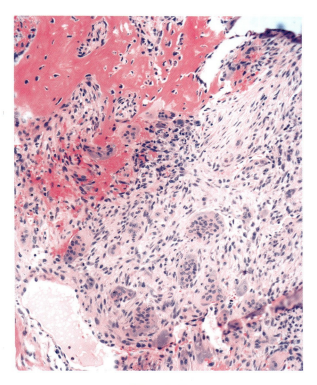

Figure 2-43

CENTRAL (INTRAOSSEOUS) GIANT CELL GRANULOMA

These tumors are histologically similar/identical to peripheral (mucosal) lesions except that central lesions are localized within bone, as seen here. In order to exclude osseous involvement, clinical and radiologic correlation is required.

pre-existing bone lesion. Lesions that have been associated with ABC include giant cell tumor (most common), unicameral bone cyst, osteosarcoma, chondroblastoma, nonossifying fibroma, osteoblastoma, fibrous dysplasia, and giant cell granuloma. The most common sites of occurrence for ABCs are the long bones, where they involve the metaphysis. Approximately 2 percent of ABCs occur in the head and neck (168). The most common site in the head and neck is the jaw, with the mandible (body > ramus > angle > symphysis > condylar process) more common than the maxilla. ABC tends to occur in the first two decades of life. It presents as a slowly or rapidly enlarging mass with associated swelling and pain; additional symptoms include, depending on the site of occurrence, headache, visual disturbances (diplopia, decreased vision), proptosis, loosening of teeth, nasal obstruction, paresthesia, limitation of motion, fracture, and

Non-Neoplastic Diseases of the Head and Neck

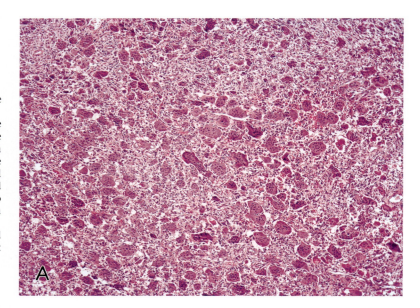

Figure 2-44

GIANT CELL TUMOR (OSTEOCLASTOMA)

A: The multinucleated giant cells are diffusely and evenly distributed.

B: The multinucleated giant cells are large and have numerous nuclei that are round to oval; nucleoli tend to cluster in the center of the giant cells. Around the giant cells is the mononuclear cell stromal component composed of plump, ovoid cells with nuclei similar in appearance to those seen in the giant cells. There is an absence of cytologic atypia.

C: Mitotic figures (arrow) are seen and in any given case may be numerous but atypical mitotic figures are not present.

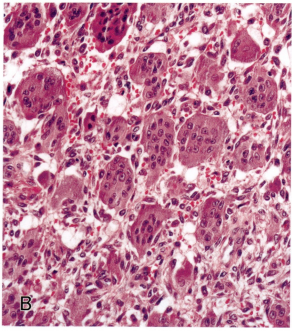
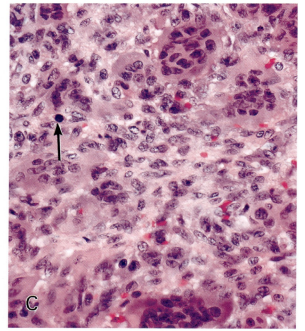

facial or abducens nerve paralysis. Occurrence in the sinonasal tract or nasopharynx may result in a soft tissue mass. The radiologic findings of ABC include an expansile, uni- or multilocular radiolucency surrounded peripherally by a thin shell of periosteal bone.

Histologically, ABCs are blood or blood-tinged serous fluid-filled cysts. The cysts lack an endothelial lining and may be lined by fibroblasts, histiocytes, and multinucleated giant cells (fig. 2-45). The intercystic stroma is fibrous, well vascularized, with mixed chronic inflammatory cells, extravasated erythrocytes, and hemosiderin. Almost all ABCs have areas in which the lesion is more or less solid and characterized by a loose arrangement of spindle cells; mitotic activity is increased (on average 1 to 3 mitoses per 10 high-power fields) but atypical mitoses are not identified. Osteoid (lace-like), reactive bony trabeculae, and osteoclastic giant

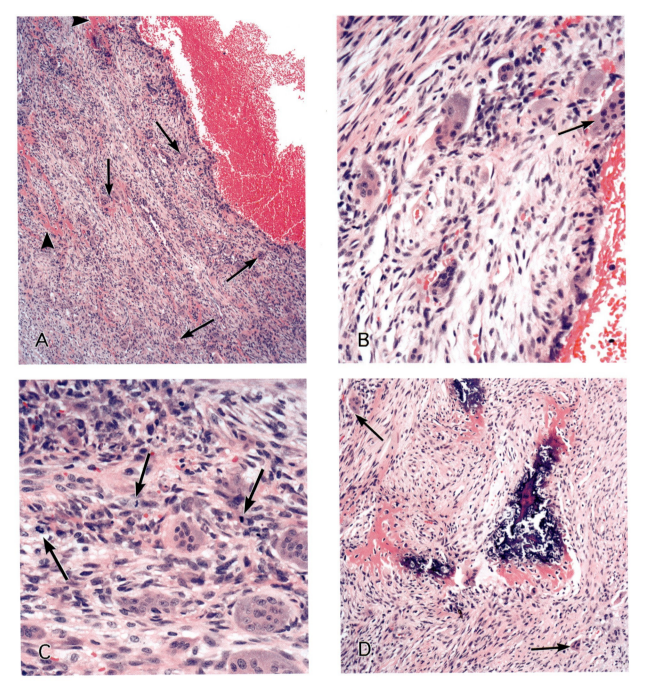

Figure 2-45

ANEURYSMAL BONE CYST

A: The blood-filled cyst (upper right) has more solid areas characterized by spindle cell proliferation, scattered multinucleated giant cells (arrows), and lace-like osteoid (arrowheads).

B: Higher magnification shows the blood-filled cyst (bottom right) lined by fibroblasts as well as giant cells (arrow); the solid area is composed of spindle cells and scattered multinucleated giant cells.

C: Increased mitotic activity is present (arrows) but atypical mitoses are not identified.

D: Mineralized/calcified matrix (so-called blue bone) is a characteristic finding and is seen in association with osteoid, (lace-like) reactive bony trabeculae set in a fibroblastic stroma with scattered multinucleated giant cells (arrows).

cells are identified. Mineralized/calcified matrix (so-called "blue bone") is characteristically present in ABCs (fig. 2-45). A variant of ABC is characterized by a firm and fleshy lesion, completely solid microscopically and lacking cystic cavities; this is referred to as solid ABC. The solid areas are composed of a spindle cell proliferation with giant cells and osteoid production, similar in appearance to the solid areas of a "conventional" ABC. There are histologic similarities to giant cell granulomas but a differentiating feature is the presence of cysts, a feature not typically seen in giant cell granuloma.

The treatment for ABCs include curettage or surgical resection. The rate of local recurrence following curettage of the jaw ranges from 20 to 38 percent. Recurrent lesions should also be managed conservatively.

Treatment and Prognosis. For central giant cell gnathic and sinonasal lesions, conservative but complete surgical resection or curettage is the treatment of choice (169,170). The central lesions may behave in a locally aggressive manner. Recurrence rates vary and are reported from 11 to near 50 percent. Radiation treatment generally is not indicated.

For peripheral lesions, conservative but complete surgical resection includes the entire depth of the lesion with curettage of subjacent bone. Peripheral lesions recur in 10 percent of cases (171). Large lesions displacing teeth have been reported (172), but characteristically, peripheral giant cell granuloma does not display aggressive behavior (171).

ORAL FIBROSING LESIONS

Oral Submucous Fibrosis

Oral submucous fibrosis is a unique, chronic progressive and irreversible generalized fibrosis of oral soft tissues that may be confused with fibromatosis. This lesion has been associated with chewing areca nut (betel quid), a habit found in rural India (173–175). Symptoms include increasing rigidity and progressive inability to open the mouth, referred to as trismus; this causes difficulties in swallowing, speaking, and eating (173, 176). Oral submucous fibrosis typically involves the buccal mucosa, lips, retromolar areas, and soft palate.

Histologically, in more advanced lesions, there is a dense submucosal collagen deposition

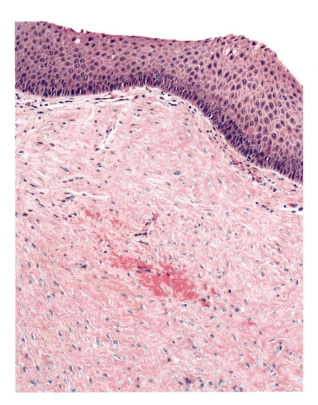

Figure 2-46

ORAL SUBMUCOUS FIBROSIS

The submucosal hyalinization replaces the submucosal soft tissues. The overlying epithelium is unremarkable here, although in other examples it may be atrophic or show the presence of intraepithelial dysplasia.

characterized by thick bands of hyalinization with replacement of the submucosal soft tissues (fig. 2-46). Hyalinization of minor salivary gland acini can be found. The epithelium is often atrophic but epithelial dysplasia can be present. Up to 10 percent of patients with oral submucous fibrosis develop squamous cell carcinoma (177,178). The development of squamous cell carcinoma is linked to the presence of tobacco as a component of betel quid.

There is no effective treatment for oral submucous fibrosis. Oral dysplasia and/or carcinoma associated with oral submucous fibrosis are treated as any other dysplasia or carcinoma.

Gingival Fibromatosis

General Features. *Gingival fibromatosis (hereditary gingival fibromatosis, idiopathic gingival fibromatosis)* presents in early childhood, appearing as generalized fibromatosis or as a papular lesion (papulosis or papular gingival fibromatosis) linked to such conditions as acanthosis nigricans, Cowden syndrome, and tuberous sclerosis (179). *Drug-related gingival hyperplasia (drug-induced fibrous hyperplasia)* is an abnormal growth of gingival tissue linked to the use of a wide variety of systemic medications (180) and initially becomes noticeable three or more months following the use of the medication. A strong association has been noted with use of cyclosporine, phenytoin, and nifedipine. A localized and more common form of gingival fibromatosis is *symmetric fibromatosis of the tuberosity*.

Microscopic Features. The histologic findings of gingival fibromatosis are similar, irrespective of clinical occurrence, and include a dense or moderately dense, avascular, submucosal, collagenized connective tissue with scattered chronic inflammatory cells. There is low cellularity consisting of fibroblasts interspersed with myofibroblasts. Myxoid change may be present and rarely, calcifications are identified. The gingival epithelium may have extreme elongation of the rete ridges, including long and narrow anastomosing rete ridges extending into connective tissue. The crevicular epithelium facing the tooth surfaces usually shows degeneration, subepithelial edema, and more extensive inflammatory cell infiltration due to the gingivitis or periodontitis that is often present. The differential diagnosis includes fibromatosis and myofibroma/myofibromatosis (see below).

Differential Diagnosis. *Fibromatosis/extraabdominal fibromatosis* is a locally aggressive, nonmetastasizing (myo)fibroblastic neoplasm characterized by locally infiltrative growth. Synonyms include *desmoid-type fibromatosis, desmoid tumor, aggressive fibromatosis, extraabdominal desmoid, extraabdominal fibromatosis, tumefactive fibroinflammatory tumor,* and *inflammatory pseudotumor.*

Fibromatosis of the head and neck region occurs primarily in the soft tissues of the neck, including the supraclavicular region and the anterolateral neck. Excluding the neck, the common sites of occurrence are the sinonasal tract, nasopharynx, tongue, and oral cavity. Approximately 10 to 15 percent of fibromatoses occur in the head and neck; in children, more than one third of cases occur in the head and neck (181,182). Fibromatosis may occur spontaneously or may be associated with Gardner syndrome or Gardner-type familial adenomatous polyposis (FAP) (183,184).

Histologically, fibromatosis is poorly circumscribed, composed of uniform-appearing spindle-shaped cells with sharply defined, pale-staining nuclei, associated with and separated by abundant collagen (fig. 2-47). The cellularity varies but in general is only moderate. The cells are uniform, with tapering or plump vesicular nuclei, small nucleoli, and indistinct cytoplasm lacking hyperchromasia, pleomorphism, or mitotic activity (fig. 2-47). Variations in the nuclear appearance include the presence of stellate-appearing nuclei. A fascicular growth pattern, including broad elongated fascicles, may be present but tends to be less well defined as compared to that seen in fibrosarcoma. The stromal component is variably collagenized and may focally be myxoid or mucoid. In some examples, keloid-like collagen or extensive hyalinization are prominent. The vascularity varies but is generally not a prominent feature; the characteristic vascularity associated with some sarcomas, including a delicate plexiform pattern, is absent in fibromatosis.

Typically, these lesions are poorly circumscribed and infiltrative along the periphery into striated muscle (fig. 2-47). In the oral cavity as well as in the sinonasal tract, they may extend into bone (fig. 2-47). At the advancing edge of the tumor, lymphoid aggregates and degenerate skeletal muscle cells with bizarre sarcolemmal nuclei are commonly seen.

By immunohistochemical staining, nuclear beta-catenin is expressed by the spindle cells in 70 to 75 percent of cases (fig. 2-47), in particular those associated with FAP, but also can be seen in sporadically occurring cases (185,186). Cytogenetic abnormalities (e.g., trisomies) on chromosomes 8 and 20 have been identified, supporting the neoplastic rather than reactive nature of fibromatosis (187). Germline mutations of the *APC* gene on the long arm of chromosome 5 have been identified in patients with Gardner-type FAP. Mutations in the gene encoding β-catenin (*CTNNB1*) are identified in up to 85 percent of sporadic lesions (188,189). *APC* and *CTNNB1* mutations result in the intranuclear accumulation of β-catenin.

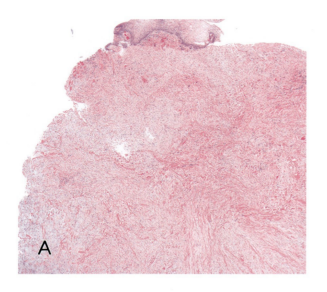
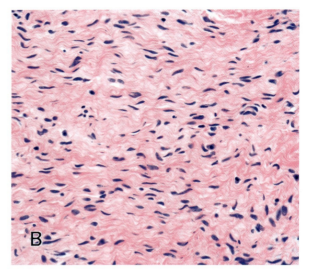
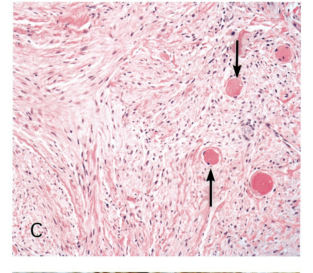
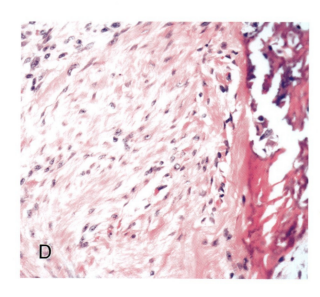
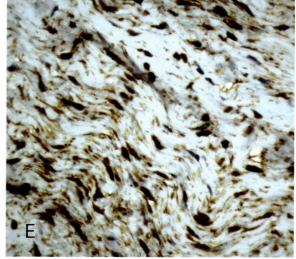

Figure 2-47

ORAL CAVITY EXTRA-ABDOMINAL (DESMOID) FIBROMATOSIS

A: A submucosal nodular or vaguely lobular, poorly circumscribed proliferation is composed of variably cellular spindle-shaped cells separated by abundant collagen.

B: At higher magnification, the proliferation is composed of bland-appearing spindle-shaped cells with associated collagenized stroma. These lesions are poorly circumscribed and infiltrative.

C,D: Infiltration includes envelopment and invasion of skeletal muscle (C; arrows) and extension into bone (D).

E: Nuclear β-catenin immunoreactivity.

The treatment of choice for fibromatosis is wide surgical excision, including several centimeters beyond the apparent macroscopic extent of the lesion. In general, the prognosis is good; however, these lesions present difficulties in management due to insinuation of the lesion into adjacent structures without clear demarcation, making complete excision difficult. As a result of the difficulties in completely excising the lesion, recurrent disease is common. Recurrence usually occurs within the first few years following surgery; those appearing within 2 years of surgery are likely related to the presence of positive margins. Radiotherapy has been used with some success in patients with residual tumor or recurrent disease. Since head and neck fibromatosis often occurs in young patients, radiotherapy should be used cautiously due to the possible complications secondary to radiation treatment. Imatinib and sorafenib have been used with varying efficacy in the treatment of primary and recurrent disease (190–192). Rarely, death is due to uncontrolled local disease. Spontaneous regression of the lesion may occur but is rare. Regression following radiotherapy may take 2 to 3 years. In extremely rare cases, transformation to an overt malignancy (fibrosarcoma) occurs and possibly relates to prior radiation therapy.

Myofibroma and *myofibromatosis* are benign neoplasms composed of myoid cells arranged around thin-walled blood vessels. The solitary type (i.e., myofibroma) is the more common, representing slightly more than half the cases (193,194). These lesions occur over a wide age range, including infants (so-called *infantile myofibromatosis*) (195). Myofibroma is most commonly seen in adults.

Myofibroma and myofibromatosis tend to occur in the head and neck region. The most common site of occurrence is in bone (mandible and skull), followed by the oral cavity, especially the buccal mucosa and tongue; less common intraoral sites of involvement include the gingiva, palate, lip, and retromolar trigone (193–196). Myofibroma/myofibromatosis may rarely involve other head and neck sites, including sinonasal tract and neck. The clinical presentation is usually that of a painless mass measuring less than 3 cm. Myofibromatosis occurs with or without visceral involvement.

The pathologic findings remain similar whether solitary or multifocal. These lesions tend to be well-circumscribed and grey-white, measuring up to 7 cm in greatest dimension (median, 2.5 cm).

The histologic features include the presence of nodular or multinodular growth, with a characteristic "zoning" appearance due to regional variation of cell types (fig. 2-48). A peripheral zone composed of plump spindle-shaped cells with elongated, cigar-shaped vesicular nuclei, small nucleoli, and pale pink cytoplasm is present, with the cells arranged in short fascicles or whorls (fig. 2-48). A central zone is composed of primitive-appearing round cells with round to polygonal to spindle-shaped, vesicular to hyperchromatic nuclei, and scant eosinophilic to clear cytoplasm. This is arranged around thin-walled, irregularly branching blood vessels showing features similar to the vascularity seen in hemangiopericytomas (glomangiomas). There is an absence of significant pleomorphism or mitotic activity. Calcification, stromal hyalinization, necrosis and intravascular growth are frequently present.

The lesional cells are reactive for vimentin and actins (smooth muscle and muscle specific) (fig. 2-48); staining for S-100 protein, desmin, and epithelial markers are negative. Ultrastructural studies have shown findings compatible with myofibroblasts, including prominent rough endoplasmic reticulum, intracytoplasmic filament bundles with dense bodies, and focal basal lamina.

Spontaneous regression may occur in solitary or multifocal lesions (195). Simple excision of solitary lesions is curative. Surgical resection of multiple lesions may be indicated in cases where there is functional impairment or where there is involvement of vital organs. Recurrence rates following surgery usually are less than 10 percent (194). Increased morbidity and mortality may be associated with (multifocal) visceral involvement. Lung involvement is associated with a poor prognosis. Death may be due to cardiopulmonary or gastrointestinal complications.

Treatment and Prognosis. For gingival (hereditary) fibromatosis, treatment includes surgical excision, including gingivectomy and gingivoplasty to recontour the tissue in order to achieve satisfactory cosmesis. The lesions

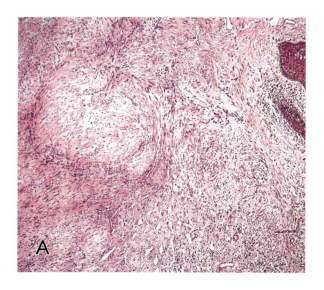
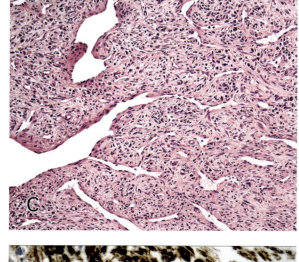
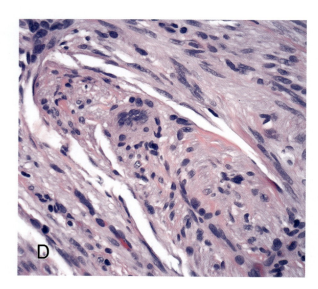
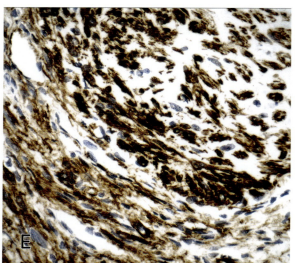

Figure 2-48

MYOFIBROMA

A: There is submucosal nodular growth.

B: The nodule is composed of spindle-shaped cells with elongated, cigar-shaped vesicular nuclei arranged in short fascicles at the periphery. Round cells with round to polygonal to spindle-shaped hyperchromatic nuclei and scant eosinophilic cytoplasm are more centrally located.

C: Irregularly branching blood vessels are similar in appearance to those associated with hemangiopericytoma.

D: Subendothelial intravascular growth.

E: Diffuse immunoreactivity for smooth muscle actin.

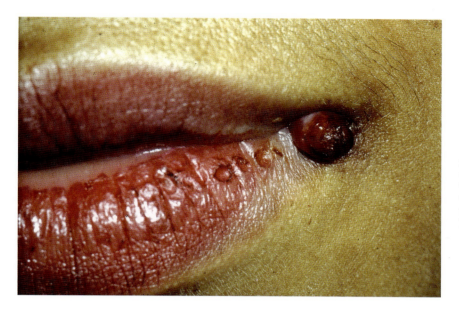

Figure 2-49

PYOGENIC GRANULOMA (LOBULAR CAPILLARY HEMANGIOMA)

In a pregnant patient (pregnancy tumor), the granuloma is a well-circumscribed red nodule with a sessile base. The patient wanted the lesion removed prior to delivery although often the lesion regresses postpartum.

may recur or progress after surgery, requiring repeated surgical resection. Improved oral hygiene greatly diminishes the risk of recurrence. Drug-related gingival hyperplasia may also be treated by gingivectomy and plaque control but discontinuation of drug use often results in cessation and even regression of gingival enlargement. Symmetrical fibromatosis of the tuberosity usually requires no treatment. Large lesions or those that interfere with function or denture placement may be removed with conservative surgical excision; recurrence has not been reported.

VASCULAR LESIONS

Pyogenic Granuloma (Lobular Capillary Hemangioma)

Definition. *Pyogenic granuloma* (PG) is a polypoid capillary hemangioma-like growth. The terminology of pyogenic granuloma is unfortunate since it is neither pus-forming nor a granulomatous process. Pyogenic granuloma is a long-used term retaining some usefulness; a commonly used modern synonym is *lobular capillary hemangioma*.

Clinical Features. PG affects both genders and occurs over a wide age range. In the oral cavity, most lesions occur on the gingiva, although other sites, including the tongue, buccal mucosa, and lip, may be affected. PG is generally a well-circumscribed nodule with a sessile or pedunculated base. These lesions appear bright red although some examples have normal coloration. The surface may be intact, but some are ulcerated with associated bleeding. The size varies widely, from a few millimeters up to 6 cm in diameter, although typically PGs do not exceed 3 cm. The lesion may arise suddenly and grow rapidly, thus causing concern for a malignant process.

PGs that arise in pregnant females are referred to as *pregnancy tumor*. These lesions share the clinical and pathologic features of PG except that they often arise in the third month of pregnancy, usually occur on the gingiva (fig. 2-49), increase in size until parturition, and following delivery may subside or disappear. Those cases in which complete regression does not occur may grow with a subsequent pregnancy, thereby suggesting a hormonal influence in their development and growth (197).

Epulis granulomatosa is another type of PG appearing as a hemorrhagic gingival mass seen in association with a poorly healing bony socket following tooth extraction. *Parulis* is also a type of PG identified at the end of a fistulous tract from an underlying intraosseous dental infection. Yet another variant of PG is the *intravascular pyogenic granuloma* that predilects to the upper extremities (arm and forearm) and the neck.

Pathogenesis. The etiology of PG includes trauma and the hormonal influences associated with pregnancy. The etiology, however, is the

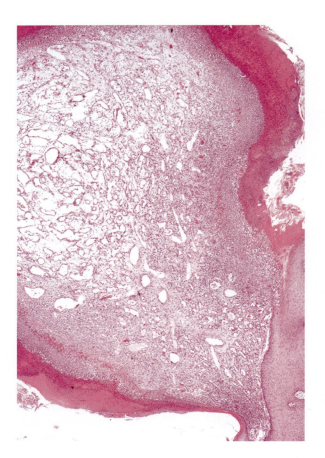 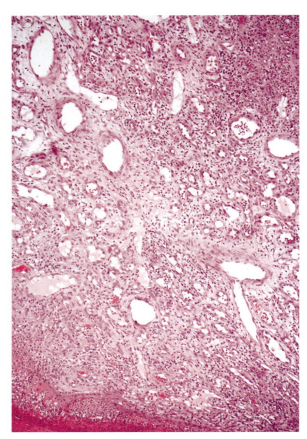

Figure 2-50

PYOGENIC GRANULOMA (LOBULAR CAPILLARY HEMANGIOMA)

Left: Polypoid submucosal vascular proliferation with surface ulceration.
Right: Higher magnification shows proliferation of nonanastamosing, capillary-sized vessels.

subject of debate, including the consideration that the underlying process is neoplastic and that these lesions are in fact lobular capillary hemangiomas (198).

Microscopic Findings. PG is a submucosal capillary-sized vascular proliferation of various-caliber endothelial-lined vascular spaces (fig. 2-50), often but not always arranged in lobules or clusters (fig. 2-51). The capillary-sized vascular spaces have distinct lumens, often angular to slit-like, which may be compressed and indistinct. The endothelial cells may be plump or inconspicuous; spindling is not a characteristic feature. The endothelial cells are bland in appearance, typically lacking cytologic atypia or mitoses (fig. 2-51). The vascular component is separated by fibrous to fibromyxoid stroma, including uniform-appearing spindle-shaped cells lacking pleomorphism. Usually there is absent to minimal mitotic figures, however, in any given lesion increased mitotic figures (but not atypical mitoses) may be seen (fig. 2-51), and in the setting of increased mitotic activity in an otherwise histologically typical lesion, the designation of *"active" pyogenic granuloma* can be used. A mixed chronic inflammatory cell reaction is present. The vascular component is usually of capillary caliber, but may range up to cavernous type spaces, but does not anastomose. Uncommonly, foci of papillary endothelial hyperplasia may be present.

PGs are almost exclusively exophytic and broad based, generally not extending into the underlying submucosal tissues. The overlying surface epithelium may be intact and unremarkable, may be atrophic, and frequently, is

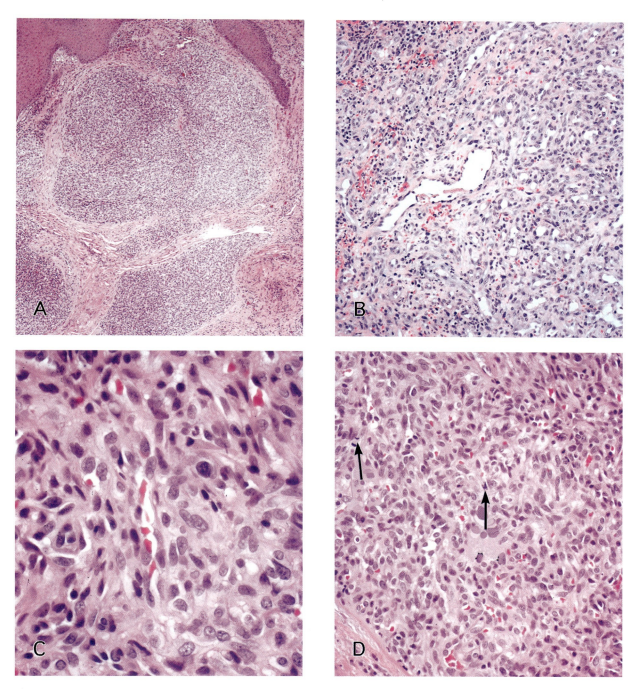

Figure 2-51

PYOGENIC GRANULOMA (LOBULAR CAPILLARY HEMANGIOMA)

A: This submucosal vascular proliferation is arranged into lobules and separated by intervening fibrous bands.

B: The vascular component is capillary sized, but may vary in size and shape; however, there is an absence of interconnecting or anastomosing vessels as is seen in angiosarcoma.

C: The cellular area includes plump nuclei but overall there is an absence of significant nuclear pleomorphism and mitotic activity.

D: The increased mitotic activity (arrows) confers the designation of "active" pyogenic granuloma but there is an absence of atypical mitoses.

ulcerated. The ulceration may be associated with infiltration of neutrophils, plasma cells, lymphocytes, and fibrinoid necrosis. Those PGs that are subjected to repeated trauma (e.g., gingival lesions) may over time become sclerotic and form a peripheral fibroma.

The histology of intravascular PGs is similar to that of nonintravascular PGs except that the former are attached to the wall of an endothelial-lined blood vessel via a fibrovascular stalk.

Differential Diagnosis. The differential diagnosis of PG includes other vascular lesions, including reactive processes (e.g., granulation tissue) and vascular neoplasms. If the mitotic activity is increased, a possible diagnosis of malignancy (e.g., Kaposi sarcoma and angiosarcoma) is suggested.

In contrast to PGs, polypoid granulation tissue tends to have a radial arrangement of vessels, with the vascular component oriented perpendicular to the surface. The patchy hypercellular lobularity of PG is lacking.

PG is almost always an exophytic nodule, whereas Kaposi sarcoma (KS) may present in either a nodular or a macular form. In contrast to the broad base of PG, the nodular form of KS is usually an infiltrative lesion with a significant component of spindle cells lining bizarre-shaped vessels. Extravasated red blood cells, hyaline globules, and hemosiderin deposits are characteristic features of KS. Evidence of KS-associated herpesvirus/human herpes virus-8 (HHV8) supports the diagnosis of KS and should not be present in PG (199).

Treatment and Prognosis. Conservative surgical removal of the lesion and any obvious source of irritation is the treatment of choice, with about a 16 percent recurrence rate (198). Although some cases of spontaneous regression have been reported (198), particularly when the source of irritation is removed, the possibility of a more serious process, such as a metastatic lesion or malignancy, masquerading as PG, mandates biopsy and histopathologic diagnosis (198).

Congenital Epulis (Congenital Granular Cell Tumor)

Definition. *Congenital epulis* is a rare, congenital, soft tissue tumor of the alveolar ridge in newborns. Synonyms include *congenital gingival granular cell tumor* and *congenital granular cell epulis*.

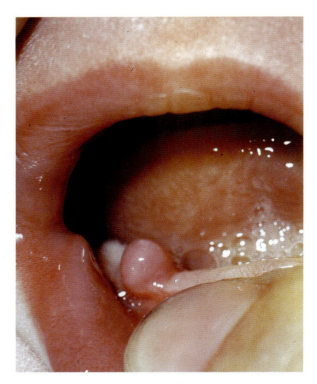

Figure 2-52

CONGENITAL EPULIS

A newborn with a 1-cm sessile nodule on the mandibular alveolar ridge.

Clinical Features. Congenital epulis is a rare lesion that is usually detected at birth, but may be diagnosed during intrauterine development. There is a marked female predilection (200). The lesion is typically a solitary mass of the anterior maxillary alveolar ridge, but multiple lesions have been reported to involve the tongue and gingiva (fig. 2-52). Large tumors may cause airway obstruction or feeding difficulty.

Pathogenesis. Owing to the absence of S-100 protein reactivity, this tumor is felt to originate from a non-neural cell of origin, but the histogenesis remains uncertain. Some authorities believe it to be a non-neoplastic (hamartomatous) lesion.

Microscopic Findings. Congenital epulis is usually a nodular growth of the alveolar ridge. The nodule is surfaced by attenuated stratified squamous epithelium. Immediately subjacent to the epithelium is a solid mass of large, rounded eosinophilic cells with granular cytoplasm and

Oral Cavity and Jaw

congenital epulis are not reactive for S-100 protein, a finding that contrasts with the granular cell tumor, but may show the presence of CD68. Despite the female predominance of these lesions, estrogen and progesterone receptors have not been demonstrated (201).

Differential Diagnosis. The distinctive clinical and pathologic correlation of this lesion usually limits the differential diagnostic considerations. The pigmented dendritic cells that characterize melanotic neuroectodermal tumor of infancy are not present in congenital epulis of the newborn. Although this lesion carries the same name as granular cell tumor, the latter is a neoplasm thought to be of modified Schwann cell origin. Findings in granular cell tumor that are not typically seen in congenital epulis include the presence of pseudoepitheliomatous hyperplasia and S-100 protein staining (Table 2-5).

Treatment and Prognosis. The treatment is surgical excision, generally performed shortly after birth; the lesion also may regress (202). Recurrence has not been reported, even following incomplete removal.

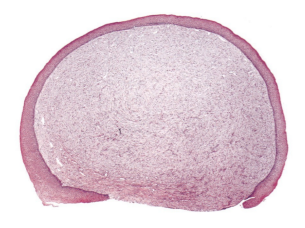
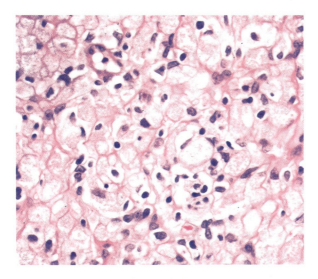

Figure 2-53

CONGENITAL EPULIS

Top: The polypoid lesion is characterized by a submucosal cellular proliferation with overlying intact squamous epithelium.

Bottom: The submucosal cellular proliferation includes enlarged cells with granular cytoplasm. The cells are similar to those seen in granular cell tumor, however, S-100 protein immunoreactivity is absent.

round to oval, slightly basophilic nuclei. The stroma may be scant to fibrous, with small-caliber vascular channels (fig. 2-53). Rarely, small islands of odontogenic epithelium are seen. The lesion is usually circumscribed, but not encapsulated. The underlying bone is not involved.

Special Stains. Immunohistochemical studies help differentiate congenital epulis from granular cell tumor (201). The granular cells of

BENIGN FIBRO-OSSEOUS LESIONS OF CRANIOFACIAL BONES

Gnathic benign fibro-osseous lesions include fibrous dysplasia and ossifying fibroma (and variants thereof). Ossifying fibroma is a neoplastic lesion and is not discussed except in the differential diagnosis of fibrous dysplasia. Gnathic fibro-osseous lesions may be histologically indistinguishable, therefore, the diagnosis and differentiation rests on the clinical-radiologic-histopathologic correlation. In the head and neck, benign fibro-osseous lesions occur most often in relation to gnathic (maxillary and mandibular) bones. For completion, the psammomatoid ossifying fibroma is included in this discussion although it predilects to the sinonasal tract.

Fibrous Dysplasia

Definition. *Fibrous dysplasia* is an idiopathic non-neoplastic bone disease in which normal medullary bone is replaced by structurally weak fibro-osseous tissue. Three variants of fibrous dysplasia are identified: monostotic, polyostotic, and McCune-Albright syndrome.

Table 2-5

DIFFERENTIAL DIAGNOSIS OF GRANULAR CELL TUMOR AND CONGENITAL EPULIS OF THE NEWBORN

	Congenital Epulis	Granular Cell Tumor
Age/gender	less than 1 year/marked female predominance	adults/slight female predominance
Site	anterior alveolar ridge	tongue or any oral mucosa or salivary gland
Immunohistochemistry	S-100 protein nonreactive	S-100 protein reactive
Pseudoepitheliomatous hyperplasia	no	sometimes
Vascularity	delicate, marked capillary network	not prominent

Monostotic Fibrous Dysplasia. Monostotic fibrous dysplasia involves only a single osseous site and represents more than 75 percent of all cases of fibrous dysplasia (203,204). There is no gender predilection or it is slightly more common in women, and it frequently occurs in older children and young adults (i.e., second and third decades of life) (205). It most commonly affects the ribs, femur, and tibia; the head and neck bones are involved in up to 25 percent of cases (203). In the head and neck, the most common sites of involvement are (in descending order of frequency) maxilla (zygomatic process), mandible (region of premolar and molar teeth), frontal bone, ethmoid and sphenoid bones, and temporal bone.

Polyostotic Fibrous Dysplasia. Polyostotic fibrous dysplasia involves two or more bones and represents 20 to 25 percent of all cases of fibrous dysplasia (203). It is more common in females than males, and tends to occur in the first decade of life. It may be limited to a few bones in one anatomic region or may be diffuse, affecting virtually every bone in the skeleton. In more than half the cases, osseous involvement includes the long bones of the extremities, pelvic bones, ribs, metacarpals, metatarsals, and the humerus; craniofacial or jaw involvement occurs in up to 50 percent of patients (203).

McCune-Albright Syndrome. This syndrome is defined by the triad of polyostotic fibrous dysplasia, endocrine dysfunction, and cutaneous pigmentation. It is the least common variant of fibrous dysplasia, representing 1 to 3 percent of all cases (203). It tends to occur in the first decade of life. The endocrine dysfunction includes hyperthyroidism or sexual precocity, the latter predominantly identified in females.

Rarely, fibrous dysplasia is associated with soft tissue myxomas (203,206). This association is more common with polyostotic fibrous dysplasia and McCune-Albright syndrome. The myxomas appear years (decades) after the bone lesions, are most common in the thigh (intramuscular), and often are multiple with a tendency to occur near to abnormal bones.

Clinical Features. Regardless of type, most patients affected by fibrous dysplasia are under 30 years of age. Craniofacial symptoms include painless, asymmetric, nonmobile swelling associated with functional disturbances; displacement or malocclusion of teeth, failure of tooth eruption in children; headaches, proptosis, nasal obstruction, especially for sinonasal tract lesions; and hearing loss (conductive). Laboratory findings include normal serum calcium and phosphorous levels, and alkaline phosphatase may be elevated.

Radiologic imaging may include the presence of a poorly defined expansile osseous lesion with a thin intact cortex or cortex of lesional bone (fig. 2-54). Predominantly fibrous lesions are radiolucent. Predominantly osseous lesions are radiodense. Those lesions with an equal admixture of fibrous and osseous components have a ground-glass appearance. Usually no periosteal reaction is seen unless there is an associated fracture.

Pathogenesis. Guanine nucleotide-binding protein/α-subunit (*GNAS*) mutations that induce the activation of G-protein α-subunit participate in the pathogenesis of fibrous dysplasia (207). *GNAS* mutations are found in 86 percent of fibrous dysplasia cases (208). The mutations occur postzygotically and ultimately lead to high levels of cAMP, excess bone resorption, and fibrous

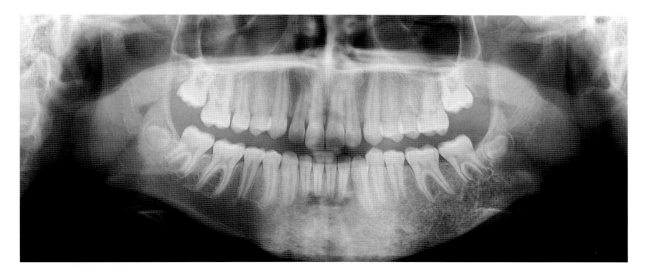

Figure 2-54

FIBROUS DYSPLASIA

A homogeneous radiolucency/radiopacity with diffuse borders extends from the right premolar region to the left third molar. There is a loss of the inferior cortex of the mandible.

replacement of bone marrow (209). *GNAS* mutations are absent in ossifying fibromas, cemento-ossifying fibromas, and cemento-ossifying dysplasias (207,210) and are reported to be absent in odontogenic myxomas (211).

Gross Findings. The lesions are tan-white to yellow, soft, rubbery, and gritty or firm.

Microscopic Findings. The fibrous tissue component is nondescript and of variable cellularity, lacking significant pleomorphism. Increased mitotic activity can be identified but atypical mitoses are not found. The osseous component includes irregularly shaped trabeculae of osteoid and immature (woven) bone arising metaplastically from the fibrous stroma (fig. 2-55). The osseous component is poorly oriented with misshapen bony trabeculae, increased cellularity, and irregular margins, and forms odd geometric patterns including "C"- or "S"-shaped configurations (fig. 2-55). The trabeculae typically lack osteoblastic rimming. Multinucleated giant cells, macrophages, increased vascularity, and calcification may be seen. Under polarized light, the bone appears woven rather than lamellar; however, lamellar bone can be seen in fibrous dysplasia and its presence does not exclude the diagnosis.

Differential Diagnosis. The differential diagnosis primarily includes ossifying fibroma and psammomatoid ossifying fibroma (relative to sinonasal tract lesions) (Table 2-6). Gnathic fibro-osseous lesions (fibrous dysplasia and ossifying fibromas) may be histologically indistinguishable, therefore, the diagnosis and differentiation rests on the clinical-radiologic-histopathologic correlation.

Ossifying fibroma (OF) is a benign, well-demarcated, slow-growing fibro-osseous neoplasm composed of fibrocellular tissue admixed with varying amounts of mineralized material (i.e., bone, cementum). Radiologically, OFs are well-circumscribed lesions with smooth contours (fig. 2-56). Their appearance varies based on the maturity of the tumor: completely radiolucent (immature lesion); completely radiopaque (mature lesion); and mixed radiolucent and radiopaque (increased mineralization with age results in radiopaque foci admixed with radiolucent areas). Histologically, OFs are well-delineated, demarcated or encapsulated lesions composed of randomly distributed mature (lamellar) bone spicules rimmed by osteoblasts admixed with a fibrous stroma (fig. 2-57). While the osseous component is generally described as mature, the central portion may be woven bone with lamellar bone at the periphery. The fibrous stroma may be densely cellular. Mitotic figures are rare to absent. Lesions with associated

Figure 2-55
FIBROUS DYSPLASIA

A: Histologically, fibrous dysplasia is characterized by a variable admixture of fibrous tissue and osseous components.

B,C: The osseous component includes immature (woven) bone in which the trabeculae form odd geometric patterns typically lacking prominent osteoblastic rimming; the fibrous tissue component is nondescript without pattern and of variable cellularity. Differentiating fibrous dysplasia from ossifying fibroma often requires radiologic correlation to determine whether the fibro-osseous lesion is circumscribed, as seen in ossifying fibroma, or has ill-defined margins, as seen in fibrous dysplasia.

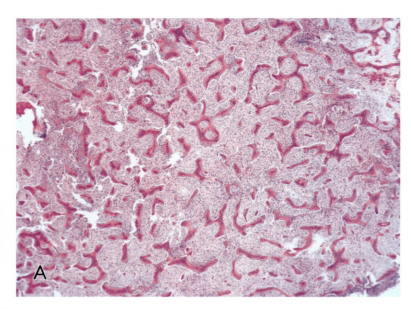

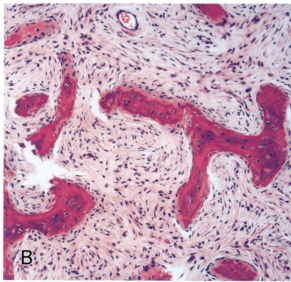

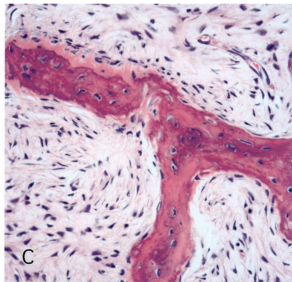

cementum are referred to as cementifying fibroma and those with cementum and bone are referred to as cemento-ossifying fibroma (figs. 2-58, 2-59). Unlike fibrous dysplasia, guanine nucleotide-binding protein/α-subunit (*GNAS*) mutations are absent in ossifying fibromas, cemento-ossifying fibromas, and cemento-ossifying dysplasias (207,210). Differentiation of ossifying fibroma from fibrous dysplasia is important since the treatment differs for these lesions (see below for the treatment of fibrous dysplasia). For ossifying fibromas, surgical excision is the treatment of choice. The well-circumscribed nature of this lesion allows for easy surgical removal. The prognosis is excellent following complete excision, and recurrences are rare.

Psammomatoid (active) ossifying fibroma (POF) is a variant of ossifying fibroma that typically occurs in the sinonasal tract and potentially may behave aggressively, with locally invasive and destructive capabilities (212). POF generally occurs in younger age groups (first and second decades), but can occur over a wide age range, including older individuals. The presenting

Table 2-6

BENIGN FIBRO-OSSEOUS LESIONS: CLINICOPATHOLOGIC COMPARISON

	FD[a]	OF	POF
Gender/age	MFD: F=M; 2nd-3rd decades; PFD: F>M; 1st decade	F>M; 2nd-4th decades	F=M; younger age groups (1st-2nd decades), but may occur in older individuals
Location	No specific site of involvement	Most common in the mandible (posterior or molar region)	Ethmoid sinus; supraorbital frontal region
Focality	MFD (75-80%); PFD (20-25%); MAS (1-3%)	Single site	Single site or involvement of multiple (contiguous) sites/sinuses
Radiology	Poorly defined expansile osseous lesion with a thin intact cortex; predominantly fibrous lesions are radiolucent; predominantly osseous lesions are radiodense; lesions with an equal admixture of fibrous and osseous components have a ground-glass appearance	Well-circumscribed or sharply demarcated lesion with smooth contours	Lytic or mixed lytic/radiopaque osseous and/or soft tissue mass varying from well-demarcated to invasive with bone erosion
Histology	Fibrous tissue component is nondescript and of variable cellularity; osseous component includes irregularly shaped trabeculae of osteoid and immature (woven) bone that is poorly oriented, with misshapen bony trabeculae with odd geometric patterns including "C"- or "S"-shaped configurations; the trabeculae typically lack osteoblastic rimming	Randomly distributed mature (lamellar) bone spicules rimmed by osteoblasts admixed with a fibrous stroma; central portions may be woven bone with lamellar bone at the periphery	Bony spicules and distinctive mineralized or calcified "psammomatoid" bodies or ossicles admixed with a fibrous stroma; psammomatoid bodies vary from a few in number to a dense population of innumerable spherical bodies; osteoclasts are present within the ossicles, and osteoblasts can be seen along their peripheral aspects; the bony trabeculae vary in appearance and include odd shapes with a curvilinear pattern; the trabeculae are composed of lamellar bone with associated osteoclasts and osteoblastic rimming
Syndromes	MAS (1-3%)	No known association	No known association
Genetic Mutations	*GNAS* mutation	None known	None known
Treatment	Disease may stabilize at puberty and, in children, therapy should be delayed if possible until after puberty; surgical resection indicated in cases with compromise of function, progression of deformity, associated pathologic fracture(s), or the development of a malignancy	Surgical resection	Surgical resection
Prognosis	Good prognosis; recurrence rates are low and death due to extension into vital structures rarely occurs	Excellent	Good following complete excision; recurrence(s) often occur due to incomplete excision; may behave in an aggressive manner with local destruction and potential invasion into vital structures
Malignant transformation	Malignant transformation (osteosarcoma) occurs in less than 1%; dismal prognosis	Not known to not occur	Not known to occur

[a]FD = fibrous dysplasia; OF = ossifying fibroma; POF = psammomatoid ossifying fibroma; MFD = monostotic fibrous dysplasia; PFD = polyostotic fibrous dysplasia; MAS = McCune-Albright syndrome; *GNAS* = guanine nucleotide-binding protein/α-subunit mutations.

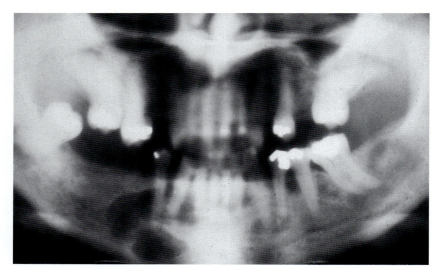

Figure 2-56

OSSIFYING FIBROMA

An ossifying fibroma involving the right anterior portion of the mandible produces a sharply defined lytic lesion.

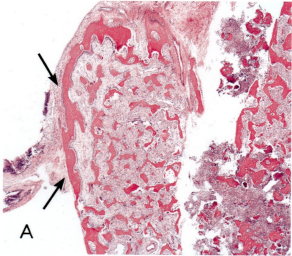

Figure 2-57

OSSIFYING FIBROMA

A: Histologically, ossifying fibroma is characterized by an admixture of mature (lamellar) bone and a fibrous stroma; along the superficial aspect the lesion has a circumscribed margin (arrows).

B,C:. The bony spicules are rimmed by osteoblasts that are more prominently present in ossifying fibroma than fibrous dysplasia. The fibrous stroma is similar to that seen in fibrous dysplasia. The overlapping features with fibrous dysplasia suggest radiologic correlation is required in rendering the diagnosis.

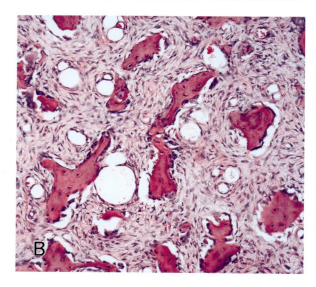
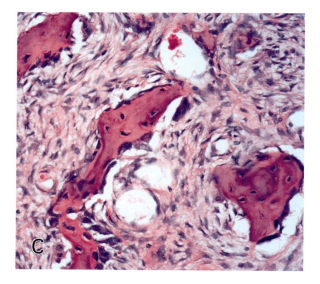

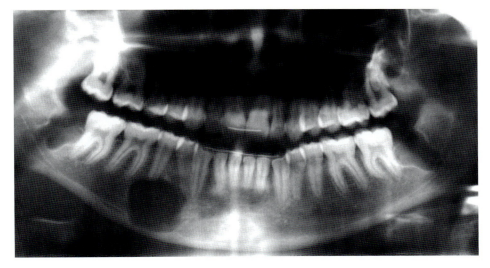

Figure 2-58

CEMENTO-OSSIFYING FIBROMA

A panoramic radiograph shows a well-demarcated radiolucency in the right mandibular premolar region.

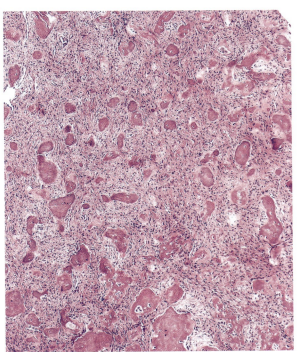 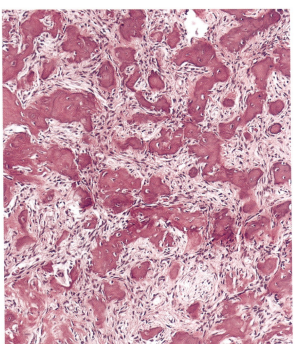

Figure 2-59

CEMENTO-OSSIFYING FIBROMA

Left: The cellular background of spindle cells has islands and trabeculae of woven and lamellar bone and acellular, basophilic cementum-like material.
Right: Islands and trabeculae of woven bone, lamellar bone, and cementum-like material are present.

symptoms include facial swelling, nasal obstruction, pain, sinusitis, headache, and proptosis. POF occurs in any area of the sinonasal tract but is most frequent in the ethmoid sinus and supraorbital frontal region (ethmoid > nasal cavity > maxillary sinus > frontal sinus); the orbit may also be involved (212). The radiologic features include a lytic or mixed lytic/radiopaque osseous or soft tissue mass varying from well demarcated to invasive with bone erosion.

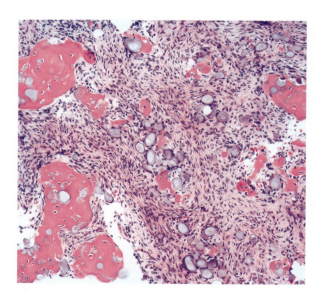 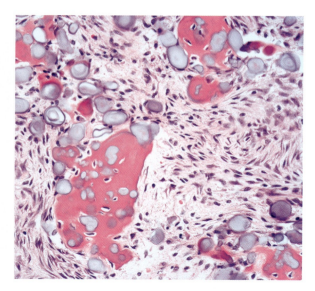

Figure 2-60

PSAMMOMATOID OSSIFYING FIBROMA

Left, right: The benign fibro-osseous lesion is characterized by the presence of spherical mineralized or calcified "psammomatoid" ossicles.

The histology of POF is that of a benign fibro-osseous proliferation composed of bony spicules and spherules admixed with a fibrous stroma. The most distinctive component is the presence of mineralized or calcified "psammomatoid" bodies or ossicles (fig. 2-60), which vary from a few in number to a dense population of innumerable spherical bodies. These ossicles are blue to black, centrally surrounded by a pink rim and with concentric laminations. The ossicles vary from small, with a round to oval shape, to large and irregularly shaped, and are present within the bony trabeculae as well as within the adjacent cellular stroma. The bony trabeculae vary in appearance and include odd shapes with a curvilinear pattern. The trabeculae are composed of lamellar bone with associated osteoclasts and osteoblastic rimming. Transition zones between the spherical ossicles and bony trabeculae are seen. The nonosseous component includes a cellular stroma with fascicular to storiform growth, composed of round to polyhedral to spindle-shaped cells with prominent basophilic nuclei and inapparent cytoplasmic borders. Mitotic figures can be seen but mitotic activity is not prominent and atypical mitoses are not present. Cellular pleomorphism may be present but anaplasia and necrosis are not identified. Giant cells can be seen among the psammomatoid ossicles or scattered throughout the nonosseous stromal component. Osteoid formation may be focally present.

Complete surgical excision is the treatment of choice. The prognosis is good following complete excision but, if margins are involved, recurrences often occur and the tumors behave in an aggressive manner, with local destruction and potential invasion into vital structures.

Treatment and Prognosis. Conservative surgical excision is the preferred treatment for fibrous dysplasia and is indicated only in cases with compromise of function, progression of deformity, pain, associated pathologic fracture(s), or the development of a malignancy. The disease may stabilize at puberty and, in children, therapy should be delayed if possible until after puberty. Recurrence rates are low and death due to extension into vital structures rarely occurs. Radiation treatment is not used because of the risk of inducing malignant change.

Malignant transformation occurs in less than 1 percent of cases, but when it occurs is most often an osteosarcoma (213–215) and less often a fibrosarcoma or chondrosarcoma (213,216). Malignant transformation is most common in the craniofacial bones (maxilla and mandible), tends to develop in bone affected by fibrous dysplasia, occurs spontaneously or in patients treated by prior radiation, is identified more often in association with the monostotic type, and has a tendency to occur years to decades following development of fibrous dysplasia. The treatment is similar to that of a primary malignant bone tumor. The prognosis for patients with malignant transformation is poor, with a tendency for metastasis to the lung resulting in short survival periods.

Cemento-Osseous Dysplasia

The *cemento-osseous dysplasias* are a group of heterogeneous bone diseases that represent various pathologic processes that all manifest by replacement of normal bone with fibrous tissue and calcified product (217,218). Although there are some histologic specific features, the most unambiguous distinctions come from oral radiographic images. Without radiographs, "benign fibro-osseous lesion" is sometimes the appropriate descriptive diagnosis. A complete discussion of the subject is not possible here; most lesions are diagnosed and treated in a dental setting, generally without biopsy. Therefore, only a cursory description of some of the various entities that are unique to the oral region will follow. Although the term dysplasia is firmly entrenched in the literature, these lesions have no tendency to transform to malignancy and are considered to be non-neoplastic. The etiology is unknown, but these lesions are limited to the jaw and may arise from pluripotential cells or other cells linked to an odontogenic origin found only within the jaw.

Grossly, multiple small, dark, gritty pieces are typically present in the biopsy material. The histologic appearance is variable, and interpretation is heavily dependent on a clinical, pathologic, and radiographic correlation as well as adequate biopsy size. As with other cemento-osseous lesions, cementum-like or ossified material of variable density is dispersed in fibrous connective tissue, without atypia. The types of cemento-osseous dysplasia include focal, periapical, and florid.

Focal Cemento-Osseous Dysplasia (FoCD). FoCD is a solitary non-neoplastic lesion of bone with a predilection for the posterior mandible (219). Middle-aged African-American females are most often affected, although the predilection has varied with the studied population. The radiographic appearance may overlap with that of small ossifying fibroma and may be frequently biopsied for diagnosis (220).

Periapical Cemento-Osseous Dysplasia (PCD). PCD is a non-neoplastic lesion of bone occurring in the anterior mandible. Prevalent in middle-aged, African-American females (221), PCD is an asymptomatic lesion that is typically detected on routine radiographic examination of anterior mandibular teeth. When tested, the involved teeth are vital, and there is no clinical swelling. The lesion may be solitary or multiple. Over time, the radiographic appearance typically progresses from radiolucent toward radiopaque. Because the lesions initially appear at the apex of the involved tooth as a radiolucent, well-circumscribed area, the dentist may mistake the lesion for inflammatory pulpal origin, leading to misdiagnosis or mismanagement (222).

Florid Cemento-Osseous Dysplasia (FloCD). Very similar to PCD, this lesion involves two or more quadrants of the jaw. It is prevalent in middle-aged African-American females (221).

A clinical, pathologic, and radiographic correlation is the key to accurate diagnosis of fibro-osseous lesions. Cemento-osseous dysplasias usually occur above the inferior alveolar canal, but share this area with ossifying fibroma, odontoma, cementoblastoma, and idiopathic osteosclerosis. Other radiopaque lesions that occur in the jaw but are infrequently biopsied include condensing osteitis and idiopathic osteosclerosis. Cementoblastoma has a unique radiographic appearance, with fusion to the involved tooth root. Odontoma is radiopaque but is composed of dentin, pulp, and occasionally, enamel. Osteoma is radiopaque but easily recognizable microscopically as benign vital bone.

Once a diagnosis of a cemento-osseous dysplasia is made, no treatment is necessary unless symptoms develop. Periodic radiographic observation is prudent since lesions may progress from focal to florid and may be associated with simple bone cysts or aneurysmal bone cysts (223,224).

PIGMENTED LESIONS

The diversity of non-neoplastic oral pigmentations ranges from physiologic to exogenous to endogenous.

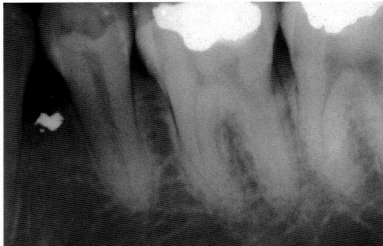

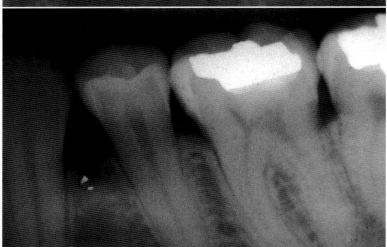

Figure 2-61

AMALGAM TATTOO

Top: Preoperative radiograph shows a focus of radiopaque material anterior to first premolar tooth.

Bottom: Postoperative radiograph shows removal of most of the radiopaque material, although a visible portion remains.

Exogenous Pigmentations

Exogenous pigmentations include *foreign body material* and *oral tattoo*, which is most commonly associated with amalgam, although any implanted, pigmented material may result in "tattoo" such as graphite, coal, metal, and plant material.

Amalgam or other metal tattoos may be observed on radiograph if the metal fragments are of sufficient density (fig. 2-61). The macules may be black, blue, or gray and the borders well defined or diffuse (225). The borders may change over time and may be asymetrical (fig. 2-62). These features may make the clinical distinction from melanoma virtually impossible. Any mucosal surface may be affected by tattoo, but the palate is more often involved in pencil implant. Amalgam tattoo has been used for forensic identification.

In amalgam tattoo, the chunks of foreign material range from black fine granules to large chunks identified within the submucosa (fig. 2-63). On routinely stained slides, amalgam and lead show up as black and brown material (figs. 2-63, 2-64). Amalgam silver salts stain the reticular fibers of collagen and therefore appear as a linear deposition of fine granules that follow the collagen fibrils around vascular channels, nerve sheaths, and other connective tissues (figs. 2-63, 2-64) (226). Graphite lacks this affinity for reticulin fibers. The foreign material usually evokes only mild inflammation, although cases with foreign body giant cell reaction and associated marked chronic inflammation may be seen (fig. 2-65) (226).

Oral Cavity and Jaw

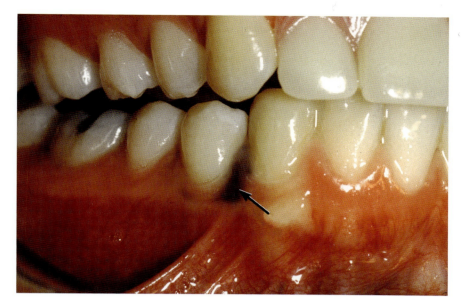

Figure 2-62

AMALGAM TATTOO

A black macule has asymmetrical borders.

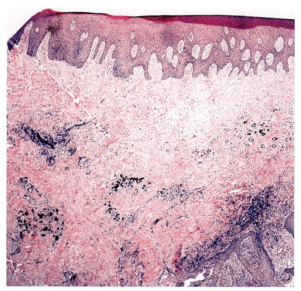 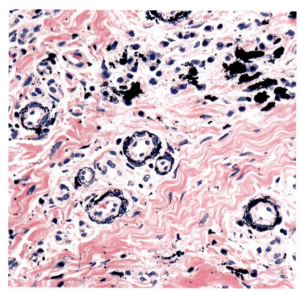

Figure 2-63

AMALGAM TATTOO

Left: Black deposits in the submucosa.
Right: Numerous solid fragments (chunks) of black deposits (amalgam) in the submucosa are surrounded by inflammatory cells and encircle blood vessels.

Graphite is distinguished from amalgam by birefringence after ammonium sulfide treatment. Amalgam is differentiated from melanin by the Fontana stain for melanin and melanin bleach, and from hemosiderin by an iron stain. Amalgam is not reactive with melanocytic-associated immunohistochemical markers (e.g., S-100 protein, HMB45, Melan A, tyrosinase, MITF1, SOX10).

The most significant clinical differential diagnostic issue is the separation of melanoma from foreign body reaction. Atypical melanocytes are not seen in foreign body tattoo. The histologic differential may include blue nevus

Non-Neoplastic Diseases of the Head and Neck

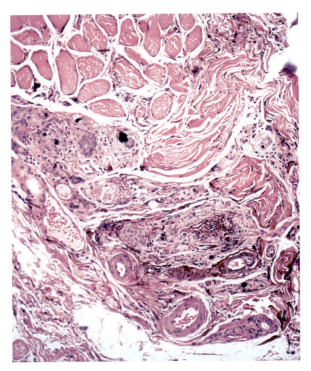 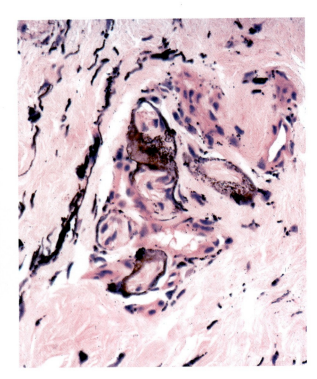

Figure 2-64

AMALGAM TATTOO

Left: The amalgam appears brown here, and extends into skeletal muscle.
Right: Brown amalgam encircles blood vessels.

and oral melanotic macule. The pigmentation in blue nevus is melanin based and therefore may be distinguished from foreign body pigmentation by special stains. Melanotic macule has increased melanin in the basal layer alone or in conjunction with melanophage histiocytes in the lamina propria.

A biopsy to exclude melanoma is generally adequate therapy for a pigmented macule. Although amalgam tattoo has been reported to cause local and systemic disease, the evidence is equivocal (227).

Endogenous Pigmentations

Endogenous pigmentations include the byproducts of red blood cells or melanocytes.

Melanotic Macule. Melanotic macule is a mucosal lesion similar to a freckle or ephelis of the skin, but an association with sun exposure is less clear since the lesion may occur on the lips or the intraoral mucosa. Some authors prefer to separate labial melanotic macule from intraoral melanotic macule.

Melanotic macule is a solitary, small, tan to brown, homogenous, symmetrical, nonpalpable pigmentation of the oral mucosa (fig. 2-66) (228). It occurs at any age, but is more common in adulthood (228). Labial melanotic macule is more common in the lower lip of adult women (229).

The hallmark histologic findings include an increase in melanin and perhaps melanocytes in the basal and parabasal layers of the surface epithelium, the latter otherwise without other significant histopathologic findings (fig. 2-67). The melanocytes are seen as individual cells without a tendency to nest or migrate throughout the surface epithelium. There is an absence of nuclear atypia and mitotic activity. Melanin accumulates in the cell body of the keratinocytes and is scarce in the dendritic cells of the upper layers of the epithelium. Melanin accumulation may be more prominent at the tips of the rete ridges (fig. 2-68). Melanin incontinence and melanophage activity may be seen in the lamina propria (fig. 2-69). Nevus cells are

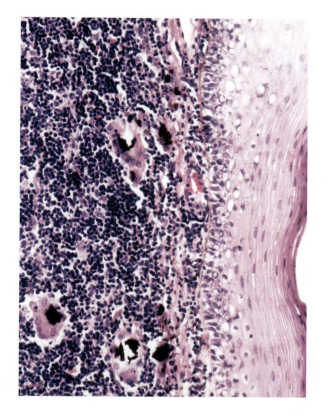 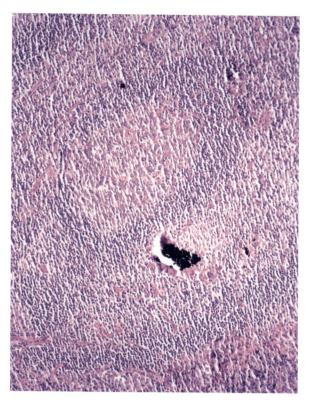

Figure 2-65

AMALGAM TATTOO

Left: Submucosal deposition of black amalgam within multinucleated giant cells are surrounded by a dense lymphoplasmacytic cell infiltrate.

Right: Foreign body giant cell reaction to the amalgam deposits is surrounded by a prominent lymphocytic cell infiltrate including germinal centers.

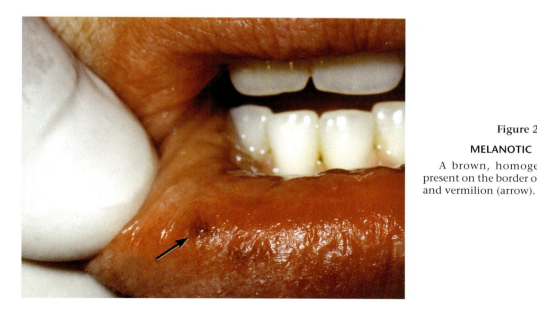

Figure 2-66

MELANOTIC MACULE

A brown, homogeneous macule is present on the border of the labial mucosa and vermilion (arrow).

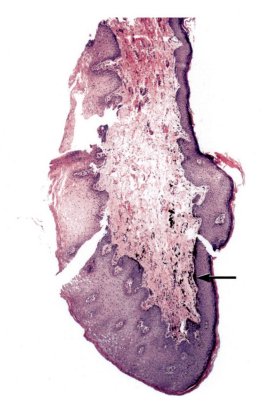 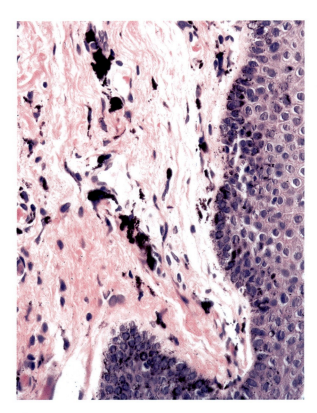

Figure 2-67

MELANOTIC MACULE

Left: Low magnification of a lip biopsy shows increased melanin pigment in the basal layer and lamina propria (arrow).
Right: Higher magnification shows the presence of focal but prominent melanin accumulation in the basal layer of epithelial cells and melanophages in the lamina propria, without the atypia or nesting that might suggest melanoma. Dendritic cells are absent in the epithelium.

not present. Fontana stain and melanin bleach identify the pigment as melanin (fig. 2-70).

The clinical differential diagnosis usually hinges on the exclusion of early melanoma, which corresponds to the absence of melanocytic atypia or pleomorphism. The combination of increased melanin in the basal layer with melanin incontinence supports the diagnosis of a melanotic macule. Melanin accumulation in the connective tissue areas alone, without an increase in basilar melanin, is better termed *melanin incontinence*. Melanin accumulation in the dendritic cells of the spinous layer of the epithelium is more characteristic of melanoacanthoma, although acanthosis and spongiosis may be seen in both melanoacanthoma and melanotic macule. Medication associated with pigmentation of the mucosa may histologically mimic a melanotic macule, and clinical correlation may be required to differentiate between melanotic macule and melanin pigmentation secondary to medicinal use.

A biopsy to exclude melanoma is generally considered appropriate therapy. Cryosurgery, laser surgery, and simple excision may be used, providing that tissue is preserved for histologic examination. Clinical diagnosis and follow-up with reassurance is adequate therapy for labial melanotic macule (230).

Black Hairy Tongue

Definition. *Black hairy tongue*, or *hairy tongue*, is a reactive condition resulting in an exaggerated form of filiform papillae on the dorsal surface of the tongue.

Clinical Features. Black hairy tongue is common, particularly in smokers (231). The midline dorsal mobile tongue is most often affected and

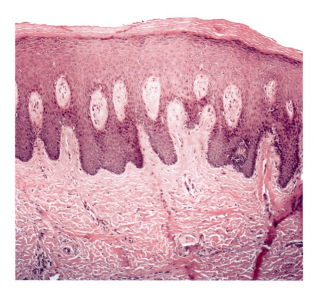 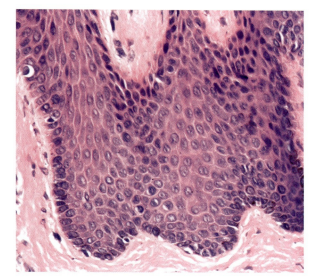

Figure 2-68

MELANOTIC MACULE

Left, right: There is focal increase in the melanin in the basal layer, particularly along the tips of the rete ridges.

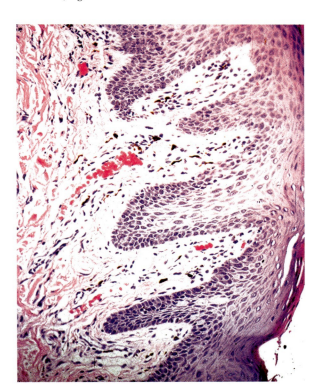 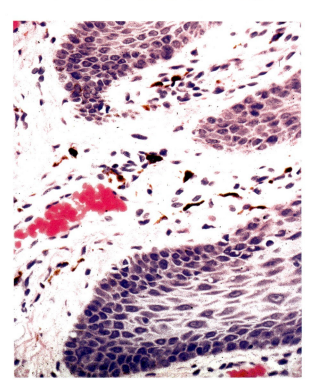

Figure 2-69

MELANOTIC MACULE

Left: Low magnification of a lip biopsy shows only faint melanin accumulation in the basal layer and prominent melanin incontinence in the lamina propria.

Right: Higher magnification shows that the melanophages in the lamina propria are devoid of nesting or cytologic atypia.

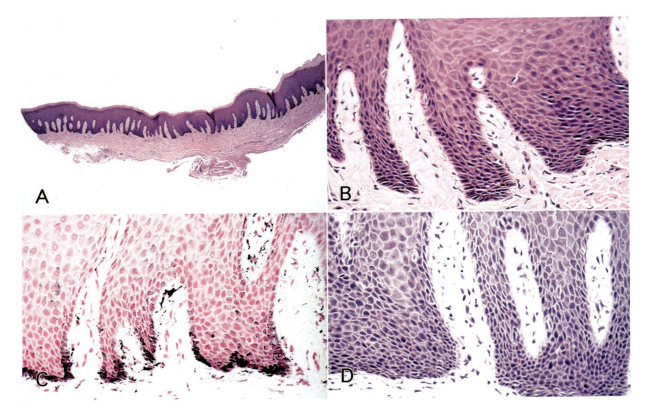

Figure 2-70

MELANOTIC MACULE

A: Melanin bleach is useful for defining the pigment seen in the basal layer.
B: Higher magnification shows the deposits in the basal layer of the epithelium.
C: A Fontana stain highlights the black pigment.
D: Melanin bleach removes the black pigment.

may be stained yellow, brown, or black (fig. 2-71). Elongation of the filiform papillae results in the hairy appearance, which may range from a coating to a shaggy, matted manifestation. The condition is often asymptomatic, but patients may be concerned about the appearance of their tongue. The condition is generally diagnosed clinically, but occasionally, is biopsied for confirmation.

Pathogenesis. Although the exact etiology is unknown, black hairy tongue is associated with a number of predisposing factors. Smoking, medications (e.g., bismuth salicylate containing medication, antibiotics), microorganisms (e.g., bacteria, fungi), chemical irritants, and poor oral hygiene are among the factors implicated in the development of black hairy tongue (232). There is no association with EBV.

Microscopic Findings. Hyperkeratosis of the filiform papillae, arranged into tall orthokeratin spires, is the hallmark of hairy tongue. The height of the orthokeratin spires is generally 3 to 4 times the width (233). There may be superficial colonies of bacteria and fungal elements, easily seen in cytologic scrapings, admixed with benign squamous cells (fig. 2-72). The mucosa may be chronically inflamed, but is not usually acanthotic, and the features of epithelial dysplasia should not be seen.

Differential Diagnosis. Although similar in name, black hairy tongue bears no relationship to oral hairy leukoplakia other than the "hairy" appearance (see earlier in this chapter). Hyperorthokeratosis may also be seen in verruca vulgaris, but a wart should be a focal lesion, not a diffuse covering of the dorsal tongue as is seen in black hairy tongue. Frictional keratosis is not as pronounced and is not common on the dorsal tongue.

Oral Cavity and Jaw

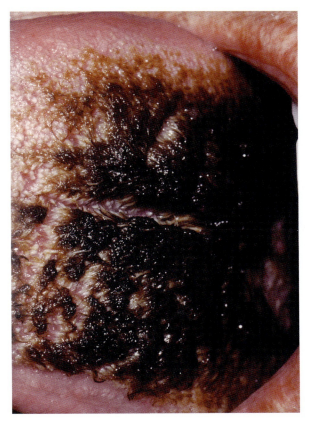

Figure 2-71
BLACK HAIRY TONGUE
A smoker's dorsal tongue with thick black coating.

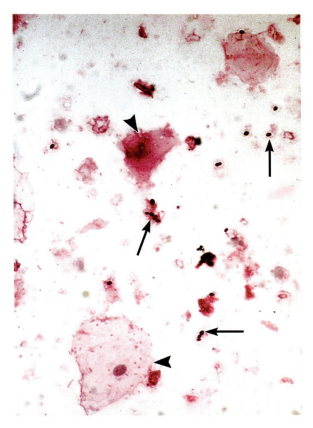

Figure 2-72
BLACK HAIRY TONGUE
Cytology specimen from tongue scraping in a patient with black hairy tongue shows fungal elements (spores; arrows) and benign keratinocytes (arrowheads).

Treatment and Prognosis. Improved oral hygiene, tongue brushing, and reduced tobacco use diminish black hairy tongue. For cases that are modulated by specific medical agents, the clinician may offer alternative agents.

Myospherulosis

Definition. *Myospherulosis* is a reactive fibroconnective lesion resulting from the placement of foreign body material.

Clinical Features. Myospherulosis is not unique to the oral tissues, but has been described in the sinonasal tract, ear/temporal bone, eyelid, skin, breast, and other locations (234). The placement of petrolatum-based products, usually as a vehicle for antibiotics, is associated with the development of the lesion (235). The exact mechanism is believed to be the interaction of the foreign material, most often the petrolatum-based product, and red blood cells; water soluble base materials seem not to be implicated. In some cases, that history may not be known since the lesions take years to become clinically evident. It is more common in the mandible, and may follow third molar extraction. The lesion may be symptomatic or may be discovered on routine radiographic examination.

The bony lesions are well circumscribed, solitary, radiolucent areas, usually at the site of a previous extraction (fig. 2-73). The surgical findings usually describe black, oily particles. Oral sites include mainly extraction sites, but also lower lip, graft site, and others.

Microscopic Findings. Dense fibroconnective tissue and a chronic inflammatory infiltrate are the background for the myospherulosis within which are cystic foci with pigmented (foreign) material (fig. 2-74). The inflammatory

177

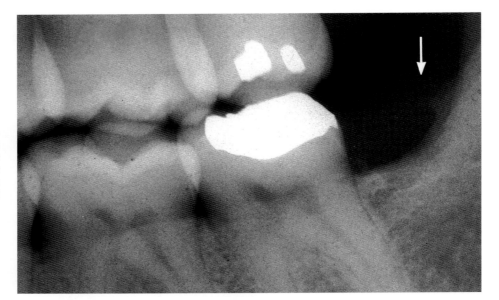

Figure 2-73

MYOSPHERULOSIS

The bite wing radiograph shows an ovoid 1-cm radiolucent area posterior to the second molar (arrow). The patient had a history of a previous third molar extraction.

population includes foreign body giant cells, lymphocytes, plasma cells, and macrophages. Cyst-like spaces containing brown spherules are the hallmark of the diagnosis and may be associated with giant cells (foreign body giant cell reaction) (fig. 2-74). True cyst lining is not a feature of the lesion. The spherules are red blood cells altered by the lipid product but retaining the golden brown color of hemoglobin and may be mistaken for infectious agents (fig. 2-75). Special stains for microorganisms are negative. The myospherules are positive for hemoglobin by immunohistochemistry.

Differential Diagnosis. The differential diagnosis of myospherulosis includes an infectious agent. Histochemical staining assists in excluding an infectious etiology.

Treatment and Prognosis. Biopsy confirms the diagnosis and is usually followed by complete resolution of the lesion.

ODONTOGENIC CYSTS

Odontogenic cysts are epithelial-lined cysts derived from the various components of the dental apparatus within the jaw bone. A thorough coverage of odontogenic cysts is beyond the scope of this text; the reader is referred to other texts that cover the full clinicopathologic spectrum of odontogenic cystic lesions (236). The following discussion is limited to the dentigerous cyst, glandular odontogenic cyst, lateral periodontal cyst, and periapical cyst, four common lesions that can be seen in daily practice. Odontogenic keratocyst (keratocystic odontogenic tumor) is a controversial entity in terms of whether it should be classified as a neoplasm or non-neoplastic odontogenic cyst. Odontogenic keratocyst is discussed within the differential diagnosis of dentigerous cyst.

Dentigerous Cyst

Definition. *Dentigerous cyst* is a developmental odontogenic cyst caused by the accumulation of fluid between the layers of the reduced enamel epithelium and the crown of the tooth, causing a separation of the follicle from the crown. It is also termed *follicular cyst*.

Clinical Features. Dentigerous cyst is the most common developmental odontogenic cyst, representing up to approximately 25 percent of all odontogenic cysts (236). It is more common in men than in women, and is most frequent in the second to fourth decades of life. Dentigerous cysts are always associated with the crown of an impacted or unerupted tooth. Permanent teeth are affected, most frequently the mandibular third molar, followed by the maxillary canines and third molars, and the mandibular second premolars.

The symptoms relate to the continuous expansion of the cyst and include displacement of teeth and facial asymmetry. With progression and expansion of the lesion to include bone, pain, numbness, and paresthesia may develop due to pressure

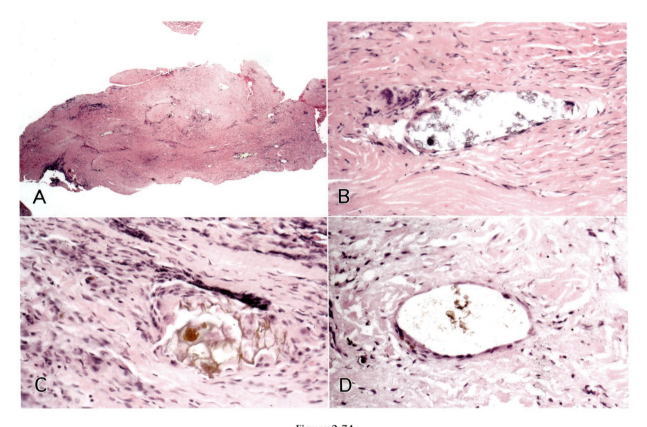

Figure 2-74

MYOSPHERULOSIS
A: Inflamed fibroconnective tissue with cystic foci and pigmented (foreign) material.
B: The cyst-like spaces lack lining cells and contain brown spherules.
C,D: Small cystic spaces contain spherules with associated giant cells (foreign body giant cell reaction).

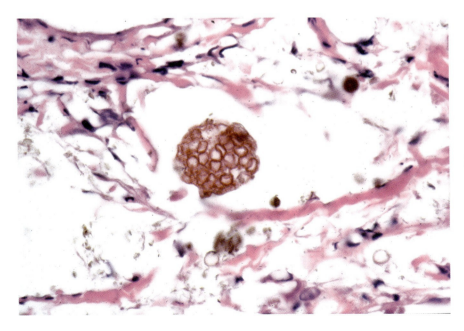

Figure 2-75

MYOSPHERULOSIS

The spherules are red blood cells altered by the lipid product but retaining the golden brown color of hemoglobin, and may be mistaken for an infectious agent. Special stains for microorganisms are negative.

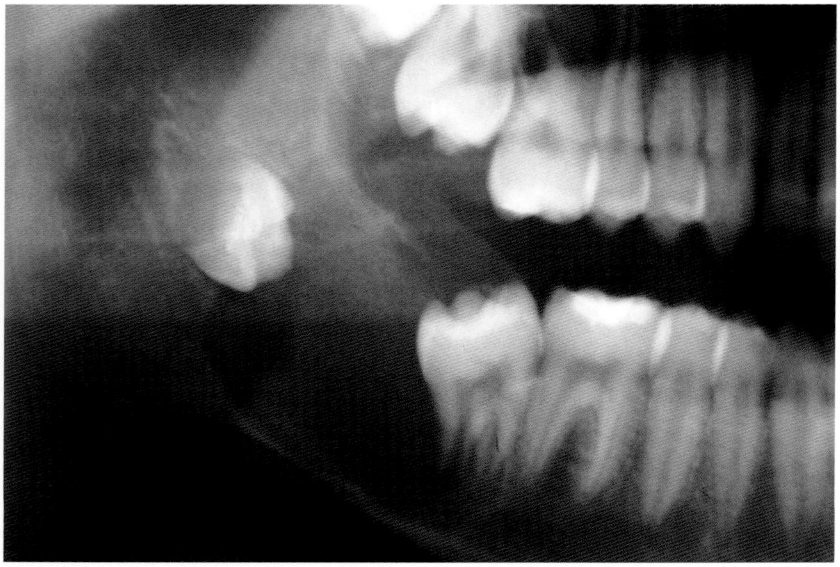

Figure 2-76

DENTIGEROUS CYST

A large unilocular radiolucent lesion envelopes the crown of the tooth.

on nerves. Superimposed infection may result in a partially erupted tooth causing swelling and pain. Dentigerous cysts typically are solitary, but rarely, may be multifocal (236,237).

The radiologic features include the presence of a well-defined, unilocular radiolucency surrounded by thin line of sclerotic bone (fig. 2-76). Three radiologic variations have been identified: central, lateral, and circumferential (236,238). Central lesions symmetrically envelop the crown of the tooth. Lateral lesions are asymmetric, with development by the follicle to one side of crown. In circumferential lesions, the entire tooth is encircled by radiolucency.

Gross Findings. Dentigerous cysts appear as a unilocular, smooth-walled cyst.

Microscopic Findings. In a *noninflamed dentigerous cyst*, the histologic features include a cyst lining that resembles reduced enamel epithelium, composed of two to three layers of flat cuboidal epithelium (fig. 2-77). The cyst wall is composed of thin fibroconnective that may be fibrous or fibromyxomatous, and may include nests and cords of odontogenic epithelium, foci of dystrophic calcifications, and under normal situations is devoid of an inflammatory cell component. Other less common findings identified in the epithelial component are mucus-containing cells (goblet cells or mucocytes), ciliated cells, and rarely, sebaceous cells (236).

In *inflamed dentigerous cysts*, the epithelial component may become thicker (hyperplastic), may be squamous in appearance, and may show downward expansion of the rete ridges (fig. 2-78). The cyst wall may show the presence of a mixed chronic inflammatory cell infiltrate, cholesterol clefts/granulomas, and a foreign body giant cell reaction. Rushton body formation appears as hyalinized, eosinophilic, angulated, linear or curved foci within the epithelium (fig. 2-78). Rushton bodies are of unknown origin and are not specific to dentigerous cysts; they are seen in other developmental and inflamed cysts including periapical (radicular) cysts and odontogenic keratocyst.

Dentigerous cysts are devoid of keratinization but rarely may show limited foci of surface keratinization. Occasionally, they may be orthokeratinized but lack the characteristic features of odontogenic keratocyst; the presence of more extensive surface keratinization may represent an odontogenic keratocyst (see under differential diagnosis).

Differential Diagnosis. The differential diagnosis includes an enlarged dental follicle (239). Dental follicles are characterized by a copious myxoid-appearing stroma with scattered identifiable epithelial (odontogenic cell) nests (fig. 2-79); the latter may be limited in extent. Other diagnostic considerations include periapical cyst, calcifying odontogenic cyst, unicystic ameloblastoma, odontogenic adenomatoid tumor, and squamous odontogenic tumor (240).

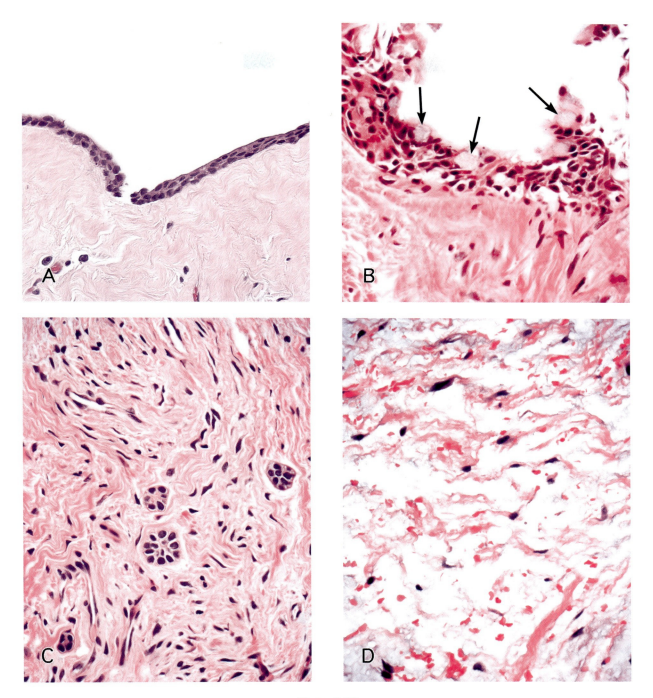

Figure 2-77

DENTIGEROUS CYST, NONINFLAMED

A: Noninflamed dentigerous cyst is lined by a thin layer of nonkeratinizing epithelium. The presence of a flat epithelium lacking rete ridges is similar to the epithelium seen in an odontogenic keratocyst (OKC) but the absence of features associated with OKC, including corrugated-appearing epithelium, basal epithelial cells with hyperchromatic nuclei and nuclear palisading, and separation of epithelial lining from underlying connective tissue allows for differentiating dentigerous cyst from OKC,

B: Mucous cells (arrows) are seen in the cyst lining epithelium.

C: Epithelial odontogenic rests in the cyst wall.

D: The fibromyxomatous stroma in dentigerous cyst may be misinterpreted as odontogenic myxoma.

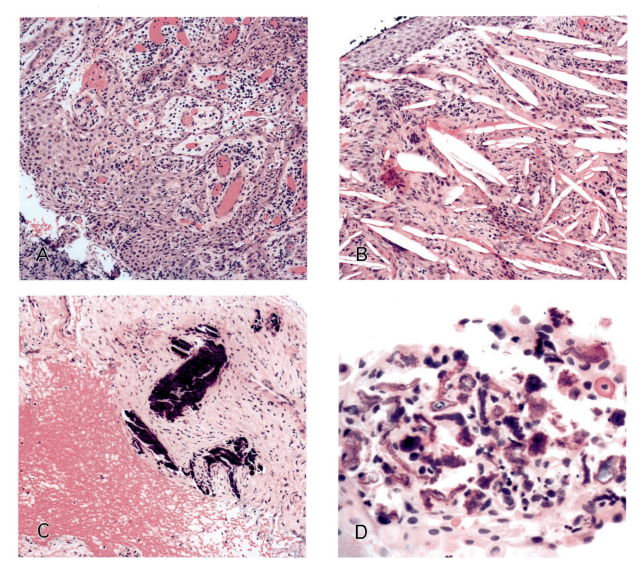

Figure 2-78

DENTIGEROUS CYST, INFLAMED

A: In an inflamed dentigerous cyst, the epithelial component becomes thicker (hyperplastic) and has a more squamous appearance.

B,C: Cholesterol granuloma formation (B) and dystrophic calcifications (C), also seen in the noninflamed cysts, are in the cyst wall.

D: Rushton body formation appears as hyalinized, eosinophilic, angulated, linear or curved foci within the epithelium; these formations are not unique to dentigerous cyst and can be seen in other odontogenic lesions (e.g., radicular cyst, odontogenic keratocyst).

In addition, the differential diagnosis includes odontogenic keratocyst (OKC), also referred to as keratocystic odontogenic tumor. OKC is a distinctive intraosseous, unicystic or multicystic tumor of odontogenic epithelial origin with specific clinical behavior and histopathologic features, including potentially aggressive (infiltrative) growth and an association with nevoid basal cell carcinoma syndrome.

OKCs tend to be more common in men than in women; occur over a wide age range but are most common in the second to third decades

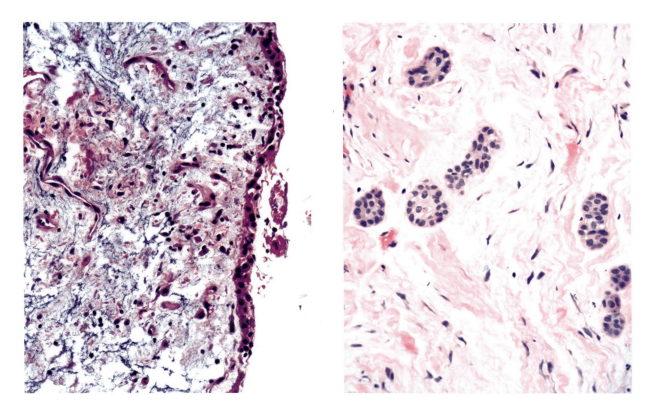

Figure 2-79

DENTAL FOLLICLE

Left: Reduced enamel epithelium and myxomatous stroma.
Right: Nests of odontogenic epithelium within the stroma may suggest a diagnosis of dentigerous cyst.

of life. OKCs affect the mandible more often than the maxilla (2 to 1); in the mandible, the most common location is in the posterior aspect, specifically the third molar and ramus area. The radiographic features are highly suggestive of the diagnosis but not diagnostic and include a well-defined or demarcated, round or ovoid unilocular radiolucency, with smooth to corticated margins. More than 80 percent of OKCs are unilocular. An unerupted or impacted tooth is part of the lesion in up to 40 percent of cases. In such instances, the radiologic appearance may suggest a diagnosis of dentigerous cyst. Resorption of the roots of teeth adjacent to OKC is uncommon and, if present, may be more suggestive of dentigerous or radicular cyst.

Histologically, the lining epithelium of OKC is composed of flat stratified squamous epithelium of 5 to 10 cell layers, with surface keratinization, including the presence of nuclei (parakeratosis). Characteristically, the epithelium has a corrugated (undulating or wavy) appearance (fig. 2-80). Additional findings include the absence of rete ridges, the presence of basal epithelial cells with hyperchromatic nuclei and nuclear palisading, and the separation of the epithelial lining from the underlying connective tissue, which is a common finding. Desquamated keratin (keratinaceous debris) can be found in the cyst lumens. An inflammatory cell component is typically absent to mild.

In the presence of intense inflammation, the characteristic features of the epithelial layers as described above may be absent and rete ridges may be present. Satellite cysts, including epithelial rests or small microcysts, may be present within the cyst wall. There may be mineralization/dystrophic calcification of the fibrous connective tissue cyst wall; cholesterol accumulation in the form of cholesterol clefts; epithelial hyaline bodies (Rushton bodies) appearing as hyalinized, eosinophilic, angulated, linear or curved foci within epithelium; melanin

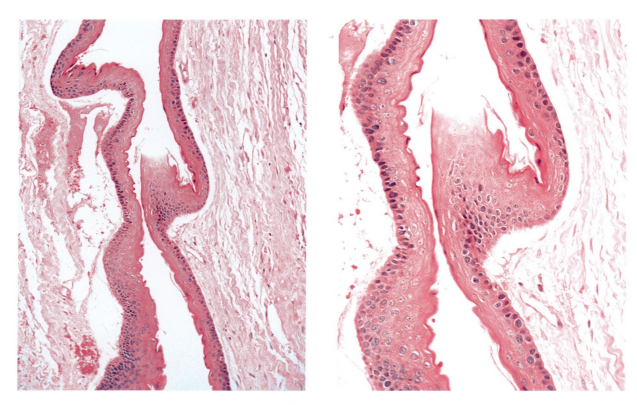

Figure 2-80

ODONTOGENIC KERATOCYST

Left, right: OKC is composed of flat stratified squamous epithelium of 5 to 10 cell layers with a characteristic corrugated (undulating or wavy) appearance. The findings include surface keratinization, parakeratosis, absence of rete ridges, basal epithelial cells with hyperchromatic nuclei, and nuclear palisading separating the epithelium from the connective tissue.

pigment and melanocytes; respiratory-type epithelium; mucocytes; and sebaceous glands.

The lesions associated with the nevoid basal cell carcinoma syndrome tend to show more satellite cysts, solid islands of epithelial proliferation, rests of odontogenic epithelium within the fibrous capsule, and foci of calcifications. Most OKCs harbor chromosomal abnormalities (loss of heterozygosity), supporting a neoplastic nature (241).

The treatment of choice for OKC is complete surgical excision of the lesion in one piece. This may prove difficult given the friable nature of the cyst wall. OKCs have the potential to be locally destructive and invade adjacent soft tissues and bone. They tend to recur, with the reported frequency varying from approximately 5 percent to more than 60 percent (242). Recurrence may be a function of inadequate surgical removal of the entire cyst including the cyst lining. Recurrence is more common in association with mandibular lesions, especially those located in the posterior body and ascending ramus. Multiple recurrences are not unusual. Usually, recurrence occurs within 5 years of the initial diagnosis, but may occur 10 or more years later. For this reason, long-term follow-up, including periodic radiologic imaging, is advocated.

Other than the tendency to recur, the overall prognosis is very good. Occasional cases may not be controllable by surgery but behave in a progressive manner with destructive growth, including extension to the skull base. Rare examples are associated with malignant transformation (squamous cell carcinoma) (242).

Treatment and Prognosis. The usual treatment for dentigerous cyst is careful enucleation of the cyst and removal of the involved tooth (238). Larger cysts are managed by marsupialization (236,243). Recurrence is uncommon and generally relates to incomplete excision. Dentigerous cysts may rarely give rise to various odontogenic tumors including ameloblastoma, mucoepidermoid carcinoma, and squamous cell carcinoma (236,238,244).

Eruption Cyst

Eruption cyst is a variant of dentigerous cyst. It is a dilation of the normal follicular space. It develops secondary to the accumulation of blood or fluid between the tooth crown and an erupting or permanent tooth and the overlying mucosa (236).

Eruption cysts occur almost exclusively in infants and young children. They are more common with deciduous mandibular central incisors, maxillary incisors, and first molars. They present as a bluish, firm to fluctuant swelling of the alveolar ridge overlying the erupted tooth. They are usually asymptomatic but if inflamed may be painful and tender. Eruption cysts are not detectable by radiology as these cysts develop outside bone.

The histologic findings include the presence of a cyst lined by nonkeratinized stratified squamous epithelium with a chronic inflammatory cell infiltrate in the cyst wall. Eruption cysts usually resolve spontaneously with eruption of the associated tooth.

Glandular Odontogenic Cyst

Definition. *Glandular odontogenic cyst* is a rare developmental odontogenic cyst that may show glandular or salivary features and aggressive behavior. It is also termed *sialo-odontogenic cyst*.

Clinical Features. The glandular odontogenic cyst occurs most commonly in the fifth to sixth decades of life. Most lesions occur in the anterior region of the mandible and may cross the midline (fig. 2-81). The lesion ranges from less than 1 cm to large destructive lesions involving most of the jaw (245–247).

Microscopic Findings. Squamous epithelium of various thickness lines the glandular odontogenic cyst. The superficial cells are cuboidal to columnar, with eosinophilic cytoplasm and frequently with mucin-producing cells (goblet cells) resulting in a hobnail surface outline ("hobnail cells") (fig. 2-82). The surface cells often have cilia. Intraepithelial microcysts or duct-like spaces are seen and are lined by a single layer of cuboidal to columnar cells,

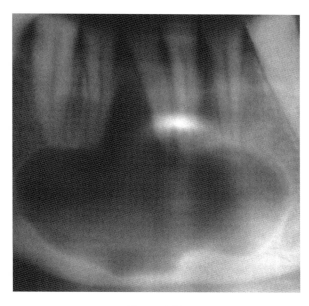

Figure 2-81

GLANDULAR ODONTOGENIC CYST

An expansile cyst in the anterior mandible crosses the midline.

similar to surface cells. The microcysts may be lined by goblet cells, may contain mucous pools and eosinophilic material, or may appear to be empty. In areas, the microcysts open onto the surface of the lining epithelium.

The hobnail cells may show apocrine snouting, characterized by "pinching off" of the surface, similar to the decapitation secretion seen in cells that line apocrine gland ducts. Clear or vacuolated cells may be present in the basal or parabasal layers; such cells contain glycogen. Papillary projections or "tufting" into the cyst lumen may be seen. The papillary projections sometimes are formed by several microcysts opening onto the surface of the cyst lining, but may also be formed independent of the microcyst. Epithelial spheres or plaque-like thickenings with a swirled appearance may be focally identified (fig. 2-82); such foci are histologically similar to those seen in association with lateral odontogenic cyst and botryoid odontogenic cyst.

Differential Diagnosis. There is some diagnostic overlap between the features of glandular odontogenic cyst and those of an interosseous low-grade cystic mucoepidermoid carcinoma. Examination of multiple sections, however, usually permits the differentiation of these lesions.

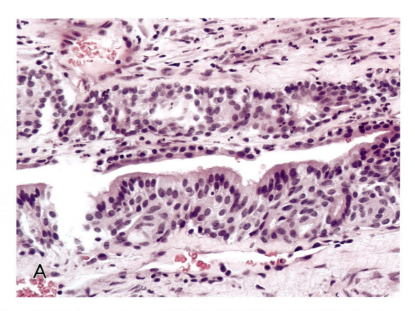

Figure 2-82

GLANDULAR ODONTOGENIC CYST

A: The cyst is lined by stratified squamous epithelium which has surface columnar and cuboidal cells. Intraepithelial microcysts or duct-like spaces are present.

B: Mucous (goblet) cells are present singly or in small clusters (arrows).

C: Epithelial spheres or plaque-like thickenings have a swirled or whorled appearance (arrow); similar epithelial swirls are seen in lateral odontogenic cyst and botryoid odontogenic cyst.

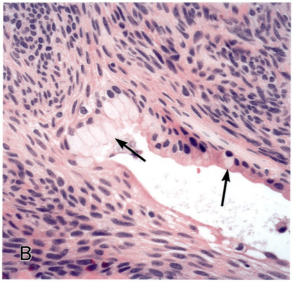

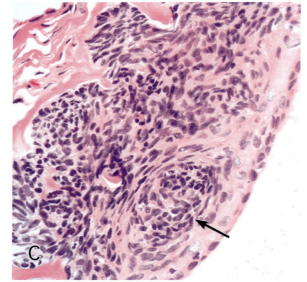

It is reported that glandular odontogenic cysts do not show *MAML2* gene rearrangements which are often found in central mucoepidermoid carcinoma (248).

Treatment and Prognosis. This cyst shows a propensity for recurrence, which occurs in 25 to 30 percent of cases (236). Because of the probability of recurrence, some authors advocate en block resection.

Lateral Periodontal Cyst

Lateral periodontal cyst is an uncommon type of developmental odontogenic cyst occurring along the lateral surface of a tooth. It is also called *botryoid odontogenic cyst*.

The lateral periodontal cyst is often asymptomatic and detected only during a radiographic examination. It is common in the fifth through seventh decades of life, with 75 to 80 percent occurring in the mandibular premolar-lateral incisor area (249). Those cysts occurring in the maxilla occur in the same tooth region (250). Most of lesions are unicystic and are less than 1 cm in diameter.

The epithelial lining is usually squamous, only one to three cell layers. Some cysts show focal nodular thickening of the lining, which is composed chiefly of clear cells (fig. 2-83).

Conservative enucleation of the cyst is the treatment of choice. Recurrence is unusual but has been reported in the botryoid variant cysts (251).

Periapical Cyst

Definition. *Periapical cyst* is an inflammatory odontogenic lesion in which the epithelium at the apex of a nonvital tooth is stimulated by inflammation to form a true epithelial-lined cyst. Synonyms include *radicular cyst*, *apical cyst*, *apical periodontal cyst*, and *dental cyst*.

Clinical Features. Periapical cyst is the most common cyst of the jaw (252). There is no gender predilection, and while it may occur at any age it most commonly occurs in the third decade of life. Periapical cysts may affect any tooth, but are most common in the maxilla.

Most patients are asymptomatic unless there is exacerbation by an acute inflammatory reaction. Symptoms associated with the affected tooth include pain during mastication and sensitivity to percussion. Multiple cysts may develop in the same patient. There is no association with any syndromes. Radiographic features include the presence of a well-circumscribed, unilocular radiolucency of variable size surrounding the apex of the involved tooth (252).

Pathogenesis. Periapical cysts develop as a sequela of a pre-existing periapical granuloma; however, the progression from a periapical granuloma to a periapical cyst is not inevitable. Periapical granuloma, also referred to as chronic apical periodontitis, represents a mass of granulation tissue at the apex of a nonvital tooth resulting from the escape of inflammatory cells and bacterial products from a necrotic pulp, usually caused by dental caries (252). Periapical granulomas may develop following resolution of a periapical abscess.

Microscopic Findings. When not inflamed, the cyst is lined with nonkeratinizing stratified squamous epithelium without hyperplastic changes (fig. 2-84). In the presence of inflammation, the epithelial lining of the cyst may be hyperplastic, with acanthosis and spongiosis (fig. 2-84). Infrequently, a variable number of mucocytes are seen. Those cysts that approximate a paranasal sinus may be lined, in

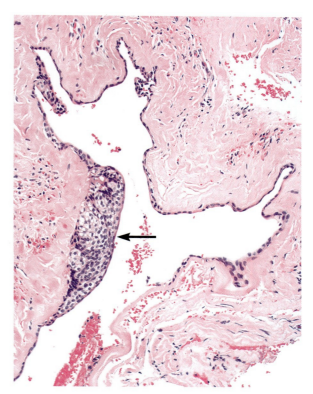

Figure 2-83

LATERAL PERIODONTAL CYST

Focal nodular epithelial thickenings (arrow) are present.

part or in total, by pseudostratified respiratory epithelium. The cyst lumen is filled with fluid and cellular debris. The cyst wall consists of dense fibroconnective tissue with an admixed acute and chronic inflammatory cell infiltrate. Additional histologic findings in the cyst lumen, epithelium, or cyst wall include mineralization/dystrophic calcification, cholesterol clefts with multinucleated giant cells (cholesterol granulomas), and hemorrhage (recent and remote in the form of hemosiderin deposition). Rushton (hyaline) bodies appear as small circumscribed pools of eosinophilic material in the cyst wall that may be surrounded by an inflammatory cell infiltrate, including neutrophils, lymphocytes, plasma cells, and multinucleated giant cells, as well as dystrophic calcification.

Periapical granulomas are composed of granulation tissue with associated mixed acute and chronic inflammation and surrounded by fibrous connective tissue. Among the chronic

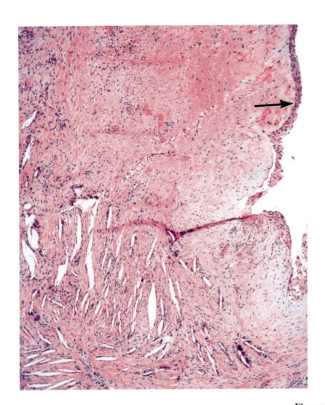 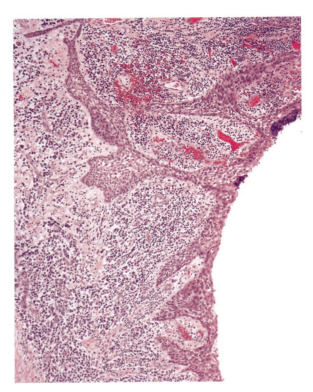

Figure 2-84

PERIAPICAL (RADICULAR) CYST

Left: Noninflamed cysts are lined by nonkeratinizing stratified squamous epithelium without hyperplastic changes (arrow). Cholesterol granuloma formation is present in the cyst wall.

Right: Inflamed cysts are lined by hyperplastic (proliferating) squamous epithelium.

inflammatory cells seen are mature plasma cells with intracytoplasmic eosinophilic globules representing immunoglobulins (Russell bodies) and foamy (lipid-laden) histiocytes. Scattered epithelial nests (rests of Malassez) may be present within the granulation tissue. Cholesterol granulomas, fresh hemorrhage, and hemosiderin deposition may be present. Scattered small foci of neutrophilic accumulation (abscess) may be found but do not reach a level diagnostic for a periapical abscess. *Periapical abscess* represents the accumulation of neutrophils at the apex of a nonvital tooth.

Differential Diagnosis. The differential diagnosis includes a variety of odontogenic and nonodontogenic cysts, as well as a periapical scar. Periapical scar is the area in bone in which a defect is created by a periapical inflammatory lesion and filled in with dense collagenous tissue (252–254). The features seen in association with a periapical scar are similar to those of periapical cyst and granuloma: involvement of a nonvital tooth, asymptomatic presentation, and presence of a sharply delineated radiolucency. Histologically, periapical scars consist of collagenous stroma with sparse inflammatory cells. The diagnosis of a periapical scar is suspected in the presence of a history of a previous periapical lesion, and radiographic imaging shows evidence of root canal filling.

Treatment and Prognosis. The treatment for both periapical cysts and periapical granulomas is the same and includes curettage following extraction of the involved tooth or conservative nonsurgical endodontic therapy, with or without extraction of the root apex. Recurrence is rare. Incomplete excision, however, may result in a residual (periapical) cyst. Residual (periapical) cyst is the designation used for periapical cysts that remain in the jaw after extraction of the associated tooth (252). The potential complications of both periapical cysts and periapical granulomas is the formation of an abscess, which in turn may progress into osteomyelitis. There is no known progression of a periapical cyst or granuloma to an ameloblastoma.

SELECTIVE AUTOIMMUNE, ALLERGIC, SYSTEMIC, AND CUTANEOUS-TYPE DISEASES AFFECTING THE ORAL CAVITY

The oral cavity may be involved by a wide variety of autoimmune, systemic, and cutaneous-type diseases. This section is limited to a few such diseases that occur in the oral cavity. The reader is referred to more detailed texts for further discussion (255,256).

Granulomatosis with Polyangiitis

Granulomatosis with polyangiitis (GPA), formerly referred to as *Wegener granulomatosis,* is a non-neoplastic, idiopathic aseptic necrotizing disease with a predilection for the upper/lower respiratory tract and the genitourinary system. It is characterized by the presence of vasculitis and destructive properties. This classic definition calls for involvement of the head and neck region, the lung, and the kidney. Most patients do not exhibit this classic clinical triad simultaneously at the time of initial presentation, and the initial biopsy material may originate from lesions of the upper aerodigestive tract in the absence of a clinical suspicion of GPA. The oral manifestations of GPA include an ulcerative lesion and gingivitis. For a more complete discussion see chapter 1.

Lichen Planus

Definition. *Lichen planus* (LP) is an immunologically mediated mucocutaneous disorder that often presents as a chronic dermatologic disease, but also commonly affects the oral mucosa.

Clinical Features. After cutaneous LP, oral LP is the next most common site of occurrence, and up to 35 percent of patients have only oral manifestations (257,258). Oral LP is more common in women than in men and is a disease of middle-aged people; pediatric LP is uncommon (259). Oral LP occurs in several forms: reticular, papular, plaque-like, atrophic, erosive, and bullous (260–263).

The reticular and erosive forms of oral LP are the most common forms. The *reticular form* of LP most commonly affects the posterior buccal mucosa and may be bilateral; other sites of involvement include the tongue (lateral and dorsal), gingiva, palate, and lip vermilion border. Sites of involvement may be concurrent. The designation as reticular is because the lesions have a characteristic pattern of interlacing white lines (so-called Wickham striae); reticular LP of the dorsal tongue, however, appears as a keratotic plaque. Patients are usually asymptomatic.

The *erosive form* of oral LP is often symptomatic, with patients complaining of associated pain. The lesion appears as an atrophic, erythematous area with central ulceration. Peripheral to the ulcer, interlacing white striations (Wickham striae) may be seen. Gingival involvement may result in desquamative gingivitis, necessitating biopsy to exclude other diseases (e.g., cicatrial pemphigoid). In severe cases, there may be epithelial separation, resulting in bullous LP.

Pathogenesis. The pathogenesis of LP is unknown but evidence points to a cell-mediated immune response (264). Many medications have been implicated in lesions that clinically simulate LP, with similar histologic findings; these lesions are referred to as lichenoid drug eruptions, and more specifically, relative to the oral mucosa, have been termed lichenoid mucositis. Lichenoid drug eruptions, including lichenoid mucositis, appear to represent a systemic anaphylactic reaction (265).

Microscopic Findings. The histopathologic findings of LP include epithelial hyperplasia (acanthosis) or atrophy, hyperkeratosis (parakeratosis and orthokeratosis), a saw-tooth configuration of the rete ridges, and a characteristic dense, band-like chronic inflammatory cell infiltrate at the interface of the epithelium and submucosa (interface mucositis) (fig. 2-85). Additional changes include hydropic degeneration (liquifaction) of the basal cell layer and dyskeratotic basal keratinocytes referred to as Civatte bodies (fig. 2-85). The chronic inflammatory cell infiltrate is predominantly composed of mature T lymphocytes. These overall findings are not specific or pathognomonic but need to be correlated with the clinical picture in order to correctly diagnose the lesion.

Differential Diagnosis. Histologically, there are numerous pathologic process with a lichenoid inflammatory reaction, including but not limited to lichenoid drug eruptions (260). The list of the medications association with

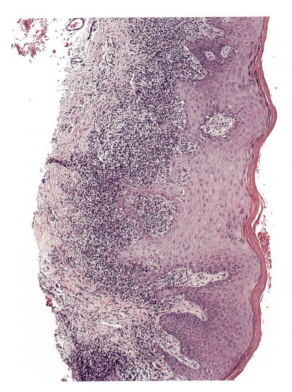 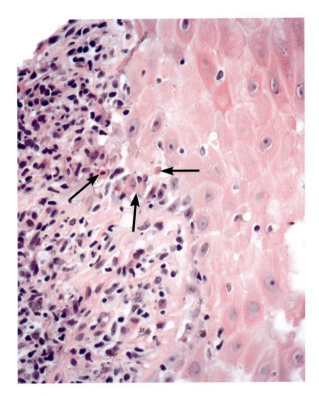

Figure 2-85

LICHEN PLANUS

Left: The histopathologic findings of lichen planus include hyperkeratotic and hyperplastic squamous epithelium with saw-toothed rete ridges and a band-like (lichenoid) inflammatory cell infiltrate at the interface of the epithelium and submucosa (interface mucositis).

Right: Degeneration of the basal layer of the epithelium with degenerating keratinocytes (arrows) and subjacent lymphocytic cell infiltrate.

lichenoid drug eruption is extensive; a partial list includes antibiotics (ketoaconazole, streptomycin, tetracycline), antihypertensive drugs (chlorothiazide, methyldopa, propranolol, spironolactone), nonsteroidal anti-inflammatory medication (naproxan, indomethacin, ibuprofen), antimalarials, and sulfonyureas (257). Once identified, discontinuation of the drug usually leads to clearing of the lesions over a period of several weeks.

Treatment and Prognosis. The treatment for oral LP is predicated on the extent of the disease. The reticular form of LP does not necessarily require treatment since it is often asymptomatic and undergoes spontaneous remission in over 50 percent of cases. Superimposed fungal infection (e.g., candidiasis) requires antifungal therapy. For limited oral erosive LP, topical corticosteroids are used. For extensive oral erosive LP, systemic corticosteroids are used; close monitoring for secondary oral candidiasis is required. Whether the erosive form of LP can undergo malignant transformation is still debatable and inconclusive (266,267), and the development of squamous cell carcinoma in the setting of LP may be more coincidental than causative. There is, however, increasing literature suggesting a premalignant potential for oral LP (268,269).

Aphthous Stomatitis

Definition. *Aphthous stomatitis* (AS) is a painful ulcerative disorder of unattached oral mucous membrane. The etiology is unknown and there is a tendency to recur. Synonyms include *canker sore* and *recurrent aphthous stomatitis*.

Clinical Features. AS is one of the more common recurrent ulcerative processes to affect the oral mucosa. There are three clinical forms: *minor*

AS, major AS, and herpetiform AS. The most common clinical form is the minor AS, seen in up to 80 percent of patients. Ulcers of the minor AS form occur more commonly in women than in men, and often begin in childhood or adolescence (270). The ulcers occur as a solitary lesion or in groups, tend to measure less than 1 cm in greatest dimension, and heal within 7 to 10 days without scarring. They tend to occur on nonkeratinized mucosa, with the buccal and labial mucosae representing the more common sites of occurrence. They may involve the tongue (ventral surface), floor of mouth, and soft palate. Involvement of keratinizing mucosa, such as the gingiva, hard palate, dorsal tongue, and lip vermilion border usually occurs as extension from an ulcer on an adjacent nonkeratinizing surface and rarely occurs as an isolated lesion at these keratinizing sites.

The ulcers are painful, with the level of pain often out of proportion to the size of the lesion. The ulcers are covered by a white to yellow, mucopurulent exudate that is removable and is surrounded by an erythematous halo. The recurrence rate of these ulcers vary from one every few years to several in a month. The designation of "recurrent aphthous stomatitis" should be reserved for recurrent ulcers confined to the mouth and seen in the absence of systemic disease (270).

Major AS occurs in a minority of patients (approximately 10 percent), the onset is usually after puberty, and ulcers recur over decades. These ulcers are also painful but are larger and deeper than the ulcers of minor AS; occur over movable mucosa with soft palate, lip, and tonsillar regions most commonly affected; and may take several weeks to heal, with the resolution of the healing process resulting in submucosal scarring. The number of ulcers varies from a single ulcer to as many as 10 ulcers.

The ulcers of herpetiform AS are more common in women than in men, occur in adulthood, tend to be smaller (1 to 2 mm) but are typically multiple. They may coalesce into larger irregular ulcers, most often on nonkeratinizing movable mucosa. They take up to 10 days to heal and have a higher frequency of recurrence over shorter periods of time. Due to their resemblance to the ulcers of herpes simplex virus, they have been termed herpetiform.

There are no specific laboratory findings associated with or diagnostic of AS. In contrast to such lesions as granulomatosis with polyangiitis (formerly Wegener granulomatosis), serum antineutrophil cytoplasmic antibodies (ANCA) and proteinase 3 levels are not elevated.

Pathogenesis. The etiology of AS includes trauma, stress, allergies, familial (genetic) predisposition, nutritional deficiencies, medications, and infections (257,270–272). AS has been associated with a number of systemic diseases, including Behçet disease, inflammatory bowel disease, celiac disease, Reiter disease, and immunocompromised conditions (e.g., AIDS/HIV disease) (270).

Microscopic Findings. The histologic findings are nonspecific. Early ulcers show central ulceration with associated fibrinopurulent exudates; deep to the ulcers, there is increased vascularity and a mixed nonspecific acute and chronic inflammation of the submucosa. Since the histology is nonspecific and not diagnostic for AS, the diagnosis requires clinical correlation. Biopsies are necessary in order to exclude other diagnoses.

Differential Diagnosis. The differential diagnosis includes a wide variety of other oral cavity ulcerative lesions, including (but not limited to) infections, vasculitic processes, and neoplasms. Special stains for microorganisms may be required to exclude an infectious etiology. The histologic findings of AS should allow for differentiating it from vasculitic lesions and neoplasms.

The differential diagnosis also include oral-related aphthoid ulceration caused by systemic diseases and other autoimmune processes. Features such as persistent diarrhea, which are suggestive of systemic disease, should raise the possibility of inflammatory bowel disease (i.e., Crohn disease or ulcerative colitis) (270). Weight loss or other signs of malabsorption may suggest gluten-sensitive enteropathy.

Behçet syndrome is another disease that clinically may resemble AS. In contrast to AS, Behçet syndrome involves extraoral sites (genital ulceration, uveitis, retinitis and conjunctivitis) (257,270). It is rare for patients apparently presenting with recurrent aphthous stomatitis subsequently to be found to have Behçet syndrome (270). Joint pain and swelling, or urethritis suggests the possibility of a syndrome of reactive arthritis (formerly known as Reiter syndrome), which is an associated condition.

Oral ulcers are seen in association with HIV infection. A detailed clinical history, including laboratory analysis (if warranted), should allow for a diagnosis of HIV infection and differentiation from the ulcers associated with AS.

Treatment and Prognosis. Solitary AS ulcers are usually self-limiting and require no therapy. Topical steroids have been used for minor AS ulcers. Low-dose systemic corticosteroids have been used for patients whose ulcers are not responsive to topical steroids. Close monitoring for secondary oral candidiasis is required. For major ulcers, intralesional corticosteroid therapy may prove effective.

RADIATION-ASSOCIATED CHANGES

Definition. *Radiation-associated injury* to the upper aerodigestive tract, including the oral cavity, pharynx, and larynx, is a fairly common occurrence because radiation treatment is the initial therapeutic modality for malignant neoplasms of these sites (273). Radiation therapy is predominantly, but not exclusively, used to treat squamous cell carcinoma of these sites.

Clinical Features. The gender and demographics of patients with radiation-associated changes typically follow those associated with upper aerodigestive tract squamous cell carcinoma, which more often affects men than women and occurs in a wide range of adult ages.

Early clinical manifestations associated with radiation include mucositis, aguesia (loss of taste), xerostomia (dry mouth), mucosal ulceration, and laryngeal edema. Delayed complications include persistent ulcers, persistent laryngeal edema, persistent xerostomia, and necrosis of soft tissue and bone (osteoradionecrosis) (273). Osteonecrosis of the jaw is a severe complication of radiotherapy for oral malignant neoplasms and more commonly occurs in the mandible than the maxilla (273). Acute changes occur from days to weeks (usually 6 weeks) following treatment; chronic changes are seen from 6 to 7 weeks to years following therapy (273). Biopsies are taken following radiation therapy to primarily exclude the possibility of recurrent carcinoma.

Microscopic Findings. Radiation to mucosal sites causes alterations in the surface epithelium, minor salivary glands, fibroblasts, skeletal muscle, and endothelial cells. Radiation-induced changes may be acute or chronic. During the acute postirradiation phase (days to weeks), biopsies are seldom obtained. Acute changes associated with radiation therapy include submucosal edema, degenerative changes of the basal layer of the surface epithelium, and ectatic changes of minor salivary gland ducts and acini.

Biopsies taken in the later (chronic) postirradiation period show variable histologic changes, including a thinner than normal surface epithelium, surface ulceration, squamous epithelial atypia, atrophy of minor salivary gland acini, pseudoepitheliomatous proliferation of minor salivary glands, squamous metaplasia of minor salivary glands with or without dyskeratosis and cytologic atypia, submucosal fibrosis, vascular alterations characterized by telangiectatic capillaries often with prominent (plump) endothelial cells, myointimal proliferation, foamy histiocytes within the intima and thrombosis, as well as atypical (bizarre) fibroblasts, and bizarre striated muscle degeneration.

Characteristically, the atypical (bizarre) fibroblasts, referred to as radiation fibroblasts, are at least twice as large as normal fibroblasts. They have large, hyperchromatic nuclei with a "smudged" appearance and have abundant basophilic-appearing cytoplasm with irregular, angulated ends (fig. 2-86). Usually, radiation fibroblasts appear isolated within the submucosa and lack the clustering or nested appearance often (but not always) seen in association with recurrent/persistent squamous cell carcinoma.

The histologic changes of osteonecrosis are nonspecific and show the typical features associated with bone necrosis, including loss of osteoblasts, fibrous replacement of bone marrow, reduction of bone marrow vasculature, and acute osteomyelitis. Infected osteoradionecrosis (IORN) typically occurs in a patient with oral squamous cell carcinoma treated with radiation who develops osteoradionecrosis. It is characterized by fragments of necrotic bone intimately associated with bacterial colonies showing findings consistent with *Actinomyces* infection as well as an associated neutrophilic cell infiltrate (fig. 2-87). Actinomycosis of the jaw is a rare disease described in patients with IORN and bisphosphonate-associated osteonecrosis (BON) (274–276).

In IORN, a benign squamous epithelial proliferation representing pseudocarcinomatous

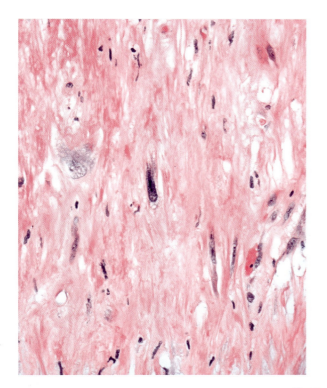 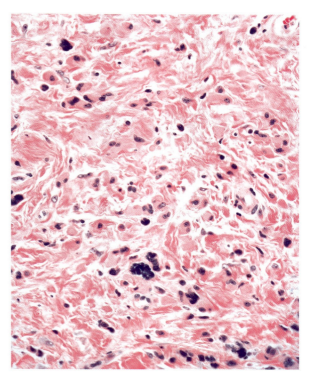

Figure 2-86

POSTRADIATION CHANGES

Left: Atypical (bizarre) fibroblasts (radiation fibroblasts) are characterized by enlarged and hyperchromatic nuclei with a "smudged" appearance and basophilic-appearing cytoplasm with irregular, angulated ends. Usually, radiation fibroblasts appear isolated within the submucosa and lack the clustering or nested appearance often seen in association with squamous cell carcinoma.

Right: Bizarre degenerated striated muscle cells.

hyperplasia (PCH) (277,278) or pseudoepitheliomatous hyperplasia (PEH) may be present. Since gnathic bone lies close to the epithelial structures of both the gum and periodontium, PCH/PEH is strongly associated with the occurrence of fistula. Mandibular involvement is much more common than involvement of the maxilla. The critical issue is whether epithelium represents PCH/PEH or invasive carcinoma. The histologic features favoring PCH/PEH include fragments of squamous epithelium in the medullary space directly applied to necrotic bone trabeculae and bland-appearing squamous cells lacking the cytomorphologic features of squamous cell carcinoma. Often, PCH/PEH is characterized by a more mature epithelial layer covering bone trabeculae without intervening stroma, and a basal-type epithelial layer surrounding a central fibrovascular core. Invasive squamous cell carcinoma tends to include tumoral islands within a centro-medullary area, surrounded by stroma with the cytomorphologic features of malignancy.

Differential Diagnosis. The key diagnostic and differential diagnostic issue is to not misdiagnose radiation-induced alterations for squamous cell carcinoma (persistent, recurrent, new) or vice versa. Certainly, the knowledge that the patient has received radiation therapy would assist in at least alerting the pathologist that radiation-induced changes may be present. Unfortunately, detailed clinical information to include essential information such as prior radiotherapy is often lacking and the surgical pathologist may not be apprised of such a possibility. This is problematic, especially in the setting of intraoperative consultation/frozen section diagnosis. Not infrequently, the pathologist is tasked to analyze

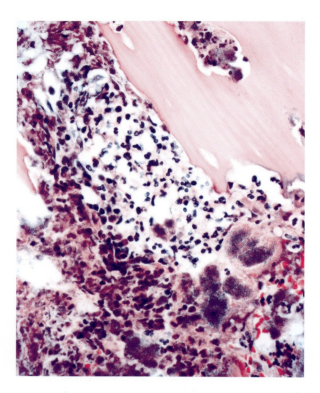 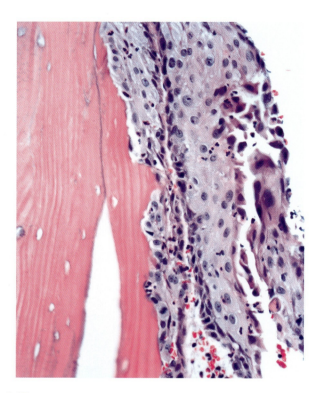

Figure 2-87

INFECTED OSTEORADIONECROSIS AND PSEUDOCARCINOMATOUS HYPERPLASIA

Left: Infected osteoradionecrosis includes necrotic bone and an associated neutrophilic infiltrate with bacterial colonies consistent with *Actinomyces* species.

Right: In pseudocarcinomatous hyperplasia, the squamous epithelium from an oral cavity fistula is directly applied to bone; the squamous epithelium consists of bland cells lacking the cytomorphologic features of carcinoma.

tissue at the time of frozen section to determine whether the changes reflect those of postradiation alterations or squamous cell carcinoma. The retention of the lobular configuration of the minor salivary glands, presence of "smudged" nuclei of the atypical fibroblasts, and absence of cohesive cellular grouping of the atypical fibroblasts scattered in scar formation or inflammatory tissue assist in distinguishing radiation change from carcinoma.

REFERENCES

Embryology, Anatomy, and Histology

1. Moore KL, Persaud TV. The respiratory system. In: Moore KL, Persaud TV, eds. The developing human: clinically oriented embryology, 7th ed. Philadelphia: Saunders; 2003:242-253.
2. Hollinshead WH. The jaws, palate, and tongue. In: Hollinshead WH, ed. Anatomy for surgeons, vol. 1, 3rd ed. Philadelphia: Harper & Row; 1982:325-387.
3. Standring S. Oral cavity. In: Standring S, ed. Gray's anatomy. The anatomical basis of clinical practice, 40th ed. Edinburgh: Elsevier Churchill Livingstone; 2008:499-525.
4. Pantanowitz L, Balogh K. Mouth, nose, and paranasal sinuses. In: Mills SE, ed. Histology for pathologists, 4th ed. Philadelphia: Lippincott Williams & Wilkins; 2012:433-459.
5. Ide F, Mishima K, Saito I. Melanin pigmentation in the juxtaoral organ of Chievitz. Pathol Int 2003;53:262-263.

Hamartomas and Choristomas, Fordyce's Granules

6. Dilley DC, Siegel MA, Budnick S. Diagnosing and treating common oral pathologies. Pediatr Clin North Am 1991;38:1227-1264.
7. Halperin V, Kolas S, Jeffries KR, Huddleston SD, Robinson HB. The occurrence of Fordyce spots, benign migratory glossitis, median rhomboid glossitis and fissured tongue in 2,478 dental patients. Oral Surg Oral Med Oral Pathol 1953;6:1072-1077.
8. Miles AE. Sebaceous glands in the lip and cheek mucosa of man. Br Dent J 1958;105:235-248.
9. Daley TD. Intraoral sebaceous hyperplasia. Diagnostic criteria. Oral Surg Oral Med Oral Pathol 1993;75:343-347.
10. Alawi F, Siddiqui A. Sebaceous carcinoma of the oral mucosa: case report and review of the literature. Oral Surg Oral Med Oral Pathol Oral Radiol Endod 2005;99:79-84.
11. Wang H, Yao J, Solomon M, Axiotis CA. Sebaceous carcinoma of the oral cavity: a case report and review of the literature. Oral Surg Oral Med Oral Pathol Oral Radiol Endod 2010;110:e37-40.

Ectopic Thyroid Tissue

12. Baughman RA. Lingual thyroid and lingual thyroglossal tract remnants. A clinical and histopathologic study with a review of the literature. Oral Surg Oral Med Oral Pathol 1972;34:781-799.
13. Kansal P, Sakati N, Rifai A, Woodhouse N. Lingual thyroid. Diagnosis and treatment. Arch Intern Med 1987;147:2046-2048.
14. Katz AD, Zager WJ. The lingual thyroid. Its diagnosis and treatment. Arch Surg 1971;102:582-585.
15. Kumar V, Nagendhar Y, Prakash B, Chattopadhyay A, Vepakomma D. Lingual thyroid gland: clinical evaluation and management. Indian J Pediatr 2004;71:e62-64.
16. Nienas FW, Gorman CA, Devine KD, Woolner LB. Lingual thyroid. Clinical characteristics of 15 cases. Ann Intern Med 1973;79:205-210.
17. Barnes TW, Olsen KD, Morgenthaler TI. Obstructive lingual thyroid causing sleep apnea: a case report and review of the literature. Sleep Med 2004;5:605-607.
18. Abdallah-Matta MP, Dubarry PH, Pessey JJ, Caron P. Lingual thyroid and hyperthyroidism: a new case and review of the literature. J Endocrinol Invest 2002;25:264-267.
19. Willinsky RA, Kassel EE, Cooper PW, et al. Computed tomography of lingual thyroid. J Comput Assist Tomogr 1987;11:182-183.
20. Goldstein B, Westra WH, Califano J. Multifocal papillary thyroid carcinoma arising in a lingual thyroid: a case report. Arch Otolaryngol Head Neck Surg 2002;128:1198-1200.
21. Perez JS, Munoz M, Naval L, Blasco A, Diaz FJ. Papillary carcinoma arising in lingual thyroid. J Craniomaxillofac Surg 2003;31:179-182.
22. Seoane JM, Cameselle-Teijeiro J, Romero MA. Poorly differentiated oxyphilic (Hurthle cell) carcinoma arising in lingual thyroid: a case report and review of the literature. Endocr Pathol 2002;13:353-360.

Oral Choristoma

23. Bajay P. Shubha BS, Agarwal K, Aggarwal C, Glial choristoma. Indian J Pediatr 2002;69:437-439.
24. Kadkade P, Planksy T, Bent JP, Prasad M. Radiology quiz case 2. Heterotopic gastrointestinal cyst of the oral cavity. Arch Otolaryngol Head Neck Surg 2004;130:373-375.
25. Wetmore RF, Bartlett SP, Pepsin B, Todd NW. Heterotopic gastric mucosa of the oral cavity: a rare entity. Int J Pediatr Otorhinolayngol 2002;66:139-142.
26. Matsushita K, Tahara M, Sato H, Nakamura E, Fujiwara T. Cartilaginous choristoma deep in the upper midline oral vestibule. Br J Oral Maxillofac Surg 2004;42:436-438.
27. Wacrenier A, Fayoux P, Augusto D, Laussel AC, Gosseling B, Leroy X. Gastric heterotopia in the nasopharynx. Int J Pediatr Otorhinolayngol 2002;64:65-67.
28. Krolls SO, Jacoway JR, Alexander WN. Osseous choristomas (osteomas) of intraoral soft tissues. Oral Surg Oral Med Oral Pathol 1971;32:588-595.

29. Chou LS, Hansen LS, Daniels TE. Choristomas of the oral cavity; a review. Oral Surg Oral Med Oral Pathol 1991;72:584-593.
30. Kaminagakura E, Andrade CR, Rangel AL, et al. Sebaceous adenoma of oral cavity: report of case and comparative proliferation study with sebaceous gland hyperplasia and Fordyce's granules. Oral Dis 2003;9:323-327.

Exostoses

31. Kolas S, Halperin V, Jefferis K, Huddleston S, Robinson HB. The occurrence of torus palatinus and torus mandibularis in 2,478 dental patients. Oral Surg Oral Med Oral Pathol 1953;6:1134-1141.
32. Bouquot JE, Gundlach KK. Oral exophytic lesions in 23,616 white Americans over 35 years of age. Oral Surg Oral Med Oral Pathol 1986;62:284-291.
33. Jainkittivong A, Langlais RP. Buccal and palatal exostoses: prevalence and concurrence with tori. Oral Surg Oral Med Oral Pathol Oral Radiol Endod 2000;90:48-53.

Oral Lymphoepithelial Cyst

34. Buchner A, Hansen LS. Lymphoepithelial cysts of the oral cavity. A clinicopathologic study of thirty-eight cases. Oral Surg Oral Med Oral Pathol 1980;50:441-449.
35. Hu JA, Li YN, Li SY. [Oral lymphoepithelial cyst: report of 3 cases.] Shanghai Kou Qiang Yi Xue 2005;4:197-199. [Chinese]
36. Proctor B, Proctor C. Congenital lesions of the head and neck. Otolaryngol Clin North Am 1970;3:221-248.

Nasopalatine Duct Cyst

37. Allard RH, van der Kwast WA, van der Waal I. Nasopalatine duct cyst. Review of the literature and report of 22 cases. Int J Oral Surg 1981;10:447-461.
38. Daley TD, Wysocki GP, Pringle GA. Relative incidence of odontogenic tumors and oral and jaw cysts in a Canadian population. Oral Surg Oral Med Oral Pathol 1994;77:276-280.
39. Elliott KA, Franzese CB, Pitman KT. Diagnosis and surgical management of nasopalatine duct cysts. Laryngoscope 2004;114:1336-1340.
40. Swanson KS, Kaugers GE, Gunsolley JC. Nasopalatine duct cyst: an analysis of 334 cases. J Oral Maxillofac Surg 1991;49:268-271.
41. Nortje CJ, Wood RE. The radiologic features of the nasopalatine duct cyst. An analysis of 46 cases. Dentomaxillofac Radiol 1988;17:129-132.
42. Takagi R, Ohashi Y, Suzuki M. Squamous cell carcinoma in the maxilla probably originating from a nasopalatine duct cyst: report of case. J Oral Maxillofac Surg 1996;54:112-115.

Fungal Disease, Candidiasis

43. Epstein JB, Polsky B. Oropharyngeal candidiasis: a review of its clinical spectrum and current therapies. Clin Ther 1998;20:40-57.
44. Fotos PG, Vincent SD, Hellstein JW. Oral candidosis. Clinical, historical, and therapeutic features of 100 cases. Oral Surg Oral Med Oral Pathol 1992;74:41-49.
45. Holmstrup P, Axéll T. Classification and clinical manifestations of oral yeast infections. Acta Odontol Scand 1990;48:57-59.
46. Lehner T. Oral thrush, or acute pseudomembranous candidiasis: a clinicopathologic study of forty-four cases. Oral Surg Oral Med Oral Pathol 1964;18:27-37.
47. Flaitz CM, Hicks MJ. Oral candidiasis in children with immune suppression: clinical appearance and therapeutic considerations. ASDC J Dent Child 1999;66:161-166.
48. Terai H, Shimahara M. Atrophic tongue associated with Candida. J Oral Pathol Med 2005;34:397-400.
49. Carter LC. Median rhomboid glossitis: review of a puzzling entity. Compendium 1990;11:446-451.
50. Kolokotronis A, Kioses V, Antoniades D, Mandraveli K, Doutsos I, Papanayotou P. Median rhomboid glossitis. An oral manifestation in patients infected with HIV. Oral Surg Oral Med Oral Pathol 1994;78:36-40.
51. van der Waal I, Beemster G, van der Kwast WA. Median rhomboid glossitis caused by Candida? Oral Surg Oral Med Oral Pathol 1979;47:31-35.
52. Wright BA. Median rhomboid glossitis: not a misnomer. Review of the literature and histologic study of twenty-eight cases. Oral Surg Oral Med Oral Pathol 1978;46:806-814.
53. Sitheeque MA, Samaranayake LP. Chronic hyperplastic candidosis/candidiasis (candidal leukoplakia). Crit Rev Oral Biol Med 2003;14:253-267.
54. Allen CM. Diagnosing and managing oral candidiasis. J Am Dent Assoc 1992;123:77-82.

Human Papillomavirus

55. Syrjanen S, Puranen M. Human papillomavirus infections in children: the potential role of maternal transmission. Crit Rev Oral Biol Med 2000;11:259-274.
56. Begum S, Cao D, Gillison M, Zahurak M, Westra WH. Tissue distribution of human papillomavirus 16 DNA integration in patients with tonsillar carcinoma. Clin Cancer Res 2005;11:5694-5699.
57. Chaturvedi AK, Engels EA, Pfeiffer RM, et al. Human papillomavirus and rising oropharyngeal cancer incidence in the United States. J Clin Oncol 2011;29:4294-4301.

58. Dyson N, Howley PM, Münger K, Harlow E. The human papillomavirus-16 E7 oncoprotein is able to bind the retinoblastoma gene product. Science 1989;243:934-937.
59. Al-Bakkal G, Ficarra G, McNeill K, Eversole LR, Sterrantino G, Birek C. Human papilloma virus type 16 E6 gene expression in oral exophytic epithelial lesions as detected by in situ rtPCR. Oral Surg Oral Med Oral Pathol Oral Radiol Endod 1999;87:197-208.
60. McKaig RG, Baric RS, Olshan AF. Human papillomavirus and head and neck cancer: Epidemiology and molecular biology. Head Neck 1998;20:250-265.
61. Steinberg BM. Human papillomavirus and head and neck cancer. In: Harrison LB, Sessions RB, Hong WK. Head and neck caner. A multidisciplinary approach. Second edition. Philadelphia; Lippincott Williams & Wilkins; 2004:973-984.

Cytomegalovirus

62. Brantsaeter AB, Liestol K, Goplen AK, Dunlop O, Bruun JN. CMV disease in AIDS patients: incidence of CMV disease and relation to survival in a population-based study from Oslo. Scand J Infect Dis 2002;34:50-55.
63. Eversole LR. Viral infections of the head and neck among HIV-seropositive patients. Oral Surg Oral Med Oral Pathol 1992;73:155-163.
64. Klatt EC, Shibata D. Cytomegalovirus infection in the acquired immunodeficiency syndrome. Clinical and autopsy findings. Arch Pathol Lab Med 1988;112:540-544.
65. Lalwani AK, Snyderman NL. Pharyngeal ulceration in AIDS patients secondary to cytomegalovirus infection. Ann Otol Rhinol Laryngol 1991;100:484-487.
66. Victoria JM, Guimaraes AL, da Silva LM, Kalapothakis E, Gomez RS. Polymerase chain reaction for identification of herpes simplex virus (HSV-1), cytomegalovirus (CMV) and human herpes virus-type 6 (HHV-6) in oral swabs. Microbiol Res 2005;160:61-65.
67. Abdel-Haq N, Chearskul P, Al-Tatari H, Asmar B. New antiviral agents. Indian J Pediatr 2006;73:313-321.
68. Biron KK. Antiviral drugs for cytomegalovirus diseases. Antiviral Res 2006;71:154-163.

Herpes Virus

69. Eversole LR. Inflammatory diseases of the mucous membranes. Part 1. Viral and fungal infections. J Calif Dent Assoc 1994;22:52-57.

Gonorrhea

70. Barlow D. The diagnosis of oropharyngeal gonorrhea. Genitourin Med 1997;73:16-17.
71. Bruce AJ, Rogers RS 3rd. Oral manifestations of sexually transmitted diseases. Clin Dermatol 2004;22:520-527.
72. Hutt DM, Judson FN. Epidemiology and treatment of oropharyngeal gonorrhea. Ann Intern Med 1986;104:655-658.
73. Siegel MA. Syphilis and gonorrhea. Dent Clin North Am 1996;40:368-383.
74. Workowski KA, Berman S, Centers for Disease Control and Prevention. Sexually transmitted disease treatment guidelines, 2010. MMWR Recomm Rep 2010;59:1-110.

Syphilis

75. Pletcher SD, Cheung SW. Syphilis and otolaryngology. Otolaryngol Clin North Am 2003;36:595-605.
76. Carey JC. Congenital syphilis in the 21st century. Curr Womens Health Rep 2003;3:299-302.
77. Fiumara NJ, Lessell S. Manifestations of late congenital syphilis. An analysis of 271 patients. Arch Dermatol 1970;102:78-83.
78. Simmank KC, Pettifor JM. Unusual presentation of congenital syphilis. Ann Trop Paediatr 2000;20:105-107.
79. Wendel GD Jr, Sheffield JS, Hollier LM, Hill JB, Ramsey PS, Sanchez PJ. Treatment of syphilis in pregnancy and prevention of congenital syphilis. Clin Infect Dis 2002;35:S200-209.
80. Barrett AW, Villarroel Dorrego M, Hodgson TA, et al. The histopathology of syphilis of the oral mucosa. J Oral Pathol Med 2004;33:286-291.

Verruca Vulgaris

81. Eversole LR, Laipis PJ, Green TL. Human papillomavirus type 2 DNA in oral and labial verruca vulgaris. J Cutan Pathol 1987;14:319-325.
82. Green TL, Eversole LR, Leider AS. Oral and labial verruca vulgaris: clinical, histological, and immunohistochemical evaluation. Oral Surg Oral Med Oral Pathol 1986;62:410-416.

Condyloma Acuminatum

83. Neville BW, Damm DD, Allen CM, Bouquot JE. Epithelial pathology. In: Neville BW, Damm DD, Allen CM, Chi AC, eds. Oral & maxillofacial pathology, 4th ed. St. Louis: Elsevier; 2016:334-335.
84. Leigh JE, Shetty K, Fidel PL, Jr. Oral opportunistic infections in HIV-positive individuals: review and role of mucosal immunity. AIDS Patient Care STDS 2004;18:443-456.
85. Butler S, Molinari JA, Plzia RA, Chandrasekar P, Vewnkat H. Condyloma acuminatum in the oral cavity: four cases and a review. Rev Infect Dis 1988;10:544-550.

86. Nash M, Lucente FE, Srinivasan K, Gould WJ. Condylomatous lesions of the upper aerodigestive tract. Laryngoscope 1987;97:1410-1416.
87. Henley JD, Summerlin DJ, Tomich CE. Condyloma acuminatum and condyloma-like lesions of the oral cavity: a study of 11 cases with an intraductal component. Histopathology 2004;44:216-221.
88. Zunt SL, Tomich CE. Oral condyloma acuminatum. J Dermatol Surg Oncol 1989;15:591-594.
89. Eversole LR, Laipis PJ, Merrell P, Choi E. Demonstration of human papillomavirus DNA in condyloma acuminatum. J Oral Pathol 1987;16:626-672.
90. Garlick JA, Taichman LB. Human papillomavirus infection of the oral mucosa. Am J Dermatopathol 1991;13:386-395.
91. Kui LL, Xiu HZ, Ning LY. Condyloma acuminatum and human papilloma virus infection in the oral mucosa of children. Pediatr Dent 2003;25:149-153.
92. Syrjänen S. PL7 Oral viral infections that could be transmitted oro-genitally. Oral Dis 2006;12(suppl 1):2.
93. Syrjänen S, Puranen M. Human papillomavirus infections in children: the potential role of maternal transmission. Crit Rev Oral Biol Med 2000;11:259-274.

Focal Epithelial Hyperplasia

94. Archard HO, Heck JW, Stanley HR. Focal epithelial hyperplasia: an unusual oral mucosal lesion found in Indian children. Oral Surg Oral Med Oral Pathol 1965;20:201-212.
95. Witkop CJ Jr, Niswander JD. Focal epithelial hyperplasia in central and south american indians and ladinos. Oral Surg Oral Med Oral Pathol 1965;20:213-217.
96. Bassioukas K, Danielides V, Georgiou I, Photos E, Zagorianakou P, Skevas A. Oral focal epithelial hyperplasia. Eur J Dermatol 2000;10:395-397.
97. Cohen PR, Hebert AA, Adler-Storthz K. Focal epithelial hyperplasia: Heck disease. Pediatr Dermatol 1993;10:245-251.
98. Eversole LR. Papillary lesions of the oral cavity: relationship to human papillomaviruses. J Calif Dent Assoc 2000;28:922-927.
99. Harris AM, van Wyk CW. Heck's disease (focal epithelial hyperplasia): a longitudinal study. Community Dent Oral Epidemiol 1993;21:82-85.
100. Flaitz CM. Focal epithelial hyperplasia: a multifocal oral human papillomavirus infection. Pediatr Dent 2000;22:153-154.
101. Jayasooriya PR, Abeyratne S, Ranasinghe AW, Tilakaratne WM. Focal epithelial hyperplasia (Heck's disease): report of two cases with PCR detection of human papillomavirus DNA. Oral Dis 2004;10:240-243.
102. Moerman M, Danielides VG, Nousia CS, Van Wanzeele F, Forsyth R, Vermeersch H. Recurrent focal epithelial hyperplasia due to HPV13 in an HIV-positive patient. Dermatology 2001;203:339-341.
103. Viraben R, Aquilina C, Brousset P, Bazex J. Focal epithelial hyperplasia (Heck disease) associated with AIDS. Dermatology 1996;193:261-262.

Oral Hairy Leukoplakia

104. Conant MA. Hairy leukoplakia. A new disease of the oral mucosa. Arch Dermatol 1987;123:585-587.
105. Sciubba JJ. Opportunistic oral infections in the immunosuppressed patient: oral hairy leukoplakia and oral candidiasis. Adv Dent Res 1996;10:69-72.
106. Sciubba J, Brandsma J, Schwartz M, Barrezueta N. Hairy leukoplakia: an AIDS-associated opportunistic infection. Oral Surg Oral Med Oral Pathol 1989;67:404-410.
107. Schiodt M, Greenspan D, Daniels TE, Greenspan JS. Clinical and histologic spectrum of oral hairy leukoplakia. Oral Surg Oral Med Oral Pathol 1987;64:716-720.
108. Hille JJ, Webster-Cyriaque J, Palefski JM, Raab-Traub N. Mechanisms of expression of HHV8, EBV and HPV in selected HIV-associated oral lesions. Oral Dis 2002;8(Suppl 2):161-168.
109. Mabruk MJ, Flint SR, Toner M, et al. In situ hybridization and the polymerase chain reaction (PCR) in the analysis of biopsies and exfoliative cytology specimens for definitive diagnosis of oral hairy leukoplakia (OHL). J Oral Pathol Med 1994;23:302-308.
110. Walling DM, Ling PD, Gordadze AV, Montes-Walters M, Flaitz CM, Nichols CM. Expression of Epstein-Barr virus latent genes in oral epithelium: determinants of the pathogenesis of oral hairy leukoplakia. J Infect Dis 2004;190:396-399.
111. de la Rosa-Garcia E, Mondragon-Padilla A, Irigoyen-Camacho ME, Bustamante-Ramirez MA. Oral lesions in a group of kidney transplant patients. Med Oral Patol Oral Cir Bucal 2005;10:196-204.
112. King GN, Healy CM, Glover MT, et al. Prevalence and risk factors associated with leukoplakia, hairy leukoplakia, erythematous candidiasis, and gingival hyperplasia in renal transplant recipients. Oral Surg Oral Med Oral Pathol 1994;78:718-726.
113. Lozada-Nur F, Robinson J, Regezi JA. Oral hairy leukoplakia in nonimmunosuppressed patients. Report of four cases. Oral Surg Oral Med Oral Pathol 1994;78:599-602.

114. Miranda C, Lozada-Nur F. Oral hairy leukoplakia in an HIV-negative patient with systemic lupus erythematosus. Compend Contin Educ Dent 1996;17:408-410.
115. Schiodt M, Norgaard T, Greenspan JS. Oral hairy leukoplakia in an HIV-negative woman with Behçet's syndrome. Oral Surg Oral Med Oral Pathol Oral Radiol Endod 1995;79:53-56.
116. Zakrzewska JM, Aly Z, Speight PM. Oral hairy leukoplakia in a HIV-negative asthmatic patient on systemic steroids. J Oral Pathol Med 1995;24:282-284.
117. Coogan MM, Greenspan J, Challacombe SJ. Oral lesions in infection with human immunodeficiency virus. Bull World Health Organ 2005;83:700-706.

Verruciform Xanthoma

118. Philipsen HP, Reichart PA, Takata T, Ogawa I. Verruciform xanthoma—biological profile of 282 oral lesions based on a literature survey with nine new cases from Japan. Oral Oncol 2003;39:325-336.
119. Travis WD, Davis GE, Tsokos M, et al. Multifocal verruciform xanthoma of the upper aerodigestive tract in a child with a systemic lipid storage disease. Am J Surg Pathol 1989;13:309-316.
120. Neville B. The verruciform xanthoma. A review and report of eight new cases. Am J Dermatopathol 1986;8:247-253.
121. Allen CM, Kapoor N. Verruciform xanthoma in a bone marrow transplant recipient. Oral Surg Oral Med Oral Pathol 1993;75:591-594.
122. Jensen JL, Liao SY, Jeffes EW 3rd. Verruciform xanthoma of the ear with coexisting epidermal dysplasia. Am J Dermatopathol 1992;14:426-430.
123. Helm KF, Hopfl RM, Kreider JW, Lookingbill DP. Verruciform xanthoma in an immunocompromised patient: a case report and immunohistochemical study. J Cutan Pathol 1993;20:84-86.
124. Visintini E, Rizzardi C, Chiandussi S, Biasotto M, Melato M, Di Lenarda R. Verruciform xanthoma of the oral mucosa. Report of a case. Minerva Stomatol 2006;55:639-645.
125. de Andrade BA, Agostini M, Pires FR, et al. Oral verruciform xanthoma: a clinicopathologic and immunohistochemical study of 20 cases. J Cutan Pathol 2015;42:489-495.
126. Drummond JF, White DK, Damm DD, Cramer JR. Verruciform xanthoma within carcinoma in situ. J Oral Maxillofac Surg 1989;47:398-400.
127. Mannes KD, Dekle CL, Requena L, Sangueza OP. Verruciform xanthoma associated with squamous cell carcinoma. Am J Dermatopathol 1999;21:66-69.

Inflammatory Papillary Hyperplasia

128. Bhaskar SN, Beasley JD, Cutright DE. Inflammatory papillary hyperplasia of the oral mucosa: report of 341 cases. J Am Dent Assoc 1970;81:949-982.
129. Moskona D, Kaplan I. Oral lesions in elderly denture wearers. Clin Prev Dent 1992;14:11-14.

Pseudoepitheliomatous Hyperplasia

130. Abu Eid R, Landini G. Morphometry of pseudoepitheliomatous hyperplasia: objective comparison to normal and dysplastic oral mucosae. Anal Quant Cytol Histol 2005;27:232-240.
131. Gacek MR, Gacek RR, Gantz B, McKenna M, Goodman M. Pseudoepitheliomatous hyperplasia versus squamous cell carcinoma of the external auditory canal. Laryngoscope 1998;108(Pt 1):620-623.
132. Rousseau A, Cornet M, Carnot F, Brasnu D, Bruneval P, Badoual C. [Mycoses of the head and neck.] Ann Pathol 2005;25:104-116. [French]
133. Courville P, Wechsler J, Thomine E, et al. Pseudoepitheliomatous hyperplasia in cutaneous T-cell lymphoma. A clinical, histopathological and immunohistochemical study with particular interest in epithelial growth factor expression. The French Study Group on Cutaneous Lymphoma. Br J Dermatol 1999;140:421-426.
134. Takeda Y, Sasou S, Obata K. Pleomorphic adenoma of the minor salivary gland with pseudoepitheliomatous hyperplasia of the overlying oral mucosa: report of two cases. Pathol Int 1998;48:389-395.
135. Grauwin MY, Mane I, Cartel JL. Pseudoepitheliomatous hyperplasia in trophic ulcers in leprosy patients. A 28-case study. Lepr Rev 1996;67:203-207.
136. Zarovnaya E, Black C. Distinguishing pseudoepitheliomatous hyperplasia from squamous cell carcinoma in mucosal biopsy specimens from the head and neck. Arch Pathol Lab Med 2005;129:1032-1036.

Proliferative Verrucous Leukoplakia

137. Gillenwater AM, Vigneswaran N, Fatani H, Saintigny P, El-Naggar AK. Proliferative verrucous leukoplakia (PVL): a review of an elusive pathologic entity! Adv Anat Pathol 2013;20:416-423.
138. Carrard VC, Brouns ER, van der Waal I. Proliferative verrucous leukoplakia; a critical appraisal of the diagnostic criteria. Med Oral Patol Oral Cir Bucal 2013;18:e411-413.
139. Arduino PG, Bagan J, El-Naggar AK, Carrozzo M. Urban legends series: oral leukoplakia. Oral Dis 2013;19:642-659.

140. Cabay RJ, Morton TH Jr, Epstein JB. Proliferative verrucous leukoplakia and its progression to oral carcinoma: a review of the literature. J Oral Pathol Med 2007;36:255-261.
141. Bagan JV, Jimenez Y, Murillo J, et al. Lack of association between proliferative verrucous leukoplakia and human papillomavirus infection. J Oral Maxillofac Surg 2007;65:46-49.
142. Campisi G, Giovannelli L, Ammatuna P, et al. Proliferative verrucous vs conventional leukoplakia: no significantly increased risk of HPV infection. Oral Oncol 2004;40:835-840.
143. Navarro CM, Sposto MR, Sgavioli-Massucato EM, Onofre MA. Transformation of proliferative verrucous leukoplakia to oral carcinoma: a ten years follow-up. Med Oral 2004;9:229-233.
144. Hansen LS, Olson JA, Silverman S Jr. Proliferative verrucous leukoplakia. A long-term study of thirty patients. Oral Surg Oral Med Oral Pathol 1985;60:285-298.

Peripheral Ossifying Fibroma

145. Buchner A, Hansen LS. The histomorphologic spectrum of peripheral ossifying fibroma. Oral Surg Oral Med Oral Pathol 1987;63:452-461.
146. Childers EL, Morton I, Fryer CE, Shokrani B. Giant peripheral ossifying fibroma: a case report and clinicopathologic review of 10 cases from the literature. Head Neck Pathol 2013;7:356-360.
147. Cuisia ZE, Brannon RB. Peripheral ossifying fibroma—a clinical evaluation of 134 pediatric cases. Pediatr Dent 2001;23:245-248.
148. Carrera Grano I, Berini Aytes L, Escoda CG. Peripheral ossifying fibroma. Report of a case and review of the literature. Med Oral 2001;6:135-141.

Peripheral Odontogenic Fibroma

149. Buchner A, Ficarra G, Hansen LS. Peripheral odontogenic fibroma. Oral Surg Oral Med Oral Pathol 1987;64:432-438.
150. Ficarra G, Sapp JP, Eversole LR. Multiple peripheral odontogenic fibroma, World Health Organization type, and central giant cell granuloma: a case report of an unusual association. J Oral Maxillofac Surg 1993;51:325-328.
151. Neville BW, Damm DD, Allen CM, Bouquot JE. Peripheral odontogenic fibroma. In: Neville BW, Damm DD, Allen CM, Chi AC, eds. Oral & maxillofacial pathology, 4th ed. St. Louis: Elsevier; 2016:678.
152. Ritwik P, Brannon RB. Peripheral odontogenic fibroma: a clinicoapthologic study of 151 cases and review of the literature with special emphasis on recurrence. Oral Surg Oral Med Oral Pathol Oral Radiol Endod 2010;110:357-363.

Irritation Fibroma

153. Giunta JL. Gingival fibrous nodule. Oral Surg Oral Med Oral Pathol Oral Radiol Endod 1999;88:451-454.
154. Hedin CA, Gerner L, Larsson A. The retrocuspid papilla and factor XIIIa: an epidemiologic and histomorphologic study. Scand J Dent Res 1994;102:290-294.
155. Cutright DE. The histopathologic findings in 583 cases of epulis fissuratum. Oral Surg Oral Med Oral Pathol 1974;37:401-411.
156. Buchner A, Merrell PW, Hansen LS, Leider AS. The retrocuspid papilla of the mandibular lingual gingiva. J Periodontol 1990;61:585-589.

Giant Cell Fibroma

157. Bakos LH. The giant cell fibroma: a review of 116 cases. Ann Dent 1992;51:32-35.
158. Houston GD. The giant cell fibroma. A review of 464 cases. Oral Surg Oral Med Oral Pathol 1982;53:582-587.
159. Gonsalves WC, Chi AC, Neville BW. Common oral lesions: Part II. Masses and neoplasia. Am Fam Physician 2007;75:509-512.

Giant Cell Lesions

160. Chaparro-Avendano AV, Berini-Aytes L, Gay-Escoda C. Peripheral giant cell granuloma. A report of five cases and review of the literature. Med Oral Patol Oral Cir Bucal 2005;10:48-57.
161. Jundt G. Central giant cell lesion. In: Barnes L, Eveson JW, Reichart P, Sidransky D, eds. World Health Organization Classification of Tumours. Pathology and genetics of head and neck tumours. Lyon, France: IARC Press; 2005:324.
162. de Lange J, Van den Akker HP. Clinical and radiological features of central giant-cell lesions of the jaw. Oral Surg Oral Med Oral Pathol Oral Radiol Endod 2005;99:464-470.
163. Regezi JA. Odontogenic cysts, odontogenic tumors, fibroosseous, and giant cell lesions of the jaws. Mod Pathol 2002;15:331-341.
164. Kartsogiannis V, Zhou H, Horwood NJ, et al. Localization of RANKL (receptor activator of NF kappa B ligand) mRNA and protein in skeletal and extraskeletal tissues. Bone 1999;25:525-534.
165. Roux S, Orcel P. Bone loss. Factors that regulate osteoclast differentiation: an update. Arthritis Res 2000;2:451-456.
166. Atkins GJ, Haynes DR, Graves SE, et al. Expression of osteoclast differentiation signals by stromal elements of giant cell tumors. J Bone Miner Res 2000;15:640-649.

167. Ju JH, Cho ML, Jhun JY, et al. Oral administration of type-II collagen suppresses IL-17-associated RANKL expression of CD4+ T cells in collagen-induced arthritis. Immunol Lett 2008;117:16-25.
168. Matt BH. Aneurysmal bone cyst of the maxilla: case report and review of the literature. Int J Pediatr Otorhinolaryngol 1993;25:217-226.
169. Rawashdeh MA, Bataineh AB, Al-Khateeb T. Long-term clinical and radiological outcomes of surgical management of central giant cell granuloma of the maxilla. Int J Oral Maxillofac Surg 2006;35;60-66.
170. Yamaguchi T, Dorfman HD. Giant cell reparative granuloma: a comparative clinicopathologic study of lesions in gnathic and extragnathic sites. Int J Surg Pathol 2001;9:189-200.
171. Lester SR, Cordell KG, Rosebush MS, Palaiologou AA, Maney P. Peripheral giant cell granulomas: a series of 279 cases. Oral Surg Oral Med Oral Pathol Oral Rradiol 2014;118:475-482.
172. Vered M, Buchner A, Dayan D. Giant cell granuloma of the jawbones—a proliferative vascular lesion? Immunohistochemical study with vascular endothelial growth factor and basic fibroblast growth factor. J Oral Pathol Med 2006;35:613-619.

Oral Submucous Fibrosis

173. Hazarey VK, Erlewad DM, Mundhe KA, Ughade SN. Oral submucous fibrosis: study of 1000 cases from central India. J Oral Pathol Med 2007;36:12-17.
174. Rajendran R. Oral submucous fibrosis: etiology, pathogenesis, and future research. Bull World Health Organ 1994;72:985-996.
175. Tilakaratne WM, Klinikowski MF, Saku T, Peters TJ, Warnakulasuriya S. Oral submucous fibrosis: Review on aetiology and pathogenesis. Oral Oncol 2005;42:561-568.
176. Cox SC, Walker DM. Oral submucous fibrosis. A review. Aust Dent J 1996;41:294-299.
177. Murti PR, Bhonsle RB, Pindborg JJ, Daftary DK, Gupta PC, Mehta FS. Malignant transformation rate in oral submucous fibrosis over a 17-year period. Community Dent Oral Epidmiol 1985;13:340-341.
178. Yang YH, Chen CH, Chang JS, Lin CC, Cheng TC, Shieh TY. Incidence rates of oral cancer and oral pre-cancerous lesions in a 6-year follow-up study of a Taiwanese aboriginal community. J Oral Pathol Med 2005;34:596-601.

Gingival Fibromatosis

179. Neville BW, Damm DD, Allen CM, Bouquot JE. Gingival fibromatosis. In: Neville BW, Damm DD, Allen CM, Chi AC, eds. Oral & maxillofacial pathology, 4th ed. St. Louis: Elsevier; 2016:151-153.
180. Neville BW, Damm DD, Allen CM, Bouquot JE. Drug-related gingival hyperplasia (drug-related gingival overgrowth). In: Neville BW, Damm DD, Allen CM, Chi AC, eds. Oral & maxillofacial pathology, 4th ed. St. Louis: Elsevier; 2016:148-151.
181. Flucke U, Tops BB, van Diest PJ, Slootweg PJ. Desmoid-type fibromatosis of the head and neck region in the paediatric population: a clinicopathological and genetic study of seven cases. Histopathology 2014;64:769-776.
182. Peña S, Brickman T, StHilaire H, Jeyakumar A. Aggressive fibromatosis of the head and neck in the pediatric population. Int J Pediatr Otorhinolaryngol 2014;78:1-4.
183. Coffin CM, Hornick JL, Zhou H, Fletcher CD. Gardner fibroma: a clinicopathologic and immunohistochemical analysis of 45 patients with 57 fibromas. Am J Surg Pathol 2007;31:410-416.
184. Colombo C, Foo WC, Whiting D, et al. FAP-related desmoid tumors: a series of 44 patients evaluated in a cancer referral center. Histol Histopathol 2012;27:641-649.
185. Amary MF, Pauwels P, Meulemans E, et al. Detection of beta-catenin mutations in paraffin-embedded sporadic desmoid-type fibromatosis by mutation-specific restriction enzyme digestion (MSRED): an ancillary diagnostic tool. Am J Surg Pathol 2007;31:1299-1309.
186. Bhattacharya B, Dilworth HP, Iacobuzio-Donahue C, et al. Nuclear beta-catenin expression distinguishes deep fibromatosis from other benign and malignant fibroblastic and myofibroblastic lesions. Am J Surg Pathol 2005;29:653-659.
187. Bridge JA, Sreekantaiah C, Mouron B, Neff JR, Sandberg AA, Wolman SR. Clonal chromosomal abnormalities in desmoid tumors: implications for histogenesis. Cancer 1992;69:430-436.
188. Huss S, Nehles J, Binot E, et al. β-catenin (CTNNB1) mutations and clinicopathological features of mesenteric desmoid-type fibromatosis. Histopathology 2013;62:294-304.
189. Le Guellec S, Soubeyran I, Rochaix P, et al. CTNNB1 mutation analysis is a useful tool for the diagnosis of desmoid tumors: a study of 260 desmoid tumors and 191 potential morphologic mimics. Mod Pathol 2012;25:1551-1558.
190. Duffaud F, Le Cesne A. Imatinib in the treatment of solid tumours. Target Oncol 2009;4:45-56.
191. Gounder MM, Lefkowitz RA, Keohan ML, et al. Activity of Sorafenib against desmoid tumor/deep fibromatosis. Clin Cancer Res 2011;17:4082-4090.

192. Penel N, Le Cesne A, Bui BN, et al. Imatinib for progressive and recurrent aggressive fibromatosis (desmoid tumors): an FNCLCC/French Sarcoma Group phase II trial with a long-term follow-up. Ann Oncol 2011;22:452-457.
193. Beham A, Badve S, Suster S, Fletcher CD. Solitary myofibroma in adults: clinicopathological analysis of a series. Histopathology 1993;22:335-341.
194. Foss RD, Ellis GL. Myofibromas and myofibromatosis of the oral region: a clinicopathologic analysis of 79 cases. Oral Surg Oral Med Oral Pathol Oral Radiol Endod 2000;89:57-65.
195. Beck JC, Devaney KO, Weatherly RA, Koopmann CF Jr, Lesperance MM. Pediatric myofibromatosis of the head and neck. Arch Otolaryngol Head Neck Surg 1999;125:39-44.
196. Lingen MW, Mostofi RS, Solt DB. Myofibromas of the oral cavity. Oral Surg Oral Med Oral Pathol Oral Radiol Endod 1995;80:297-302.

Pyogenic Granuloma

197. Cardoso JA, Spanemberg JC, Cherubini K, Figueiredo MA, Salum FG. Oral granuloma gravidarum: a retrospective study of 41 cases in southern Brazil. J Appl Oral Sci 2013;21:215-218.
198. Mills SE, Cooper PH, Fechner RE. Lobular capillary hemangioma: the underlying lesion of pyogenic granuloma: a study of 73 cases from the oral and mucous membranes. Am J Surg Pathol 1980;4:471-479.
199. Gordon-Nunez MA, de Vasconceles Carvalho M, Benevenuto TG, Lopes MF, Silva LM, Galvão HC. Oral pyogenic granuloma: a retrospective analysis of 293 cases in a Brazilian population. J Oral Maxillofac Surg 2010;68:2185-2188.

Congenital Epulis

200. Childers EL, Fanburg-Smith JC. Congenital epulis of the newborn: 10 new cases of a rare oral tumor. Am Diagn Pathol 2011;15:157-161.
201. Vered M, Dobriyan A, Buchner A. Congenital granular cell epulis presents an immunohistochemical profile that distinguishes it from the granular cell tumor of the adult. Virchows Arch 2009;454;303-310.
202. Bhatia SK, Goyal A, Ritwik P, Rai S. Spontaneous regression of a congenital epulis in a newborn. J Clin Pediatr Dent 2013;37:297-299.

Fibrous Dysplasia

203. Barnes L. Fibrous dysplasia. In: Barnes L, ed. Surgical pathology of the head and neck. Second edition, revised and expanded. New York; Marcel Dekker; 2001:1090-1095.
204. Henry A. Monostotic fibrous dysplasia. J Bone Joint Surg Br 1969;51:300-306.
205. Jundt G. Fibrous dysplasia. In: Barnes L, Eveson JW, Reichart P, Sidransky D, eds. World Health Organization Classification of Tumours. Pathology and genetics of head and neck tumours. Lyon, France; IARC Press, 2005:321-322.
206. Miettinen M, Hockerstedt K, Reitamo J, Totterman S. Intramuscular myxoma—a clinicopathological study of twenty-three cases. Am J Clin Pathol 1985;84:265-272.
207. Tabareau-Delalande F, Collin C, Gomez-Brouchet A, et al. Diagnostic value of investigating GNAS mutations in fibro-osseous lesions: a retrospective study of 91 cases of fibrous dysplasia and 40 other fibro-osseous lesions. Mod Pathol 2013;26:911-921.
208. Shi RR, Li XF, Zhang R, Chen Y, Li TJ. GNAS mutational analysis in differentiating fibrous dysplasia and ossifying fibroma of the jaw. Mod Pathol 2013;26:1023-1031.
209. Farugi T, Dhawan N, Bahl J, et al. Molecular phenotypic aspects and therpeutic horizens of rare genetic bone disorders. Biomed Res Int 2014;2014:670842.
210. Patel MM, Wilkey JF, Abdelsayed R, D'Silva NJ, Malchoff C, Mallya SM. Analysis of GNAS mutations in cemento-ossifying fibromas and cemento-osseous dysplasias of the jaws. Oral Surg Oral Med Oral Pathol Oral Radiol Endod 2010;109:739-743.
211. Friedrich RE, Scheuer HA, Assaf AT, Grob T, Zustin J. Odontogenic myxomas are not associated with GNAS1 mutations. Anticancer Res 2012;32:2169-2172.
212. Wenig BM, Vinh TN, Smirniotopoulos JG, Fowler CB, Houston GD, Heffner DK. Aggressive psammomatoid ossifying fibromas of the sinonasal region: a clinicopathologic study of a distinct group of fibro-osseous lesions. Cancer 1995;76:1155–1165.
213. Ruggieri P, Sim FH, Bond JR, Unni KK. Malignancies in fibrous dysplasia. Cancer 1994;73:1411-1424.
214. Taconis WK. Osteosarcoma in fibrous dysplasia. Skeletal Radiol 1988;17:163-170.
215. Yabut SM Jr, Kenan S, Sissons HA, Lewis MM. Malignant transformation of fibrous dysplasia. A case report and review of the literature. Clin Orthop 1988;228:281–289.
216. Blackwell JB. Mesenchymal chondrosarcoma arising in fibrous dysplasia of the femur. J Clin Pathol 1993;46:961-962.

Cemento-Osseous Dysplasias

217. Su L, Weathers DR, Waldron CA. Distinguishing features of focal cemento-osseous dysplasia and cemento-ossifying fibromas I. A pathologic spectrum of 316 cases. Oral Surg Oral Med Oral Pathol 1997;84:301-309.

218. Su L, Weathers DR, Waldron CA. Distinguishing features of focal cemento-osseous dysplasia and cemento-ossifying fibromas II. A pathologic spectrum of 316 cases. Oral Surg Oral Med Oral Pathol 1997;84:540-549.
219. Summerlin DJ, Tomich CE. Focal cemento-osseous dysplasia: a clinicpathologic study of 221 cases. Oral Surg Oral Med Oral Pathol 1994;78:611-620.
220. MacDonald-Jankowski DS. Fibro-osseous lesions of the face and jaws. Clin Radiol 2004;5911-5925.
221. Alsufyani NA, Lam EW. Osseous (cemento-osseous) dysplasia of the jaws: clinical and radiographic analysis. J Can Dent Assoc 2011;77:b70.
222. Bhattacharyya I, Islam N, Cohen D. Diagnostic discussion. Periapical cemento-osseous dysplasia. Todays FDA 2015;27:52-57.
223. Mahomed F, Altini M, Meer S, Coleman H. Cemento-osseous dysplasia with associated simple bone cysts. J Oral Maxillofac Surg 2005;63:1549-1554.
224. Peacock ME, Krishna R, Gustin JW, Stevens MR, Arce RM, Abdelsayed RA. Retrospective study on idiopathic bone cavity and its association with cementoosseous dysplasia. Oral Surg Oral Med Oral Pathol Oral Radiol 2015;119:e246-251.

Exogenous Pigmentation

225. Hussaini HM, Waddell JN, West LM, et al. Silver solder "tattoo" a novel form of oral pigmentation identified with the use of field emission scanning electron microscopy and electron dispersive spectrography. Oral Surg Oral Med Oral Pathol Radiol Endod 2011;112e6-10.
226. Buchner A, Hansen LS. Amalgam pigmentation (amalgam tattoo) of the oral mucosa. A clinicopathologic study of 268 cases. Oral Surg Oral Med Oral Pathol 1980;49:139-147.
227. Parizi JL, Nai GA. Amalgam tattoo: a cause of sinusitis? J Appl Oral Sci 2010;18:100-104.

Endogenous Pigmentation

228. Buchner A, Merrell PW, Carpenter WM. Relative infrequency of solitary melanocytic lesions of the oral mucosa. J Oral Pathol Med 2004;33:550-557.
229. Kaugars GE, Heise AP, Riley WT, Abbey LM, Svirsky JA. Oral melanotic macules. A review of 353 cases. Oral Surg Pral Med Oral Pathol 1993;76:59-61.
230. Shen ZY, Liu W, Bao ZX, Zhou ZT, Wang LZ. Oral melanotic macule and primary oral malignant melanoma: epidemiology, location involved, and clinical implications. Oral Surg Oral Med Oral Pathol Oral Radiol Endod 2011;112:e21-25.

Black Hairy Tongue

231. Ioffreda MD, Gordon CA, Adams DR, Naides SJ, Miller JJ. Black tongue. Arch Dermatol 2001;137:968-969.
232. Thompson DF, Kessler TL. Drug-induced black hairy tongue. Pharmacotherapy 2010;30:585-593.
233. Manabe M, Lim HW, Wintzer M, Loomis CA. Architectural organization of filiform papillae in normal and black hairy tongue epithelium: dissection of differentiation pathways in a complex human epithelium according to their patterns of keratin expression. Arch Dermatol 1999;135:177-181.

Myosperulosis

234. Sarkar S, Gangane N, Sharma S. Myospherulosis of maxillary sinus—a case report with review of the literature. Indian J Pathol 1998;41:491-493.
235. Dunlap CL, Barker BF. Myospherulosis of the jaws. Oral Surg Med Oral Pathol 1980;50:238-243.

Odontogenic Cysts, Dentigerous Cyst

236. Neville BW, Damm DD, Allen CM, Bouquot JE. Odontogeinc cysts and tumors. In: Neville BW, Damm DD, Allen CM, Chi AC, eds. Oral & maxillofacial pathology, 4th ed. St. Louis: Elsevier; 2016:632-650.
237. Ko KS, Dover DG, Jordan RC. Bilateral dentigerous cysts—report of an unusual case and review of the literature. J Can Dent Assoc 1999;65:49-51.
238. Verbin RS. Dentigerous cyst. In: Barnes L, ed. Surgical pathology of the head and neck. Second edition, revised and expanded. New York; Marcel Dekker; 2001:1442-1447.
239. Kim J, Ellis GL. Dental follicular tissue: misinterpretation as odontogenic tumors. J Oral Maxillofac Surg 1993;51:762-767.
240. Dunsche A, Babendererde O, Luttges J, Springer IN. Dentigerous cyst versus unicystic ameloblastoma—differential diagnosis in routine histology. J Oral Pathol Med 2003;32:486-491.
241. Henley J, Summerlin DJ, Tomich C, Zhang S, Cheng L. Molecular evidence supporting the neoplastic nature of odontogenic keratocyst: a laser capture microdissection study of 15 cases. Histopathology 2005;47:582-586.
242. Robinson RA, Vincent SD. Tumors and cysts of the jaws. AFIP Atlas of Tumor Pathology, 4th Series, Fascicle 16. Washington, DC: American Registry of Pathology; 2012:72-77.
243. Motamedi MH, Talesh KT. Management of extensive dentigerous cysts. Br Dent J 2005;198:203-206.
244. Roofe SB, Boyd EM Jr, Houston GD, Edgin WA. Squamous cell carcinoma arising in the epithelial lining of a dentigerous cyst. South Med J 1999;92:611-614.

Glandular Odontogenic Cysts

245. Fowler CB, Brannon RB, Kessler HP, Castle JT, Kahn MA. Glandular odontogenic cyst: analysis of 46 cases with special emphasis on microscopic criteria for diagnosis. Head Neck Pathol 2011;5:364-375.
246. Gardner DG, Kessler HP, Morency R, Schaffner DL. The glandular odontogenic cyst: an apparent entity. J Oral pathol 1988;17:359-366.
247. Kaplan I, Anavi Y, Hrshberg A. Glandular odontogenic cyst: a challenge in diagnosis and treatments. Oral Dis 2008;14:575-581.
248. Bishop JA, Yonescu R, Batista D, Warnock GR, Westra WH. Glandular odontogenic cysts (GOCs) lack MAML2 rearrangements; a finding to discredit the putative nature of GOC as a precursor to central mucoepidermoid carcinoma. Head Neck Pathol 2014;8:287-290.

Lateral Periodontal Cyst

249. Wysocki GP, Brannon RB, Gardner DG, Sapp P. Histogenesis of the lateral periodontal cyst and the gingival cyst of the adult. Oral Surg Oral Med Oral Pathol 1980;50:327-334.
250. Siponen M, Neville BW, Damm DD, Allen CM. Multifocal lateral periodontal cysts: a report of 4 cases and review of the literature. Oral Surg Oral Med Oral Pathol Oral Radiol Endod 2011;111:225-233.
251. Gurol M, Burkes EJ Jr, Jacoway J. Botryoid odontogenic cyst: analysis of 33 cases. J Periodontal 1995;66:1069-1075.

Periapical Cyst

252. Verbin RS. Inflammatory cysts. In: Barnes L, ed. Surgical pathology of the head and neck, 2nd ed, revised and expanded. New York: Marcel Dekker; 2001:1465-1472.
253. Abbott PV. The periapical space—a dynamic interface. Aust Endod J 2002;28:96-107.
254. Gallini G, Merlini C, Martelossi L, Benetti C. [Inflammatory odontogenic lesions of the jaws.] Dent Cadmos 1991;59:80-94. [Italian]

Autoimmune, Allergic, Systemic, and Cutaneous-Type Diseases Affecting the Oral Cavity

255. Müller S. Noninfectious vesiculoerosive and ulcerative lesions of the oral mucosa. In: Barnes L, ed. Surgical pathology of the head and neck, 2nd ed., revised and expanded. New York; Marcel Dekker; 2001:301-341.
256. Neville BW, Damm DD, Allen CM, Bouquot JE. Allergies and immunologic diseases. In: Neville BW, Damm DD, Allen CM, Chi AC, eds. Oral & maxillofacial pathology, 4th ed. St. Louis; Elsevier; 2016:303-326.

Lichen Planus

257. Müller S. Oral manifestations of dermatologic disease: a focus on lichenoid lesions. Head Neck Pathol 2011;5:36-40.
258. Neville BW, Damm DD, Allen CM, Bouquot JE. Dermatologic diseases. In: Neville BW, Damm DD, Allen CM, Chi AC, eds. Oral & maxillofacial pathology, 4th ed. St. Louis: Elsevier; 2016:729-734.
259. Laeijendecker R, Van Joost T, Tank B, Oranje AP, Neumann HA. Oral lichen planus in childhood. Pediatr Dermatol 2005;22:299-304.
260. Batsakis JG, Cleary KR, Cho KJ. Lichen planus and lichenoid lesions of the oral cavity. Ann Otol Rhinol Laryngol 1994;103:495-497.
261. Ingafou M, Leao JC, Porter SR, Scully C. Oral lichen planus: a retrospective study of 690 British patients. Oral Dis 2006;12:463-468.
262. Vincent SD, Fotos PG, Baker KA, Williams TP. Oral lichen planus: the clinical, historical, and therapeutic features of 100 cases. Oral Surg Oral Med Oral Pathol 1990;70:165-171.
263. Xue JL, Fan MW, Wang SZ, Chen XM, Li Y, Wang L. A clinical study of 674 patients with oral lichen planus in China. J Oral Pathol Med 2005;34:467-472.
264. Thornhill MH. Immune mechanisms in oral lichen planus. Acta Odontol Scand 2001;59:174-177.
265. Jainkittivong A, Langlais RP. Allergic stomatitis. Semin Dermatol 1994;13:91-101.
266. Bornstein MM, Kalas L, Lemp S, Altermatt HJ, Rees TD, Buser D. Oral lichen planus and malignant transformation: a retrospective follow-up study of clinical and histopathologic data. Quintessence Int 2006;37:261-271.
267. Müller S, Waldron CA. Premalignant lesions of the oral cavity. In: Barnes L, ed. Surgical pathology of the head and neck, 2nd ed, revised and expanded. New York; Marcel Dekker; 2001:342-368.
268. Mignogna MD, Fedele S, Lo Russo L, Mignogna C, de Rosa G, Porter SR. Field cancerization in oral lichen planus. Eur J Surg Oncol 2007;33:383-389.
269. van der Meij EH, Mast H, van der Waal I. The possible premalignant character of oral lichen planus and oral lichenoid lesions: A prospective five-year follow-up study of 192 patients. Oral Oncol 2007;43:742-748.

Aphthous Stomatitis

270. Scully C. Clinical practice. Aphthous ulceration. N Engl J Med 2006;355:165-172.
271. Scully C. Are viruses associated with aphthae and oral vesiculoerosive disorders? Br J Oral Maxillofac Surg 1993;31:173-177.

272. Vincent SD, Lilly GE. Clinical, historic, and therapeutic features of aphthous stomatitis. Literature review and open clinical trial employing steroids. Oral Surg Oral Med Oral Pathol 1992;74:79-86.

Radiation-Associated Changes

273. Fajardo LP. Radiation injury. In: Barnes L, ed. Surgical pathology of the head and neck. Second edition, revised and expanded. New York; Marcel Dekker; 2001:2171-2190.
274. Hansen T, Kunkel M, Springer E, Walter C, Weber A, Siegel E, Kirkpatrick CJ. Actinomycosis of the jaws—histopathological study of 45 patients shows significant involvement in bisphosphonate-associated osteonecrosis and infected osteoradionecrosis. Virchows Arch 2007;451:1009-1017.
275. Hansen T, Wagner W, Kirkpatrick CJ, Kunkel M. Infected osteoradionecrosis of the mandible: follow-up study suggests deterioration in outcome for patients with Actinomyces-positive bone biopsies. Int J Oral Maxillofac Surg 2006;35:1001-1004.
276. Hansen T, Kunkel M, Weber A, James Kirkpatrick C. Osteonecrosis of the jaws in patients treated with bisphosphonates—histomorphologic analysis in comparison with infected osteoradionecrosis. J Oral Pathol Med 2006;35:155-160.
277. Noh SJ, Cho NP, Kang MJ. Intraosseous pseudocarcinomatous hyperplasia associated with chronic osteomyelitis of the mandible: report of two cases. J Oral Maxillofac Surg 2014;72:440-444.
278. Warter A, Walter P, Meyer C, Barrière P, Galatir L, Wilk A. Mandibular pseudocarcinomatous hyperplasia. Histopathology 2000;37:115-117.

3 PHARYNX

By Dr. Bruce M. Wenig

EMBRYOLOGY, ANATOMY, AND HISTOLOGY

The pharynx is a 12- to 14-cm long musculomembranous tube shaped like an inverted cone that extends from the cranial base to the lower border of the cricoid cartilage (level of the 6th cervical vertebra) (1). The pharynx is limited superiorly by the posterior part of the body of the sphenoid bone and the basilar part of the occipital bone, and inferiorly by the esophagus with which it is continuous. The pharynx lies behind and communicates with the nasal, oral, and laryngeal cavities via the nasopharynx, oropharynx, and hypopharynx (laryngopharynx), respectively, its three anatomic divisions (1). The hypopharynx is often included as part of the larynx, but given the differences in embryology from the larynx and the inclusion of hypopharyngeal cancers in the AJCC staging system of pharyngeal and not laryngeal cancers (2), the hypopharynx, including the piriform sinus, is included in this section on the pharynx rather than the larynx.

Embryology

The primitive pharynx is derived from the foregut, developing from both the branchial arches and pharyngeal pouches (3). The embryologic pharynx is of endodermal derivation (3). At its cephalic end, the embryologic pharynx is in direct continuity with the ectoderm forming the stomodeum (3). The embryologic pharynx and stomodeum are separated from the buccopharyngeal membrane, the latter lined by ectoderm along its exterior surface and endoderm along its interior surface. In its embryologic development, the buccopharyngeal membrane ruptures (approximately 3rd week of gestation), resulting in contact between the stomodeum and the foregut (3).

In contrast to the mucosa of the nasal cavity and paranasal sinuses (so-called Schneiderian membrane), which is of ectodermal derivation, the lining of the pharynx, including the nasopharynx, oropharynx, and hypopharynx, is predominantly of endodermal origin. The palatine tonsils develop from the 2nd pharyngeal pouch and the tubotympanic recess (which forms the eustachian tube and tympanic cavity) from the 1st pharyngeal pouch (3).

Anatomy

The pharynx consists of three functionally and structurally distinct subparts: the nasopharynx, oropharynx, and hypopharynx (fig. 3-1). The oropharynx includes the soft palate, tonsillar pillars, palatine tonsils, posterior tonsillar pillars, uvula, and the base of tongue including the lingual tonsils. The Waldeyer tonsillar tissue ring is a component of the pharynx formed by a ring or oblique wreath of extranodal lymphoid tissue at the upper end of the pharynx consisting of the palatine tonsils, nasopharyngeal tonsils (adenoids), base of tongue (lingual tonsils), and adjacent submucosal lymphatics. The nasopharyngeal tonsils (adenoids) lie posteriorly and laterally to the nasopharynx. The orifice of eustachian tube lies along the lateral aspects of the nasopharyngeal wall.

Anatomic Borders

Oropharynx. The oropharynx represents the portion of the pharynx that extends from the superior surface of the soft palate to the superior surface of the hyoid bone (or floor of the ventricle). The anterior border is continuous with the mouth through the oropharyngeal isthmus; the posterior border is on a level with the 2nd and 3rd cervical vertebrae; and the superior border is the horizontal plane of the palate.

The superior portion of the anterior oropharynx is bounded by the opening of the mouth into the oropharynx, referred to as the fauces. The lateral walls of the fauces are composed of the two tonsillar pillars. Between these pillars

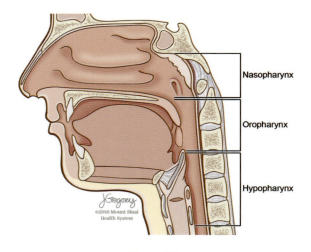

Figure 3-1

ANATOMY OF PHARYNX

The regions of the pharynx including nasopharynx, oropharynx and hypopharynx, are seen. (Courtesy of J. Gregory, Mount Sinai Health System.)

lie the palatine tonsils in the tonsillar fossa. The anterior tonsillar pillar is the palatoglossal arch, which curves downward and forward from the soft palate to the tongue. The posterior tonsillar pillar, or palatopharyngeal arch, extends downward from the posterolateral border of the soft palate laterally along the pharyngeal wall.

The inferior border of the oropharynx is the horizontal plane of the hyoid bone (upper border of the epiglottis) marked by the opening of the piriform sinus at the level of the tip of the epiglottis. The lateral border is the palatopharyngeal arch.

Nasopharynx. The nasopharynx is situated behind the nasal cavity and above the soft palate. It begins anteriorly at the posterior choana and extends along the plane of the airway to the level of the free border of the soft palate. The anterior border is continuous with the nasal cavities through the choanae. The posterior border is continuous with the roof and is further supported by the 1st cervical vertebra (anterior arch of the atlas). The superior (roof) border is the base of the skull (occipital bone) and the posterior part of the body of the sphenoid bone. The inferior (floor) border is continuous with the oropharynx; during swallowing, the soft palate and uvula provide a functional floor. The soft palate is the only truly mobile portion of the nasopharynx. The lateral border contains the pharyngeal orifice of the

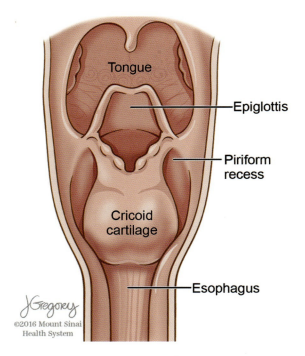

Figure 3-2

HYPOPHARYNX

The hypopharynx includes the piriform sinus (or recess), which expands bilaterally and forward around the sides of the larynx and lies between the larynx and the thyroid cartilage. (Courtesy of J. Gregory, Mount Sinai Health System.)

eustachian tube, which in the posterior portion has a submucosal cartilaginous elevation called the torus tubarius, behind which is a shallow depression called the fossa of Rosenmüller.

Hypopharynx. The superior border is just above the level of the hyoid bone. The inferior border is the lower border of the cricoid cartilage. The anterior border is the mucosa on the medial surface of the thyroid cartilage. The lateral borders attach to the hyoid bone and thyroid cartilage. The medial border is the larynx and its appendages.

The piriform sinus (fig. 3-2) is the part of the hypopharynx that expands bilaterally and forward around the sides of the larynx, and lies between the larynx and the thyroid cartilage. The piriform sinus is also referred to as the piriform recess and piriform fossa. Piriform means pear-shaped from Latin pirum, "pear," and forma, "shape"; pyriform means flame-shaped from the Greek word for "fire." The piriform sinus is pear shaped and not flame shaped, and although both spellings have been used for this anatomic site, the correct spelling based on anatomic shape is piriform.

Parapharyngeal Space. The pharyngeal space, also referred to as the lateral pharyngeal space, lies deep to the tonsil and lateral to the pharynx (1,4). The parapharyngeal space is roughly pyramidal in shape. The base of the pyramid is formed superiorly by the base of the skull, with the apex of the pyramid formed inferiorly by the attachment of the cervical fascia to the hyoid bone. The pharyngeal superior constrictor muscle lies medial to the parapharyngeal space. Lateral to the parapharyngeal space are the pterygoid lamina, inner surface of the mandibular ramus, and the deep lobe of the parotid gland. Posteriorly, the parapharyngeal space lies in direct continuity with the retropharyngeal space, the latter representing loose connective tissue lying behind the pharynx and anterior to the prevertebral fascia of the vertebral column.

The parapharyngeal space includes the internal carotid artery, internal jugular vein, glossopharyngeal (IX) nerve, hypopharyngeal (XII) cranial nerve, cervical sympathetic chain, vagal body, carotid body, and lymph nodes (1). The parapharyngeal space is involved by a variety of disease processes, either originating from the structures within it (e.g., nerve sheath tumor, paragangliomas, primary lymphomas) or secondarily extending from adjacent structures (e.g., tonsillar abscess, parotid neoplasm), metastases to its lymph nodes from head and neck primary malignant tumors, or, less commonly, from primary malignant neoplasms originating from outside the head and neck region.

Histology

Oropharynx. The epithelial lining of the oropharynx is stratified squamous epithelium, which normally does not have a keratin layer (fig. 3-3) (5). The submucosa contains the minor salivary glands, which are mixed seromucous but predominantly mucous glands.

The palatine and lingual tonsils are epithelial-lined structures (fig. 3-3) considered to represent extranodal lymphoid tissue. They are characterized by the presence of a prominent lymphoid component, including germinal centers, but, in contrast to lymph nodes, do not have a subcapsular sinus or sinusoids. Unlike the adenoids, the palatine and lingual tonsils have 10 to 20 (tonsillar) crypts formed by the invagination of the free surface mucosa; these narrow tubular epithelial diverticuli branch within the tonsils and frequently are packed with plugs of shed epithelial cells, lymphocytes, and bacteria, which may calcify. Actinomycotic colonies (*Actinomyces israellii*) are commensal microorganisms that may be found within the tonsillar crypts (fig. 3-3).

The tonsillar crypts are lined by specialized stratified squamous epithelium, known as reticulated epithelium (fig. 3-4), which lacks the orderly laminar structure of the surface stratified squamous epithelium of the tonsils including loss of cellular polarity and surface maturation (6,7). As the stratified squamous epithelium of the tonsillar surface extends into the tonsillar crypts, a dense lymphoid infiltrate, as well as macrophages, penetrates the reticulated epithelium, obscuring the junction between the epithelial and lymphoid components (fig. 3-4).

The basal lamina of the reticulated epithelium is discontinuous and, therefore, porous, facilitating migration of lymphocytes and dendritic cells, the latter representing potent antigen-processing cells. The intimate association of epithelial cells and lymphocytes facilitates direct transport of antigen (e.g., human papillomavirus [HPV], human immunodeficiency virus [HIV]) from the external environment to the tonsillar lymphoid cells (7). The reticulated epithelial cells are functionally similar to microfold (M) cells of the gastrointestinal tract, although lymphoid tissue elsewhere depends on direct antigen delivery through afferent lymphatic vessels, but such afferent vessels are absent from the tonsils.

The total surface area of the reticulated epithelium is large, owing to the complex branched nature of the tonsillar crypts. The reticulated epithelium is characterized by numerous (intraepithelial) blood vessels (6,7) that can be further delineated by vascular endothelial cell immunomarkers (such as CD31). The discontinuous basal lamina of the reticulated epithelium and the numerous intraepithelial blood vessels explain why any carcinoma arising from the crypt epithelium, especially HPV-associated cancers, should be interpreted as invasive carcinoma rather than carcinoma in situ. Metastatic carcinomas to the cervical neck may originate from very small crypt carcinomas (1 to 2 mm) that

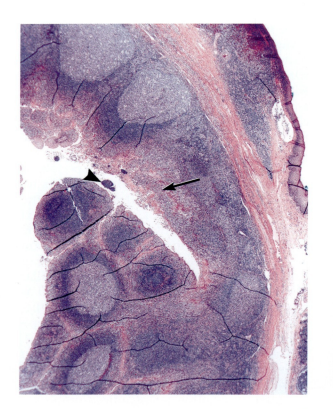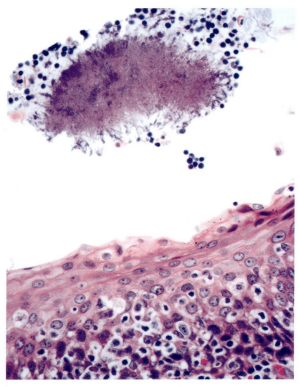

Figure 3-3

OROPHARYNGEAL TONSILS

Left: At low-power magnification, the lingual (as well as palatine) tonsils are lined by surface nonkeratinizing squamous epithelium (upper right) that includes tonsillar crypts (arrow) formed by invagination of the surface mucosa (not shown). The crypts appear as narrow tubular epithelial diverticuli branching within the tonsils. They frequently contain actinomycotic colonies (so-called sulfur granules [top]).

Right: Higher magnification of the actinomycotic colonies ("sulfur granules"). These represent microorganisms normally found within tonsillar crypts.

Figure 3-4

TONSILLAR CRYPT RETICULATED EPITHELIUM

A: Transition from the stratified squamous epithelium of the tonsillar surface (lower left) into the tonsillar crypts lined by the reticulated epithelium (arrows). A dense lymphoid infiltrate obscures the junction between epithelial and lymphoid components. Like the adenoids, the palatine and lingual tonsils contain a prominent submucosal lymphoid component, including germinal centers, with orientation of the mantle lymphocytes toward the surface epithelium.

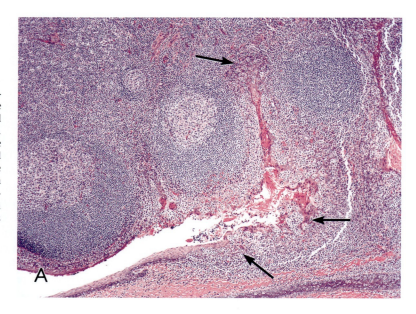

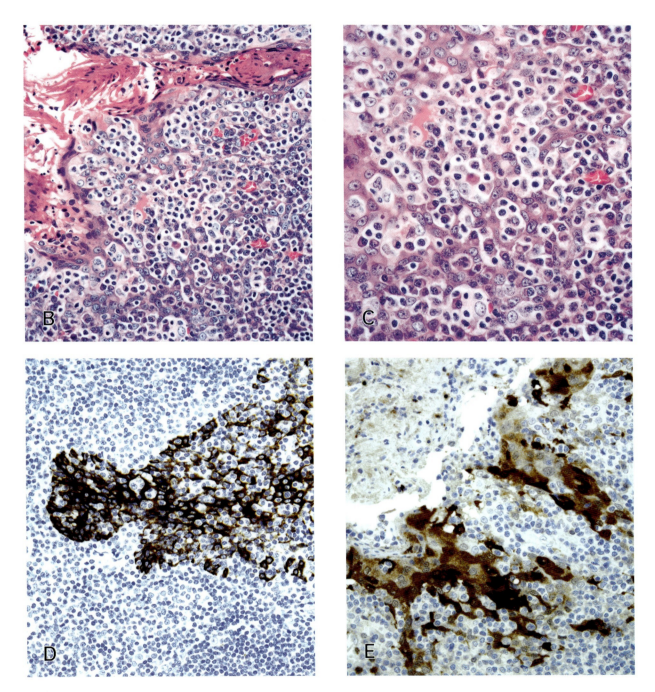

Figure 3-4, continued

B: The basal lamina of reticulated epithelium is discontinuous and porous, facilitating migration of mature lymphocytes and plasma cells (and dendritic cells), which penetrate the reticulated epithelium and obscure the junction between the epithelial and lymphoplasmacytic components.

C: Reticulated epithelial cells are basaloid appearing, with vesicular nuclei, an increased nuclear to cytoplasmic ratio, absence of keratinization, absence of intercellular bridges, and loss of a distinct cytoplasmic border.

D: Cytokeratin (AE1/AE3) staining highlights the epithelial cells while the lymphoplasmacytic cell infiltrate lacks such staining.

E: Patchy (negative) p16 immunoreactivity may be seen in normal (non-neoplastic) tonsillar crypt epithelium. There is no evidence of carcinoma.

histologically appear to be wholly confined to the crypt epithelium without apparent evidence of invasion into the submucosa. The reticulated epithelial cells are basaloid appearing, with vesicular nuclei, an increased nuclear to cytoplasmic ratio, absence of keratinization, absence of intercellular bridges, and loss of a distinct cytoplasmic border (fig. 3-4). HPV-associated squamous cell carcinomas originating from tonsillar crypt epithelium are nonkeratinizing and may be viewed as "poorly differentiated"; however, such cancers are in fact differentiated, originating and recapitulating the features of its cell of origin, which is the specialized tonsillar crypt reticulated epithelium (8). p16 immunoreactivity may be seen in normal (non-neoplastic) tonsillar crypt epithelium (fig. 3-4) and is not evidence of the presence of HPV-associated intraepithelial dysplasia or carcinoma.

The minor salivary glands of the palatine tonsils (as well as the uvula and soft palate) are mixed seromucous glands but are predominantly mucous, and can be seen embedded in the underlying muscle. The minor salivary glands at the lingual tonsils/base of the tongue are pure mucous.

Nasopharynx. The epithelium of the nasopharynx varies from stratified squamous type in the lower and posterior regions, to ciliated pseudostratified (respiratory) columnar type near the choanae and adjacent roof of the nasopharynx, to intermediate ("transitional") type in the junctional zones in the roof and lateral walls (fig. 3-5). Although these types of epithelia may be associated with a specific part of the nasopharyngeal region, this is not constant, so that any site may be covered by any type of epithelium.

The intermediate epithelium is seen at the junction between squamous and respiratory-type epithelium (similar epithelium is identified in the larynx). The intermediate epithelium includes basaloid nuclei with minimal cytoplasm, an appearance that may suggest intraepithelial dysplasia (fig. 3-5). The presence of smooth rather than coarse nuclear chromatin, smooth rather than irregular nuclear contours, generally limited nuclear pleomorphism, and absence of increased mitotic activity should allow distinction from intraepithelial dysplasia. Also, in the nasopharynx, isolated foci of intraepithelial dysplasia occurring in the absence of an invasive carcinoma are rarely seen. Unlike the oral cavity and glottic portion of the larynx, where intraepithelial dysplastic lesions may result in clinical symptoms warranting biopsy, intraepithelial dysplasia of the pharynx typically does not cause symptoms, so that it is extremely uncommon for the pathologist to identify isolated intraepithelial dysplastic alterations of the pharynx without an association with invasive carcinoma. When confronted with foci histologically suspicious for intraepithelial dysplasia in a routine specimen from the nasopharynx, it is likely intermediate (transitional) epithelium. The submucosa of the nasopharynx contains minor salivary glands as well as a prominent lymphoid component.

The nasopharyngeal tonsils, also known as the adenoids, represent extranodal lymphoid tissue characterized by an epithelium that is infiltrated by many small lymphoid cells (so-called lymphoepithelium) that expand and disrupt the epithelium to produce a reticulated pattern (fig. 3-6). This results in a blurred interface between the epithelium and submucosa. The cells are basaloid appearing, with uniform vesicular nuclei and typically lack keratinization, but abrupt areas of keratinization may be present. The epithelial component is cytokeratin positive (fig. 3-6). In nonendemic populations, normal nasopharyngeal mucosa is typically negative for the presence of Epstein-Barr virus (EBV) as seen by in situ hybridization for EBV-encoded RNA (EBER) (fig. 3-6). The lymphoid component may include the presence of germinal centers but lacks a capsule, sinusoids or epithelial crypts.

Hypopharynx. The epithelium is nonkeratinizing stratified squamous epithelium. Seromucous glands are seen throughout the submucosa. The oropharyngeal epithelium is not characterized by lymphoepithelium or reticulated epithelium.

CLASSIFICATION

The classification of non-neoplastic lesions of the pharynx is seen in Table 3-1.

DEVELOPMENTAL CYSTIC LESIONS: NASOPHARYNGEAL CYSTS

Nasopharyngeal cysts are divided into congential cysts and acquired cysts. Congenital cysts of the nasopharynx include Rathke pouch cyst, Thornwaldt cyst, and dermoid cyst. Acquired

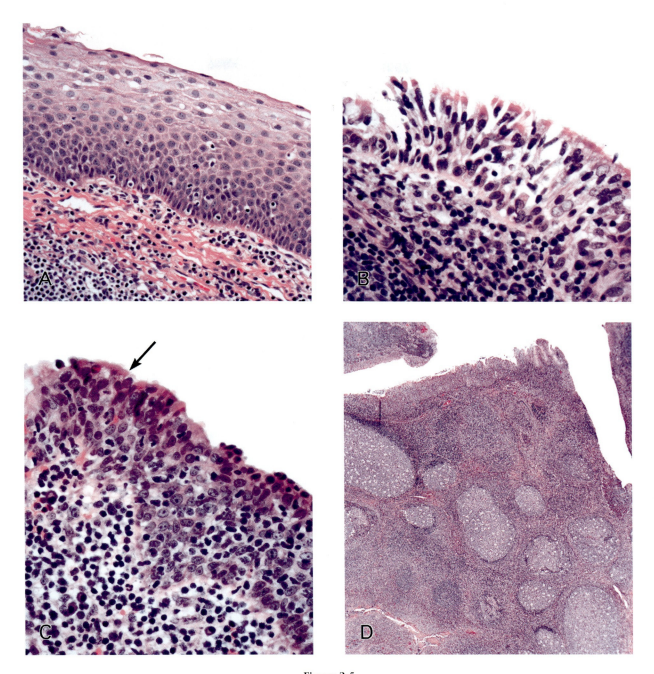

Figure 3-5

NORMAL NASOPHARYNGEAL HISTOLOGY

A,B: Areas of the nasopharynx are lined by nonkeratinizing stratified squamous epithelium (A) or ciliated columnar (respiratory)-type epithelium (B).

C: Intermediate ("transitional") epithelium lies between the squamous and respiratory-type epithelium. It is characterized by cells with basaloid nuclei, smooth nuclear contours and limited nuclear pleomorphism, and no increased mitotic activity. The surface cilia is preserved (arrow). Such features should allow for distinction from intraepithelial dysplasia, the latter rarely seen as an isolated finding in nasopharyngeal biopsies in the absence of an invasive carcinoma.

D: The nasopharyngeal tonsils, also referred to as adenoids, are extranodal lymphoid tissues lined by squamous or respiratory epithelium, with a submucosal lymphoid cell population including variably sized germinal centers containing clear tangible bodies. Unlike the palatine tonsils, epithelial-lined crypts are not present.

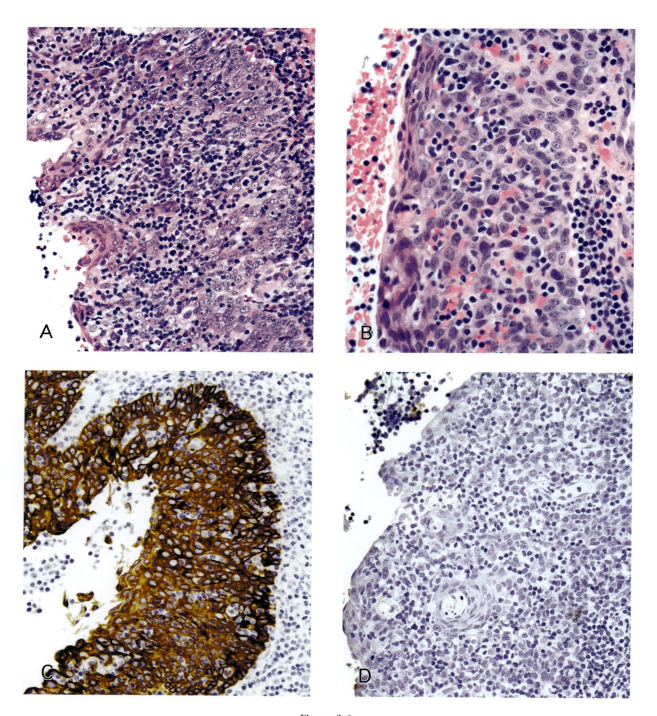

Figure 3-6

NASOPHARYNGEAL "LYMPHOEPITHELIUM"

A: The epithelium is characterized by basaloid-appearing cells with uniform, vesicular nuclei infiltrated by small lymphoid cells that expand and disrupt the epithelium and produce a reticulated pattern.

B: At higher magnification, the epithelial cells are composed of uniform, vesicular nuclei and small eosinophilic nucleoli.

C: Cytokeratin (AE1/AE3) staining highlights the epithelial cells while the lymphoid cells lack such staining.

D: In nonendemic populations, the nasopharyngeal mucosa is negative for the Epstein-Barr virus (EBV) (in situ hybridization for EBV-encoded RNA).

Table 3-1

CLASSIFICATION OF NON-NEOPLASTIC LESIONS OF THE PHARYNX (NASOPHARYNX, OROPHARYNX, AND HYPOPHARYNX)

Nasopharyngeal Cysts
  Rathke pouch cyst
  Thornwaldt cyst
  Dermoid cyst
  Retention cysts
  Others

Hamartomas, Choristomas, and Teratomatous Lesions
  Nasopharyngeal hamartoma
  Heterotopic CNS[a] tissue
  Nasopharyngeal dermoid
  Lymphangiomatous polyp
  Salivary gland anlage tumor

Infectious and Related Diseases/Lesions
  Viral (HPV, EBV, HIV, CMV, HSV), including infectious mononucleosis, HIV-associated lymphoid hyperplasia of Waldeyer ring, others
  Fungal
  Bacterial including gonorrhea, syphilis, bacillary angiomatosis, others
  Protozoal
  Sarcoidosis
  Others

Reactive, Inflammatory, and Tumor-Like Lesions
  Tangier disease
  Others

[a]CNS = central nervous system; HPV = human papilloma-virus; EBV = Epstein-Barr virus; HIV = human immunodeficiency virus; CMV = cytomegalovirus; HSV = herpes simplex virus.

Table 3-2

NON-NEOPLASTIC CYSTIC LESIONS OF THE NASOPHARYNX AND OROPHARYNX

Developmental
  Rathke pouch cyst
  Thornwaldt cyst
  Dermoid cyst
  Others

Nondevelopmental (Acquired)
  Midline and lateral retention cysts

retention cysts of the nasopharynx of seromucinous gland and lymphoid crypt origin, and can occur in midline or lateral locations (9–13). Acquired cysts of the nasopharynx include midline and lateral retention cysts. Developmental cystic lesions are delineated in Table 3-2.

Rathke Pouch Cyst

Definition. *Rathke pouch cyst* is the congenital cystic dilatation of the Rathke cleft due to failure of the lumen between the anterior lobe of the pituitary gland and the pars intermedia to obliterate. It is also termed *Rathke cleft cyst*.

Embryology. The Rathke pouch is an ectodermally derived outpocketing arising from the roof of the primitive oral cavity and lying superior to the buccopharyngeal membrane that develops around the 3rd week of gestation, and grows toward the brain (fig. 3-7) (14). The Rathke pouch ultimately forms the anterior lobe of the pituitary gland (9). By the 5th week of gestation, this pouch has elongated and become constricted at its attachment to the oral epithelium. It comes into contact with the infundibulum, which ultimately develops into the posterior lobe of the pituitary gland. The posterior part of the Rathke pouch develops into the pars intermedia. The lumen between the anterior lobe and the pars intermedia gradually obliterates. If the lumen does not close, however, a cleft is formed (Rathke cleft) that may become cystic and develop into a Rathke cyst (14).

Clinical Features. Rathke pouch cysts represent approximately 2 percent of all lesions of the sella turcica (15). Typically, Rathke pouch cyst is an asymptomatic, congenital lesion that is incidentally found in routine autopsies. Symptomatic cysts occur but are uncommon (16). Symptomatic cysts are more common in women than men, and occur over a wide age range, but are most common in the fourth decade of life (16). Symptoms include headaches, visual disturbances, nausea, vomiting, and pituitary-related abnormalities (galactorrhea, amenorrhea, diabetes insipidus, and meningeal irritation) (16–18). The sudden onset of severe headache or a sudden increase in headache severity may occur and is associated with hemorrhage into the cyst, a presentation that mimics the clinical syndrome of pituitary tumor apoplexy, leading to the designation of Rathke pouch cyst apoplexy (19,20). Serum prolactin may be increased (15,21). A rare association with Klinefelter syndrome has been reported (22). Rathke pouch cyst and pituitary adenoma as a hybrid lesion has occurred (20,23–25), including in a patient with acromegaly (26).

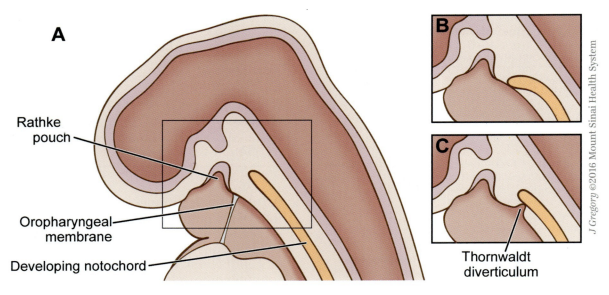

Figure 3-7

EMBRYOLOGIC DEVELOPMENT OF RATHKE POUCH AND THORNWALDT CYST

A: Sagittal illustration of the developing pharynx including the level of the oropharyngeal membrane which separates the ectodermally derived mucosa from the endodermally derived mucosa. The location of the developing notochord is shown in the mesoderm that eventually will become the clivus.

B: Sagittal drawing shows the normal ventral migration of the notochord to touch the pharyngeal mucosa.

C: Sagittal drawing shows Tornwaldt sinus or pit that develops if the notochord attaches to the pharyngeal mucosa and drags it dorsally as the notochord migrates back to its normal location. (Courtesy of J. Gregory, Mount Sinai Health System.)

Radiographically, the cyst is well-circumscribed, round or lobulated, and lacks calcifications (fig. 3-8). The best imaging clue is a nonenhancing, noncalcified, intrasellar or suprasellar cyst with an intracystic nodule (27). In Rathke pouch cysts with intracystic nodules, the cyst fluid shows low signal intensity to isointensity relative to the intensity of the nodules on T1-weighted images, and isointensity to high signal intensity on T2-weighted images (28). The cyst content is usually similar to cerebrospinal fluid; more complex cysts may show increased density, with septa partitioning the cystic portion. The absence of calcifications assists in differentiating a Rathke pouch cyst from a craniopharyngioma, which is characterized by the presence of calcifications (29). Nevertheless, rare examples of Rathke cyst are associated with mineralization (30). Most lesions have intrasellar and suprasellar components, although lesions confined to the sella turcica, suprasellar lesions, and intrasphenoidal lesions occur (16).

Microscopic Findings. The cysts are lined by cuboidal to columnar epithelium, with or without cilia (fig. 3-9); goblet cells and foci of squamous epithelium may be present. Mineralization (calcifications), cholesterol granulomas, and xanthomatous cells may be seen (fig. 3-9).

The epithelial cells are reactive for cytokeratin and epithelial membrane antigen (EMA), with variable reactivity for S-100 protein, chromogranin, glial fibrillary acidic protein (GFAP), and pituitary peptide markers (31,32).

Treatment and Prognosis. Drainage of the cyst with partial removal of the cyst wall (for diagnosis) via a transphenoidal approach is the treatment of choice (33). More recently, endoscopic endonasal removal of Rathke cysts has been reported (34–36). The recurrence rate is 5 percent (16).

Thornwaldt Cyst

Definition. *Thornwaldt cyst* is a developmental anomaly of the posterior superior nasopharynx in which the pharyngeal to notochord contact persists, creating a potential space for in-growth of pharyngeal tissue. When infected, this is referred to as *Thornwaldt disease* or *syndrome* (37).

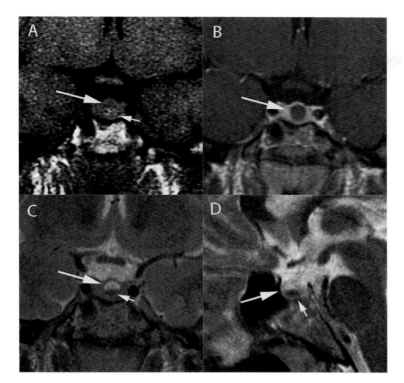

Figure 3-8

RATHKE POUCH CYST

A: Coronal T1-weighted image of the sella shows a cystic mass in the center of the adenohypophysis (large arrow). There is a slightly hyperintense nodule at the inferior aspect of the cyst (small arrow).

B: The postcontrast coronal T1-weighted image shows that no components of the lesion enhance (arrow).

C,D: Coronal (C) and sagittal (D) T2-weighted images show hyperintense signal of the fluid component of the cyst (large arrows) and hypointense signal of the nodule (small arrows). (Courtesy of Dr. D. E. Meltzer, New York, NY.)

Synonyms include *pharyngeal bursa* and *Thornwaldt bursa*. It is also spelled as *Tornwaldt cyst*.

Embryology. The pharyngeal bursa is a sac-like depression on the posterosuperior nasopharyngeal wall that forms around the 6th week of gestation when the cephalic portion of the notochord comes into close contact with the foregut (fig. 3-7). This contact between the pharynx and the notochord is usually transient but may persist in adults (38); the pharyngeal respiratory epithelium may grow and create a potential space that may be walled off, creating the Thornwaldt cyst.

Clinical Features. Thornwaldt cyst is uncommon. There is no gender predilection and these cysts occur at any age, although most are diagnosed in the second to fourth decades of life. The cyst is asymptomatic but when infected, symptoms include drainage of purulent material into the nasopharynx, headaches, otalgia and fullness of the ear, halitosis, and neck soreness or stiffness (39,40). The cysts are located in the midline of the posterior nasopharyngeal wall but may be found slightly off midline. They usually extend upward and backward toward the occipital bone. Thornwaldt cyst lies caudal to the location of Rathke pouch cyst.

Radiographically, Thornwaldt cysts appear as a mass high on the posterior nasopharyngeal wall. Air may be seen extending from the midline posterior nasopharynx toward the occipital tubercle (41,42). On computerized tomography (CT) scan, the cyst may contain fluid of similar density to cerebrospinal fluid, which does not enhance after contrast. Calcifications may be identified.

The endoscopic appearance of these lesions is that of a submucosal, firm and smooth mass. The adjacent mucosa may be erythematous (43).

Microscopic Findings. The cysts are submucosal. The lining includes ciliated respiratory epithelium. Squamous metaplasia is present in an infected cyst.

Differential Diagnosis. The differential diagnosis includes Rathke pouch cyst, which is localized to the area of the sella turcica, in contrast to Thornwaldt cyst, which is located in the posterior pharynx.

Treatment and Prognosis. Surgical excision is the treatment of choice. Incomplete excision

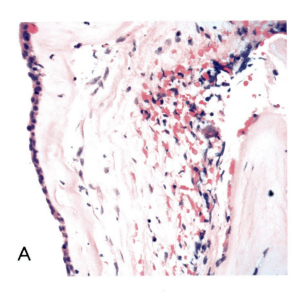
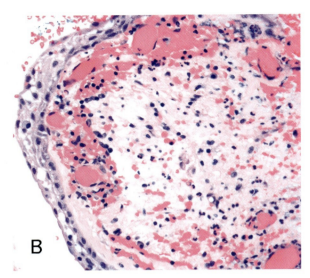
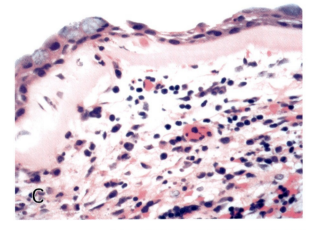

Figure 3-9

RATHKE POUCH CYST

A–C: Histologically, the cyst lining variably includes cuboidal cells (A), squamous cells (B), and goblet (mucous) cells (C) (arrowheads).
D: Submucosal hemorrhage and cholesterol granuloma formation without calcifications are also found.
E: Associated calcifications may be present, as here.

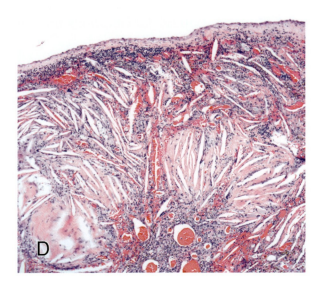
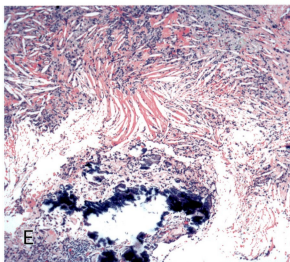

results in recurrence. Antibiotic therapy is given preoperatively for those with infected cysts.

PHARYNGEAL HAMARTOMAS, CHORISTOMAS, AND TERATOMATOUS LESIONS

Hamartoma is a non-neoplastic developmental anomaly caused by the excessive growth of normal cells or tissue indigenous to its site of occurrence. Hamartomatous lesions occur in all head and neck sites, but tend to predilect to the nasal cavity, paranasal sinuses, and the nasopharynx. *Choristoma* (heterotopia, ectopia, aberrant rest) is a non-neoplastic developmental anomaly of essentially normal tissue but with the tissue elements being foreign to its anatomic location.

Nasopharyngeal Hamartomas

Clinical Features. Hamartomas of the nasopharynx are uncommon. Reports of nasopharyngeal hamartomas are often included with nasal hamartomas, so that a true incidence of hamartomas exclusively limited to the nasopharynx cannot be determined. There is no gender predilection. Nasopharyngeal hamartomas occur in adults and children. In adults, the clinical presentation includes nasal obstruction, difficulty breathing, postnasal drainage, and epistaxis (44–47); in pediatric patients, the clinical presentation includes noisy breathing, stridor, feeding difficulties, and transient cyanosis (48).

Gross Findings. Nasopharyngeal hamartomas are described as polypoid to cauliflower-like, circumscribed and lobulated masses partially or completely filling the nasopharynx. They are 1 to 4 cm in greatest dimension.

Microscopic Findings. Hamartomas may be comprised of epithelial and/or mesenchymal components. Epithelial hamartomas include minor salivary gland elements (seromucous glands, ducts, acini) or, less commonly, epithelial elements (squamous or columnar cells). Epithelial hamartomas may be histologically identical to the respiratory epithelial adenomatoid hamartoma and seromucinous hamartoma of the sinonasal tract (see chapter 1) (49). Mesenchymal hamartomatous elements may include blood vessels, fibrous stroma, and lymphoid tissue (46,50). Metaplastic components such as bone may be present.

Differential Diagnosis. The differential diagnosis primarily includes a teratoma. The absence of cellular elements of all three germ cell layers, which characterizes a teratoma, allows for distinguishing a hamartomatous lesion from teratoma. Schneiderian-type inverted papillomas may originate in the nasopharynx (51) but the characteristic histology of inverted papillomas allows for differentiation from a hamartoma. The absence of an infiltrative growth pattern separates malignant neoplasms of both epithelial and mesenchymal derivation from a hamartoma.

Treatment and Prognosis. Simple excision is curative.

Pharyngeal/Nasopharyngeal Central Nervous System Heterotopias

The *heterotopia* consists of central nervous system (CNS) tissue as a mass lesion in the nasopharynx, without connection to the cranial cavity. This is a rare lesion that occurs in neonates and infants. It presents with airway obstruction (52–55). CNS heterotopias may occur in association with congenital anomalies (53–60). Radiographic evaluation may assist in the diagnosis and in determining the extent of the lesion (61).

Histologically, these lesions are similar to heterotopic CNS tissue of the nasal cavity. Heterotopic CNS tissue in the nasopharynx may appear polypoid, with identifiable CNS tissue seen within the submucosa (fig. 3-10). The CNS tissue is immunoreactive for GFAP (fig. 3-10). In contrast to the nasal lesions, those of the nasopharynx may include the presence of ependymal elements, choroid plexus (52), and intracytoplasmic melanin (54,62). Rarely, the heterotopic CNS tissue has given rise to an oligodendroglioma (63). Simple excision is curative.

Nasopharyngeal Dermoid, or Teratoid, Lesions

Definition. *Nasopharyngeal dermoid*, or *teratoid*, *lesions* represent a developmental (congenital) anomaly predominantly composed of skin (ectodermal derived) but also may include well-formed cartilage (mesodermal derived); the absence of endodermal-derived structures and the presence of limited heterogeneity of tissue types argue against inclusion as a teratoma. The fact that these lesions contain skin, a tissue type not normally found in the nasopharynx, suggests that they may be better classified as

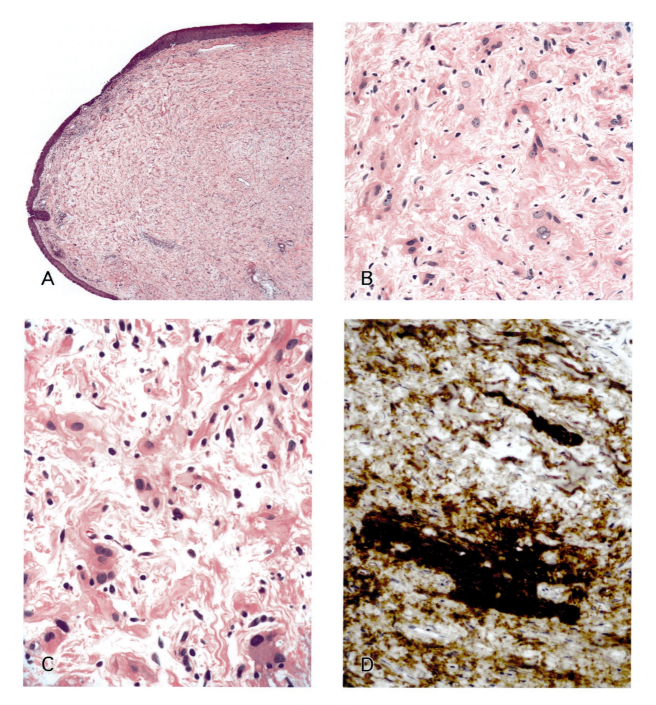

Figure 3-10

NASOPHARYNGEAL HETEROTOPIC CENTRAL NERVOUS SYSTEM TISSUE

A: A polypoid lesion has intact surface respiratory and squamous epithelia and a submucosal, fibrous and variably cellular proliferation effacing the normal submucosal structures.

B: At higher magnification, the submucosal tissue is composed of astrocytes and neuroglial fibers with associated fibrous and variably vascularized tissue.

C: Irregularly shaped neuroglial cells are composed of round to oval nuclei and abundant eosinophilic-appearing cytoplasm.

D: Confirmation of a neuroglial origin is seen by the presence of immunoreactivity for glial fibrillary acidic protein (GFAP).

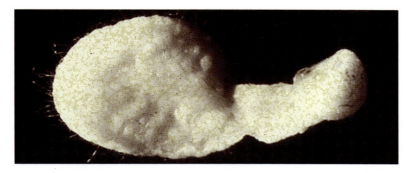

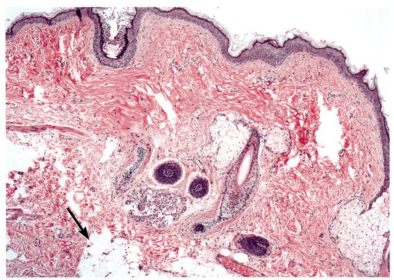

Figure 3-11

NASOPHARYNGEAL DERMOID CYST (HAIRY POLYP)

Top: Resection specimen of a polypoid solid mass with identifiable hairs on the surface of the lesion.

Bottom: The dermoid cyst consists of skin (keratinizing squamous epithelium), cutaneous adnexal structures including hair follicles and sebaceous glands, and mature adipose tissue (arrow). Although not illustrated here, cartilage and bone may be present.

a choristoma rather than a hamartoma, and possibly of first branchial arch origin (54,64,65). Some authors argue that these lesions are best classified as a subset of benign teratoma (66). The lesion is also known as *hairy polyp*.

Clinical Features. Nasopharyngeal dermoids occur in newborns or infants, who present with difficulties in breathing, swallowing, or sucking (54,67–75). There is no gender predilection although some reports indicate a female predilection (67), while others report a male predilection (76). Nasopharyngeal dermoids may occur as an isolated lesion or may be associated other congenital anomalies or malformations (64,77,78). Concurrent lesions of the pharynx and other sites, including the ear region, have been reported (79), as have bilateral lesions (80). Isolated, histologically similar lesions have been identified in nonpharyngeal sites including the middle ear (81,82), eustachian tube (83,84), tongue (85), soft palate (86), and hard palate and lower lip (76).

Gross Findings. Nasopharyngeal dermoids are polypoid, predominantly solid but partially cystic lesions and may be pedunculated or sessile (fig. 3-11).

Microscopic Findings. Histologically, there is a combination of various ectodermal and mesodermal tissues, including skin (keratinizing squamous epithelium), cutaneous adnexa, cartilage, bone, muscle (striated or smooth), and fibrous or mature adipose tissue (fig. 3-11). The lesions are covered by skin, and hair follicles and sebaceous glands are present in the submucosa. In addition, elastic cartilage can be identified. Similar histologic findings identified in a lesion of the ear have suggested to some authors that these lesions are of branchial cleft origin, representing congenital accessory auricles, akin to accessory tragus (65). In addition to cartilage, other tissue types found to a varying degree include muscle (smooth and striated), fibroadipose tissue, vascular tissue, and meningothelial elements (87).

Differential Diagnosis. Given the definition of these lesions as a non-neoplastic developmental anomaly, the main entity in the differential diagnosis is teratoma. The absence of endodermally derived tissue and the wide variety of tissue types usually seen in teratoma allow for distinguishing these lesions.

Treatment and Prognosis. Simple surgical excision is curative.

Lymphangiomatous Polyp of the Tonsil

Definition. *Lymphangiomatous polyp of the tonsil* is a non-neoplastic developmental lesion composed of tissue elements native to the nasopharynx and categorized as a hamartoma (88,89). It is also known as *lymphoid polyp*.

Clinical Features. Lymphangiomatous polyps are uncommon. There is an equal gender predilection. They occur over a wide age range, from the first to the seventh decades, with a mean age of occurrence at 25 years (89), but may occur at a very young age (90). The clinical presentation includes dysphagia, sore throat, and the sensation of a mass lesion in the throat. Symptoms may be present from a few weeks to years. These lesions are unilateral, without side predilection; a rare bilateral case has been reported (91). Most are of palatine tonsil origin but occasionally they originate from the nasopharynx or from the nasopharyngeal tonsil (i.e., adenoids) (89). By clinical examination, many of these lesions are felt to be neoplasms.

Gross Findings. Most lesions are polypoid or pedunculated, with a smooth external surface (fig. 3-12) and spongy to firm consistency. On cut section a white, tan, or yellow lesion measures from 0.5 to 3.8 cm. Some lesions are sessile.

Microscopic Findings. The polyps are covered by squamous or respiratory epithelium composed of a submucosal proliferation of dilated lymphatic vascular channels and varying amounts of fibrous connective tissue (fig. 3-13). The vascular components are thin-walled and usually contain proteinaceous fluid and mature lymphocytes. Mature adipose tissue may be present and prominent fibrosis may dominate in any given lesion. Some lesions are exclusively or predominantly papillary, with a lymphoid and edematous stroma. Epithelial hyperplasia, hyperkeratosis, and dyskeratosis without epithelial dysplasia and nested epitheliotropism are

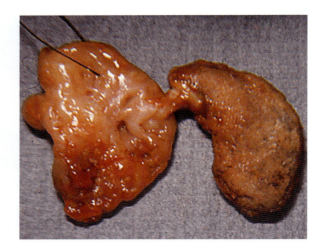

Figure 3-12

TONSILLAR LYMPHANGIOMATOUS POLYP

The polyp, attached to the tonsil (right) by a pedicle, has a solid and cystic appearance.

sometimes seen (89). The latter includes the presence of mature lymphocytes packed into rounded intramucosal spaces.

Special stains are not required for the diagnosis. However, immunohistochemical staining shows the presence of vascular endothelial markers, factor VIII-related antigen, CD31, CD34, and podoplanin (D2-40) in the endothelial and subendothelial cells of the vascular channels. Smooth muscle actin reactivity can be found within the vascular walls. The lymphoid component shows reactivity for both B-cell (CD20) and T-cell (CD3) markers.

Differential Diagnosis. The differential diagnosis includes nasopharyngeal (juvenile) angiofibroma, fibroepithelial polyps, papillomas, and lymphangioma. Nasopharyngeal (juvenile) angiofibroma is a nasopharyngeal-related lesion that occurs in adolescent males, typically presents with epistaxis due to its rich blood supply, and often attains large size with extensive growth and even bone erosion. Histologically, nasopharyngeal angiofibromas have a cellular stroma composed of stellate fibroblasts and staghorn-shaped thin-walled vascular structures, the latter typically lacking, or with an attenuated, smooth muscle component. The fibroblastic cells in angiofibroma show (nuclear) β-catenin and androgen receptor immunoreactivity. In contrast, lymphoangiomatous polyps occur in women

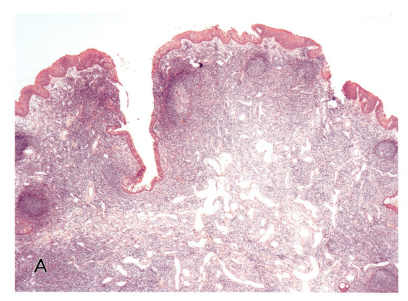
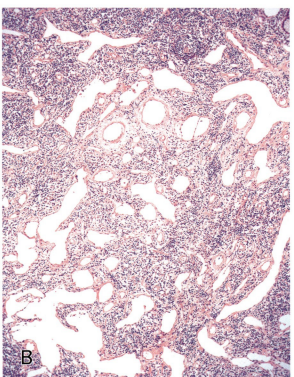
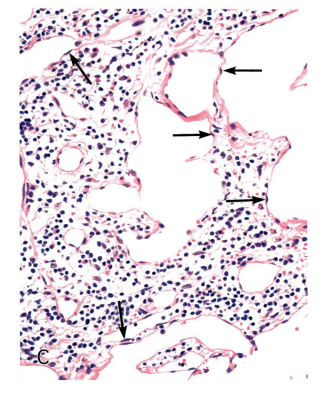

Figure 3-13

TONSILLAR LYMPHANGIOMATOUS POLYP

A: The surface squamous epithelium of this polypoid lesion appears bosselated. It overlies a submucosal proliferation of dilated lymphatic vascular channels and a lymphoid cell infiltrate including lymphoid follicles.

B: Variably shaped lymph-vascular channels with an associated lymphocytic cell infiltrate.

C: At higher magnification, the dilated spaces are lined by flattened endothelial cells (arrows).

and tend to have a paucicellular fibrous stroma with a prominent lymphoid component.

Squamous papillomas are epithelial neoplasms characterized by the presence of an exophytic surface epithelial proliferation of multilayered bland epithelial cells and lacking an associated lymphoid component. Most lack surface keratin although occasionally prominent (hyper)keratosis is identified. Rare examples of sinonasal-type papillomas may occur in the pharynx (oropharynx and nasopharynx) (92) but the histology of the lesions contrast so distinctly from lymphangiomatous polyps that differentiation is straightforward.

Lymphangiomas are neoplasms of endothelial-lined lymphatic spaces that are histologically characterized by the presence of widely dilated and irregularly appearing vascular channels. These features are not usually associated with lymphangiomatous polyps (88,89).

Treatment and Prognosis. Simple surgical excision, usually in the form of a unilateral tonsillectomy, is curative.

Salivary Gland Anlage Tumor

Definition. *Salivary gland anlage tumor* (SGAT) is a benign tumor with mixed epithelial and mesenchymal elements recapitulating the early stages in the embryology of salivary glands between the 4th and 8th week of development. SGAT is postulated to be a hamartoma of minor salivary gland derivation rather than a neoplasm since its histologic and architectural features are similar in some respects to the developing salivary gland (93). It is also known as *congenital pleomorphic adenoma*.

Clinical Features. SGAT is a rare lesion with less than 20 cases reported in the literature (93–102). There is a male predilection. It usually presents in the immediate neonatal period or in early infancy (by 6 weeks) (93). Symptoms include respiratory distress, nasal airway obstruction, and feeding difficulties. The tumor is often located at or near midline in the nasopharynx (93). The consistent midline presentation is a feature in common with other developmental anomalies in the head and neck region, including dermoid sinus, nasal glioma, and thyroglossal duct cyst. CT and magnetic resonance imaging (MRI) delineate the size of the mass and its relationship to surrounding anatomic structures (97). A case of SGAT was diagnosed in utero by fetal MRI performed secondary to the clinical finding of polyhydramnios, which identified a nasopharyngeal mass (100).

Gross Findings. The tumor is a pedunculated polyp measuring from 1.5 to 4.0 cm. There may be ulceration with hemorrhage and necrosis.

Microscopic Findings. At low magnification, the tumor is characterized by multiple submucosal solid nodules separated by less cellular stroma and a network of delicate linear and branching, small duct-like or glandular structures. Nests of solid or cystic squamous epithelium are set in a variably fibromyxoid stroma (fig. 3-14). The duct-like structures and squamous nests (with or without keratinization) tend to be more prominent toward the periphery of the more cellular stromal nodules but may be present centrally. The duct-like structures may be connected to the surface epithelium in areas. The surface is lined by a nonkeratinizing squamous mucosa.

The epithelial units within the internodular stroma blend into cellular nodules. The cellular nodules are predominantly composed of fusiform cells forming short fascicles or trabecula. The stromal cells are characterized by ovoid to spindle-shaped nuclei with uniformly dispersed nuclear chromatin and eosinophilic cytoplasm with indistinct cell borders. Mitotic figures may be present. Extensive hemorrhagic necrosis is likely the result of torsion. Rarely, bone formation may be present.

Immunohistochemically, the epithelial components are reactive for cytokeratins (pancytokeratins, CK7) and p63 (fig. 3-15); epithelial membrane antigen (EMA) is restricted to tubular structures. The mesenchymal components are reactive for vimentin, cytokeratins (AE1/AE3, CAM 5.2, CK7, OSCAR), p63, and muscle-specific actin but nonreactive for S-100 protein and GFAP. Both the epithelial and mesenchymal elements are consistently reactive for salivary gland amylase.

The proliferation rate (by Ki-67 or MIB1 staining) is variable; even within the same tumor it can vary from 1 to 30 percent. Ultrastructurally, some of the stromal-like cells manifest the features of myoepithelial cells (93).

Treatment and Prognosis. Simple excision (polypectomy) is curative. There have been no reported recurrences following complete excision.

INFECTIOUS DISEASES

Infections of the pharynx include bacterial, viral, fungal, mycobacterial, and protozoan. The breadth of infectious diseases of the pharynx is extensive. This section focuses on select and more common types.

Tonsillitis

Definition. *Tonsillitis* is a primary (bacterial) infection of the palatine tonsils. Synonyms include *chronic tonsillitis, hyperplastic tonsils, tonsils with benign lymphoid hyperplasia,* and *chronic fibrosing tonsillitis.*

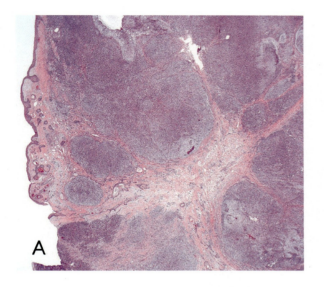
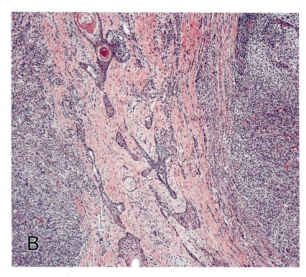
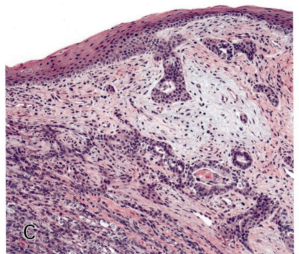

Figure 3-14

SALIVARY GLAND ANLAGE TUMOR (SGAT)

A: At low magnification, SGAT is characterized by multiple submucosal solid nodules separated by less cellular stroma and a network of delicate, linear and branching, small duct-like structures and nests of solid or cystic squamous epithelium with variable (internodular) fibromyxoid stroma.

B: Duct-like structures and squamous nests (with and without keratinization) are more prominently seen toward the periphery of (and in between) the cellular stromal nodules.

C: Focally, duct-like structures are connected to surface epithelium.

D: The cellular nodule is composed of fusiform cells forming short fascicles or a trabecular growth pattern.

E: The stromal cells are composed of ovoid to spindle-shaped nuclei with uniform, dispersed nuclear chromatin and eosinophilic cytoplasm with indistinct cell borders. A mitotic figure is present (arrow).

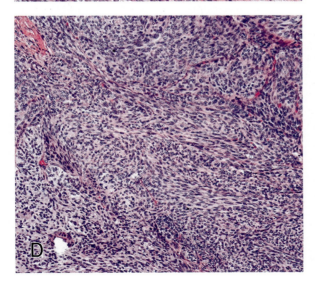
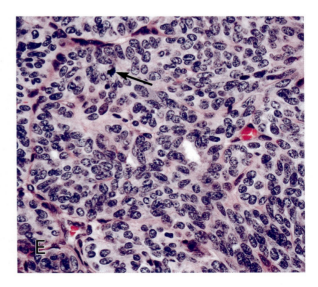

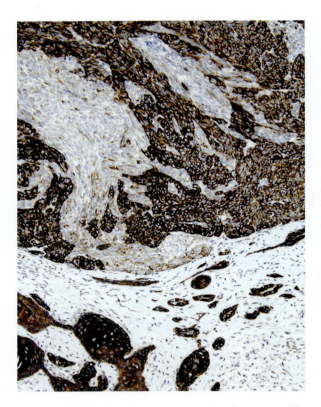 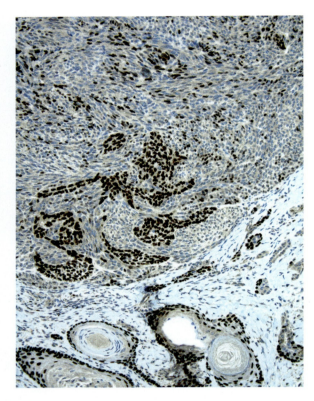

Figure 3-15

SALIVARY GLAND ANLAGE TUMOR: IMMUNOHISTOCHEMISTRY

Left: Cytokeratin (AE1/AE3) is expressed in the epithelial components (squamous nests and duct-like structures) and mesenchymal component.

Right: Variable p63 reactivity is seen in the epithelial and mesenchymal components.

Clinical Features. Tonsillitis is one of the more common diseases of the head and neck. According to the United States Vital Health Statistics report, acute pharyngotonsillitis is responsible for more than 6 million office visits each year by children younger than 15 years of age and an additional 1.8 million visits by adolescents and young adults aged 15 to 24 years (103). There is no gender predilection. Patients with acute exudative tonsillitis are typically young and include children, teenagers, and young adults.

The symptoms include rapid onset of fever, localized pain to the tonsillar region (odynophagia), and malaise; associated referred pain to the ear (otalgia) and dysphagia may be present. Involvement of the adjacent pharyngeal wall, as well as the adenoids, is common. Incubation periods tend to be short (i.e., days) and associated lymphadenopathy is common.

The etiologic agent is typically a bacterial infection, most often group A β-hemolytic streptococci, *Haemophilus influenzae,* and *Staphyloccocus aureus* (103–106); less common agents include *Corynebacterium diphtheriae* (diphtheria) and *Bordetella pertussis* (whooping cough). Viruses may cause tonsillitis, including adenoviruses and EBV (104,107–111). EBV-related oropharyngotonsillitis may occur in the absence of infectious mononucleosis (111).

On examination, the tonsils (and/or adenoids) are enlarged, hyperemic, and covered by a yellow exudate. It is not possible to differentiate the etiology of acute suppurative tonsillitis by laboratory examination, including serum C-reactive protein, peripheral white blood cell counts, and erythrocyte sedimentation rate, based on the limited clinical picture and epidemiologic factors (110). Contrast enhanced axial

CT shows diffuse enhancement and prominence of tonsillar tissue.

Microscopic Findings. An acute inflammatory infiltrate of the tonsils is hardly ever seen in surgical pathology material. The presence of neutrophils within the tonsillar crypt is not an indication of acute tonsillitis (or adenoiditis); neutrophils must be present in the parenchyma in order to consider the diagnosis. More typically, there is benign lymphoid hyperplasia characterized by enlarged and irregularly shaped germinal centers that include the presence of tingible body macrophages and identifiable mantle lymphocytes. Often, there is polarity (i.e., increased cellularity) of the mantle cell lymphocytes toward the site of the antigenic stimulation; the latter usually is from the epithelium surface of the tonsillar crypt so that there is expansion of the mantle lymphocytes on the side of the germinal center that is oriented toward the epithelium (fig. 3-16). In association with the benign lymphoid hyperplasia, there may be interfollicular expansion with increased mature plasma cells. In the presence of a viral infection, a prominent immunoblastic proliferation may be seen (see Infectious Mononucleosis). Fibrosis may or may not be present. A peritonsillar abscess, which includes the presence of pools of neutrophils (the histologic definition of an abscess), chronic inflammatory cells, or both, may be present.

Actinomycotic organisms, in the form of "sulfur granules," are saprophytes and normally found in the tonsillar crypts (see fig. 3-3). The presence of these microorganisms is not an indication of an infection. In order to consider a diagnosis of an actinomycotic infection, the microorganism must be identified within the tonsillar parenchyma, typically associated with an acute inflammatory infiltrate including abscess formation (see chapter 4 for illustrations).

The surface epithelium is usually intact and unremarkable but may be eroded (particularly in resolving acute tonsillitis). Rarely, papillary hyperplasia is present, which histologically includes the presence of surface papillary projections formed by hyperplastic lymphoid tissue (112).

Differential Diagnosis. Usually the diagnosis of tonsillitis is straightforward. The differential diagnosis includes specific infectious diseases such as HIV infection of the tonsils (and adenoids) and other specific infectious diseases, and a neoplastic proliferation (e.g., non-Hodgkin lymphoma). The presence of a mixed (heterogenous) inflammatory infiltrate lacking atypia excludes a malignant lymphoma.

Treatment and Prognosis. The treatment for bacterial infection involves the administration of antibiotics. Penicillin is the primary antibiotic used for treatment. Broad-spectrum cephalosporins (e.g., cefuroxime axetil) are very effective for persistent infection. Patients allergic to penicillin are treated with azithromycin. Antibiotic therapy can shorten the clinical course of group A β-hemolytic streptococcal pharyngotonsillitis, reduce the rate of transmission, and prevent suppurative and nonsuppurative complications, such as peritonsillar abscess and acute rheumatic fever (103).

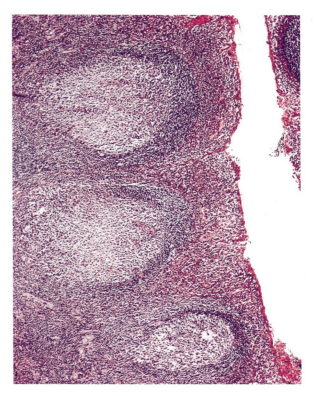

Figure 3-16

CHRONIC TONSILLITIS

The tonsillitis is characterized by the presence of benign (reactive) lymphoid hyperplasia, including submucosal, variably sized germinal centers. Often there is polarity (i.e., increased cellularity) of the mantle cell lymphocytes toward the crypt epithelium (right).

The use of surgery is controversial. Some patients have repeated (recurrent) attacks of tonsillitis. These patients may be antibiotic resistant, resulting in the recurrent attacks. For these (and perhaps other) patients, surgical management may be required (108). Patients who experience at least three episodes of tonsillitis in 3 consecutive years, five episodes in 2 years, or seven episodes in 1 year may benefit from surgery (113). Postoperative bleeding occurs in 3 to 6 percent of patients (114–123). Primary postoperative bleeding occurs within the first 24 hours after surgery and usually is related to the surgical procedure. Secondary or delayed postoperative bleeding occurs more than 24 hours after surgery and usually is related to loosening of the sutures by infection.

Post-transplant lymphoproliferative disorder (PTLD) is a life-threatening complication that may follow orthotopic liver transplantation (OLT) in children. This abnormal proliferation of lymphoid cells is related to EBV infection in immunocompromised children (124). The first symptoms are often in the ear, nose, or throat (ENT) area. Following OLT in children, nonbacterial tonsillar inflammation or hypertrophy associated with an EBV infection is often the first manifestation of PTLD (124). At the time of OLT, these patients are EBV seronegative but seroconversion occurs at the time of diagnosis or within 2 years of the diagnosis (124). Immediate tonsillectomy and immunosuppression are the proposed treatments for patients with acute tonsillitis associated with EBV seroconversion (124). Tonsillectomy, combined with tapering of immunosuppression, offers the best chance for a complete recovery.

Peritonsillar Abscess

Definition. A *peritonsillar abscess* is a collection of purulent material behind the posterior capsule of the tonsil. It is also referred to as *quinsy*.

Clinical Features. There is no gender predilection (125). Peritonsillar abscess primarily occurs in adolescents and adults (126,127), but may occur in children as well (128,129). Approximately one third of patients have a prior history (one or more episodes) of tonsillitis (130). The development of an abscess occurs over time, with gradually increasing pharyngeal (throat) discomfort occurring over days with subsequent dysphagia, odynophagia, ipsilateral otalgia, "hot potato" voice, trismus, and fever. On examination, the tonsils are enlarged and bulging, with deviation of the uvula and soft palate. Involvement is often bilateral and the abscess is typically located in the superior pole of the tonsils. Cervical adenopathy may be present.

CT scan is useful in localizing the abscess and confirming the presence of deep neck abscesses, but its accuracy has limitations (131). Intraoral ultrasound has a sensitivity and specificity of 89 to 95 percent and 79 to 100 percent, respectively, for correctly diagnosing peritonsillar abscess (132).

Pathogenesis. Etiologic agents most often include α- and β-hemolytic streptococci (126,133,134) and anaerobic bacteria (mainly *Bacteroides* sp. and *Fusobacterium nucleatum*) (129,135). Due to the prior use of antibiotics, the peritonsillar abscess is culture negative in up to 40 percent of cases (136).

Microscopic Features. The histologic findings include the presence of large (confluent) pools of neutrophils (the histologic definition of an abscess), chronic inflammatory cells, or both in the peritonsillar soft tissues (fig. 3-17).

Differential Diagnosis. Peritonsillitis is characterized by the presence of acute and chronic inflammation with granulation tissue. In contrast to peritonsillar abscess, there is no pooling of inflammatory cells.

Treatment and Prognosis. Conservative management including analgesics, antibiotics, fluids, and incision and drainage is effective for peritonsillar abscess (130,137). Incision and drainage is needed for diagnosis, for excluding the possibility of a neoplastic process, and for gathering material for culture and antibiotic sensitivity. Tonsillectomy is selectively utilized, but is also considered effective management especially in conjunction with antimicrobial therapy (137). The recurrence rate (10 to 15 percent) is low with conservative management (138).

Complications, if unrecognized or untreated, include extension of abscess into the parapharyngeal space and potentially into the wall of the carotid artery; extension of abscess superiorly to the base of skull and/or into the cranial cavity; extension inferiorly to the hypopharynx (piriform sinus) with obstruction of and possible rupture into the airway; and extension into the mediastinum via the carotid sheath

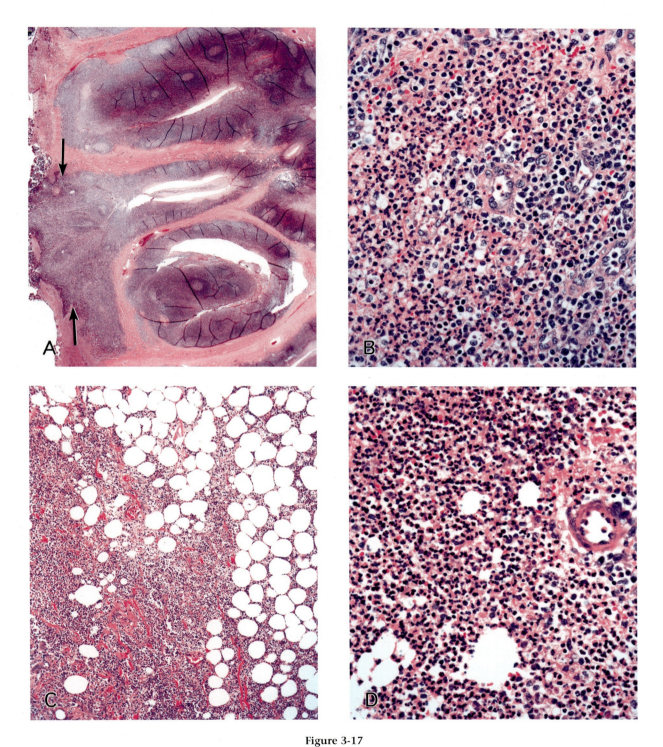

Figure 3-17

PERITONSILLAR ABSCESS

A. At low magnification, an inflammatory cell infiltrate extends into peritonsillar soft tissue (arrows).

B: At higher magnification, the infiltrate includes an admixture of acute and chronic inflammatory cells.

C,D: The inflammatory cells are almost exclusively composed of pools of polymorphonuclear leukocytes (abscess formation) that involve peritonsillar adipose tissue.

or retropharyngeal space (126,131,139). Death occurs from aspiration, airway obstruction, erosion into major blood vessels, or extension to the mediastinum (135).

Lemierre Disease/Syndrome

Lemierre disease/syndrome is a rare aggressive oropharyngeal infection that is associated with throat infection and thrombosis of the internal jugular vein or one of its tributaries, with subsequent distant septic emboli (140). Lemierre disease is caused most commonly by the bacterium *Fusobacterium necrophorum*, a Gram-negative obligate anaerobe.

Lemierre disease occurs in pediatric and adult patients. It is characterized by a history of recent pharyngitis followed by ipsilateral internal jugular vein thrombosis and metastatic abscesses. Patients present with exudative tonsillitis, sore throat, dysphagia, and unilateral neck pain (141,142). The diagnosis of septic thrombophlebitis is best confirmed by obtaining a CT scan of the neck with contrast (141).

Treatment with broad-spectrum antibiotics is considered the primary mode of therapy (e.g., prolonged course of intravenous beta-lactam antibiotic plus metronidazole) (140). Surgery is indicated for abscess formation or to resect/debride necrotic tissue. Severe complications that may lead to death include bacteremia; septic shock; septic abscesses to the lungs, joints, liver, peritoneum, kidneys, and brain; disseminated intravascular coagulopathy; encephalopathy; and pleural effusion (140,141,143).

EBV-Related Diseases and Infectious Mononucleosis

Definition. *Infectious mononucleosis* (IM) is a systemic, benign, self-limiting infectious lymphoproliferative disease primarily, but not exclusively, caused by EBV infection. EBV is an enveloped icosahedral herpesvirus with double-stranded linear DNA. EBV is strongly tropic for B lymphocytes and also for T lymphocytes. A number of non-neoplastic lesions and neoplasms are associated with EBV (Table 3-3) (144–156). The prototypic pharyngeal non-neoplastic disease associated with EBV is infectious mononucleosis; in other head and neck sites, oral hairy leukoplakia is common (see chapter 2). EBV is also associated with malignant neoplasms

Table 3-3

EPSTEIN-BARR VIRUS (EBV)-ASSOCIATED NON-NEOPLASTIC LESIONS AND NEOPLASMS

Non-Neoplastic Lesions
  Infectious mononucleosis
  Oral hairy leukoplakia
  EBV-associated hemophagocytic syndrome
  Chronic active EBV infection
  X-linked lymphoproliferative disorder

Neoplasms
  Hematolymphoid
    NK/T cell lymphoma
    Hodgkin lymphoma
    Burkitt lymphoma
    Pyothorax-associated lymphoma
  Epithelial
    Nasopharyngeal carcinoma, differentiated, non-keratinizing and undifferentiated subtypes
    Lymphoepithelial carcinomas
    Gastric adenocarcinoma
  Mesenchymal
    Smooth muscle tumors

including hematolymphoid malignancies (e.g., nasal-type NK/T-cell lymphoma, Burkitt lymphoma, Hodgkin lymphoma) and epithelial malignancies, including nasopharyngeal-type nonkeratinizing carcinomas, lymphoepithelial carcinomas (e.g., salivary glands, lung, thymus, stomach), and gastric adenocarcinoma.

Clinical Features. There is no sex predilection and IM occurs in all age groups but primarily affects adolescents and young adults. EBV is estimated to cause from 80 to 95 percent of the cases of IM (157). The clinical presentation of EBV-associated IM includes acute pharyngotonsillitis, with patients experiencing sore throat, fever, and malaise. The pharyngotonsillitis is often severe and may be exudative. The moderate to severe pharyngitis associated with IM is characterized by marked swollen and enlarged tonsils covered by dirty gray exudates. Lymphadenopathy commonly affects posterior cervical lymph nodes, but both anterior and posterior nodes may be involved. Tender lymphadenopathy, particularly of the posterior cervical lymph nodes, occurs. Systemically, there may be hepatosplenomegaly with chemical evidence of hepatitis. A prodromal period of 2 to 5 days consists of malaise and fatigue and frequently occurs prior to the onset of the full syndrome.

The diagnosis of IM is established in a patient with the typical clinical presentation and appropriate laboratory findings. Tissue confirmation of the diagnosis is usually not required. In the atypical case, where the patient presents with adenotonsillar or lymph node enlargement without fever, sore throat, or splenomegaly, a biopsy may be needed in order to establish a diagnosis and rule out a malignant process (158).

Pathogenesis. Most cases are caused by a primary EBV infection. EBV is transmitted by close human contact, frequently with saliva during kissing. There is some dispute in the literature whether the initial infection begins in oropharyngeal and nasopharyngeal epithelial cells or in B lymphocytes. EBV is strikingly lymphotrophic, targeting B lymphocytes through binding of the viral envelope glycoprotein gp350 to the complement receptor CD21 on the surface of B lymphocytes (159,160). Epithelial cells are infected by the binding of EBV to CR2-like receptor found on the surface of epithelial cells (161).

Evidence has shown that, after binding to primary B cells, most Epstein-Barr virions are not internalized but remain on the B-cell surface and from there transfer efficiently to CD21-negative epithelial cells, increasing epithelial infection (162). Transfer infection is associated with the formation of B-cell-epithelial conjugates, with gp350/CD21 complexes focused at the intercellular synapse (163); transfer involves the gp85 and gp110 viral glycoproteins but is independent of gp42, the HLA class II ligand that is essential for B-cell entry (162).

Through efficient binding to the B-cell surface, EBV simultaneously accesses both lymphoid and epithelial compartments; in particular, infection of pharyngeal epithelium by orally transmitted virus becomes independent of initial virus replication in the B-cell system (162). In most B cells, EBV establishes latent infection; in a minority of B cells, there is productive infection with lysis of infected cells and release of virions that may infect other B cells. The activated B cells disseminate in the circulation and secrete antibodies, including heterophile anti-sheep red blood cell antibodies.

By infecting B cells, EBV elicits humoral and cellular immune responses that induce the formation of new antigens including viral capsid antigen (VCA), membrane antigen (MA), early antigen (EA) (diffuse [EA-D] and restricted [EA-R]), Epstein-Barr nuclear antigen (EBNA), and lymphocyte-detected membrane antigen (LYDMA). The earliest phase of disease is characterized by infection of B cells that proliferate, develop neo-antigens, circulate, stimulate immune response, and synthesize immunoglobulin. VCA, EA, and EBNA are the viral proteins most important for serodiagnosis in immunocompetent patients.

Other microorganisms associated with mononucleosis-like syndromes include cytomegalovirus (CMV), *Toxoplasma gondii*, rubella virus, hepatitis A virus, and adenoviruses (157,164). Human herpesvirus 6 (HHV6) is also lymphotrophic and can produce heterophile-negative IM (165,166).

Laboratory Findings. There is a peripheral blood absolute lymphocytosis, with more than 60 percent lymphocytes in a total leukocyte population of over $5000/mm^3$ (164). The term mononucleosis refers to an increase in lymphocytes and not monocytes. Prominent atypical lymphocytes (Downey cells) are often more than 10 percent of the total leukocyte count. The atypical lymphocytes are mostly T-lymphocyte populations activated in response to B-cell infection and express CD8 (CD8-positive cytotoxic T cells), but also include CD16-positive NK cells (164). Cytologic alterations are not pathognomonic for IM as similar cells are found in CMV mononucleosis, toxoplasmosis, and infectious hepatitis (164). There are mild to moderate elevations of liver enzymes, including aspartate and alanine aminotransferase.

The diagnosis of IM is confirmed by serologic findings: the demonstration of serum antibodies to sheep erythrocytes (positive Paul-Bunnell heterophil antibody test) or horse erythrocytes (positive Mono-Spot test). The Mono-Spot test is a simple, rapid, highly specific and sensitive test for the heterophil antibodies of IM; false-positive tests occur but are rare (164). False-negative tests occur particularly in young children who produce heterophil antibodies in limited amounts (164).

In patients with IM exhibiting the typical clinical presentation and hematologic findings but who are heterophile antibody negative, the most likely agents are EBV and CMV. Non-EBV infectious agents causing infectious mononucleosis are not associated with a positive heterophile antibody and Mono-Spot test. In these patients, serodiagnosis is invaluable and includes an appreciable serum response to EBV viral capsid antigen (VCA) with both IgM and IgG antibodies at the time of clinical presentation; at presentation or shortly thereafter, many infected patients develop antibodies to early antigen complex (EA). During the early phase of primary infection, antibodies to EBNA are usually not demonstrable. IgM antibodies to VCA disappear within 2 to 3 months following infection; antibodies to EA disappear within 2 to 6 months, and IgG antibodies to VCA and anti-EBNA antibodies persist for life and are indicative of a chronic carrier state.

Microscopic Findings. At low magnification, there is distortion or partial effacement of the nodal/tonsillar architecture, with reactive follicular hyperplasia characterized by enlarged and irregularly shaped germinal centers (fig. 3-18). There is expansion of the interfollicular areas with a polymorphous proliferation of small lymphocytes, transformed lymphocytes, immunoblasts, plasma cells, and Reed-Sternberg-like cells (fig. 3-18). The presence of immunoblasts may result in a mottled appearance.

The lymphocytic and immunoblastic proliferation often displays marked cytologic atypia, with one or more prominent nucleoli, increased mitotic activity, and phagocytosis. The immunoblasts may cluster or occasionally form sheets effacing portions of the tissue and simulating a malignant lymphoma; immunoblasts are occasionally binucleated, simulating the appearance of the Reed-Sternberg cells of Hodgkin lymphoma (167,168). Necrosis may be seen and is usually focal, characterized by individual cell necrosis, although larger confluent zones of necrosis and infarction may be present (169,170). A vascular proliferation with prominent endothelial cells is always present. With nodal involvement, at least some subcapsular sinuses are patent and contain a polymorphous lymphoid infiltrate similar to the interfollicular infiltrate.

Histochemical stains for microorganisms are negative. Immunohistochemical studies show B-cell (e.g., CD20) and T-cell (e.g., CD3) reactivity (fig. 3-19) without immunoreactivity for CD15 (Leu-M1). Immunoblasts may stain with CD30 (171,172). Immunoreactivity can be seen for EBV latent membrane protein (LMP) (fig. 3-19), including in the Reed-Sternberg-like cells (172). In situ hybridization for EBV-encoded RNA (EBER) (fig. 3-19) is more specific and sensitive than EBV LMP.

Cytogenetic and molecular genetic evaluations show an absence of gene rearrangements. Polymerase chain reaction (PCR) analysis may detect the presence of virus (generation of proteins containing EBV-encoded polypeptide sequences) and represents a more reliable and sensitive means for detecting the presence of virus than serodiagnosis (173,174).

Differential Diagnosis. The differential diagnosis of IM includes non-Hodgkin malignant lymphomas, especially large cell or immunoblastic lymphoma (B-cell lineage) and anaplastic CD30-positive large cell lymphoma; Hodgkin disease; and HIV-associated changes (see later in chapter). The markedly atypical interfollicular cellular proliferation can easily be misinterpreted as a non-Hodgkin lymphoma (160,175,176). Attention to the clinical history, especially the typical demographics associated with IM, should suggest the diagnosis. Confirmatory laboratory analysis and absence of immunohistochemical and molecular biologic confirmation of a neoplastic process assist in avoiding the potential trap of misdiagnosing IM for a lymphoma. Primary Hodgkin lymphoma of the tonsils or mucosal sites of the upper aerodigestive tract is exceedingly rare; when Hodgkin disease involves these sites, it usually does so secondarily following primary nodal disease (177).

Treatment and Prognosis. IM is associated with a favorable clinical course, often with resolution of symptoms within 4 to 6 weeks, although fatigue may last longer, resolving over a period of several months. Therapy is supportive, including rest and fluid intake (178).

Rarely, serious and potentially fatal complications develop and include hepatic dysfunction with jaundice, elevated hepatic enzyme levels, and rarely, liver failure (179); splenic rupture, secondary to splenic involvement with massive splenomegaly (180,181); respiratory failure (182,183); nephritis, renal failure, or hemolytic uremic syndrome (184–186); and life-threatening thrombocytopenia and bleeding diathesis (187). IM has been linked to an increased risk of developing Hodgkin lymphoma and multiple sclerosis (188–191) and potential progression to non-Hodgkin lymphomas (192).

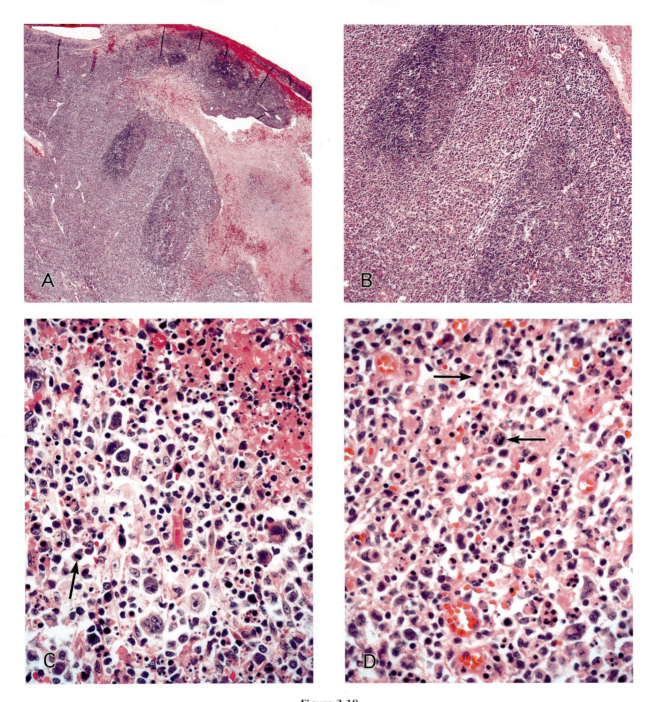

Figure 3-18
INFECTIOUS MONONUCLEOSIS

A,B: Seen are distortion and partial effacement of the tonsillar architecture with preservation of germinal centers and interfollicular expansion by a cellular proliferation. Confluent areas of necrosis are seen in the center right and upper right of each image, respectively.

C,D: At higher magnification, the interfollicular areas include a proliferation of immunoblasts, plasma cells, Reed-Sternberg-like cells, and lymphocytes. The lymphocytes show marked nuclear atypia with prominent nucleoli, increased mitotic activity (arrows) that may include atypical forms, and necrosis (confluent foci and individual cell). Out of context with the clinical history and laboratory findings, these histologic features suggest a diagnosis of malignant lymphoma.

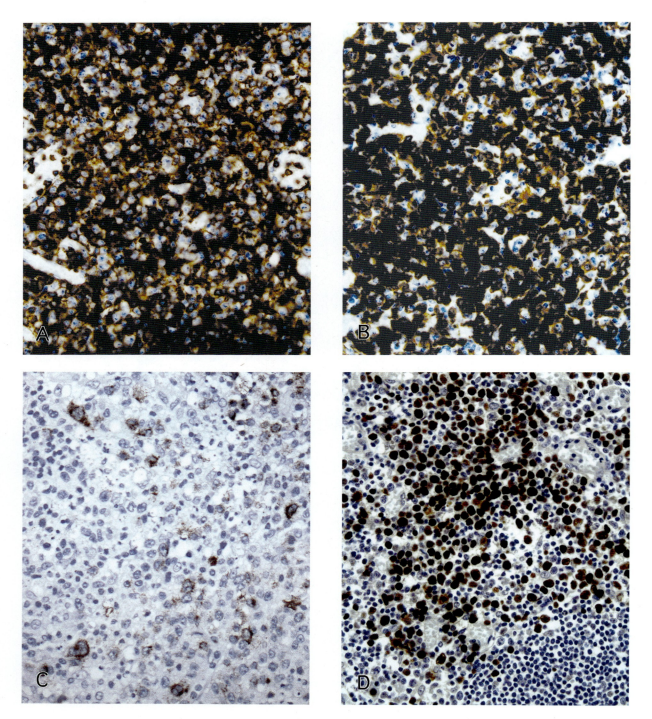

Figure 3-19

INFECTIOUS MONONUCLEOSIS

A,B: The atypical lymphoid cells express CD20 (B-cell marker) (A) and CD3 (T-cell marker) (B). Reactivity for both CD20 and CD3 is indicative of a polyclonal (benign) cell proliferation.

C: Also expressed is immunoreactivity for EBV latent membrane protein (cytoplasmic staining).

D: In situ hybridization is positive for EBV-encoded RNA (EBER; nuclear staining). (C is courtesy of Dr. A. T. Turk, New York, NY.)

The most serious complications arise in individuals with X-linked lymphoproliferative disease (XLP), also referred to as Duncan disease. XLP is caused by mutations in *SH2D1A* and *XIAP (BIRC4)*; it may also occur in rare instances with no identified underlying genetic cause (193). XLP occurs in males with mutations in the signaling lymphocyte-activation molecule-associated protein that regulates T and NK cells (193). The mutation has been mapped to chromosome Xq24-25 coding for cell surface receptor on T and NK cells but not B cells. These patients are immunosuppressed and possess a rare, familial, fatal form of combined immunodeficiency (193). The three most commonly recognized phenotypes of SH2D1A-related XLP are: 1) hemophagocytic lymphohistiocytosis (HLH), also referred to as hemophagocytic syndrome; 2) dysgammaglobulinemia; and 3) lymphoproliferative disorders (malignant lymphoma), which are typically high-grade B-cell lymphomas, non-Hodgkin type, often extranodal, and in particular involving the intestine (194). Regardless of clinical phenotype, the only curative treatment is allogeneic hematopoietic cell transplantation which should be considered in most patients as early as possible (195).

Human Papillomavirus

Human papillomavirus (HPV) represents a large group of small, double-stranded, circular DNA viruses. The viruses include cottontail rabbit papillomavirus (CRPV) and human papillomavirus (HPV). HPV is a sexually transmitted disease, although direct maternal transmission has been suggested (196). HPV is strongly epitheliotropic and is associated with both non-neoplastic and neoplastic lesions (197).

The non-neoplastic pharyngeal diseases associated with HPV include verrucae (verruca vulgaris, or common wart, and condyloma acuminatum) and a rare pharyngeal lesion that is associated with low-risk viruses including types 6 and 11 (198,199). More than 100 types of HPV are associated with benign and malignant epithelial neoplasms. HPV-associated benign neoplasms include squamous papilloma associated with low-risk viruses including types 6 and 11. HPV-associated malignant neoplasms include oropharyngeal carcinomas associated with high-risk viruses including types 16 and 18.

The role of HPV in neoplastic proliferations may stem from its function as a promoter in the multistep process of carcinogenesis in squamous cells of the upper aerodigestive tract. Two viral oncoproteins of high-risk HPVs, E6 and E7, promote tumor progression by the inactivation of p53 and retinoblastoma tumor suppressor gene products, respectively (200). These viral oncoproteins are capable of disrupting the cell-cycle regulatory pathways in the genetic progression to squamous cell carcinoma. Dysfunction of the retinoblastoma gene product results in abnormal cell proliferation and the development of malignant tumors (197,200). A discussion of pharyngeal neoplasms is beyond the scope of this text.

Human Immunodeficiency Virus Infection and Acquired Immunodeficiency Syndrome

The clinical syndrome of *acquired immunodeficiency syndrome* (AIDS) is characterized by opportunistic infection(s) and/or neoplasia, with an associated immunodeficiency. AIDS-related pathology may be seen in every organ system as a result of infection by the *human immunodeficiency virus* (HIV)-1, the causative agent of AIDS. The head and neck represents a microcosm of the entire body with respect to the manifestations of AIDS. Virtually every conceivable pathologic process associated with HIV infection and AIDS can be found within the head and neck, including a wide variety of opportunistic infections, reactive lymphoproliferative processes, and hematolymphoid and nonlymphoid neoplasms (Table 3-4). These pathologic changes may be the initial manifestations of HIV infection or AIDS, or they may represent a component of systemic disease.

Pathogenesis. Infection with the HIV-1 initiates a series of events within the host immune system that ultimately leads to the destruction of cellular immunity. The resultant immunosuppression renders the host susceptible to the opportunistic infections and tumors that are the hallmark of AIDS.

HIV-1 is a human retrovirus of the lentivirus genus. The virus is a membrane-bound, double-stranded RNA characterized by the presence of a unique enzyme, reverse transcriptase, at its core. Reverse transcriptase allows the viral RNA to be transcribed "backwards" into DNA and then

Table 3-4

HUMAN IMMUNODEFICIENCY VIRUS (HIV) AND ACQUIRED IMMUNODEFICIENCY SYNDROME (AIDS)-RELATED PATHOLOGY OF THE HEAD AND NECK

Opportunistic Infections
  Viral
    Cytomegalovirus
    Herpes
    Others
  Bacteria
    Mycobacteria (*M. tuberculosis; M. avium intracellulare*)
    Others
  Fungal
    Cryptococcus neoformans
    Aspergillus
    Others
  Protozoal
    Toxoplasma gondii
    Pneumocystis jiroveci (formerly *carinii*)
    Cryptosporidium
    Microsporidium

Benign Lesions
  Lymphadenopathy
  Extranodal lymphoid proliferation (adenotonsillar disease)
  HIV salivary gland disease
  Bacillary angiomatosis

Nonhematolymphoid Malignancies
  Kaposi sarcoma
  Malignant lymphomas
  Carcinomas
  Other

inserted into the host genome (201,202). HIV preferentially infects CD4-positive (helper) T-cell lymphocytes and other cells of the immune system that bear both the CD4 receptor and one of two chemokine receptors (CCR-5 and CXCR-4) on their surface. These cells include CD4-positive lymphocytes, dendritic cells, and macrophages. HIV is transmitted through blood, sexual (body fluids) routes, and maternofetal routes.

The overwhelming majority of early cases of HIV infection and AIDS in the United States and Europe were reported in men who had sex with men (homosexual and bisexual); although this remains the major risk group (53 percent), intravenous drug users (36 percent) and women (18 percent) are the two groups with the highest increase in rates of AIDS in the United States (203). Most cases in Africa and Asia are heterosexually transmitted because infected females are usually at peak reproductive ages; the incidence of vertical transmission is also high. Prior to the screening of blood products for HIV in 1984, recipients of contaminated blood and blood products (hemophiliacs) were at much higher risk of acquiring the infection. This mode of transmission continues to be a threat in areas of the world where the blood supply is not screened. More than 30 million persons are infected with HIV-1 worldwide. The World Health Organization (WHO) estimates that there are 16,000 new infections worldwide every day; 44,000 new HIV-1 infections were predicted in the United States for 1998 (204).

Spectrum of Disease. HIV-1 causes a spectrum of disease manifestations. With initial infection, the constellation of findings are caused directly by infection with HIV-1 and the patient's immune response. The transient, primary, symptomatic illness is associated with high-titer viremia and a vigorous response to the invading virus. The flu-like viral syndrome is characterized by fever, fatigue, pharyngitis, lymphadenopathy including tonsillar and adenoidal enlargement, and a maculo-papular rash. Due to the abundance of lymphoid tissue in the head and neck, including lymph nodes and extranodal lymphoid tissues (e.g., Waldeyer tonsillar ring and related to the parotid gland), this anatomic region often manifests findings related to infection.

During primary HIV infection there is a peak in viral load, which then decreases and levels out at what is known as the "set point"; this viral set point is prognostically significant. Individuals with a low viral set point are more likely to progress slowly to AIDS (over 10 years); individuals with a high viral set point are likely to progress rapidly to AIDS (less than 5 years). During primary infection, the immune system responds vigorously to the virus, at which time the patient is not immunodeficient and does not have AIDS; as the disease proceeds, especially if untreated, the virus begins to destroy the cellular arm of the patient's immune system. As CD4-positive cells of the immune system are destroyed, the patient loses the ability to fight off the myriad pathogens that are ubiquitous in our world.

AIDS is the immunodeficiency that results from HIV-1 infection; patients with AIDS are infected by pathogenic microorganisms as well as

Table 3-5

CENTERS FOR DISEASE CONTROL (CDC) CLASSIFICATION SYSTEM FOR HIV-INFECTED ADULTS AND ADOLESCENTS

CD4+ T-Cell Categories	A Asymptomatic, Acute, or PGL[a]	B[b] Symptomatic, B conditions	C AIDS Indicator Conditions
1 = ≥ 500/mL or 29%	A1	B1	C1
2 = 200-499/mL or 14-28%	A2	B2	C2
3 = < 200/ml or immunologic AIDS	A3[c]	B3	C3

[a]PGL = progressive generalized lymphadenopathy; AIDS = acquired immunodeficiency syndrome.
[b]Category B symptomatic conditions are defined as those occurring in an HIV-infected adolescent or adult that meet at least one of the following criteria: they are attributed to HIV infection or indicate a defect in cell-mediated immunity and they are considered to have a clinical course or management that is complicated by HIV infection. Examples include, but are not limited to, the following: bacillary angiomatosis; oropharyngeal candidiasis (thrush); vulvovaginal candidiasis, persistent or resistant; pelvic inflammatory disease (PID); cervical dysplasia (moderate or severe)/cervical carcinoma in situ; hairy leukoplakia, oral; herpes zoster (shingles), involving two or more episodes or at least one dermatome; idiopathic thrombocytopenic purpura; constitutional symptoms, such as fever (>38.5°C) or diarrhea lasting >1 month; and peripheral neuropathy.
[c]Persons under subcategories A3, B3, C1, C2, and C3 are reportable as AIDS cases in the United States and territories (effective 01 January, 1993).

opportunistic infections. The diagnosis of HIV-1 infection is conceptually simple: like most infections, it begins when the pathogen invades the host. The diagnosis of AIDS is much less clearcut. AIDS is a diagnosis of criteria. In the United States, the diagnosis is made by fulfilling criteria developed by the Centers for Disease Control and Prevention (CDC). The CDC classification system is based on three clinical categories (A, B, and C) and three CD4-T-cell count categories (1, 2, and 3) (Table 3-5) (205). The HIV-1 viral load, which has become a critical tool in diagnosing and managing patients with HIV-1 infection, is not included in the CDC criteria.

Early diagnosis is critical since effective initiation of antiretroviral therapy, if administered in the earliest phase of infection, has a major positive impact on prognosis and long-term survival. Indicators of HIV disease and AIDS are listed in Table 3-6.

The clinical staging and case definition of HIV for resource-constrained settings were developed by the WHO in 1990 and revised in 2007. Staging is based on the clinical findings that guide the diagnosis, evaluation, and management of HIV/AIDS, and it does not require a CD4 cell count. The staging system is used in many countries to determine eligibility for antiretroviral therapy, particularly in settings in which CD4 testing is not available. The clinical stages are categorized as 1 through 4, progressing from primary HIV infection to advanced HIV/AIDS (Table 3-6). These stages are defined by specific clinical conditions or symptoms. For the purpose of the WHO staging system, adolescents and adults are defined as individuals aged 15 years or older. The surveillance case definition for HIV infection and AIDS is listed in Table 3-7 (206,207). The WHO case definition for HIV infection and AIDS is listed in Table 3-8. Patients diagnosed with advanced HIV infection (including AIDS) not previously reported should be reported according to a standard case definition. Advanced HIV infection is diagnosed based on clinical or immunologic (CD4) criteria among people with confirmed HIV infection (Table 3-9). AIDS case reporting for surveillance is no longer required if primary HIV infection or advanced HIV infection is reported.

HIV-Related Lymphoid Changes of Nasopharyngeal and Palatine Tonsils

Clinical Features. HIV infection may first present clinically as enlargement of the lymphoid tissues of Waldeyer ring, including the tonsils, and particularly, nasopharyngeal lymphoid tissue (adenoids). These tissues are a major site of viral replication (208). The lymphoid enlargement may be unilateral and raise concern for a possible diagnosis of lymphoma. Such a clinical scenario prompts excision of the enlarged tissues. Concurrent (unilateral) cervical

Table 3-6

INDICATORS OF HIV DISEASE AND AIDS

Clinical Stage 1
    asymptomatic HIV infection
    persistent generalized lymphadenopathy
    acute (primary) HIV infection with accompanying illness or history of acute HIV infection

Clinical Stage 2
    moderate unexplained weight loss (<10% of presumed or measured body weight)
    recurrent respiratory infections (sinusitis, tonsillitis, otitis media, and pharyngitis)
    herpes zoster
    angular cheilitis
    recurrent oral ulceration
    papular pruritic eruptions
    seborrheic dermatitis
    fungal nail infections

Clinical Stage 3
    unexplained severe weight loss (>10% of presumed or measured body weight)
    unexplained chronic diarrhea for >1 month
    unexplained persistent fever for >1 month (>37.6°C, intermittent or constant)
    persistent oral candidiasis (thrush)
    oral hairy leukoplakia
    pulmonary tuberculosis (current)
    severe presumed bacterial infections (e.g., pneumonia, empyema, pyomyositis, bone or joint infection, meningitis, bacteremia)
    acute necrotizing ulcerative stomatitis, gingivitis, or periodontitis
    unexplained anemia (hemoglobin <8 g/dL)
    neutropenia (neutrophils <500 cells/μL)
    chronic thrombocytopenia (platelets <50,000 cells/μL)

Clinical Stage 4
    HIV wasting syndrome, as defined by the CDC (see Table 3-9)
    Pneumocystis pneumonia
    recurrent severe bacterial pneumonia
    chronic herpes simplex infection (orolabial, genital, or anorectal site for >1 month or visceral herpes at any site)
    esophageal candidiasis (or candidiasis of trachea, bronchi, or lungs)
    extrapulmonary tuberculosis
    Kaposi sarcoma
    cytomegalovirus infection (retinitis or infection of other organs)
    central nervous system toxoplasmosis
    HIV encephalopathy
    cryptococcosis, extrapulmonary (including meningitis)
    disseminated nontuberculosis mycobacteria infection
    progressive multifocal leukoencephalopathy
    Candida of the trachea, bronchi, or lungs
    chronic cryptosporidiosis (with diarrhea)
    chronic isosporiasis
    disseminated mycosis (e.g., histoplasmosis, coccidioidomycosis, penicilliosis)
    recurrent nontyphoidal *Salmonella* bacteremia
    lymphoma (cerebral or B-cell non-Hodgkin)
    invasive cervical carcinoma
    atypical disseminated leishmaniasis
    symptomatic HIV-associated nephropathy
    symptomatic HIV-associated cardiomyopathy
    reactivation of American trypanosomiasis (meningoencephalitis or myocarditis)

Table 3-7
SURVEILLANCE CASE DEFINITION FOR HIV INFECTION AND AIDS[a]

I. In adults, adolescents, or children aged greater than or equal to 18 months[b], a reportable case of HIV infection must meet at least one of the following criteria:
Laboratory criteria
    positive result on a screening test for HIV antibody (e.g., repeatedly reactive enzyme immunoassay), followed by a positive result on a confirmatory (sensitive and more specific) test for HIV antibody (e.g., Western blot or immunofluorescence antibody test)
or
    positive result or report of a detectable quantity on any of the following HIV virologic (nonantibody) tests:
        HIV nucleic acid (DNA or RNA) detection (e.g., DNA polymerase chain reaction [PCR] or plasma HIV-1 RNA)[c]
        HIV p24 antigen test, including neutralization assay;
        HIV isolation (viral culture)
or
Clinical or other criteria (if the above laboratory criteria are not met)
    diagnosis of HIV infection, based on the laboratory criteria above, that is documented in a medical record by a physician
or
    conditions that meet criteria included in the case definition for AIDS

II. In a child aged less than 18 months, a reportable case of HIV infection must meet at least one of the following criteria:
Laboratory criteria
    Definitive: positive results on two separate specimens (excluding cord blood) using one or more of the following HIV virologic (nonantibody) tests:
        HIV nucleic acid (DNA or RNA) detection[d]
        HIV p24 antigen test, including neutralization assay, in a child greater than or equal to 1 month of age
        HIV isolation (viral culture)
or
    Presumptive: a child who does not meet the criteria for definitive HIV infection but who has:
        positive results on only one specimen (excluding cord blood) using the above HIV virologic tests and no subsequent negative HIV virologic or negative HIV antibody tests
or
        clinical or other criteria (if the above definitive or presumptive laboratory criteria are not met)
        diagnosis of HIV infection, based on the laboratory criteria above, that is documented in a medical record by a physician
or
        conditions that meet criteria included in the 1987 pediatric surveillance case definition for AIDS (17,19)

III. A child aged less than 18 months born to an HIV-infected mother will be categorized for surveillance purposes as not infected with HIV if the child does not meet the criteria for HIV infection but meets the following criteria:
Laboratory criteria
    Definitive:
        at least two negative HIV antibody tests[b] from separate specimens obtained at greater than or equal to 6 months of age
or
        at least two negative HIV virologic tests[b] from separate specimens, both of which were performed at greater than or equal to 1 month of age and one of which was performed at greater than or equal to 4 months of age
and no other laboratory or clinical evidence of HIV infection (i.e., has not had any positive virologic tests, if performed, and has not had an AIDS-defining condition)
or
    Presumptive: a child who does not meet the above criteria for definitive "not infected" status but who has:
        one negative EIA[e] HIV antibody test performed at greater than or equal to 6 months of age and NO positive HIV virologic tests, if performed
or
        one negative HIV virologic test[b] performed at greater than or equal to 4 months of age and NO positive HIV virologic tests, if performed
or
        one positive HIV virologic test with at least two subsequent negative virologic tests[d], at least one of which is at greater than or equal to 4 months of age; or negative HIV antibody test results, at least one of which is at greater than or equal to 6 months of age

Table 3-7, continued

III. continued:
   and
      no other laboratory or clinical evidence of HIV infection (i.e., has not had any positive virologic tests, if performed, and has not had an AIDS-defining condition)
   or
      clinical or other criteria (if the above definitive or presumptive laboratory criteria are not met)
         determined by a physician to be "not infected", and a physician has noted the results of the preceding HIV diagnostic tests in the medical record
   and
      no other laboratory or clinical evidence of HIV infection (i.e., has not had any positive virologic tests, if performed, and has not had an AIDS-defining condition)

IV. A child aged less than 18 months born to an HIV-infected mother will be categorized as having perinatal exposure to HIV infection if the child does not meet the criteria for HIV infection (II) or the criteria for "not infected with HIV" (III)

[a]From MMWR 1999;48(RR-13):1-27,29-13.
[b]Children aged greater than or equal to 18 months but less than 13 years are categorized as "not infected with HIV" if they meet the criteria in III.
[c]In adults, adolescents, and children infected by other than perinatal exposure, plasma viral RNA nucleic acid tests should NOT be used in lieu of licensed HIV screening tests (e.g., repeatedly reactive enzyme immunoassay). In addition, a negative (i.e., undetectable) plasma HIV-1 RNA test result does not rule out the diagnosis of HIV infection.
[d]HIV nucleic acid (DNA or RNA) detection tests are the virologic methods of choice to exclude infection in children aged less than 18 months. Although HIV culture can be used for this purpose, it is more complex and expensive to perform and is less well standardized than nucleic acid detection tests. The use of p24 antigen testing to exclude infection in children aged less than 18 months is not recommended because of its lack of sensitivity.
[e]EIA = enzyme immunoassay.

Table 3-8
WORLD HEALTH ORGANIZATION (WHO) CASE DEFINITION FOR HIV INFECTION

Adults and children 18 months or older
HIV infection is diagnosed based on:
   positive HIV antibody testing (rapid or laboratory-based enzyme immunoassay). This is confirmed by a second HIV antibody test (rapid or laboratory-based enzyme immunoassay) relying on different antigens or of different operating characteristics
and/or
   positive virological test for HIV or its components (HIV-RNA or HIV-DNA or ultrasensitive HIV p24 antigen) confirmed by a second virological test obtained from a separate determination

Children younger than 18 months
HIV infection is diagnosed based on:
   positive virological test for HIV or its components (HIV-RNA or HIV-DNA or ultrasensitive HIV p24 antigen) confirmed by a second virological test obtained from a separate determination taken more than four weeks after birth
   positive HIV antibody testing is not recommended for definitive or confirmatory diagnosis of HIV infection in children until 18 months of age

adenopathy may be present. The histopathologic features (see below) suggest the possibility of HIV infection, but serologic evaluation is confirmatory.

Primary HIV infection results in a spectrum of histopathologic changes (209). The clinical presentation includes nasal congestion, airway obstruction, sore throat (pharyngitis), otalgia, facial weakness, fever, and a nasopharyngeal or tonsillar mass (209). Patients may be known to be HIV infected or the HIV-related enlargement of tonsils and/or adenoids occurs in patients who are not known to be HIV infected or at risk for HIV infection (209). The risk factors for HIV infection include homosexuality, blood transfusions, and intravenous drug abuse.

Table 3-9
CRITERIA FOR DIAGNOSIS OF ADVANCED HIV (INCLUDING AIDS[a])

Clinical criteria for diagnosis of advanced HIV in adults and children with confirmed HIV infection:
   presumptive or definitive diagnosis of any stage 3 or stage 4 condition
and/or
   immunologic criteria for diagnosing advanced HIV in adults and children 5 years or older with confirmed HIV infection: CD4 count less than 350/mm^3 of blood in an HIV-infected adult or child
and/or
   immunologic criteria for diagnosing advanced HIV in a child younger than 5 years of age with confirmed HIV infection:
      %CD4+ <30 among those younger than 12 months
      %CD4+ <25 among those aged 12–35 months
      %CD4+ <20 among those aged 36–59 months

[a]AIDS in adults and children is defined as: clinical diagnosis (presumptive or definitive) of any stage 4 condition with confirmed HIV infection; or immunologic diagnosis in adults and children with confirmed HIV infection and >5 years of age, first-ever documented CD4 count less than 200 per mm^3 or %CD4+ <15; or among children with confirmed HIV infection aged 12–35 months first ever documented %CD4 <20; or among children with confirmed HIV infection and less than 12 months of age first ever documented %CD4 <25.

Microscopic Findings. The presence of the HIV in nasopharyngeal and tonsillar tissues causes a unique constellation of diagnostic histopathologic features, including florid follicular hyperplasia, follicle lysis, and productively HIV-infected multinucleated giant cells of probable dendritic cell origin (209,210). The histomorphologic changes in HIV-induced tonsillar and adenoidal enlargement vary with the progression of disease. In the early stages of infection, there is florid follicular hyperplasia, with and without follicular fragmentation, as well as follicle lysis with areas of follicular involution (fig. 3-20). Additional findings include the presence of monocytoid B-cell hyperplasia, paracortical and interfollicular zone expansion with immunoblasts and plasma cells, interfollicular clusters of high endothelial venules, intrafollicular hemorrhage, and the presence of multinucleated giant cells (211). The giant cells characteristically cluster adjacent to or within the adenoidal surface epithelium or the tonsillar crypt epithelium (fig. 3-21) (209,212).

Patients with more advanced stages of disease have the histologic features of lymphoid obliteration seen in the terminal stages of HIV infection or AIDS. There is effacement of nodal architecture, loss of the normal lymphoid cell population with replacement by a benign plasma cell infiltrate, and increased vascularity (209). The multinucleated giant cells characteristically seen in the early and chronic stages of disease are not identified in the more advanced stages of HIV infection.

Special Studies. Special stains for microorganisms (other than HIV) are negative. Immunoreactivity for HIV p24 (gag protein), an indicator of active HIV infection, is consistently identified in the early and chronic stages of disease (209). Anti-HIV p24 reactivity is seen within the follicular dendritic cell network of the germinal centers, in scattered interfollicular lymphocytes, in the multinucleated giant cells, and within the intraepithelial cells of the crypt epithelium (fig. 3-22) (209). The HIV p24-positive intraepithelial cells are S-100 protein (a dendritic cell marker) positive and their morphologic appearance correlates with the appearance of dendritic cells (210). Reactivity with both B-cell (CD20) and T-cell markers or subsets (CD3) is seen within the germinal centers and in the interfollicular regions, as well as in scattered intraepithelial cells.

In more advanced stages of disease, characterized by loss of germinal centers and the presence of a predominant plasma cell infiltrate, there is an absence of lymphoid cell markers (CD45, CD3). In these cases, the plasma cell infiltrate shows reactivity with kappa and lambda light chains, indicative of a benign proliferation. Surface and crypt epithelia are cytokeratin reactive. Immunoreactivity with EBV-LMP, herpes simplex virus (HSV), or CMV is not present.

Evidence of HIV RNA by in situ hybridization is seen in the follicular dendritic cell network,

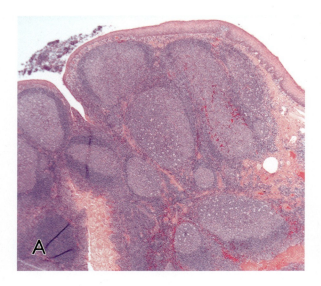
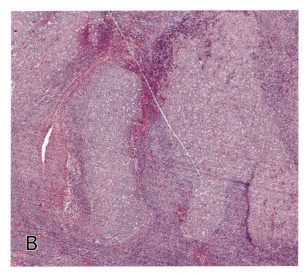

Figure 3-20

HUMAN IMMUNODEFICIENCY VIRUS (HIV) INFECTION OF WALDEYER TONSILLAR TISSUES

A: Early histologic manifestations of HIV infection include the presence of florid follicular hyperplasia, characterized by enlarged and irregularly shaped germinal centers, with loss or attenuation of mantle lymphocytes. Some germinal centers approximate the surface epithelium.

B: Irregular-shaped germinal centers within the deeper submucosa of the tonsil shows attenuated to partially absent mantle cell lymphocytes.

C,D: There is follicle lysis, in which germinal centers are variably infiltrated by small lymphocytes, creating a "moth eaten" appearance, as well as the absence of clearly defined mantle zones.

E: Monocytoid B-cell hyperplasia is seen in the chronic phase of HIV-infected tonsils.

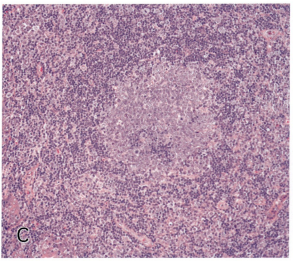
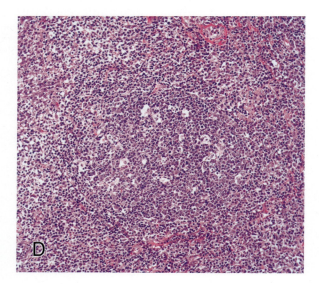
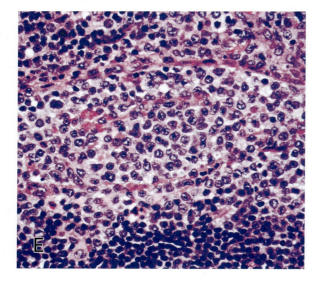

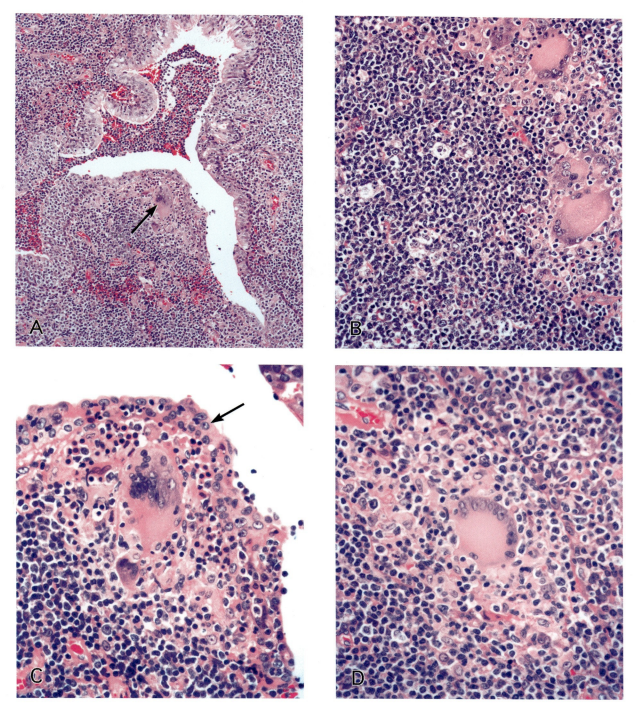

Figure 3-21

MULTINUCLEATED GIANT CELLS (MGC)

A,B: In association with tonsillar HIV infection, MGCs represent an important diagnostic clue. Characteristically, the MGCs localize/cluster near (or within) the crypt epithelium (arrow) (A) and may localize to germinal centers (B).

C,D: MGCs approximate the tonsillar crypt epithelium (arrow) (C) and lie within the reticulated epithelium (lymphoepithelium) (D), which may be difficult to appreciate by light microscopy because of the benign lymphoplasmacytic cells and may require cytokeratin staining (not shown) for identification.

Non-Neoplastic Diseases of the Head and Neck

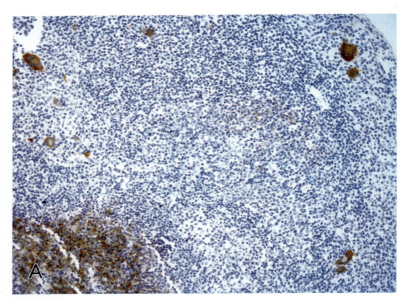

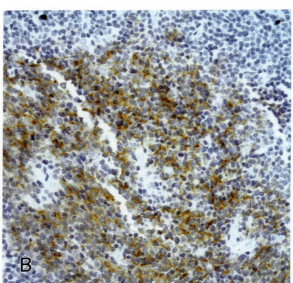
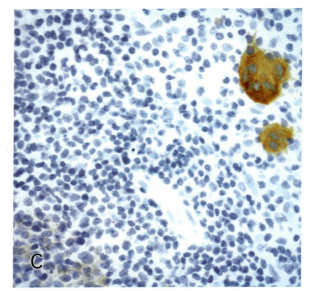

Figure 3-22

HIV p24 CORE ANTIGEN

A: At low magnification, p24 expression is present in a germinal center (lower left) and scattered multinucleated giant cells, confirming the presence of HIV infection.

B,C: At higher magnification, HIV p24 immunoreactivity is seen within follicular dendritic cells (B) and in multinucleated giant cells (C).

in the multinucleated giant cells, and in mature lymphocytes localized to the germinal centers, interfollicular zones, and within the surface or crypt epithelia (209). The strongest signal is present in the multinucleated giant cells.

Differential Diagnosis. The differential diagnosis includes other infectious diseases, infectious-related proliferative processes (e.g., infectious mononucleosis), and malignant lymphoma.

Treatment and Prognosis. There is no specific treatment for the tonsillar and adenoidal enlargement related to HIV infection other than excision for symptomatic relief or to exclude a possible diagnosis of malignancy. Early initiation of antiretroviral therapy has reduced HIV-associated morbidity and has significantly prolonged life and the disease-free interval (213). Antiretroviral therapy can reliably reduce viral loads to levels below 50 copies/mL when the circulating virus is susceptible to available drugs. When viral loads are reduced to low levels, further immune decline is usually prevented and immune function is usually improved. Most patients with effective virologic suppression demonstrate improvement in the CD4 count but a few patients will not show benefit for unknown reasons.

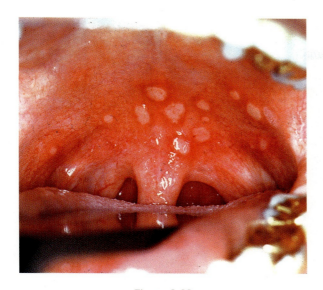

Figure 3-23

CYTOMEGALOVIRUS (CMV) INFECTION OF THE PALATE

Multiple, discrete, oval mucosal lesions are seen.

Recognition of HIV infection in Waldeyer tonsillar ring, an initial manifestation of disease, is essential for the initiation of antiretroviral therapy.

AIDS-Related Opportunistic Infectious Diseases

A number of opportunistic infections of the upper aerodigestive tract, including viruses, bacteria, fungi, and protozoa, occur in association the immune compromised state caused by HIV or secondary to AIDS. Among the more common viruses that infect head and neck sites in this setting are cytomegalovirus and the herpes viruses (simplex and zoster).

Cytomegalovirus

Clinical Features. *Cytomegalovirus* (CMV) is the most common opportunistic pathogen recognized at autopsy in AIDS patients (214–216). Additional clinical settings for CMV infection of the head and neck include immune compromised patients following stem cell or solid organ transplantation. In general, CMV infection involving the head and neck is not common, but may involve the pharyngeal region (217,218).

Gross Findings. CMV appears as a single or multiple, oval, tan-white, ulcerated lesion with a hyperemic rim, with or without an associated exudate (fig. 3-23).

Microscopic Findings. Histologic findings include mucosal ulceration, necrosis, and cytomegaly. Cytopathic findings include nucleomegaly and characteristic intranuclear or intracytoplasmic inclusions, typically in nonepithelial cells (endothelial cells and fibroblasts) rather than in squamous cells. The inclusions are intranuclear basophilic Cowdry type B inclusions (so-called owl eye inclusions) and ill-defined amphophilic cytoplasmic inclusions (fig. 3-24).

Identification of CMV is facilitated by immunohistochemical staining and in situ hybridization (fig. 3-24). DNA sequencing analysis by PCR confirms CMV (219). The multiplex polymerase chain reaction (M-PCR) assay is a rapid, sensitive, and economical method for the detection of CMV as well as HSV-1, HSV-2, and EBV in a single PCR tube (220).

Differential Diagnosis. The differential diagnosis primarily includes other viral inclusion diseases such as herpesvirus-associated diseases. Immunohistochemical stains allow for distinction among these viral inclusion diseases.

Treatment and Prognosis. Given the occurrence of CMV in the head and neck in association with immune compromised diseases/states, treatment is usually with systemic antiviral agents (e.g., valganciclovir and ganciclovir) (221, 222). The overall prognosis is dependent on the underlying disease state and the ability to control the local/systemic infection. In AIDS patients, CMV infection generally resolves when CD4 counts exceed $100/mm^3$ but is a grave prognostic sign if counts do not recover to those levels.

Herpes Simplex Virus

Definition. *Herpes simplex viruses* (HSV) are large, enveloped, double-stranded DNA viruses that are members of the family Herpesviridae. Two distinct subtypes of HSV are identified: type 1 referred to as the "oral" type and type 2 referred to as the "genital" type. The virus type, however, is not a reliable indicator of the anatomic site affected, especially with changing sexual habits, and the distinction between HSV-1 and HSV-2 is no longer relevant.

Clinical Features. Because of its tendency to infect cells of ectodermal origin (skin or mucous membranes), HSV is a frequent cause of mucocutaneous disease in the HIV-positive patient (223). Head and neck manifestations are those

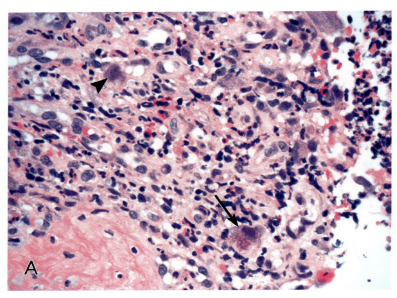

Figure 3-24

CYTOMEGALOVIRUS INFECTION

A: The mesenchymal cells show cytomegaly with characteristic intranuclear (arrowhead) and intracytoplasmic (arrow) inclusions.

B,C: CMV immunoreactivity (B) and in situ hybridization for CMV (C) confirm the diagnosis by showing intranuclear and intracytoplasmic positivity.

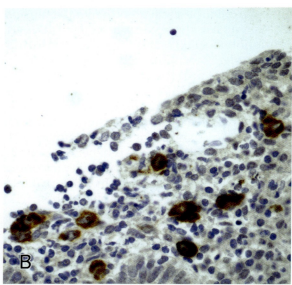
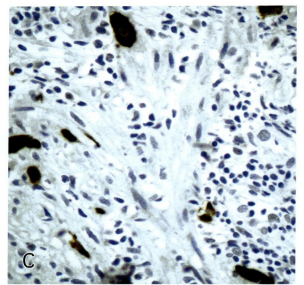

of an ulcerated lesion that involves the intraoral region, nasal cavity, lip, external ear, pharynx, and tonsil; in addition, enlargement and tenderness of cervical and submental lymph nodes may be seen. In the pharynx, HSV appears as a vesicular lesion that bleeds easily and may be covered with a black crust or as shallow tonsillar ulcers covered with gray exudates.

Herpes zoster (HZ) infection occurs as varicella (chicken pox) or as dermatomal zoster (shingles); the latter, while not specific for HIV infection, appears to be related to HIV infection and may represent an early marker for the immunosuppression associated with HIV infection. HZ can localize to any dermatome, is neurotropic, and can cause unremitting pain. HZ infection of the pharynx may be associated with cranial neuropathies (224). Head and neck manifestations include involvement of the 8th cranial nerve or geniculate ganglion (Ramsay-Hunt syndrome), producing severe ear pain, hearing loss, vertigo, and facial nerve paralysis (225).

Gross Findings. HSV infection appears as single or multiple, oval, tan-white, ulcerated lesions with a hyperemic rim, with or without associated exudates.

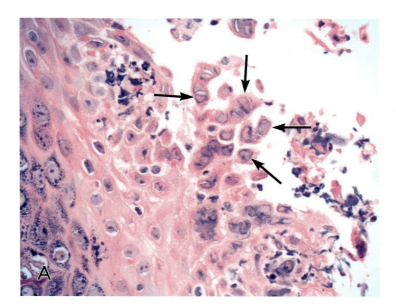

Figure 3-25

HERPES SIMPLEX VIRUS (HSV) INFECTION

A: In the pharynx, intranuclear eosinophilic inclusions (Cowdry cells; arrows) are seen within degenerating (squamous) epithelial cells, imparting a ground-glass appearance.

B: A multinucleated giant cell (arrow) is characterized by presence of syncytial cells with intranuclear inclusions and the tendency of nuclei to mold to one another. Balloon degeneration of epithelial cells with intranuclear inclusions is seen within degenerating epithelial cells (arrowheads).

C: In situ hybridization for HSV confirms the diagnosis by showing intranuclear positivity.

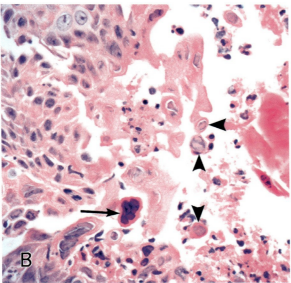
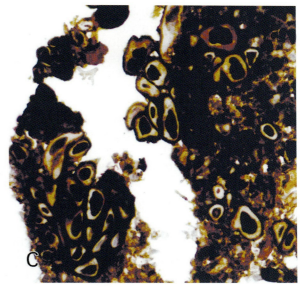

Microscopic Findings. The intraepidermal vesicle formation of HSV infection is marked by acantholysis and balloon degeneration of epithelial cells (fig. 3-25). In mucosal sites, there is focal ulceration, intraepithelial vesicles, acantholysis, neutrophilic infiltrate, necrosis, balloon degeneration of epithelial cells, and intranuclear inclusions within the degenerating epithelial cells. The diagnostic cytopathic features include nuclear molding, multinucleated giant cells, and eosinophilic inclusions (fig. 3-25). The edge of the ulcer and sloughed squamous cells are the best sites for identifying the characteristic cytopathic changes. Multinucleated giant cells may be numerous. In HZ infection the intranuclear inclusions are indistinguishable from those seen in herpes simplex.

Identification of CMV may be facilitated by immunohistochemical staining or in situ hybridization (fig. 3-25). DNA sequencing analysis by PCR can be used to confirm or identify HSV (219). The M-PCR assay is a rapid, sensitive, and economical method for detection of HSV-1 and HSV-2 as well as EBV and CMV in a single PCR tube (220). HZ is characterized by varicella zoster virus (VZV) DNAemia at onset and for many weeks thereafter, and VZV DNA is present in the oropharynx shortly after the onset of HZ (226). Detection of VZV DNA in blood and saliva facilitates the diagnosis of HZ.

Differential Diagnosis. The differential diagnosis of HSV infection primarily includes other viral inclusion diseases such as CMV. Immunohistochemical stains allow distinction.

Treatment and Prognosis. The treatment for herpetic infection includes antiviral chemotherapy with acyclovir, ganciclovir, and foscarnet.

Measles Infection

Measles, an acute childhood illness caused by RNA paramyxovirus (also referred to as *rubeola*), may infect the pharynx (e.g., tonsils) of immune competent individuals. Measles is highly contagious and transmitted by oral and respiratory secretions. The availability of live measles virus vaccine has made this disease less common in the United States. Following a prodromal period, a generalized rash develops beginning on the face and spreading to the trunk and extremities. The rash usually resolves within 10 days. Immunosuppressed patients may not develop the characteristic rash.

Histologically, tonsillar involvement results in reactive follicular hyperplasia with interfollicular Warthin-Finkeldey-type giant cells. These are characterized by multiple nuclei arranged in grape-like clusters (fig. 3-26).

Fungus Infections

Many fungi, including *Candida* species, secondarily infect HIV-positive patients. In the head and neck, the single most important fungal pathogen is *Candida*. The oral cavity is primarily targeted in *Candida* infection (*oral candidiasis* [*thrush*] and *oral hairy leukoplakia*) but infections of the pharynx also occur (227,228).

Oropharyngeal histoplasmosis is closely associated with immunosuppression, especially in patients with AIDS. Oropharyngeal histoplasmosis may represent the initial manifestation of disseminated histoplasmosis (229).

Bacteria and Spirochetes

Bacterial infections of mucosal sites of the head and neck are common but generally represent a clinical diagnosis and virtually never a surgical disease. In immunocompromised patients, however, infection by opportunistic microorganisms potentially results in tissue sampling for diagnostic purposes. HIV-infected/AIDS patients may experience an increased incidence of mucosal gonorrhea and syphilis, including pharyngeal infection (230–235).

Gonorrhea. Gonorrhea is a localized and systemic disease caused by *Neisseria gonorrhoeae*, a pyogenic Gram-negative diplococcus. Otolaryngic manifestations include gonococcal pharyngitis, which generally is asymptomatic but may present with sore throat, tonsillar hypertrophy, or cervical adenopathy (236–244). The microorganism infects mucosal and glandular structures.

To confirm the diagnosis, Gram stains of smears made from purulent material from the infected site demonstrate the presence of Gram-negative diplococci in the polymorphonuclear leukocytes. Gram stains, however, may be unreliable due to the presence of other organisms, so that samples must be cultured on appropriate media (chocolate agar) for identification. DNA amplification testing for the identification of oropharyngeal *N. gonorrhoeae* offers additional and greater sensitivity than standard cultures (245). The differential diagnosis includes nonspecific inflammatory reactions.

Ceftriaxone is the drug of choice for the routine treatment of gonorrhea. All patients with gonorrhea are treated with an oral regimen active against *Chlamydia trachomatis*, usually azithromycin. Dual therapy may enhance the efficacy of treatment for pharyngeal gonorrhea and using more than one drug may retard antimicrobial resistance to *N. gonorrhea*. Such treatment is warranted even in persons who test negative for *C. trachomatis*.

Syphilis. Syphilis is a systemic venereal disease caused by *Treponemal pallidum*, a member of the family Spirochaetaceae which includes *T. pertenue* (yaws) and *T. carateum* (pinta). The clinical stages of syphilis are *primary, secondary, tertiary*, and *congenital*, any of which can affect virtually every site in the head and neck and cause an array of clinical manifestations. Involvement of the head and neck may result in 1) tonsillar involvement manifesting as a painless solitary chancre which appears at the site of inoculation in the primary stage; chancres may clinically mimic a neoplasm; 2) skin lesions and lymphadenopathy (seen in

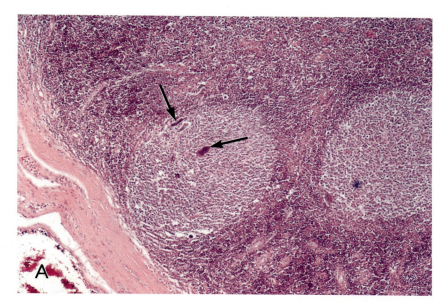
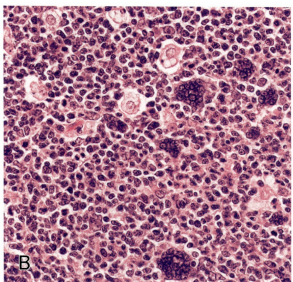
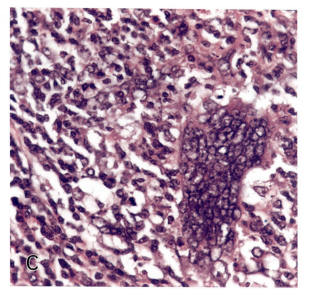

Figure 3-26
MEASLES TONSILLITIS
A: There is reactive follicular hyperplasia, with interfollicular multinucleated (Warthin-Finkeldey type) giant cells (arrows).
B,C: Higher magnification of the interfollicular multinucleated giants.

90 percent of the patients in the secondary or disseminated stage); and 3) pharyngotonsillitis (fig. 3-27), which may be a presenting symptom in secondary syphilis. Mucosal involvement produces "mucous patches" which are highly contagious (230,232,234,247,242,246). Other head and neck symptoms in the secondary stage include rhinitis, laryngitis, pharyngitis, cranial nerve deficits, sensorineural deafness, labyrinthitis, and glossitis.

The tertiary stage of syphilis typically involves the central nervous system (neurosyphilis) and aorta (cardiovascular syphilis). Localized, nonprogressive lesions, however, may develop in mucosal otolaryngic sites and are termed "benign tertiary syphilis" or "gummas"; the gummatous reaction represents a pronounced immunologic reaction of the host.

There are two types of serologic test for syphilis: the nontreponemal (nonspecific) serologic tests and the treponemal (specific) serologic tests (247). These tests are most reactive in the secondary stage of the disease. Nontreponemal (nonspecific) serologic tests detect antibodies to lipoprotein material and cardiolipin released from cells damaged by treponemes. They screen

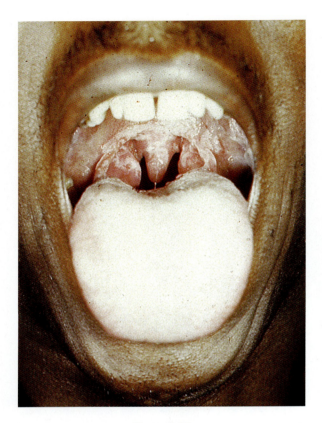

Figure 3-27
SYPHILITIC PHARYNGOTONSILLITIS
A diffuse white exudate overlies the soft palate, uvula, and tonsils.

for disease and monitor the course of disease. They include venereal disease research laboratory (VDRL), rapid plasma regain (RPR), unheated serum reagin (USR), and toluidine red unheated serum (TRUST) tests (247). Treponemal (specific) serologic tests detect the presence of antibodies to treponemal antigens, are used to confirm a positive nontreponemal screening test, and confirm infection in patients with a negative nontreponemal test in late or latent disease stages, which can occur in up to 30 percent of patients with tertiary syphilis. These include the fluorescent treponemal antibody absorption test (FTA-ABS), the microhemagglutination-*T. palladium* test (MHA-TP) which is preferred owing to its relative simplicity, and the enzyme immunoassay (EIA) which is increasingly used for screening (247).

Congenital syphilis develops via transplacental infection. The manifestations are primarily mucocutaneous and osseous, and include in decreasing frequency, frontal bossing, short maxilla, high palatal arch, saddle nose, mulberry molars, Hutchinson incisors, sternoclavicular thickening, interstitial keratitis, rhagades, and 8th nerve deafness (248–251).

Mucosal infection results in surface ulceration with associated fibrinoid necrosis (fig. 3-28). An inflammatory infiltrate, predominantly composed of plasma cells with scattered admixed histiocytes, lymphocytes, and polymorphonuclear leukocytes, is present in the submucosa. This inflammatory infiltrate has a tendency to involve small blood vessels, which display endothelial cell proliferation ("plasma cell endarteritis") (fig. 3-28). Concentric layers are produced that markedly narrow the lumen of the affected vessel, resulting in obliterative endarteritis (252). Obliterative endarteritis, coupled with the inflammatory infiltrate produced by the spirochetes, represents the histologic hallmark of the disease.

Organisms can be demonstrated in the chancre by Warthin-Starry staining. They appear as elongated, thin rod-like structures (fig. 3-28). A variety of techniques, including darkfield examination of smears and immunohistochemistry (fig. 3-28), are used to detect organisms (247). The differential diagnosis includes nonspecific inflammatory reactions.

The treatment of choice for syphilis remains penicillin G and other β-lactam antibiotics administered in a single intramuscular injection. For persons allergic to penicillin, doxycycline or tetracycline are effective alternatives. Although at present unproven, syphilitic involvement of the oral mucosa has been considered a precancerous lesion.

REACTIVE, INFLAMMATORY, AND TUMOR-LIKE LESIONS

Tangier Disease

Definition. *Tangier disease* is a high density lipoprotein (HDL) deficiency syndrome. It is characterized by severe plasma deficiency or absence of HDL and apolipoprotein A-I (apoA-I, the major HDL apolipoprotein), and by the accumulation of cholesteryl esters in tissue macrophages (xanthomatous cells) and prevalent atherosclerosis (253).

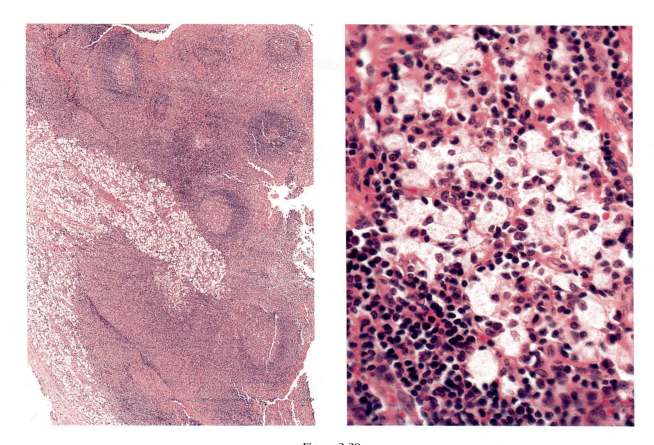

Figure 3-30

TANGIER DISEASE

Left, right: Xanthomatous cells are deposited in the tonsillar parenchyma. These cells are similar in appearance to the histiocytic cells seen in sinus histiocytosis with massive lymphadenopathy (Rosai-Dorfman disease), but in contrast to those cells, the cells in Tangier disease are not immunoreactive for S-100 protein.

therapy (253). Due to its ability to deplete cells of cholesterol and to raise plasma HDL levels, ABCA1 has become a promising therapeutic target for preventing cardiovascular disease. The prognosis is good; however, coronary artery disease is common in patients over the age of 40 years of age.

REFERENCES

Embryology, Anatomy, and Histology

1. Standring S. Pharynx. In: Standring S, ed. Gray's anatomy. The anatomical basis of clinical practice. 40th ed. Edinburgh: Elsevier Churchill Livingstone; 2008:561-575.
2. Edge SB, Byrd DR, Compton CC, Fritz AG, Greene FL, Trotti A III, eds. Pharynx (including base of tongue, soft palate, and uvula). In: AJCC cancer staging manual, 7th ed. New York: Springer; 2010:41-53.
3. Moore KL, Persaud TV. The pharyngeal apparatus. In: Moore ML, Persaud TV, ed. The developing human: clinically oriented embryology, 7th ed. Philadelphia: Saunders, Elsevier; 2003:201-240.
4. Hollinshead WH. The pharynx and larynx. In: Hollinshead WH, ed. Anatomy for surgeons, vol. 1, 3rd ed. Philadelphia: Harper & Row; 1982:389-441.
5. Mills SE. Larynx and pharynx. In: Mills, SE, ed. Histology for pathologists, 4th ed. Philadelphia: Lippincott, Williams & Wilkins; 2012:461-475.
6. Perry ME, Jones MM, Mustafa Y. Structure of the crypt epithelium in human palatine tonsils. Acta Otolaryngol Suppl 1988;454:53-59.
7. Perry ME. The specialised structure of crypt epithelium in the human palatine tonsil and its functional significance. J Anat 1994;185(Pt 1):111-127.
8. Westra WH. The morphologic profile of HPV-related head and neck squamous carcinoma: Implications for diagnosis, prognosis, and clinical management. Head Neck Pathol 2012:6(Suppl 1):S48-54.

Developmental Cysts

9. Muro-Cacho C, Patel NJ, Klotch DW, Dussia E. Nasopharyngeal cysts. Am J Otolaryngol 2000;21:108-111.
10. Plaza Mayor G, Martínez San Millán J, Barberá Durán R, Pérez Martínez C, Folgué Calvo L, Denia Lafuente A. [Nasopharyngeal cysts. Report of four cases and literature review.] An Otorrinolaringol Ibero Am 1999;26:607-619. [Spanish]
11. Benke TT, Zitsch RP 3rd, Nashelsky MB. Bilateral oncocytic cysts of the nasopharynx. Otolaryngol Head Neck Surg 1995;112:321-324.
12. Nicolai P, Luzzago F, Maroldi R, Falchetti M, Antonelli AR. Nasopharyngeal cysts. Report of seven cases with review of the literature. Arch Otolaryngol Head Neck Surg 1989l;115:860-864.
13. Singh KP, Pahor AL. Congenital cyst of the nasopharynx. J Laryngol Otol 1977;91:75-79.

Rathke Pouch Cyst

14. Moore KL, Persaud TV. The nervous system. In: Moore ML, Persaud TV, ed. The developing human: clinically oriented embryology, 7th ed. Philadelphia: Saunders, Elsevier; 2003:429-463.
15. Ross DA, Norman D, Wilson CB. Radiologic characteristics and results of surgical management of Rathke's cysts in 43 patients. Neurosurgery 1992;30:173-179.
16. Voelker JL, Campbell RL, Muller J. Clinical, radiographic, and pathological features of symptomatic Rathke's cleft cysts. J Neurosurg 1991;74:535-544.
17. Kumar M, Dutta D, Shivaprasad KS, et al. Diabetes insipidus as a presenting manifestation of Rathke's cleft cyst. Indian J Endocrinol Metab 2013;17(Suppl 1):S127-129.
18. Wait SD, Garrett MP, Little AS, Killory BD, White WL. Endocrinopathy, vision, headache, and recurrence after transsphenoidal surgery for Rathke cleft cysts. Neurosurgery 2010;67:837-843
19. Chaiban JT, Abdelmannan D, Cohen M, Selman WR, Arafah BM. Rathke cleft cyst apoplexy: a newly characterized distinct clinical entity. J Neurosurg. 2011;114:318-324.
20. Gessler F, Coon VC, Chin SS, Couldwell WT. Co-existing rathke cleft cyst and pituitary adenoma presenting with pituitary apoplexy: report of two cases. Skull Base Rep 2011;1:99-104.
21. Isono M, Kamida T, Kobayashi H, Shimomura T, Matsuyama J. Clinical features of symptomatic Rathke's cleft cyst. Clin Neurol Neurosurg 2001;103:96-100.
22. Gotoh M, Nakano J, Midorikawa S, Niimura S, Ono Y, Mizuno K. Multiple endocrine disorders and Rathke's cleft cyst with Klinefelter's syndrome: a case report. Endocr J 2002;49:523-529.
23. Babu R, Back AG, Komisarow JM, Owens TR, Cummings TJ, Britz GW. Symptomatic Rathke's cleft cyst with a co-existing pituitary tumor; Brief review of the literature. Asian J Neurosurg 2013;8:183-187.
24. Karavitaki N, Scheithauer BW, Watt J, et al. Collision lesions of the sella: co-existence of craniopharyngioma with gonadotroph adenoma and of Rathke's cleft cyst with corticotroph adenoma. Pituitary 2008;11:317-323.
25. Sumida M, Migita K, Tominaga A, Iida K, Kurisu K. Concomitant pituitary adenoma and Rathke's cleft cyst. Neuroradiology 2001;43:755-759.
26. Gupta V, Grossman A, Kapadia A, Thorat K. Acromegaly associated with a symptomatic Rathke's cyst. Indian J Endocrinol Metab 2011;15:140-142.
27. Osborn AG, Preece MT. Intracranial cysts: radiologic-pathologic correlation and imaging approach. Radiology 2006;239:650-664.

28. Byun WM, Kim OL, Kim DS. MR imaging findings of Rathke's cleft cysts: significance of intracystic nodules. AJNR Am J Neuroradiol 2000;21:485–488
29. Shin JL, Asa SL, Woodhouse LJ, Smyth HS, Ezzat S. Cystic lesions of the pituitary: clinicopathological features distinguishing craniopharyngioma, Rathke's cleft cyst, and arachnoid cyst. J Clin Endocrinol Metab 1999;84:3972-3982.
30. Nakasu Y, Nakasu S, Nakajima M, Itoh R, Matsuda M. Atypical Rathke's cleft cyst associated with ossification. AJNR Am J Neuroradiol 1999;20:1287-1289.
31. Inoue T, Matsushima T, Fukui M, Iwaki T, Takeshita I, Kuromatsu C. Immunohistochemical study of intracranial cysts. Neurosurgery 1988;23:576-581.
32. Uematsu Y, Rojas-Corona RR, Llena JF, Hirano A. Epithelial cysts in the central nervous system, characteristic expression of cytokeratins in an immunohistochemical study. Acta Neurochir (Wien) 1990;107:93-101.
33. Im SH, Wang KC, Kim SK, et al. Transsphenoidal microsurgery for pediatric craniopharyngioma: special considerations regarding indications and method. Pediatr Neurosurg 2003;39:97-103.
34. Alfieri A, Schettino R, Tarfani A, Bonzi O, Rossi GA, Monolo L. Endoscopic endonasal removal of an intra-suprasellar Rathke's cleft cyst: case report and surgical considerations. Minim Invasive Neurosurg 2002;45:47-51.
35. Kim EY, Park HS, Kim JJ, et al. Endoscopic transsphenoidal approach through a widened nasal cavity for pituitary lesions. J Clin Neurosci 2001;8:437-41.
36. Madhok R, Prevedello DM, Gardner P, Carrau RL, Snyderman CH, Kassam AB. Endoscopic endonasal resection of Rathke cleft cysts: clinical outcomes and surgical nuances. J Neurosurg 2010;112:1333-1339.

Thornwaldt Cyst

37. Miyahara H, Matsunaga T. Tornwaldt's disease. Acta Otolaryngol Suppl 1994;517:36-39.
38. Hollender AR. The nasopharynx: a study of 140 autopsy specimens. Laryngoscope 1946;56:282-304.
39. Boucher RM, Hendrix RA, Guttenplan MD. The diagnosis of Thornwaldt's cyst. Trans Pa Acad Ophthalmol Otolaryngol 1990;42:1026-1030.
40. Miller RH, Sneed WF. Thornwaldt's bursa. Clin Otolaryngol Allied Sci 1985;10:21-25.
41. Skinner LJ, Colreavy MP, Griffin JF, Burns HP. Radiology quiz case. Thornwaldt cyst. Arch Otolaryngol Head Neck Surg 2003;129:1137-1138.
42. Weismann JL. Thornwaldt cyst. Am J Otolaryngol 1992;13:381-385.
43. Yanagisawa E, Yanagisawa K. Endoscopic view of Thornwaldt cyst of the nasopharynx. Ear Nose Throat J 1994;73:884-885.

Nasopharyngeal Hamartomas

44. Baillie EE, Batsakis JG. Glandular (seromucinous) hamartoma of the nasopharynx. Oral Surg 1974;38:760-762.
45. Graeme-Cook F, Pilch BZ. Hamartomas of the nose and nasopharynx. Head Neck 1992;14:321–327.
46. Park SK, Jung H, Yang YI. Mesenchymal hamartoma in nasopharynx: a case report. Auris Nasus Larynx. 2008;35:437-439.
47. Zarbo RJ, McClatchey KD. Nasopharyngeal hamartoma: report of a case and review of the literature. Laryngoscope 1983;93:494-497.
48. Birt BD, Knight-Jones EB. Respiratory distress due to nasopharyngeal hamartoma. Br Med J 1969;3:281-282.
49. Metselaar RM, Stel HV, van der Baan S. Respiratory epithelial adenomatoid hamartoma in the nasopharynx. J Laryngol Otol 2005;119:476-478.
50. Owens D, Alderson D, Garrido C. Nasopharyngeal hamartoma: importance of routine complete nasal examination. J Laryngol Otol 2004;118:558-560.
51. Sulica RL, Wenig BM, Debo RF, Sessions RB. Schneiderian-type papillomas of the nasopharynx. Ann Otol Rhinol Laryngol 1999;108:392-397.

Pharyngeal/Nasopharyngeal Central Nervous System Heterotopias

52. Buccoliero AM, Caldarella A, Noccioli B, Fiorini P, Taddei A, Taddei GL. Brain heterotopia in pharyngeal region. A morphological and immunohistochemical study. Pathol Res Pract 2002;198:59-63.
53. Cohen AH, Abt AB. An unusual cause of neonatal respiratory obstruction: heterotopic pharyngeal brain tissue. J Pediat 1970;76:119-122.
54. Heffner DK. Problems in pediatric otorhinolaryngic pathology. III. Teratoid and neural tumors of the nose, sinonasal tract, and nasopharynx. Int J Pediatr Otorhinolaryngol 1983;6:1-21.
55. Seibert RW, Seibert JJ, Jimenez JF, Angtuaco EJ. Nasopharyngeal brain heterotopia—a cause of upper airway obstruction in infancy. Laryngoscope 1984;94:818-819.
56. Forte V, Friedberg J, Thorner P, Park A. Heterotopic brain in the parapharyngeal space. Int J Pediatr Otorhinolaryngol 1996;37:253-260.
57. Lassaletta Atienza L, Lopez-Rios Moreno F, Madero S, Villafruela MA, Alvarez Vicent JJ. [Heterotopic brain tissue in the pharynx.] Acta Otorrinolaringol Esp 1999;50:232-235. [Spanish]
58. Ruff T, Diaz JA. Heterotopic brain in the nasopharynx. Otolaryngol Head Neck Surg 1986;94:254-256.
59. Uemura T, Yoshikawa A, Onizuka T, Hayashi T. Heterotopic nasopharyngeal brain tissue associated with cleft palate. Cleft Palate Craniofac J 1999;36:248-251.

60. Zarem HA, Gray GF Jr, Morehead D, Edgerton MT. Heterotopic brain in the nasopharynx and soft palate: report of two cases. Surgery 1967;61:483-486.
61. Braun M, Boman F, Hascoet JM, Chastagner P, Brunet A, Simon C. Brain tissue heterotopia in the nasopharynx. Contribution of MRI to assessment of extension. J Neuroradiol 1992;19:68-74.
62. Momose F, Hashimoto K, Shioda S. Heterotropic brain tissue in the oropharynx. Report of a case. Oral Surg Oral Med Oral Pathol 1989;68:682-685.
63. Bossen EH, Hudson WR. Oligodendroglioma arising in heterotopic brain tissue of the soft palate and nasopharynx. Am J Surg Pathol 1987;11:571-574.

Nasopharyngeal Dermoid

64. Burns BV, Axon PR, Pahade A. 'Hairy polyp' of the pharynx in association with an ipsilateral branchial sinus: evidence that the 'hairy polyp' is a second branchial arch malformation. J Laryngol Otol 2001;115:145-148.
65. Heffner DK, Thompson LD, Schall DG, Andersen V. Pharyngeal dermoids ("hairy polyps") as accessory auricles. Ann Otol Rhinol Laryngol 1996;105:819–824.
66. Ferlito A, Devaney KO. Developmental lesions of the head and neck. Terminology and biologic behavior. Ann Otol Rhinol Laryngol 1995;104:913-918.
67. Cone BM, Taweevisit M, Shenoda S, Sobol S, Schemankewitz E, Shehata BM. Pharyngeal hairy polyps: five new cases and review of the literature. Fetal Pediatr Pathol 2012;31:184-189.
68. Coppit GL 3rd, Perkins JA, Manning SC. Nasopharyngeal teratomas and dermoids: a review of the literature and case series. Int J Pediatr Otorhinolaryngol 2000;52:219-227.
69. Jarvis SJ, Bull PD. Hairy polyps of the nasopharynx. J Laryngol Otol 2002;116:467-469.
70. Karagama YG, Williams RS, Barclay G, Lancaster JL, Kokai GK. Hairy polyp of the oropharynx in a newborn: a case report. Rhinology 2003;41:56-57.
71. Kelly A, Bough ID Jr, Luft JD, Conard K, Reilly JS, Tuttle D. Hairy polyp of the oropharynx: case report and literature review. J Pediatr Surg 1996;31:704-706.
72. Mitchell TE, Girling AC. Hairy polyp of the tonsil. J Laryngol Otol 1996;110:101-103.
73. Van Haesendonck J, Van de Heyning PH, Claes J, et al. A pharyngeal hairy polyp causing neonatal airway obstruction: a case study. Int J Pediatr Otorhinolaryngol 1990;19:175-180.
74. Vaughan C, Prowse SJ, Knight LC. Hairy polyp of the oropharynx in association with a first branchial arch sinus. J Laryngol Otol 2012;126:1302-1304.
75. Walsh RM, Philip G, Salama NY. Hairy polyp of the oropharynx: an unusual cause of intermittent neonatal airway obstruction. Int J Pediatr Otorhinolaryngol 1996;34:129-134.
76. Tariq MU, Din NU, Bashir MR. Hairy polyp, a clinicopathologic study of four cases. Head Neck Pathol 2013;7:232-235.
77. Aughton DJ, Sloan CT, Milad MP, Huang TE, Michael C, Harper C. Nasopharyngeal teratoma ('hairy polyp'), Dandy-Walker malformation, diaphragmatic hernia, and other anomalies in a female infant. J Med Genet 1990;27:788-790.
78. Haddad J Jr, Senders CW, Leach CS, Stool SE. Congenital hairy polyp of the nasopharynx associated with cleft palate: report of two cases. Int J Pediatr Otorhinolaryngol 1990;20:127-135.
79. Simoni P, Wiatrak BJ, Kelly DR. Choristomatous polyps of the aural and pharyngeal regions: first simultaneous case. Int J Pediatr Otorhinolaryngol 2003;67:195-199.
80. Franco V, Florena AM, Lombardo F, Restivo S. Bilateral hairy polyp of the oropharynx. J Laryngol Otol 1996;110:288-290.
81. Boedts D, Moerman M, Marquet J. A hairy polyp of the middle ear and mastoid cavity. Acta Otorhinolaryngol Belg 1992;46:397-400.
82. Kieff DA, Curtin HD, Limb CJ, Nadol JB. A hairy polyp presenting as a middle ear mass in a pediatric patient. Am J Otolaryngol 1998;19:228-231.
83. Nalavenkata S, Meller C, Forer M, Patel NP. Dermoid cysts of the Eustachian tube: a transnasal excision. Int J Pediatr Otorhinolaryngol. 2013;77:588-593.
84. Nicklaus PJ, Forte V, Thorner PS. Hairy polyp of the eustachian tube. J Otolaryngol 1991;20:254-257.
85. Erdogan S, Tunali N, Canpolat T, Tuncer R. Hairy polyp of the tongue: a case report. Pediatr Surg Int 2004;20:881-882.
86. Yilmaz M, Ibrahimov M, Ozturk O, Karaman E, Aslan M. Congenital hairy polyp of the soft palate. Int J Pediatr Otorhinolaryngol 2012;76:5-8.
87. Olivares-Pakzad BA, Tazelaar HD, Dehner LP, Kasperbauer JL, Bite U. Oropharyngeal hairy polyp with meningothelial elements. Oral Surg Oral Med Oral Pathol Oral Radiol Endod 1995;79:462-468.

Lymphangiomatous Polyp

88. Heffner DK. Pathology of the tonsils and adenoids. Otolaryngol Clin N Am 1987;20:279-286.
89. Kardon DE, Wenig BM, Heffner DK, Thompson LD. Tonsillar lymphangiomatous polyps: a clinicopathologic series of 26 cases. Mod Pathol 2000;13:1128-1133.
90. Park E, Pransky SM, Malicki DM, Hong P. Unilateral lymphangiomatous polyp of the palatine tonsil in a very young child: a clinicopathologic case report. Case Rep Pediatr 2011;2011:451542.
91. Chen HH, Lovell MA, Chan KH. Bilateral lymphangiomatous polyps of the palatine tonsils. Int J Pediatr Otorhinolaryngol 2010;74:87-88.

92. Sulica L, Wenig BM, Debo R, Sessions R. Schneiderian-type papillomas of the nasopharynx.. Ann Otol Rhinol Laryngol 1999;108:392-397.

Salivary Gland Anlage Tumor

93. Dehner LP, Valbuena L, Perez-Atayde A, Reddick RL, Askin FB, Rosai J. Salivary gland anlage tumor ("congenital pleomorphic adenoma"). A clinicopathologic, immunohistochemical and ultrastructural study of nine cases. Am J Surg Pathol 1994;18:25-36.
94. Boccon-Gibod LA, Grangeponte MC, Boucheron S, Josset PP, Roger G, Berthier-Falissard ML. Salivary gland anlage tumor of the nasopharynx: a clinicopathologic and immunohistochemical study of three cases. Pediatr Pathol Lab Med 1996;16:973-983.
95. Cohen EG, Yoder M, Thomas RM, Salerno D, Isaacson G. Congenital salivary gland anlage tumor of the nasopharynx. Pediatrics 2003;112:e66-69.
96. Gauchotte G, Coffinet L, Schmitt E, et al. Salivary gland anlage tumor: a clinicopathological study of two cases. Fetal Pediatr Pathol 2011;30:116-123.
97. Herrmann BW, Dehner LP, Lieu JE. Congenital salivary gland anlage tumor: a case series and review of the literature. Int J Pediatr Otorhinolaryngol 2005;69:149-156.
98. Michal M, Sokol L, Mukensnabl P. Salivary gland anlage tumor. A case with widespread necrosis and large cyst formation. Pathology 1996;28:128-130.
99. Mogensen MA, Lin AC, Chang KW, Berry GJ, Barnes PD, Fischbein NJ. Salivary gland anlage tumor in a neonate presenting with respiratory distress: radiographic and pathologic correlation. AJNR Am J Neuroradiol 2009;30:1022-1023.
100. Radhakrishnan R, Calvo-Garcia MA, Lim FY, Elluru RG, Koch BL. Congenital salivary anlage tumor—in utero and postnatal imaging. Pediatr Radiol 2015;45:453-456.
101. Tinsa F, Boussetta K, Bousnina S, et al. Congenital salivary gland anlage tumor of the nasopharynx. Fetal Pediatr Pathol 2010;29:323-329.
102. Vranic S, Caughron SK, Djuricic S, et al. Hamartomas, teratomas and teratocarcinosarcomas of the head and neck: report of 3 new cases with clinico-pathologic correlation, cytogenetic analysis, and review of the literature. BMC Ear Nose Throat Disord 2008;8:8.

Tonsillitis

103. Brook I, Dohar JE. Management of group A beta-hemolytic streptococcal pharyngotonsillitis in children. J Fam Pract 2006;55:S1-11.
104. Barzalai A, Miron D, Sela S. Etiology and management of acute and recurrent Group A streptococcal tonsillitis. Curr Infect Dis Rep 2001;3:217-223.
105. Pichichero ME. Group A beta-hemolytic streptococcal infections. Pediatr Rev 1998;19:291-302.
106. Sidell D, Shapiro NL. Acute tonsillitis. Infect Disord Drug Targets 2012;12:271-276.
107. Cappelletty D. Microbiology of bacterial respiratory infections. Pediatr Infect Dis J 1998;17(Suppl):S55-61.
108. Endo LH, Ferreira D, Montenegro MC, et al. Detection of Epstein-Barr virus in tonsillar tissue of children and the relationship with recurrent tonsillitis. Int J Pediatr Otorhinolaryngol 2001;58:9-15.
109. Klein JO. Microbiology of diseases of the tonsil and adenoids. Ann Otol Rhinol Laryngol 1975;84 (Pt 2, Suppl 19):30-33.
110. Sun J, Keh-Gong W, Hwang B. Evaluation of the etiologic agents for acute suppurative tonsillitis in children. Zhonghua Yi Xue Za Zhi (Taipei) 2002;65:212-217.
111. Yoda K, Sata T, Kurata T, Aramaki H. Oropharyngotonsillitis associated with nonprimary Epstein-Barr virus infection. Arch Otolaryngol Head Neck Surg 2000;126:185-193.
112. Carrillo-Farga J, Abbud-Neme F, Deutsch E. Lymphoid papillary hyperplasia of the palatine tonsils. Am J Surg Pathol 1983;7:579-582.
113. Georgalas CC, Tolley NS, Narula A. Tonsillitis. BMJ Clin Evid 2009:2009.
114. Windfuhr JP, Chen YS. Post-tonsillectomy and -adenoidectomy hemorrhage in nonselected patients. Ann Otol Rhinol Laryngol 2003;112:63-70.
115. Bhattacharyya N, Kepnes LJ. Revisits and postoperative hemorrhage after adult tonsillectomy. Laryngoscope 2014;124:1554-1556.
116. Chowdhury K, Tewfik TL, Schloss MD. Post-tonsillectomy and adenoidectomy hemorrhage. J Otolaryngol 1988;17:46-49.
117. Handler SD, Miller L, Richmond KH, Baranak CC. Post-tonsillectomy hemorrhage: incidence, prevention and management. Laryngoscope 1986;96:1243-1247.
118. Ikoma R, Sakane S, Niwa K, Kanetaka S, Kawano T, Oridate N. Risk factors for post-tonsillectomy hemorrhage. Auris Nasus Larynx 2014;41:376-379.
119. Krishna P, Lee D. Post-tonsillectomy bleeding: a meta-analysis. Laryngoscope 2001;111:1358-1361.
120. Paradise JL, Bluestone CD, Colborn DK, Bernard BS, Rockette HE, Kurs-Lasky M. Tonsillectomy and adenotonsillectomy for recurrent throat infection in moderately affected children. Pediatrics 2002;110(Pt 1):7-15.
121. Myssiorek D, Alvi A. Post-tonsillectomy hemorrhage: an assessment of risk factors. Int J Pediatr Otorhinolaryngol 1996;37:35-43.

122. Seshamani M, Vogtmann E, Gatwood J, Gibson TB, Scanlon D. Prevalence of complications from adult tonsillectomy and impact on health care expenditures. Otolaryngol Head Neck Surg 2014;150:574-781.
123. Windfuhr JP. Serious complications following tonsillectomy: how frequent are they really? ORL J Otorhinolaryngol Relat Spec 2013;75:166-173.
124. Nouwen J, Smets F, Rombaux P, Hamoir M, Sokal EM. Acute tonsillitis as the first manifestation of post-transplant lymphoproliferative disorder. Ann Otol Rhinol Laryngol 2002;111:165-168.

Peritonsillar Abscess

125. Risberg S, Engfeldt P, Hugosson S. Incidence of peritonsillar abscess and relationship to age and gender: retrospective study. Scand J Infect Dis 2008;40:792-796.
126. Matsuda A, Tanaka H, Kanaya T, Kamata K, Hasegawa M. Peritonsillar abscess: a study of 724 cases in Japan. Ear Nose Throat J 2002;81:384-839.
127. Schraff S, McGinn JD, Derkay CS. Peritonsillar abscess in children: a 10-year review of diagnosis and management. Int J Pediatr Otorhinolaryngol 2001;57:213-218.
128. Baldassari C, Shah RK. Pediatric peritonsillar abscess: an overview. Infect Disord Drug Targets 2012;12:277-280.
129. Klug TE. Incidence and microbiology of peritonsillar abscess: the influence of season, age, and gender. Eur J Clin Microbiol Infect Dis 2014;33:1163-1167.
130. Herzon FS, Martin AD. Medical and surgical treatment of peritonsillar, retropharyngeal, and parapharyngeal abscesses. Curr Infect Dis Rep 2006;8:196-202.
131. Alaani A, Griffiths H, Minhas SS, Olliff J, Lee AB. Parapharyngeal abscess: diagnosis, complications and management in adults. Eur Arch Otorhinolaryngol 2005;262:345-450.
132. Powell J, Wilson JA. An evidence-based review of peritonsillar abscess. Clin Otolaryngol 2012;37:136-145.
133. Powell EL, Powell J, Samuel JR, Wilson JA. A review of the pathogenesis of adult peritonsillar abscess: time for a re-evaluation. J Antimicrob Chemother 2013;68:1941-1950.
134. Sunnergren O, Swanberg J, Mölstad S. Incidence, microbiology and clinical history of peritonsillar abscesses. Scand J Infect Dis 2008;40:752-755.
135. Brook I. Microbiology and management of peritonsillar, retropharyngeal, and parapharyngeal abscesses. J Oral Maxillofac Surg 2004;62:1545-1550.
136. Snow DG, Campbell JB, Morgan DW. The microbiology of peritonsillar sepsis. J Laryngol Otol 1991;105:553-555.
137. Herzon FS. Mosher Award thesis. Peritonsillar abscess: incidence, current management practices, and a proposal for treatment guidelines. Laryngoscope 1995;105(Suppl 74):1-17.
138. Johnson RF, Stewart MG, Wright CC. An evidence-based review of the treatment of peritonsillar abscess. Otolaryngol Head Neck Surg 2003;128:332-343.
139. McCurdy JA Jr. Peritonsillar abscess. A comparison of treatment by immediate tonsillectomy and interval tonsillectomy. Arch Otolaryngol 1977;103:414-415.

Lemierre Disease

140. Righini CA, Karkas A, Tourniaire R, et al. Lemierre syndrome: study of 11 cases and literature review. Head Neck 2014;36:1044-1051.
141. Kuppalli K, Livorsi D, Talati NJ, Osborn M. Lemierre's syndrome due to Fusobacterium necrophorum. Lancet Infect Dis 2012;12:808-815.
142. Wright WF, Shiner CN, Ribes JA. Lemierre syndrome. South Med J 2012;105:282-288.
143. Khan A, Ganesan S, Arora M, Hussain N. Life threatening complication of sore throat: Lemierre's syndrome. Indian J Pediatr 2013; 80:1059-1061.

Epstein Barr Virus and Infectious Mononucleosis

144. Cohen JI. Benign and malignant Epstein-Barr virus-associated B-cell lymphoproliferative diseases. Semin Hematol 2003;40:116-123.
145. Deyrup AT, Lee VK, Hill CE, et al. Epstein-Barr virus-associated smooth muscle tumors are distinctive mesenchymal tumors reflecting multiple infection events: a clinicopathologic and molecular analysis of 29 tumors from 19 patients. Am J Surg Pathol 2006;30:75-82.
146. Grinstein S, Preciado MV, Gattuso P, et al. Demonstration of Epstein-Barr virus in carcinomas of various sites. Cancer Res 2002;62:4876-4878.
147. Hiraki A, Fujii N, Masuda K, Ikeda K, Tanimoto M. Genetics of Epstein-Barr virus infection. Biomed Pharmacother 2001;55:369-372.
148. Iezzoni JC, Gaffey MJ, Weiss LM. The role of Epstein-Barr virus in lymphoepithelioma-like carcinomas. Am J Clin Pathol 1995;103:308-315.
149. Jenson HB, Leach CT, McClain KL, et al. Benign and malignant smooth muscle tumors containing Epstein-Barr virus in children with AIDS. Leuk Lymphoma 1997;27:303-314.
150. Jenson HB. Virologic diagnosis, viral monitoring, and treatment of Epstein-Barr Virus infectious mononucleosis. Curr Infect Dis Rep 2004;6:200-207.

151. Kanegane H, Nomura K, Miyawaki T, Tosato G. Biological aspects of Epstein-Barr virus (EBV)-infected lymphocytes in chronic active EBV infection and associated malignancies. Crit Rev Oncol Hematol 2002;44:239-249.
152. Kawa K. Epstein-Barr virus—associated diseases in humans. Int J Hematol 2000;71:108-117.
153. McClain KL, Leach CT, Jenson HB, et al. Association of Epstein-Barr virus with leiomyosarcomas in children with AIDS. N Engl J Med 1995;332:12-18.
154. Nava VE, Jaffe ES. The pathology of NK-cell lymphomas and leukemias. Adv Anat Pathol 2005;12:27-34.
155. Pattle SB, Farrell PJ. The role of Epstein-Barr virus in cancer. Expert Opin Biol Ther 2006;6:1193-1205.
156. Yachie A, Kanegane H, Kasahara Y. Epstein-Barr virus-associated T-/natural killer cell lymphoproliferative diseases. Semin Hematol 2003;40:124-132.
157. Bravender T. Epstein-Barr virus, cytomegalovirus, and infectious mononucleosis. Adolesc Med State Art Rev 2010;21:251-264
158. Salvador AH, Harrison EG Jr, Kyle RA. Lymphadenopathy due to infectious mononucleosis: its confusion with malignant lymphoma. Cancer 1971;27:1029-1040.
159. Hatton OL, Harris-Arnold A, Schaffert S, Krams SM, Martinez OM. The interplay between Epstein-Barr virus and B lymphocytes: implications for infection, immunity, and disease. Immunol Res 2014;58:268–276.
160. Strickler JG, Fedeli F, Horwitz CA, Copenhaver CM, Frizzera G. Infectious mononucleosis in lymphoid tissue. Histopathology, in situ hybridization, and differential diagnosis. Arch Pathol Lab Med 1993;117:269-278.
161. Tugizov SM, Berline JW, Palefsky JM. Epstein-Barr virus infection of polarized tongue and nasopharyngeal epithelial cells. Nat Med 2003;9:307-314.
162. Shannon-Lowe CD, Neuhierl B, Baldwin G, Rickinson AB, Delecluse HJ. Resting B cells as a transfer vehicle for Epstein-Barr virus infection of epithelial cells. Proc Natl Acad Sci USA 2006;103:7065-7070.
163. Urquiza M, Lopez R, Patino H, Rosas JE, Patarroyo ME. Identification of three gp350/220 regions involved in Epstein-Barr virus invasion of host cells. J Biol Chem 2005;280:35598-35605.
164. Hutchinson RE, Schexneider KI. Infectious mononucleosis and Epstein-Barr virus infection. In: McPherson RA, Pincus MR, eds. Henry's Clinical diagnosis and management by laboratory methods. 22nd ed. Philadelphia: Elsevier Saunders; 2011:611-614.
165. Akashi K, Eizuru Y, Sumiyoshi Y, et al. Brief report: severe infectious mononucleosis-like syndrome and primary human herpesvirus 6 infection in an adult. N Engl J Med 1993;329:168-171.
166. Steeper TA, Horwitz CA, Ablashi DV, et al. The spectrum of clinical and laboratory findings resulting from human hepresvirus-6 (HHV-6) in patients with mononucleosis-like illnesses not resulting fro, Epstein-Barr virus or cytomegalovirus. Am J Clin Pathol 1990;93:776-783.
167. Strum SB, Park JK, Rappaport H. Observations of cells resembling Reed-Sternberg cells in conditions other than Hodgkin's disease. Cancer 1970;26:176-190.
168. Tindle BH, Parker JW, Lukes RJ. "Reed-Sternberg cells" in infectious mononucleosis. Am J Clin Pathol 1972;58:607-617.
169. Kojima M, Nakamura S, Sugihara S, Sakata N, Masawa N. Lymph node infarction associated with infectious mononucleosis: report of a case resembling lymph node infarction associated with malignant lymphoma. Int J Surg Pathol 2002;10:223-226.
170. Kojima M, Nakamura S, Itoh H, Yamane Y, Miyawaki S, Masawa N. Lymph node lesion in infectious mononucleosis showing geographic necrosis containing cytologically atypically B-cells. A case report. Pathol Res Pract 2004;200:53-57.
171. Abbondanzo SL, Sato N, Straus ES, Jaffe ES. Acute infectious mononucleosis: CD30 (Ki-1) antigen expression and histologic considerations. Am J Clin Pathol 1990;93:698-702.
172. Isaacson PG, Schmid C, Pan L, Wotherspoon AC, Wright DH. Epstein-Barr virus latent membrane protein expression by Hodgkin and Reed-Sternberg-like cells in acute infectious mononucleosis. J Pathol 1992;167:267-271.
173. Gulley ML. Molecular diagnosis of Epstein-Barr virus-related diseases. J Mol Diagn 2001;3:1-10.
174. Sahin F, Gerceker D, Karasartova D, Ozsan TM. Detection of herpes simplex virus type 1 in addition to Epstein-Barr virus in tonsils using a new multiplex polymerase chain reaction assay. Diagn Microbiol Infect Dis 2007;57:47-51.
175. Childs CC, Parham DM, Berard CW. Infectious mononucleosis: The spectrum of morphologic changes simulating lymphoma in lymph nodes and tonsils. Am J Surg Pathol 1987;11:122-132.
176. Dorfman RE, Warnke R. Lymphadenopathy simulating the malignant lymphomas. Hum Pathol 1974;5:519-550.
177. Kapadia SB, Roman LN, Kingma DW, Jaffe ES, Frizzera G. Hodgkin's disease of Waldeyer's ring. Clinical and histoimmunophenotypic findings and association with Epstein-Barr virus in 16 cases. Am J Surg Pathol 1995;19:1431-1439.
178. Chan SC, Dawes PJ. The management of severe infectious mononucleosis tonsillitis and upper airway obstruction. J Laryngol Otol 2001;115:973-977.

179. Cacopardo B, Nunnari G, Mughini MT, Tosto S, Benanti F, Nigro L. Fatal hepatitis during Epstein-Barr virus reactivation. Eur Rev Med Pharmacol Sci 2003;7:107-109.
180. Badura RA, Oliveira O, Palhano MJ, Borregana J, Quaresma J. Spontaneous rupture of the spleen as presenting event in infectious mononucleosis. Scand J Infect Dis 2001;33:872-874.
181. Stockinger ZT. Infectious mononucleosis presenting as spontaneous splenic rupture without other symptoms. Mil Med 2003;168:722-724.
182. Gautschi O, Berger C, Gubler J, Laube I. Acute respiratory failure and cerebral hemorrhage due to primary Epstein-Barr virus infection. Respiration 2003;70:419-422.
183. Karachalios G, Charalabopoulos AK, Karachaliou IG, Charalabopoulos K. Infectious mononucleosis, diffuse pneumonia and acute respiratory failure in an elderly woman. Int J Clin Pract 2004;58:90-92.
184. Helin K, Ekroos H. A case of mononucleosis complicated by acute nephritis. Scand J Urol Nephrol 2002;36:152-153.
185. Lei PS, Lowichik A, Allen W, Mauch TJ. Acute renal failure: unusual complication of Epstein-Barr virus-induced infectious mononucleosis. Clin Infect Dis 2000;31:1519-1524.
186. Simonetti GD, Dumont-Dos Santos K, Pachlopnik JM, Ramelli G, Bianchetti MG. Hemolytic uremic syndrome linked to infectious mononucleosis. Pediatr Nephrol 2003;18:1193-1194.
187. Walter RB, Hong TC, Bachli EB. Life-threatening thrombocytopenia associated with acute Epstein-Barr virus infection in an older adult. Ann Hematol 2002;81:672-675.
188. Auwaerter PG. Recent advances in the understanding of infectious mononucleosis: are prospects improved for treatment or control? Expert Rev Anti Infect Ther 2006;4:1039-1049.
189. Jarrett RF. Risk factors for Hodgkin's lymphoma by EBV status and significance of detection of EBV genomes in serum of patients with EBV-associated Hodgkin's lymphoma. Leuk Lymphoma 2003;44(Suppl 3):S27-32.
190. Tselis A. Epstein-Barr virus cause of multiple sclerosis. Curr Opin Rheumatol 2012;24:424-428.
191. Xiao D, Ye X, Zhang N, et al. A meta-analysis of interaction between Epstein-Barr virus and HLA-DRB1*1501 on risk of multiple sclerosis. Sci Rep 2015;5:18083.
192. Kobbervig C, Norback D, Kahl B. Infectious mononucleosis progressing to fatal malignant lymphoma: a case report and review of the literature. Leuk Lymphoma 2003;44:1215-1221.
193. Veillette A, Pérez-Quintero LA, Latour S. X-linked lymphoproliferative syndromes and related autosomal recessive disorders. Curr Opin Allergy Clin Immunol 2013;13:614-622.
194. Hoshino T, Kanegane H, Doki N, et al. X-linked lymphoproliferative disease in an adult. Int J Hematol 2005;82:55-58.
195. Janka GE. Familial and acquired hemophagocytic lymphohistiocytosis. Eur J Pediatr 2007;166:95-109.

Human Papillomavirus

196. Syrjanen S, Puranen M. Human papillomavirus infections in children: the potential role of maternal transmission. Crit Rev Oral Biol Med 2000;11:259-274.
197. Ang KK, Sturgis EM. Human papillomavirus-assoicated head and neck cancer. In: Harrison LB, Sessions RB, Kies MS, eds. Head and neck caner. A multidisciplinary approach, 4th ed. Philadelphia; Wolters Kluwer - Lippincott Williams & Wilkins; 2014:236-251.
198. Castro TP, Bussoloti Filho I. Prevalence of human papillomavirus (HPV) in oral cavity and oropharynx. Braz J Otorhinolaryngol 2006;72:272-282.
199. Ng YT, Lau WM, Fang TJ, Hsieh JR, Chung PC. Unexpected upper airway obstruction due to disseminated human papilloma virus infection involving the pharynx in a parturient. Acta Anaesthesiol Taiwan 2010;48:87-90.
200. Dyson N, Howley PM, Münger K, Harlow E. The human papillomavirus-16 E7 oncoprotein is able to bind the retinoblastoma gene product. Science 1989;243:934-937.

AIDS and HIV

201. Hirsch M, Curran J. Human immunodeficiency viruses. In: Fields B, Knipe D, Howley P, eds. Fields Virology, Vol 2. Philadelphia: Lippincott-Raven Press; 1996:1953-69.
202. Perez KA, Saag MS, Kilby JM. Human immunodeficiency virus. In: Mandell GL, Mildvan D, eds. Atlas of AIDS, 3rd ed. Philadelphia: Current Medicine Group; 2001:23-43.
203. Frankel SS, Wenig BM. Human immunodeficiency virus and acquired immunodeficiency syndrome. In: Fu YS, Wenig BM, Abemayor E, Wenig BL, eds. Head and neck pathology with clinical correlation. New York: Churchill Livingstone; 2001:65-80.
204. Vermund SH, Drotman DP. Epidemiology, natural history and prevention. In: Mandell GL, Mildvan D, eds. Atlas of AIDS, 3rd ed. Philadelphia: Current Medicine; 2001:1-22.
205. Castro KG, Ward JW, Slotsker L, et al. 1993 revised classification system for HIV infection and expanded surveillance definition for AIDS among adolescents and adults. MMWR Recomm Rep 1992;41 [RR-17]:1-19.

206. Fleming PL, Ward JW, Janssen RS, et al. Guidelines for national human immunodeficiency virus case surveillance, including monitoring for human immunodeficiency virus infection and acquired immunodeficiency syndrome. Centers for Disease Control and Prevention. MMWR 1999;48(RR-13):1-27, 29-31.
207. Centers for Disease Control and Prevention (CDC). Revised surveillance case definition for HIV infection—United States, 2014. MMWR Recomm Rep 2014;63(RR-03):1-10.

HIV-Related Lymphoid Changes

208. Frankel SS, Tenner-Racz K, Racz P, et al. Active replication of HIV-1 at the lymphoepithelial surface of the tonsil. Am J Pathol 1997;151:89-96.
209. Wenig BM, Thompson LD, Frankel SS, et al. Lymphoid changes of the nasopharyngeal and palatine tonsils that are indicative of human immunodeficiency virus infection. A clinicopathologic study of 12 cases. Am J Surg Pathol 1996;20:572-587.
210. Frankel SS, Wenig BM, Burke AP, et al. Replication of HIV-1 in dendritic cell-derived syncytia at the mucosal surface of the adenoid. Science 1996;272:115-117.
211. Orenstein JM, Wahl SM. The macrophage origin of the HIV-expressing multinucleated giant cells in hyperplastic tonsils and adenoids. Ultrastruct Pathol 1999;23:79-91.
212. Dargent JL, Lespagnard L, Kornreich A, Hermans P, Clumeck N, Verhest A. HIV-associated multinucleated giant cells in lymphoid tissue of the Waldeyer's ring: a detailed study. Mod Pathol 2000;13:1293-1299.
213. Consolidated Guidelines on the Use of Antiretroviral Drugs for Treating and Preventing HIV Infection: Recommendations for a Public Health Approach. Geneva: World Health Organization; 2013 Jun. PubMed PMID: 24716260.

Cytomegalovirus

214. Brantsaeter AB, Liestol K, Goplen AK, Dunlop O, Bruun JN. CMV disease in AIDS patients: incidence of CMV disease and relation to survival in a population-based study from Oslo. Scand J Infect Dis 2002;34:50-55.
215. Eversole LR. Viral infections of the head and neck among HIV-seropositive patients. Oral Surg Oral Med Oral Pathol 1992;73:155-163.
216. Klatt EC, Shibata D. Cytomegalovirus infection in the acquired immunodeficiency syndrome. Clinical and autopsy finding. Arch Pathol Lab Med 1988;112:540-544.
217. French PD, Birchall MA, Harris JR. Cytomegalovirus ulceration of the oropharynx. J Laryngol Otol. 1991;105:739-742.
218. Lalwani AK, Snyderman NL. Pharyngeal ulceration in AIDS patients secondary to cytomegalovirus infection. Ann Otol Rhinol Laryngol 1991;100:484-487.
219. Victoria JM, Guimaraes AL, da Silva LM, Kalapothakis E, Gomez RS. Polymerase chain reaction for identification of herpes simplex virus (HSV-1), cytomegalovirus (CMV) and human herpes virus-type 6 (HHV-6) in oral swabs. Microbiol Res 2005;160:61-65.
220. Sahin F, Gerceker D, Karasartova D, Ozsan TM. Detection of herpes simplex virus type 1 in addition to Epstein-Barr virus in tonsils using a new multiplex polymerase chain reaction assay. Diagn Microbiol Infect Dis 2007;57:47-51.
221. Biron KK. Antiviral drugs for cytomegalovirus diseases. Antiviral Res 2006;71:154-163.
222. Einsele H, Mielke S, Grigoleit GU. Diagnosis and treatment of cytomegalovirus 2013. Curr Opin Hematol 2014;21:470-475.

Herpes Virus

223. Eversole LR. Inflammatory diseases of the mucous membranes. Part 1. Viral and fungal infections. J Calif Dent Assoc 1994;22:52-57.
224. Lin YY, Kao CH, Wang CH. Varicella zoster virus infection of the pharynx and larynx with multiple cranial neuropathies. Laryngoscope 2011;121:1627-1630.
225. Goldani LZ, da Silva LF, Dora JM. Ramsay Hunt syndrome in patients infected with human immunodeficiency virus. Clin Exp Dermatol 2009;34:e552-554.
226. Levin MJ. Varicella-zoster virus and virus DNA in the blood and oropharynx of people with latent or active varicella-zoster virus infections. J Clin Virol 2014;61:487-495.

Fungus Infections

227. Lin JN, Lin CC, Lai CH, et al. Predisposing factors for oropharyngeal colonization of yeasts in human immunodeficiency virus-infected patients: a prospective cross-sectional study. J Microbiol Immunol Infect 2013;46:129-135.
228. Thompson GR 3rd, Patel PK, Kirkpatrick WR, et al. Oropharyngeal candidiasis in the era of antiretroviral therapy. Oral Surg Oral Med Oral Pathol Oral Radiol Endod. 2010;109:488-495.
229. Antonello VS, Zaltron VF, Vial M, Oliveira FM, Severo LC. Oropharyngeal histoplasmosis: report of eleven cases and review of the literature. Rev Soc Bras Med Trop 2011;44:26-29.

Bacteria and Spirochetes

230. Ablanedo-Terrazas Y, la Barrera CA, Ruiz-Cruz M, Reyes-Terán G. Oropharyngeal syphilis among patients infected with human immunodeficiency virus. Ann Otol Rhinol Laryngol 2013;122:435-439.
231. Ditzen AK1, Braker K, Zoellner KH, Teichmann D. The syphilis-HIV interdependency. Int J STD AIDS 2005;16:642-643.

232. Ikenberg K, Springer E, Bräuninger W, et al. Oropharyngeal lesions and cervical lymphadenopathy: syphilis is a differential diagnosis that is still relevant. J Clin Pathol 2010;63:731-736.
233. Mayer KH. Sexually transmitted diseases in men who have sex with men. Clin Infect Dis 2011;53(Suppl 3):S79-83.
234. Oddó D, Carrasco G, Capdeville F, Ayala MF. Syphilitic tonsillitis presenting as an ulcerated tonsillar tumor with ipsilateral lymphadenopathy. Ann Diagn Pathol 2007;11:353-357.
235. Workowski KA. Sexually transmitted infections and HIV: diagnosis and treatment. Top Antivir Med 2012;20:11-16.

Gonorrhea and Syphilis

236. Barlow D. The diagnosis of oropharyngeal gonorrhoea. Genitourin Med 1997;73:16-17.
237. Bruce AJ, Rogers RS 3rd. Oral manifestations of sexually transmitted diseases. Clin Dermatol 2004;22:520-527.
238. Hutt DM, Judson FN. Epidemiology and treatment of oropharyngeal gonorrhea. Ann Intern Med 1986;104:655-658.
239. Manavi K, Zafar F, Shahid H. Oropharyngeal gonorrhoea: rate of co-infection with sexually transmitted infection, antibiotic susceptibility and treatment outcome. Int J STD AIDS 2010;21:138-140.
240. Reinton N, Moi H, Olsen AO, et al. Anatomic distribution of Neisseria gonorrhoeae, Chlamydia trachomatis and Mycoplasma genitalium infections in men who have sex with men. Sex Health 2013;10:199-203.
241. Rodriguez-Hart C, Chitale RA, Rigg R, Goldstein BY, Kerndt PR, Tavrow P. Sexually transmitted infection testing of adult film performers: is disease being missed? Sex Transm Dis 2012;39:989-994.
242. Siegel MA. Syphilis and gonorrhea. Dent Clin North Am 1996;40:368-383.
243. Thomson-Glover R, Brown R, Edirisinghe DN. Isolated pharyngeal Neisseria gonorrhoeae in heterosexual male contacts. Int J STD AIDS 2013;24:983-985.
244. van Liere GA, Hoebe CJ, Dukers-Muijrers NH. Evaluation of the anatomical site distribution of chlamydia and gonorrhoea in men who have sex with men and in high-risk women by routine testing: cross-sectional study revealing missed opportunities for treatment strategies. Sex Transm Infect 2014;90:58-60.
245. Page-Shafer K, Graves A, Kent C, Balls JE, Zapitz VM, Klausner JD. Increased sensitivity of DNA amplification testing for the detection of pharyngeal gonorrhea in men who have sex with men. Clin Infect Dis 2002;34:173-176.
246. Pletcher SD, Cheung SW. Syphilis and otolaryngology. Otolaryngol Clin North Am 2003;36:595-605.
247. LaSala PR, Smith MB. Spirochete infections. In: McPherson RA, Pincus MR, eds. Henry's Clinical diagnosis and management by laboratory methods, 22nd ed. Philadelphia: Elsevier Saunders; 2011:1129-1144.
248. Carey JC. Congenital syphilis in the 21st century. Curr Womens Health Rep 2003;3:299-302.
249. Fiumara NJ, Lessell S. Manifestations of late congenital syphilis. An analysis of 271 patients. Arch Dermatol 1970;102:78-83.
250. Simmank KC, Pettifor JM. Unusual presentation of congenital syphilis. Ann Trop Paediatr 2000;20:105-107.
251. Wendel GD Jr, Sheffield JS, Hollier LM, Hill JB, Ramsey PS, Sanchez PJ. Treatment of syphilis in pregnancy and prevention of congenital syphilis. Clin Infect Dis 2002;35:S200-209.
252. Barrett AW, Villarroel Dorrego M, Hodgson TA, et al. The histopathology of syphilis of the oral mucosa. J Oral Pathol Med 2004;33:286-291.

Tangier Disease

253. Puntoni M, Sbrana F, Bigazzi F, Sampietro T. Tangier disease: epidemiology, pathophysiology, and management. Am J Cardiovasc Drugs 2012;12:303-311.
254. Fasano T, Zanoni P, Rabacchi C, et al. Novel mutations of ABCA1 transporter in patients with Tangier disease and familial HDL deficiency. Mol Genet Metab 2012;107:534-541.
255. Singaraja RR, Visscher H, James ER, et al. Specific mutations in ABCA1 have discrete effects on ABCA1 function and lipid phenotypes both in vivo and in vitro. Circ Res 2006;99:389-397.
256. Maxfield FR, Tabas I. Role of cholesterol and lipid organization in disease. Science 2005;438:612-621.
257. Nofer JR, Remaley AT. Tangier disease: still more questions than answers. Cell Mol Life Sci 2005;62:2150-2160.
258. Hoffman HN, Fredrickson DS. Tangier disease (familial high density lipoprotein deficiency). Clinical and genetic features in two adults. Am J Med 1965;39:582-593.
259. Schoenberg BS, Schoenberg DG. Eponym: tangerine tonsils in Tangier: high density lipoprotein deficiency. South Med J 1978;71:453-454.
260. Neqi SI, Brautbar A, Virani SS, et al. A novel mutation in the ABCA1 gene causing an atypical phenotype of Tangier disease. J Clin Lipidol 2013;7:82-87.
261. Kolovou GD, Mikhailidis DP, Anagnostopoulou KK, Daskalopoulou SS, Cokkinos DV. Tangier disease four decades of research: a reflection of the importance of HDL. Curr Med Chem 2006;13:771-782.

4 NECK

By Dr. Bruce M. Wenig

ANATOMY

The prominent landmarks in the neck are the hyoid bone, thyroid cartilage, trachea, and sternocleidomastoid muscles. The neck is divided into the anterior and posterior triangles by the sternocleidomastoid muscles (fig. 4-1) (1,2).

Anterior Triangle. The anatomic boundaries of the anterior triangle include: the lateral limit, the anterior border of the sternocleidomastoid muscle; the medial limit, the anatomic midline of the neck; and the superior limit, the lower border of the mandible. The subdivisions of the anterior triangle include the carotid triangle, submandibular (submaxillary) triangle, inferior carotid (muscular) triangle, and submental or suprahyoid triangle. The contents of the anterior triangle include the common carotid artery with its internal and external branches, cranial nerves IX to XII, the internal jugular vein, and the superficial and deep cervical lymph nodes (1,2).

Posterior Triangle. The anatomic boundaries of the posterior triangle include: the anteromedial limit, the posterior border of the sternocleidomastoid muscle; the posterolateral limit, the anterior border of the trapezius muscle; and the inferior limit, the clavicle. The contents of the posterior triangle include the subclavian artery, external jugular vein, branches of the cervical plexus, cranial nerve XI (spinal accessory), and numerous lymph nodes, including the posterior cervical and supraclavicular lymph nodes (1,2).

Cervical Lymph Nodes. The neck is divided into six levels, encompassing the complete topographic anatomy of the neck (Table 4-1), although a seventh level (level VII) may be include. The lymph nodes are: level I, submental, submandibular nodes; level II to IV, upper, middle, and lower deep cervical nodes; level V, posterior triangle nodes; level VI, lymph nodes around the thyroid gland (referred to as the central compartment); and level VII, lymph nodes in the tracheoesophageal groove and superior mediastinum (fig. 4-2).

CLASSIFICATION

The classification of non-neoplastic lesions of the neck is seen in Table 4-2.

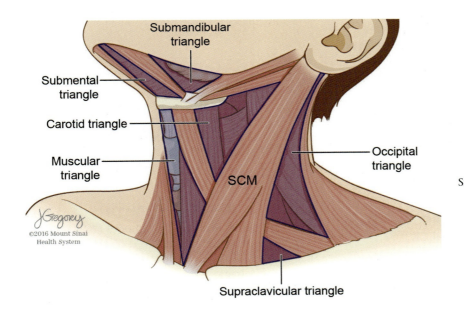

Figure 4-1

TRIANGLES OF THE NECK

(Courtesy of J. Gregory, Mount Sinai Health System.)

Table 4-1
LYMPH NODE LEVELS AND SUBLEVELS[a]

Lymph Node Level	Description
I	sublevel IA: submental—lymph nodes within the triangular boundary of the anterior belly of the digastric muscles and the hyoid bone sublevel IB: submandibular—lymph nodes within the boundaries of the anterior belly of the digastric muscle, stylohyoid muscle, and body of the mandible
II (Upper Jugular)	lymph nodes located around the upper third of the internal jugular vein and the adjacent spinal accessory nerve, extending from: above—level of the skull base below—level of the inferior border of the hyoid bone medial (anterior)—stylohyoid muscle (radiologic correlate is the vertical plane defined by the posterior surface of the submandibular gland) lateral (posterior)—posterior border of the SCM[b] sublevel IIA: nodes located anterior (medial) to the vertical plane defined by the spinal accessory nerve sublevel IIB: nodes located posterior (lateral) to the vertical plane defined by the spinal accessory nerve
III (Midjugular)	lymph nodes located around the middle third of the internal jugular vein extending from: above—inferior border of the hyoid bone below—inferior border of the cricoid cartilage medial (anterior)—lateral border of sternohyoid muscle lateral (posterior)—posterior border of the SCM
IV (Lower Jugular)	lymph nodes located around the lower third of the internal jugular vein extending from: above—inferior border of cricoid cartilage below—clavicle
V (Posterior Triangle)	lymph nodes in this group are predominantly located around the lower half of the spinal accessory nerve and the transverse cervical artery and extend from: superior—apex formed by convergence of the SCM and trapezius muscle inferior—clavicle medial (anterior)—posterior border of SCM lateral (posterior)—anterior border of trapezius muscle sublevels include V-A and V-B separated by a horizontal plane marking the inferior border border of the anterior cricoid arch: V-A: above this plane includes the spinal accessory lymph nodes V-B: below this plane includes the lymph nodes that follow the transverse cervical vessels and the supraclavicular nodes with the exception of the Virchow node which is located in level IV
VI (Anterior Compartment)	boundaries of this compartment include: superior—hyoid bone inferior—suprasternal notch lateral—common carotid arteries lymph nodes in this level include: pretracheal and paratracheal nodes precricoid (delphian) nodes perithyroidal nodes including those along the recurrent laryngeal nerves

[a]Modified from a table in reference 3.
[b]SCM = sternocleidomastoid muscle.

CYSTIC (NON-NEOPLASTIC) LESIONS OF THE NECK

Cystic lesions of the neck are a diverse group. Benign cystic lesions of the cervical neck are listed in Table 4-3.

Branchial Anomalies

Definition. *Branchial anomalies* (BA) are congenital malformations related to the branchial apparatus.

Embryology. The branchial apparatus appears around the 4th week of gestation and

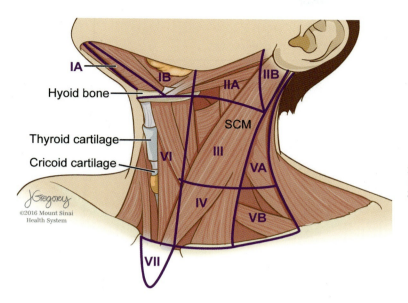

Figure 4-2

NODAL STATIONS I THROUGH VII

These are delineated in a node-negative neck. (SCM = sternocleidomastoid muscle). (Courtesy of J. Gregory, Mount Sinai Health System.)

Table 4-2
CLASSIFICATION OF NON-NEOPLASTIC LESIONS OF THE NECK
Developmental Cystic Anomalies
Branchial cleft anomalies
Thyroglossal duct cyst
Cervical thymic cyst
Bronchogenic cyst
Dermoid cyst
Others
Infectious and Related Diseases/Lesions
Bacterial and mycobacterial
Fungal
Viral
Protozoal
Sarcoidosis
Others
Reactive, Inflammatory, and Tumor-like Lesions
Mesenchymal lesions
Others

Table 4-3
NON-NEOPLASTIC CYSTIC LESIONS OF THE CERVICAL NECK
Developmental Cysts
Branchial cleft cysts
Thyroglossal duct cyst
Cervical thymic cyst
Bronchogenic cyst
Parathyroid cyst
Others

consists of a paired series of 6 arches, 5 pouches, and 5 clefts or grooves (4). The embryologic development of the head and neck structures are classified through the development of the branchial apparatus, including arches (mesoderm), clefts (ectoderm), and pharyngeal pouches (endoderm) (Table 4-4); the branchial apparatus gives rise to most of the important structures of the head and neck, including the face, oral cavity, ears, and neck (4).

Clinical Features. BAs have no gender predilection and can occur at any age, but they most commonly become evident in young adults. They predominantly occur in the lateral neck, along the anterior portion of the sternocleidomastoid muscle. They are also seen in the area around the external ear, in the external auditory canal, and in the parotid gland. Generally, BAs occur as an isolated phenomenon but may be familial or may rarely be associated with other congenital defects including malformed auricles, hearing abnormalities, patent ductus arteriosus, and tear duct atresia (5,6). *HATS syndrome,* which including hemimaxillary enlargement, asymmetry of the face, tooth abnormalities, and skin findings, is a rare developmental disorder involving the first and second branchial arches (7,8).

BAs are divided according to the branchial apparatus involved, and are further divided

Table 4-4

BRANCHIAL APPARATUS AND DERIVATIVES

	Arches (Mesoderm)	Pharyngeal Pouches (Endoderm)	Clefts (Ectoderm)

First	cartilage bar (Meckel cartilage):
	  ramus and body of mandible
	  maxilla
	  incus (body)
	  malleus (head and neck)
	  part of pinna of ear
	muscles and ligaments:
	  temporalis
	  masseter
	  pterygoids (medial and lateral)
	  digastric (anterior belly)
	  mylohyoid
	  tensor tympani
	  tensor veli palatini
	  anterior two thirds of tongue
	  spheno-mandibular ligament
	  anterior malleolar ligament
	innervation:
	  trigeminal (maxillary and mandibular divisions)
	vasculature:
	  facial artery
		epithelial lining of the middle ear cavity, inner part of the tympanic membrane, eustachian tube, mastoid air cells	epithelial lining of the external auditory canal and outer part of the tympanic membrane

Second	cartilage bar (Reichert cartilage):
	  incus (long process)
	  malleus (manubrium)
	  stapes (long process)
	  styloid process
	  hyoid (lesser horn and upper body)
	  Part of pinna of ear
	muscles and ligaments:
	  facial (auricularis, buccinator, frontalis, occipitalis, orbicularis oculi, oris platysma)
	  digastric (posterior belly)
	  stapedius
	  stylohyoid
	  stylohyoid ligament
	innervation:
	  facial
	vasculature:
	  lingual branch of external carotid artery
		epithelial lining of the tonsillar fossa and palatine tonsil	none

into cysts, sinuses, and fistulas (9–11). Cysts are epithelial lined structures that may occur as an isolated lesion or may occur in association with a sinus or fistula. Sinuses are tracts with a single opening; the opening may be to the skin, representing a branchial cleft or ectodermally-derived sinus tract (cutaneous sinus tract), or to mucosa, representing a branchial pouch or endodermally derived sinus tract (mucosal sinus tract). Fistulas are tracts with two openings, which can be cutaneous or mucosal.

Cysts present as nontender, fluctuant masses in appropriate locations; they may become inflamed and abscesses may develop, potentially associated with dysphagia, dyspnea, or stridor. Sinuses and fistulas are associated with discharge of mucoid or purulent secretions from the tract opening. Up to 10 percent of cases are bilateral (5,6).

Histogenesis. The histogenesis of BAs is controversial. Among the structures proposed as the origins for these anomalies are the branchial

Table 4-4, continued

	Arches (Mesoderm)	Pharyngeal Pouches (Endoderm)	Clefts (Ectoderm)

Third	cartilage bar:
	  hyoid (lower body and greater horn)
	muscles and ligaments:
	  stylopharyngeus
	  palatopharyngeus
	  posterior third (base or root) of tongue
	innervation:
	  glossopharyngeal
	vasculature:
	  internal carotid artery
		inferior parathyroid glands, thymus, pyriform sinus	none

Fourth	cartilage bar:
	  thyroid
	muscles and ligaments:
	  cricothyroid
	  levator palatini
	  posterior third (base) of tongue
	innervation:
	  vagus (superior laryngeal branch)
	vasculature:
	  arch of aorta
	  right subclavian artery
		superior parathyroid
		C cells of ultimobranchial body
			none

Fifth and Sixth	cartilage bar:
	  cricoid
	  arytenoids
	muscles and ligaments:
	  intrinsic muscles of larynx
	  upper esophageal muscles
	innervation:
	  vagus (recurrent laryngeal)
	vasculature:
	  pulmonary arteries
	  ductus arteriosus
		C cells of ultimobranchial body (5th pharyngeal pouch)
		6th pharyngeal pouch
			none
			
			none

apparatus, salivary gland inclusions, and the thymic duct (12,13).

First Branchial Anomalies

Clinical Features. First BAs typically occur in the area of the external ear and include cysts, sinuses, and fistulas (14–18). In comparison to second BAs, first BAs are uncommon, representing from 1 to 8 percent of all branchial apparatus defects (19). They occur in a variety of locations, including preauricular, postauricular, or infraauricular areas, at the angle of the jaw, associated with the ear lobe, in the external auditory canal, or involving the parotid gland (20). Involvement of the external auditory canal may result in otalgia or otorrhea (21). Children with first BAs often present with otologic complications, including otorrhea, otitis media, and cholesteatoma (21). Parotid involvement may result in an intraparotid or periparotid mass that may be mistaken for a parotid gland tumor (22).

The radiologic features include the presence of an ovoid cystic mass in the area around the external auditory canal or in the parotid space (fig. 4-3). Type I first branchial cleft cysts appear as cystic masses below or posterior to the pinna; type II cysts appear as a well-marginated cystic mass in the parotid space or periparotid area. Computerized tomography (CT) findings show a well-circumscribed, nonenhancing or rim-enhancing, low-density mass; in the presence of infection, a thick enhancing rim may be identified (23).

Gross Findings. Cysts represent over two thirds (68 percent) of these anomalies (17,24). First BAs appear as solitary cystic lesions without

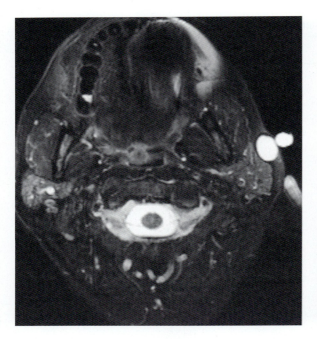

Figure 4-3

FIRST BRANCHIAL CLEFT CYST

Axial fat-suppressed FSE T2-weighted image of the neck shows a cystic type lesion superficial to the left parotid gland. (Courtesy of Dr. A. Khorsandi, New York, NY.)

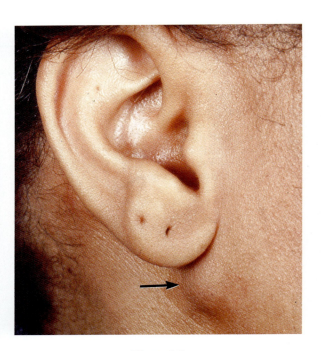

Figure 4-4

FIRST BRANCHIAL CLEFT CYST

Infra-auricular, freely movable and fluctuant mass (arrow).

an associated sinus tract (fig. 4-4). Sinuses and fistulas equally make up the remainder of these lesions. The fistula tract in first BAs may extend from the skin over or through the parotid gland and open in the external auditory canal.

Microscopic Findings. First BAs are divided into two types as defined by Work (14,25). Type I contains only ectodermal elements, including, keratinizing squamous epithelium without adnexal structures (i.e., hair follicles, sebaceous glands, sweat glands), or cartilage, thereby duplicating the membranous external auditory canal (fig. 4-5). As such, type I is a first cleft anomaly only. Typically, type I lesions are located medial, inferior, or posterior to the concha and pinna. Sinuses parallel the external auditory canal and end in a blind sac at the level of the mesotympanum. The external auditory canal is intact and hearing is normal.

Type II lesions have both ectodermal and mesodermal elements, including keratinized squamous epithelium, cutaneous adnexae, and cartilage, thereby duplicating the external auditory canal and pinna (fig. 4-5). Type II anomalies typically localize to a point just below the angle of the mandible. Sinus or fistula tracts extend upward over the angle of the mandible, through the parotid gland, toward the external auditory canal. Type II anomalies are more intimately associated with the parotid gland than type I anomalies, although parotid tissue may be found in association with type I sinus or fistula tracts (fig. 4-6). Tracts associated with type II defects may terminate short of the external auditory canal or may open up in the external auditory canal near the junction of the cartilaginous and osseous portions. Communication with the middle ear is uncommon.

For either type I or type II defects, an associated prominent lymphoid component may be identified (fig. 4-6), although in contrast to second BAs, such a lymphoid component is not usually present unless the lesion is inflamed or infected. In such circumstances, a lymphoid component may be prominent.

Olsen et al. (17) believed that there were overlapping histologic features between Work types I and II. They recommend classifying all first branchial cleft anomalies only as cysts, sinuses, or fistulas.

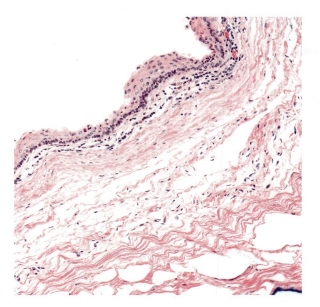 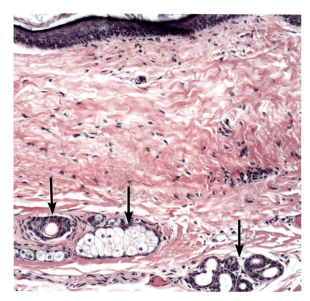

Figure 4-5

FIRST BRANCHIAL CLEFT CYST

Left: Work type I first branchial cleft cyst is composed of a keratinizing squamous epithelial lining devoid of adnexal structures.

Right: Work type II first branchial cleft cyst is characterized by a keratinizing squamous epithelial lining with associated adnexal structures within the cyst wall (arrows; from left to right include hair follicle, sebaceous cells, and eccrine glands).

Differential Diagnosis. The differential diagnosis for type I and type II defects includes epidermoid cyst and dermoid, respectively. Clinical correlation helps in the differentiation of these histologically similar-appearing lesions.

Treatment and Prognosis. Irrespective of the histology, complete surgical excision is the treatment of choice. Inadequate excision results in recurrence and increased risk of infection. Incision and drainage are indicated in cases where abscesses have developed; complete surgical excision must wait until the resolution of the infection.

Type II anomalies are often intimately associated with the parotid gland, necessitating a superficial parotidectomy to ensure complete excision. Although there is no consistent relationship between the tract and the facial nerve as it courses through the parotid gland, exposure and dissection of the nerve and its branches are required for Work type II anomalies.

Second Branchial Anomalies

Clinical Features. Second BAs account for the majority of the branchial apparatus anomalies (92 to 99 percent of all cases). Second BAs affect both genders equally, typically occur in the third to fifth decades of life, and are uncommon in patients older than 50 years of age. Fewer than 3 percent of cysts present after the age of 50 (26) so that lateral neck cysts in patients 50 years of age and older should prompt diagnostic consideration of a metastatic cystic squamous cell carcinoma.

The cysts occur along the anterior border of the sternocleidomastoid muscle, most commonly at the angle of the mandible. They present as a painless, fluctuant neck mass which may increase in size during an upper respiratory tract infection, at which time they may become painful (fig. 4-7). Cysts are much more common than fistulas (6,27).

Sinuses and fistulas are most often identified at birth or in early childhood, presenting as a small opening above the clavicle through which mucoid secretions may be expressed. These are divided into three types: 1) incomplete external, having an external (cutaneous) but no internal (pharyngeal) opening; 2) incomplete internal, having a pharyngeal but no cutaneous opening; and 3) complete, having both pharyngeal and

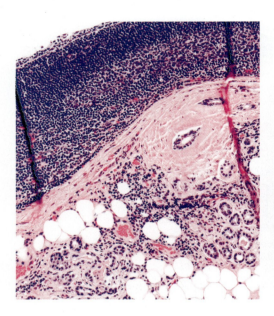
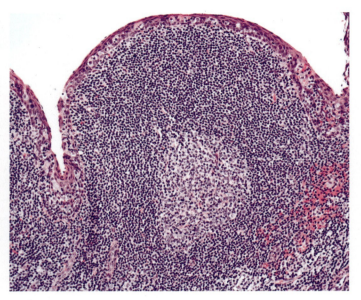

Figure 4-6

FIRST BRANCHIAL CLEFT CYSTS

Left: A benign lymphoid proliferation and parotid parenchyma are present within the cyst wall.
Right: The benign lymphoid component includes germinal centers. In contrast to second branchial anomalies, a lymphoid component is not usually present in first branchial cleft anomalies unless the lesion is inflamed or infected.

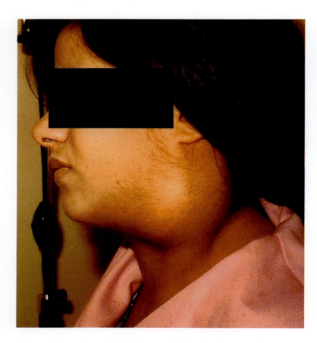

Figure 4-7

SECOND BRANCHIAL CLEFT CYST

The cyst presents along the anterior border of the sternocleidomastoid muscle as a painless, fluctuant neck mass. (Courtesy of Dr. M. Persky, New York, NY.)

cutaneous openings. The cutaneous opening is seen anywhere along the anterior border of the sternocleidomastoid muscle, from the hyoid bone to the sternum, with the epithelial tract coursing cephalad, between the internal and external carotid arteries, over cranial nerves IX and XII, deep to the posterior belly of the digastric muscle and terminating close to the middle constrictor muscle; the internal opening also may be in the pharyngeal wall or tonsillar region. Rarely, second BAs may occur in the nasopharynx (28–30).

On radiologic examination, second branchial cleft cysts appear as well-defined, low density, ovoid lesions surrounded by a thin, uniform wall (fig. 4-8) (31). Noninflamed cysts have no or minimal CT mural enhancement; infected cysts have increased CT density of the central fluid with rim enhancement and a poorly defined cyst wall. Fistulas and sinus tracts extend either toward the skin surface, supratonsillar fossa, or between the internal and external carotid arteries.

Gross Findings. The cysts are thin-walled structures filled with cheesy material or serous, mucoid, or purulent fluid. Nodular excrescences may line the cyst wall.

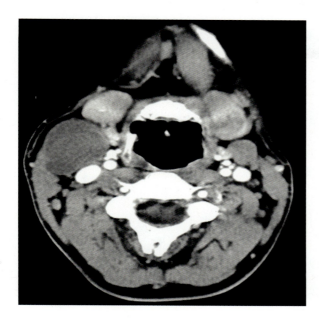

Figure 4-8

SECOND BRANCHIAL CLEFT CYST

Contrast-enhanced axial computerized tomography (CT) image shows a nonenhancing cystic lesion in the right juxtahyoid neck. This lesion is anterior to the right sternocleidomastoid muscle and the right jugular vein. (Courtesy of Dr. A. Khorsandi, New York, NY.)

Microscopic Findings. Generally, smears of noninflamed branchial cleft cysts are hypocellular. They contain anucleated and nucleated squamous cells (fig. 4-9) and a variable admixture of inflammatory cells including neutrophils (fig. 4-9) (32). The squamous component is usually sparse but may be cellular. On Giemsa staining, the anucleated squamous cells have glassy-appearing cytoplasm (referred to as "robin's egg"), and ghost-like outlines of the nuclei may be present. Parakeratotic cells have small hyperchromatic nuclei with smooth nuclear membranes (32). On Papanicolaou staining, the keratotic cells have cytoplasmic orangeophilia (not as intensely orangeophilic as seen in cervical/vaginal preparations) and markedly hyperchromatic nuclei with smooth nuclear membranes. Nuclear atypia and mitoses are typically not identified.

In inflamed branchial cleft cysts, however, significant nuclear atypia of the parakeratotic cellular component may be present, creating diagnostic problems with metastatic cystic well-differentiated keratinizing squamous cell

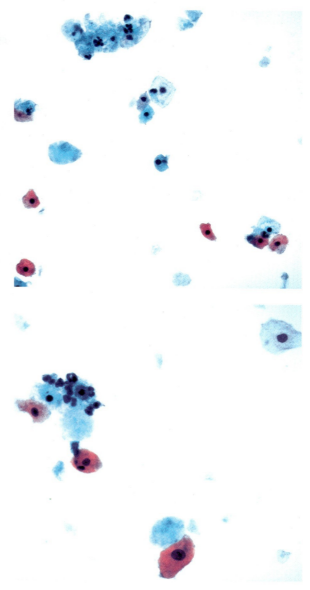

Figure 4-9

BRANCHIAL CLEFT CYST

Top, bottom: A fine-needle aspiration biopsy consists of anucleated and nucleated benign squamous cells with a variable number of associated neutrophils. See figure 4-12 for corresponding histology of the resection specimen.

carcinoma (fig. 4-10), although these cysts still tend to be dominated by anucleated squamous cells (32). The atypia in this setting tends to be degenerative, characterized by smudgy nuclei and a low nuclear to cytoplasmic ratio (33). Caution must be exercised to not overdiagnose

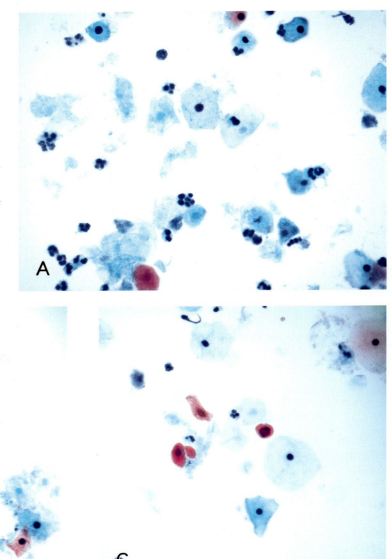

Figure 4-10

INFLAMED BRANCHIAL CLEFT CYST

A: A fine-needle aspiration biopsy shows anucleated and nucleated benign squamous cells and increased numbers of neutrophils.

B,C: Atypical squamous cells are characterized by smudgy nuclei with a low nuclear to cytoplasmic ratio. This should not be overinterpreted as squamous cell carcinoma. (See fig. 4-13 for corresponding histology of the resection specimen.)

such inflamed cysts or underdiagnose metastatic cystic squamous cell carcinoma (33).

The cysts are usually uniloculated and lined by squamous epithelium. The benign lymphoid cell component in the cyst wall may include the presence of germinal centers (fig. 4-11). The cyst lining epithelium is predominantly stratified squamous epithelium (90 percent of cases) (fig. 4-12); less frequently, a purely columnar epithelial lining or a mixed lining is seen. The cyst wall typically contains a nodular or diffuse lymphoid infiltrate in over 95 percent of cases, with identifiable subcapsular and medullary sinuses.

In inflamed cysts, acute and chronic inflammation as well as fibrosis and granulation tissue may be prominent and even replace the surface epithelium in cases associated with repeated infections. In addition, cytologic atypia may be present (fig. 4-13). Ruptured cysts may include the presence of a foreign body giant cell reaction.

Fistulas often are composed of stratified squamous epithelium associated with the external segments and columnar epithelium with the internal segments. There is no evidence of thymic (thymic cyst) or thyroid (thyroglossal duct cyst) tissue.

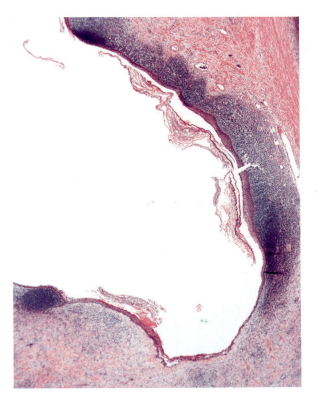 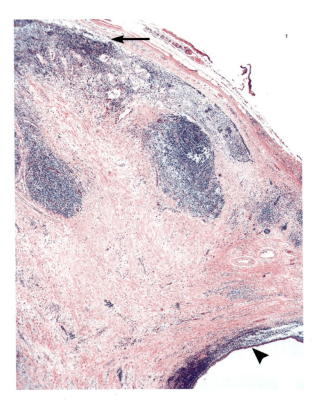

Figure 4-11

BRANCHIAL CLEFT CYST

Left: At low magnification, the branchial cleft cyst is unilocular, lined by squamous epithelium, and contains diffuse and nodular lymphoid tissue in the cyst wall.

Right: The branchial cleft cyst is lined by squamous epithelium (arrowhead) with a nodular and diffuse lymphoid infiltrate in the cyst wall that may also include identifiable subcapsular sinuses (arrow).

By immunohistochemical staining, branchial cleft cysts are reactive for cytokeratins and p63. Typically, they are p16 negative (figs. 4-12, 4-13). They can, however, exhibit focal strong p16 reactivity limited to the superficial squamous epithelium (fig. 4-14) as well as in glandular epithelium (34). p16 may be overexpressed in almost 50 percent of benign branchial cleft cysts, limiting its diagnostic utility in this setting. Molecular testing (in situ hybridization, polymerase chain reaction [PCR]) is then necessary to confirm presence of high-risk human papillomavirus (HPV) and the malignant nature of the cyst. The absence of p16 helps distinguish branchial cleft cyst from oropharyngeal nonkeratinizing squamous cell carcinoma, but it is not as useful in cases of keratinizing squamous cell carcinoma, as the latter are typically p16 negative. Branchial cleft cysts typically have a low proliferation rate (less than 5 percent) by Ki-67 (MIB1) staining compared to metastatic carcinomas. Branchial cleft cysts are negative for thyroglobulin, thyroid transcription factor 1 (TTF1), and PAX8.

Differential Diagnosis. The differential diagnosis of second BAs includes thyroglossal duct cyst, thymic cyst, metastatic cystic squamous cell carcinoma, and metastatic papillary thyroid carcinoma. See below for a discussion of thyroglossal duct cyst and thymic cyst.

The most important entity to differentiate from a branchial cleft cyst is metastatic cystic squamous cell carcinoma (HPV-associated and non-HPV-associated). In general, in fine needle aspiration biopsies, there is greater cellularity in metastatic cystic squamous cell carcinoma than in a branchial cleft cyst, and the cellular component tends to have a greater degree of nuclear atypia, including hyperchromatic and pleomorphic

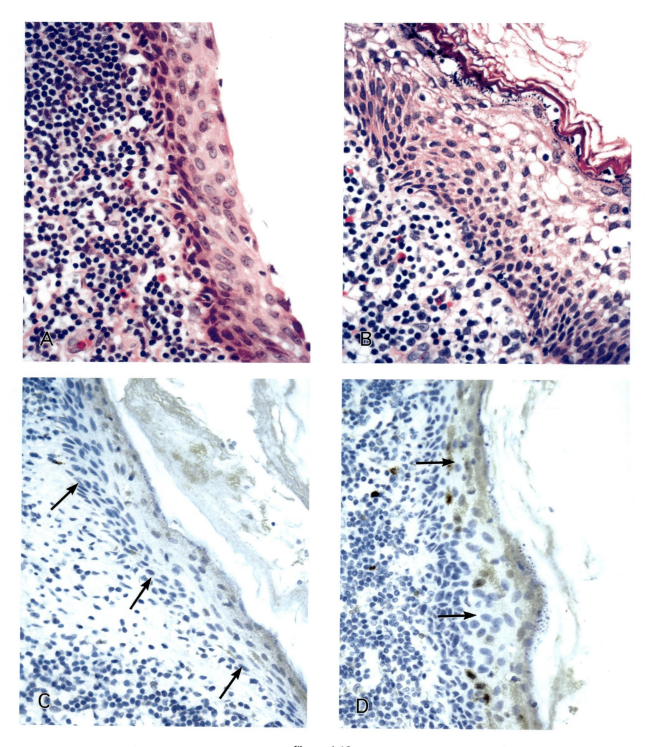

Figure 4-12

BRANCHIAL CLEFT CYST

A,B: The benign squamous epithelium lacks surface keratosis (A) or includes surface keratosis (B).

C,D: Typically, branchial cleft cysts are p16 negative (arrows) whether without surface keratosis (C) or with surface keratosis (D).

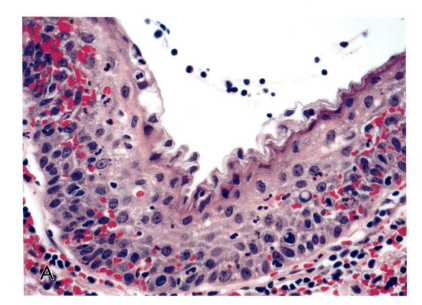

Figure 4-13

INFLAMED BRANCHIAL CLEFT CYST

A: Squamous epithelium with associated acute and chronic inflammation, and reactive epithelial cells including enlarged and hyperchromatic nuclei.

B: Atypical squamous cells include detached atypical cells (arrow).

C: Patchy p16 staining is present; such staining is negative lacking diffuse and strong reactivity in more than 70 percent of the cells.

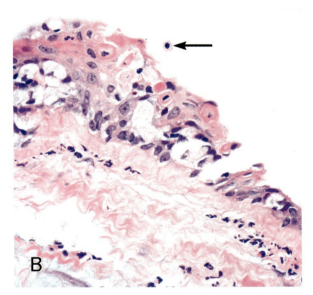

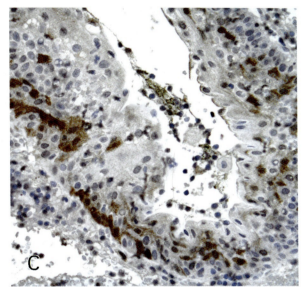

nuclei, increased nuclear to cytoplasmic ratio, and irregular nuclear membranes (fig. 4-15).

In cystic nonkeratinizing carcinoma, there is an immature cellular element characterized by an absence of keratinization and high nuclear to cytoplasmic ratio (figs. 4-16, 4-17). Necrotic debris is also present in metastatic cystic keratinizing squamous cell carcinoma. Overall, a diagnosis of carcinoma is aided by the presence of increased cellularity, with a greater degree of cytologic atypia, increased immature atypical nonkeratinized cells, and necrotic debris. Some examples of cystic metastatic squamous cell carcinoma, however, are composed of bland cytomorphologic features, but even in such cases, there are usually foci of cytologically atypical/malignant epithelial cells characterized by pleomorphic nuclei and increased mitotic activity, as well as an increased proliferation rate as determined by Ki-67 (MIB1) staining. Further, diffuse and strong (nuclear and cytoplasmic) p16 immunoreactivity may be present (figs. 4-16, 4-17).

The presence of p16 immunoreactivity represents a surrogate marker for HPV16 and confirms the diagnosis of metastatic cystic HPV-associated (nonkeratinizing) carcinoma

Non-Neoplastic Diseases of the Head and Neck

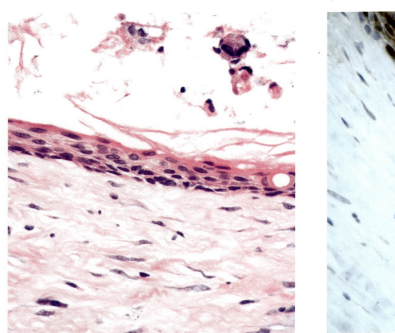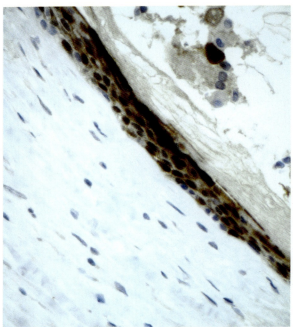

Figure 4-14

BRANCHIAL CLEFT CYST

Left: This branchial cyst is lined by typical benign squamous epithelium.
Right: Unlike most branchial cleft cysts, there is diffuse and strong p16 immunoreactivity, especially in the superficial squamous epithelium. p16 may be overexpressed in almost 50 percent of benign branchial cleft cysts. In such an occurrence, molecular testing (in situ hybridization, polymerase chain reaction [PCR]) is negative despite the p16 immunoreactivity.

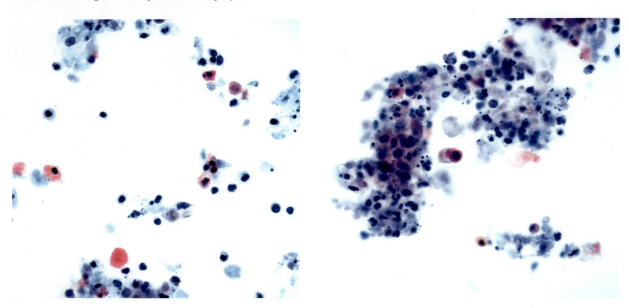

Figure 4-15

METASTATIC CYSTIC SQUAMOUS CELL CARCINOMA

Left, right: Fine-needle aspiration shows the presence of nuclear atypia, including hyperchromatic and pleomorphic nuclei, increased nuclear to cytoplasmic ratio, irregular nuclear membranes, and associated necrotic debris.

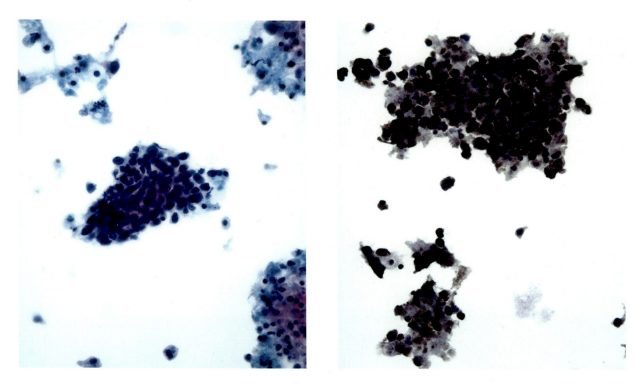

Figure 4-16

METASTATIC CYSTIC NONKERATINIZING CARCINOMA

Left: Fine-needle aspiration shows clusters of immature cells lacking keratinization and characterized by marked cytologic atypia and associated necrotic debris.

Right: The neoplastic cells are diffusely and strongly p16 immunoreactive, supporting origin from the oropharynx (i.e., tonsil or base of tongue).

of oropharyngeal origin (i.e., tonsil, base of tongue), assisting in differentiating it from a branchial cleft cyst, which should be nonreactive for p16 (34,35). As previously noted, branchial cleft cysts can exhibit focal strong p16 reactivity limited to the superficial squamous epithelium (and glandular epithelium) (34). p16 may be overexpressed in almost 50 percent of benign branchial cleft cysts. In such cases, molecular analysis, evaluating for the presence of high-risk, transcriptionally active virus, is necessary to differentiate metastatic carcinoma (HPV positive) from branchial cleft cyst (HPV negative), confirm the presence of HPV, and confirm the malignant nature of the cyst. The absence of p16 helps distinguish branchial cleft cyst from oropharyngeal nonkeratinizing squamous cell carcinoma but is not as useful in cases of keratinizing squamous cell carcinoma since the latter are typically p16 negative.

Confusion and controversy exist concerning the diagnosis of metastatic cystic squamous cell carcinoma and carcinoma arising in a branchial cleft cyst (so-called branchial cleft carcinoma or branchiogenic carcinoma). The criteria for the diagnosis of a branchiogenic carcinoma, as set forth by Martin et al. (36), include: 1) the tumor occurs along the line extending from a point anterior to the tragus along the anterior border of the sternocleidomastoid muscle to the clavicle; 2) histology supports origin from a branchial cleft-derived structure (i.e., situated in the lateral aspect of the neck); 3) histology supports carcinoma arising in the wall of an epithelial-lined cyst; and 4) a minimum of 5-year follow-up demonstrates no evidence of a primary source for this neoplasm. Despite the fulfillment of these criteria, it is highly unlikely that carcinoma arises in a branchial cleft cyst. Rather, these cystic squamous cell carcinomas

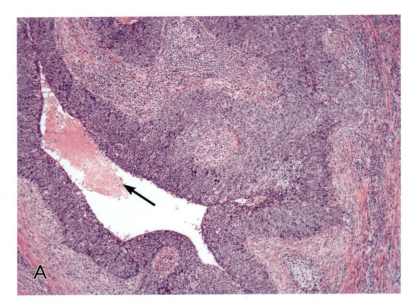

Figure 4-17

METASTATIC CYSTIC NONKERATINIZING (HPV-ASSOCIATED) SQUAMOUS CELL CARCINOMA

A: Resection specimen of a lateral neck mass shows a cystic, epithelial-lined lesion invading the cyst wall and associated intracystic necrotic debris (arrow).

B: At higher magnification, the malignant nature of the neoplastic cells are appreciated, characterized by the presence of immature basaloid cells with marked nuclear pleomorphism and increased mitotic activity.

C: The neoplastic cells are diffusely and strongly p16 immunoreactive, supporting origin from the oropharynx (i.e., tonsil or base of tongue).

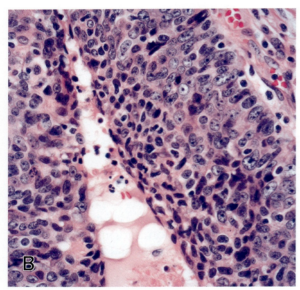

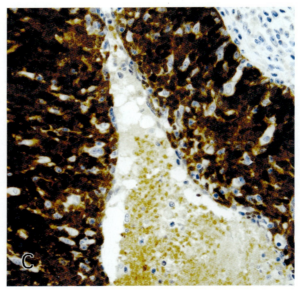

originate in a primary tumor in Waldeyer tonsillar ring (37). The neoplasm may be small (1 to 2 mm), defying clinical or imaging detection, but nevertheless is capable of resulting in large metastatic foci (centimeters). There is partial or complete replacement of the lymph node by an epithelial-lined structure with central cystic change. The epithelium varies from areas that are bland, composed of uniform cells lacking pleomorphism, crowding, or loss of polarity, to overtly malignant-appearing epithelium composed of pleomorphic cells with increased cellularity, mitoses, and a loss of polarity.

Papillary thyroid carcinoma (PTC) may metastasize as a cystic lesion in the lateral neck, suggesting a diagnosis of branchial cleft cyst. Most often, the metastasis originates from the ipsilateral thyroid lobe. Typically, metastatic PTC shows a papillary architecture, the presence of colloid-filled follicles, and diagnostic nuclear alterations. Often, however, the clinical scenario includes the absence of a suspected or known primary thyroid carcinoma that, coupled with the absence of characteristic histologic features, may result in an erroneous diagnosis of branchial cleft cyst. The histology

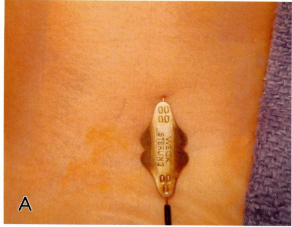
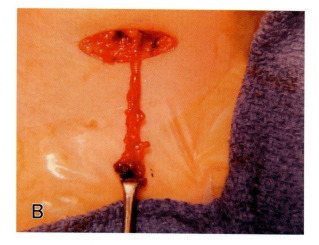
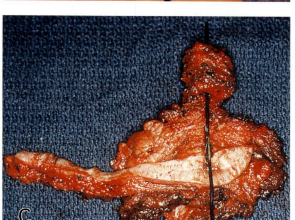

Figure 4-18

BRANCHIAL CLEFT FISTULA

A: A probe-patent fistulous tract from a second branchial cleft cyst opens through the skin in the lower neck.

B. Partially resected fistula tract.

C: Excised fistula tract, including the cutaneous end (lower right). (Courtesy of Dr. M. Persky, New York, NY.)

may include a flattened/attenuated epithelial lining without papillary architecture. Attention to the nuclear details and, perhaps most importantly, immunohistochemical staining, allows for differentiating PTC from branchial cleft cyst. In suspicious cases, thyroglobulin, TTF-1, and PAX8 reactivity are present in metastatic PTC and absent in branchial cleft cysts. Thyroglobulin reactivity is the single best marker for lesions of thyroid follicular epithelial cell origin, including PTC, and is generally absent in all other (nonfollicular epithelial cell origin) lesions, including branchial cleft cysts. TTF1 reactivity is not unique for follicular epithelial-derived lesions of the thyroid gland but can be present in other lesion types including (but not limited to) medullary thyroid carcinoma and pulmonary adenocarcinoma; however, it is absent in branchial cleft cysts. Irrespective of the histologic (nuclear) features, thyroid tissue located in lymph nodes situated lateral to the great neck vessels represents metastatic PTC.

Treatment and Prognosis. Complete surgical excision is the treatment of choice for BAs (38). Fistulas or sinus tracts may extend either toward the skin surface (fig. 4-18) or supratonsillar fossa, between the internal and external carotid arteries. Depending on the extent of the fistula tract, a tonsillectomy may be needed. A functional neck dissection may be necessary when branchial remnants are infected (39).

Third Branchial Anomalies

Clinical Features. Third BAs are rare. They present as recurrent neck abscesses associated with stridor or as recurrent episodes of acute suppurative unilateral thyroiditis (40–48). A sinus or fistula opens externally anterior to the lower third of the sternocleidomastoid muscle; if complete, the internal opening of the sinus or fistula

Non-Neoplastic Diseases of the Head and Neck

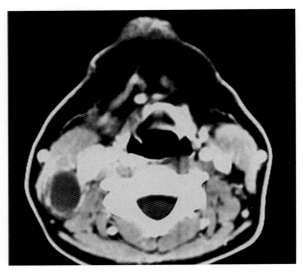

Figure 4-19

THIRD BRANCHIAL CLEFT CYST

Contrast-enhanced axial CT of the neck shows a rim-enhancing cystic lesion in the right juxtathyroid neck; this lesion is deep to the sternocleidomastoid muscle and posterior to the right jugular vein. (Courtesy of Dr. A. Khorsandi, New York, NY.)

is in the piriform sinus, following the passage of the tract along the carotid sheath and penetrating the thyrohyoid membrane cranial to the superior laryngeal nerve (48,49). Cysts occur anywhere along the sinus tract but are most commonly found in the region of the laryngeal ventricle or in the anteroinferior cervical triangle (40).

Contrast enhanced CT findings include the presence of a rounded or ovoid, sharply marginated lesion with central fluid density and a thin cyst wall without significant enhancement (fig. 4-19) (50). The cyst may contain air if it communicates with the pyriform sinus via a patent tract. Infected cysts show an enhancing thickened wall, with the cyst content of higher attenuation than an uninfected cyst. Barium or water-soluble contrast swallow may outline an associated fistula or sinus if present.

Microscopic Findings. The cysts are lined by a stratified squamous epithelium or ciliated epithelium; an associated marked lymphocytic cell infiltrate may be present. Thymic tissue, derived from the third branchial cleft pouch, may or may not be present.

Treatment and Prognosis. Complete surgical resection of a third BA (cyst, sinus, fistula) is the treatment of choice and is necessary in order to prevent recurrence (51–53). The surgical procedure may require a subtotal thyroidectomy.

Fourth Branchial Anomalies

Clinical Features. Fourth BAs are extremely rare. The clinical manifestations are similar to those of third BAs, including recurrent neck abscesses or recurrent episodes of acute suppurative unilateral thyroiditis (46,54–60). Almost all fourth BAs are sinuses that usually originate from the piriform sinus (60). Most patients present prior to the age of 20 years. Rarely, the clinical presentation includes stridor (61).

The sinus tract usually has an internal opening at the apex of the piriform sinus, caudal to the superior laryngeal nerve, then descends translaryngeally beneath the thyroid cartilage, exiting the larynx near the cricothyroid joint below the inferior constrictor muscle; it then continues superficial to the recurrent laryngeal nerve, ending in the paratracheal region or in the thyroid gland (60). Fourth branchial cleft sinus tracts extend from the piriform sinus caudal (rather than cranial as occurs in a third branchial cleft sinus tract) to the superior laryngeal nerve, exiting the larynx near the cricothyroid joint (60). Like third BAs, fourth BAs may or may not include thymic tissue.

Treatment and Prognosis. Complete surgical resection of a fourth BA is the treatment of choice and is necessary in order to prevent recurrence (62). The surgical procedure may require a subtotal thyroidectomy.

Thyroglossal Duct Cyst

Definition. *Thyroglossal duct cyst* (TGDC) is a persistent and cystic dilatation of the thyroglossal duct in the midline of the neck.

Embryology. The thyroid gland originates as a diverticulum from the floor of the pharynx during the 4th week of gestation (63). The pharyngeal attachment of the thyroid is the foramen cecum, located on the dorsal surface of the tongue immediately posterior to the circumvallate papillae, from where the gland descends into the neck. In its descent, the thyroglossal duct courses anterior to the hyoid bone, then hooks around the anteroinferior border of the hyoid to lie on its posterior surface, prior to descending into its anatomically normal place in the neck

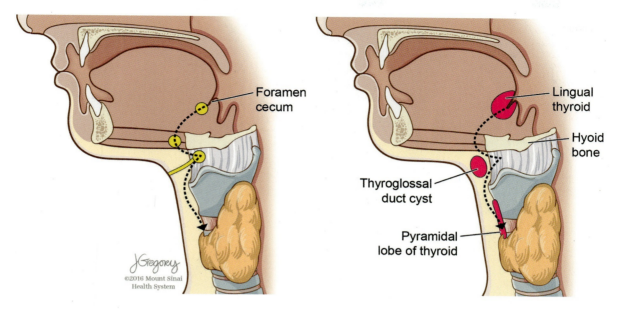

Figure 4-20

NORMAL DESCENT OF THE THYROID GLAND

Left: The thyroid gland descends from the foramen cecum, located at the base of the tongue, in a midline and caudad direction to its final location in the midline anterior aspect of the neck. The broken line indicates the course taken by the thyroglossal duct during its descent with the developing thyroid gland.

Right: Possible locations of ectopic thyroid or thyroglossal duct cysts. Most thyroglossal duct cysts are located just inferior to the hyoid bone. (Courtesy of J. Gregory, Mount Sinai Health System.)

(fig. 4-20) (64). Involution of the thyroglossal duct occurs by the 6th or 7th week of gestation. Failure of the duct to involute, however, may result in cysts, sinuses, or fistulas anywhere along its path of descent into the neck.

The pyramidal lobe of the thyroid gland represents the vestigial remnant of the thyroglossal duct. The pyramidal lobe is present in up to 40 percent of the population (65).

Clinical Features. TGDCs are twice as common as branchial cleft anomalies. There is no gender predilection. TGDCs occur over a wide age range but most patients present before the fourth decade of life (66–68). Approximately 70 percent of cases occur in the midline of the neck above the thyroid isthmus, at or below the level of the hyoid bone (67–70). A minority of cases present in the paramedian neck (68). Approximately 25 percent occur above the hyoid bone (69–71), of which a small percentage (less than 4 percent) are found at the base of the tongue (72,73). TGDCs are nearly always connected to the hyoid bone in the midline neck; uncommonly, they occur lateral to the midline but do not occur in the lateral portion of the neck (i.e., lateral to the jugular vein). Rarely, intrahyoidal TGDCs are identified (74,75).

The clinical presentation of an uninfected thyroglossal duct cyst is usually that of an asymptomatic midline neck mass. The cysts vary from soft to firm, and typically move upward on swallowing. Inflamed or infected TGDCs may be associated with tenderness and pain. In neonates, extrinsic airway compression with apnea, cyanosis, and respiratory compromise may occur (76). In comparison to children, TGDCs in adults more likely present with a complaint other than mass or infection, such as pain, dysphagia, dysphonia, and the manifestation of fistula formation (77).

Radiologic evaluation (e.g., CT, magnetic resonance imaging [MRI], ultrasound) identifies cysts mainly in the infrahyoid region (67,68). TGDCs appear as midline, round or elongated cystic lesions embedded in the infrahyoid strap muscles (fig. 4-21). Expansion or destruction of the cartilaginous structure of the hyoid bone may be seen.

Non-Neoplastic Diseases of the Head and Neck

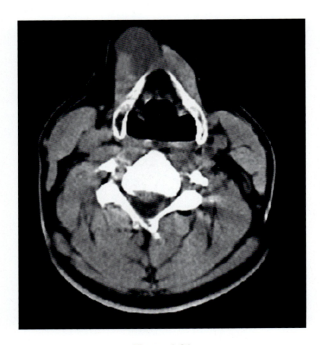

Figure 4-21

THYROGLOSSAL DUCT CYST

Noncontrast axial CT of the neck shows a cystic right paramedian lesion at the level of the thyroid cartilage. (Courtesy of Dr. A. Khorsandi, New York, NY.)

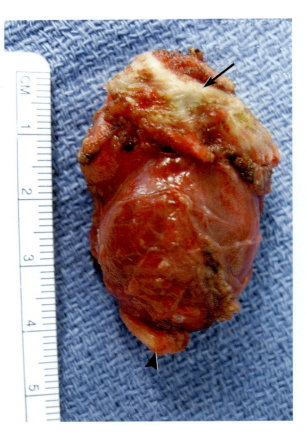

Figure 4-22

THYROGLOSSAL DUCT CYST

The cyst is located in the center of the illustration bordered on its superior aspect by the hyoid bones, appearing as a whitish structure (arrow), and at its inferior aspect by the "tail" of the pyramidal lobe of the thyroid gland (arrowhead). (Courtesy of Dr. M. Persky, New York, NY.)

The location of the cyst is important to the diagnosis. TGDCs at the level of the hyoid bone are found in the midline, abutting the hyoid bone, and may project into the pre-epiglottic space; in the infrahyoid neck, TGDCs are embedded in strap muscles; and above the hyoid bone they occur at the base of tongue or within the posterior floor of the mouth. TGDCs seldom contain enough thyroid follicular epithelial tissue to be seen on scintiscan. The presence of nodular soft tissue excrescences in a midline cystic neck mass on CT scan may suggest the possibility of a papillary carcinoma arising in a TGDC (78). However, radiologic evidence of calcifications (histologically confirmed as psammomatous calcification) can be found in association with a benign TGDC (79). The wall of the cyst may enhance if infected.

Gross Findings. TGDCs are smooth-walled cystic structures that usually measure less than 2 cm (fig. 4-22). The cystic content includes clear mucinous fluid; infected cysts contain purulent material.

Microscopic Findings. In noninflamed TGDCs, the cyst lining is respiratory (columnar) epithelium but may also include squamous epithelium (fig. 4-23). In the presence of inflammation, the cyst lining undergoes metaplastic change and is lined by squamous epithelium. Squamous metaplasia may be focal or, less commonly, extensive. The presence of thyroid tissue in the cyst wall varies and may be dependent on the extent of specimen sampling; nevertheless, thyroid tissue is found in over 60 percent of the cases (fig. 4-23). The absence of thyroid tissue does not exclude the diagnosis. The thyroid tissue may be normal, hyperplastic, and nodular or neoplastic (see below). Further, changes of chronic lymphocytic (Hashimoto) thyroiditis

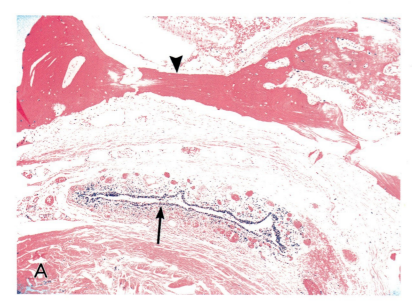
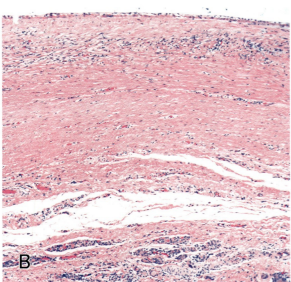
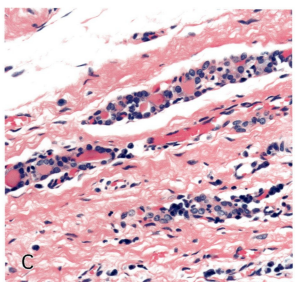

Figure 4-23

THYROGLOSSAL DUCT CYST

A: A cystic epithelial lesion (arrow) is located in proximity to the hyoid bone (arrowhead).

B: An attenuated epithelial-lined cyst (top) with thyroid follicular epithelium is seen deep in the cyst wall (bottom).

C: At higher magnification, the unremarkable colloid-filled thyroid follicles are seen. The presence of thyroid tissue in the cyst wall varies and may be dependent on the extent of specimen sampling. Thyroid tissue is found in over 60 percent of the cases.

may be identified, including nodularity, prominent lymphoplasmacytic cell infiltrate, and follicular cells characterized by the presence of oncocytes with prominent granular eosinophilic cytoplasm (so-called Hürthle cells) (fig. 4-24). Psammomatous calcifications are identified in benign TGDCs (79). Uncommonly, mucous glands are found in the wall. There are reported instances of cartilage (80) and ossification (81) in TGDCs but these findings are rare.

Fine-needle aspiration biopsy (FNAB) can be used as the initial diagnostic modality for TGDCs (82). The smears are low in cellularity, and inflammatory cells are more numerous than epithelial cells. FNAB results in an accurate preoperative diagnosis of TGDC, allowing for a Sistrunk procedure (see below) to be performed on these patients rather than an inappropriate local resection (82).

Although unnecessary for the diagnosis, immunohistochemical staining shows the thyroid tissue to be reactive for thyroglobulin, TTF1, PAX8, and CD56.

Differential Diagnosis. The differential diagnosis of TGDC includes thymic cyst, laryngocele, branchial cleft cysts, and metastatic (cystic)

Figure 4-24

THYROGLOSSAL DUCT CYST

A: Chronic lymphocytic (Hashimoto-type) thyroiditis is associated with thyroid follicular epithelium. An epithelial-lined cyst (top) containing colloid-filled follicles in its wall (bottom) is characterized by nodularity and the presence of a prominent lymphocytic cell infiltrate including lymphoid follicles and germinal centers.

B,C: Thyroid follicles are associated with a prominent lymphoplasmacytic cell infiltrate characterized by cells with prominent granular eosinophilic cytoplasm (oncocytes or so-called Hürthle cells).

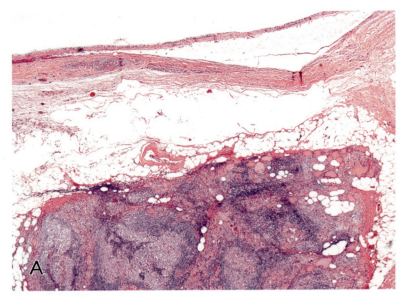
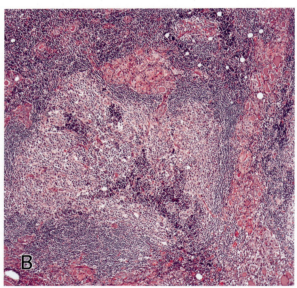
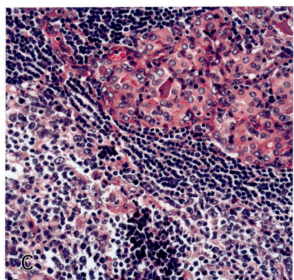

papillary thyroid carcinoma. The nuclear characteristics of the thyroid tissue in a TGDC lack the constellation of features associated with papillary thyroid carcinoma. The presence of extensive squamous metaplasia may raise concern for squamous cell carcinoma (83), but metaplastic foci are typically bland-appearing and lack the cytomorphologic features of carcinoma

Treatment and Prognosis. Surgery is the treatment of choice (67,84). The surgical procedure, referred to as the Sistrunk procedure, includes en bloc surgical resection of the cyst, the middle third of the hyoid bone (Sistrunk procedure), and the suprahyoid tract up to the foramen cecum. The Sistrunk procedure carries low rates of complications (less than 10 percent) and recurrence (less than 2 percent) (66,67,84–88). Although the Sistrunk procedure has a very high success rate, occasional patients have recurrent disease despite a competently performed operation (89). For such patients, extending the Sistrunk operation with an anterior wide local excision is recommended (89,90). If the middle third of the hyoid bone is not removed, the recurrence rate is 25 percent or more (70,88). Complications include recurrence, rupture, infection, undesirable scar, and fistula (cutaneous involvement) (85,91,92).

Neoplasms in TGDCs. Benign and malignant neoplasms may occur in the setting of a TGDC. Benign tumors include follicular adenoma (93). The development of a carcinoma in a TGDC is rare (94–98). Most carcinomas that develop in this setting are the classic type of PTC (approximately 90 percent), with rare examples of follicular variant and tall cell variant of PTC, follicular carcinoma, squamous (epidermoid) carcinoma, mucoepidermoid carcinoma, adenosquamous carcinoma, or anaplastic carcinoma (66,93,99–108). In the presence of adequate sampling and characteristic nuclear features, the diagnosis of PTC in TGDC can be established by preoperative FNAB (109). Squamous and adenosquamous carcinomas probably arise from the cyst lining rather than from the thyroid cell component.

PTC arising in a TGDC occurs more commonly in women than men, occurs over a wide age range (first to eighth decades of life), is predominantly of the classic (usual) morphologic type although variants (e.g., follicular variant, tall cell variant) may be identified, has a similar (excellent) prognosis to that of PTC, and may recur or metastasize (to cervical neck lymph nodes) but rarely is lethal (93,98,103,106,110,111). In the presence of PTC arising in a TGDC, detailed clinical evaluation of the thyroid gland proper is indicated. Ten to 15 percent of patients with TGDCs have a coexisting carcinoma in the normally situated thyroid gland (103,106,112), often representing incidental papillary microcarcinoma (fig. 4-25). There is no clear consensus regarding optimal management for PTC arising in a TGDC, but may include Sistrunk procedure alone; Sistrunk procedure with total thyroidectomy (fig. 4-26); and Sistrunk procedure with total thyroidectomy and neck dissection. C-cell–related thyroid lesions, such as medullary thyroid carcinoma, do not occur in TGDCs due to the different embryologic derivation of the C cells.

Cervical Thymic Cyst

Definition. *Cervical thymic cyst* is cervical thymic tissue sequestered from the main thymic gland during its embryologic descent. The sequestered thymic tissue may be solid (so-called accessory cervical thymic tissue) or cystic (cervical thymic cyst) (113).

Embryology. The thymus develops in the 6th week of gestation, arising primarily from the third branchial pouch (mesoderm) (63). The fourth branchial pouch provides minimal contribution to the development of the thymus (113). The thymic primordia descend in the neck along the course of the carotid sheath. Connection of the paired primordia to the pharynx is retained by the thymopharyngeal ducts. During the 8th week of gestation, the thymic primordia fuse in the midline of the neck and then descend into the mediastinum. Failure of descent or failure to involute results in thymic abnormalities, including cervical thymic cyst. Cervical thymic cysts are considered to be congenital while mediastinal thymic cysts are felt to be acquired.

Clinical Features. Cervical thymic cysts are uncommon. They occur slightly more often in men; most (67 percent) occur during the first decade of life, with the rest occurring in the second through third decades (114–117). Rarely, cervical thymic cysts occur in adults (118).

Cervical thymic cysts are found anywhere between the angle of the mandible and the sternum, including the lateral and midline neck. Most patients present with a slow-growing, painless neck mass that may transiently increase in size during a Valsalva movement; uncommonly, the clinical presentation includes dyspnea, dysphagia, hoarseness, and pain. Cervical thymic cysts are rarely (if ever) associated with a sinus or fistula.

The cervical thymic cyst may represent an isolated cystic lesion in the neck, may extend into the mediastinum, or may be in continuity with an intrathoracic thymus gland. Connections to intrathoracic structures result in abnormal radiologic findings. The appearance of a cervical thymic cyst on CT is characteristic and consists of a nonenhancing cystic mass in the lateral infrahyoid neck, in the lateral visceral space, or adjacent to the carotid space (119). The course of the descent of embryologic thymic tissue in the neck to the mediastinum indicates the potential site of deposition of an ectopic cervical thymic cyst. In a child, a cystic lesion that has an intimate relationship to the carotid sheath is likely to be a thymic cyst (120).

Gross Findings. The cysts are unilocular or multilocular, usually contain clear, serous fluid, and measure up to 15 cm in greatest dimension

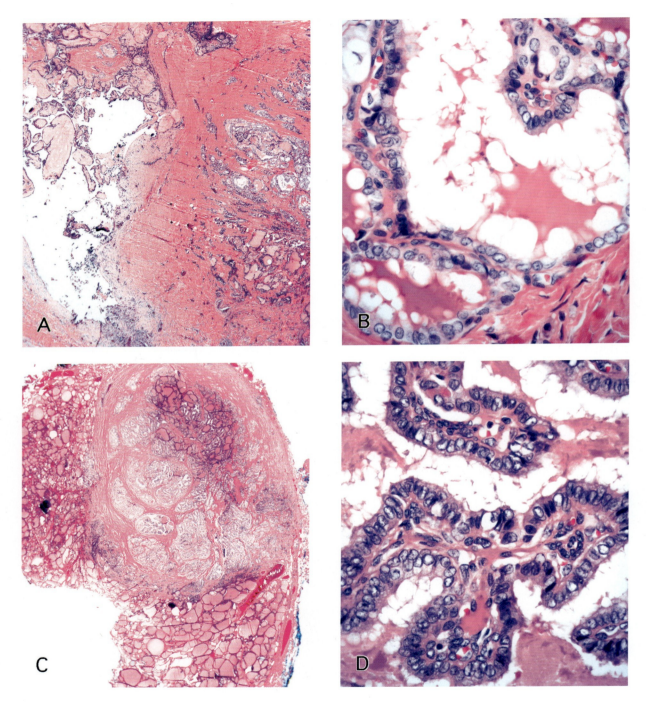

Figure 4-25

PAPILLARY THYROID CARCINOMA, CLASSIC TYPE ARISING IN A THYROGLOSSAL DUCT CYST WITH CONCURRENT PAPILLARY THYROID MICROCARCINOMA

A: Low magnification of a midline neck cyst in a papillary carcinoma in the thyroid gland proper shows an infiltrative neoplasm with papillary architecture.

B: At higher magnification, the diagnostic nuclear features of papillary thyroid carcinoma are present.

C,D: The resected thyroid gland (see fig. 4-26) shows a papillary thyroid microcarcinoma (C) that has diagnostic nuclear features (D).

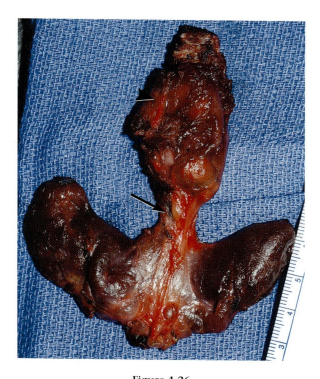

Figure 4-26

SISTRUNK PROCEDURE

A thyroglossal duct cyst (arrowhead) connected by an intact pyramidal lobe of the thyroid gland (arrow) was excised by the Sistrunk procedure, with total thyroidectomy (bottom of image). Both the thyroglossal duct cyst and the thyroid gland had foci of papillary thyroid carcinoma (see fig. 4-25). (Courtesy of Dr. M. Urken, New York, NY.)

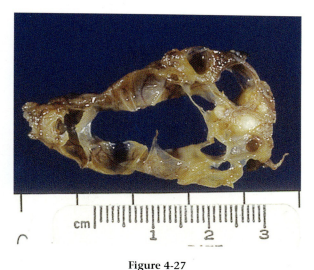

Figure 4-27

THYMIC CYST

The multilocular cyst has smooth walls and focal solid areas.

(fig. 4-27). The lining of the cyst wall is smooth or trabeculated; the cyst wall varies in thickness.

Microscopic Findings. The cyst wall is lined by cuboidal, columnar, or squamous epithelium, and by definition, the wall contains thymic tissue, including characteristic epithelial islands referred to as Hassall corpuscles, as well as lymphoid follicles (figs. 4-28, 4-29). Hassall corpuscles, the most readily identifiable histologic feature of thymic tissue (normally restricted to the thymic medulla), are characterized by keratinized epithelial (granular) cells with a concentric pattern of keratinization (fig. 4-30). The identification of thymic tissue may require extensive sampling. When cysts become infected, the surface epithelium may be replaced by fibrous tissue. Secondary alterations include the presence of foreign body giant cell reaction or cholesterol granulomas (fig. 4-30). Because the third and fourth branchial pouches give rise to the inferior and superior parathyroid glands, respectively, parathyroid parenchyma may be found in thymic cysts.

Differential Diagnosis. The primary differential diagnostic consideration is a branchial cleft cyst. Clinical and histopathologic differences should differentiate these lesions. Both cervical thymic cyst and branchial cleft cyst tend to occur in the anterior cervical triangle. In contrast to cervical thymic cysts, which typically occur in the first decade of life, have a slight female predilection, generally are not associated with sinuses or fistulas, and have thymic tissue in their walls, the branchial cleft cysts tend to occur in the third decade of life, have equal gender predilection, commonly are associated with cysts and fistulas, and have lymphoid tissue in their wall.

Treatment and Prognosis. The treatment for cervical thymic cyst is simple surgical excision, which is curative. Cervical thymic cysts have no potential to undergo malignant transformation, which is not true of mediastinal thymic cysts.

Bronchogenic Cysts

Definition. *Bronchogenic cysts,* also termed *bronchial cysts*, originate from buds or diverticula that separate from the foregut during the formation of the tracheobronchial tree (121). Bronchogenic cysts are generally extrapulmonary: most are found in the mediastinum and

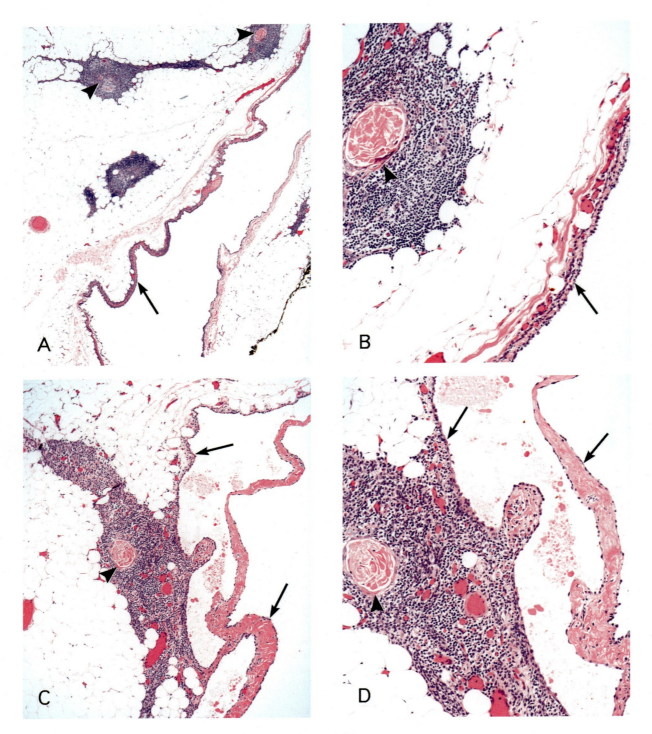

Figure 4-28

CERVICAL THYMIC CYST

A,B: A unilocular epithelial-lined cyst (arrows) has scattered clusters of lymphoid cells within the cyst wall including identifiable Hassall corpuscles (arrowheads).

C,D: A multilocular epithelial-lined cyst (arrows) has scattered clusters of lymphoid cells within the cyst wall including identifiable Hassall corpuscles (arrowheads).

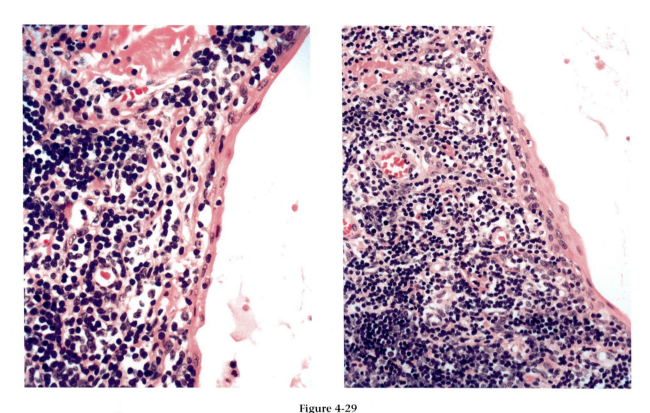

Figure 4-29

THYMIC CYST

Left, right: The epithelial lining of thymic cysts vary and include cuboidal epithelium (left) or squamous epithelium (right).

are referred to as *mediastinal bronchogenic cysts* (122,123). Only rarely do they occur in the lung (124). Bronchogenic cysts may occur outside the thoracic cavity as well, and almost invariably are found in the skin or subcutaneous tissue (125), representing the most common site of occurrence (referred to as *cutaneous bronchogenic cysts*); in the cervical neck particularly near the suprasternal notch (manubrium sterni); and much less often in the lower neck or shoulder (121,126–128).

Clinical Features. Bronchogenic cysts occur over a wide age range, from birth to the sixth decade of life. For mediastinal bronchogenic cysts, the average age of occurrence is in the third and fourth decades (122,123,129). Cutaneous bronchogenic cysts are usually discovered at or soon after birth (121). Bronchogenic cysts occur in both genders equally, although a male predilection is reported for cutaneous bronchogenic cysts (125). In the very young, mediastinal bronchogenic cysts may produce life-threatening respiratory distress, with stridor and airway obstruction (123,130–132). In adults, medistinal bronchogenic cysts are usually asymptomatic and identified by routine chest X rays. Cutaneous bronchogenic cysts appear as asymptomatic nodules that are almost never recognized as such clinically but are often mistaken for cystic hygromas (lymphangiomas), epidermoid cysts, branchial cleft cysts, dermoid cysts, teratomas, and thyroglossal duct cysts (121,133).

Radiographically, the mediastinal bronchogenic cyst is a solitary, smooth, round to ovoid cyst in the mediastinum (middle, posterior, or superior), closely associated with the trachea or major bronchi. An occasional example may be found within the wall of the bronchus (134), trachea (132,135), or esophagus (136), attached to the pericardium or even within the outflow tract of the right ventricle or the interatrial septum (132,137,138). Rare examples have

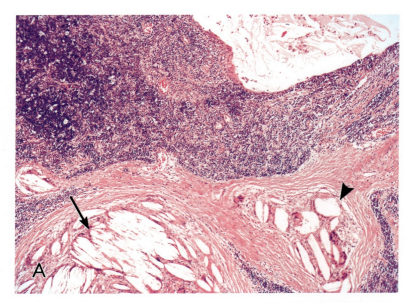

Figure 4-30

THYMIC CYST

A: Secondary alterations in thymic cysts often include the presence of cholesterol granulomas (arrow) and a foreign body giant cell reaction (arrowhead).

B: The most readily identifiable histologic feature of thymic tissue is the Hassall corpuscle (arrow).

C: Hassall corpuscles are keratinized epithelial (granular) cells with a concentric pattern of keratinization.

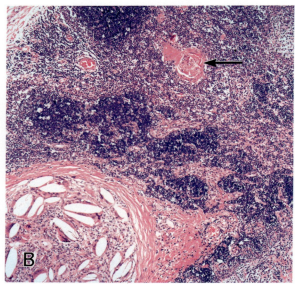
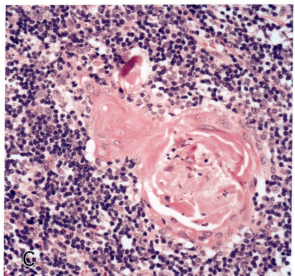

been reported in the pharyngeal region (139) or lateral neck (140,141).

Gross Findings. The cysts are typically unilocular and thin-walled, and measure up to 15 cm in greatest dimension. They have a smooth lining that on occasion may be trabeculated; the cyst content varies from serous to serosanguinous to mucoid, and if infected, purulent content.

Microscopic Findings. The cyst lining usually is ciliated respiratory epithelium, with glands within its walls (fig. 4-31) (bronchial type glands in mediastinal cysts and seromucous glands in cutaneous cysts). Cartilage (fig. 4-31) and smooth muscle are usually present. Cartilage is much less commonly found in the wall of cutaneous bronchogenic cysts (125). Squamous metaplasia of the surface epithelium may be identified.

Differential Diagnosis. The differential diagnosis includes branchial cleft cyst, thyroglossal duct cyst (TGDC), dermoid cyst, and teratoma. The presence of (sero)mucous glands, cartilage, and smooth muscle in bronchogenic cyst allows differentiation from a branchial cleft cyst and TGDC in which these components are not found. The presence of thyroid follicles in a TGDC helps differentiate it from a bronchogenic

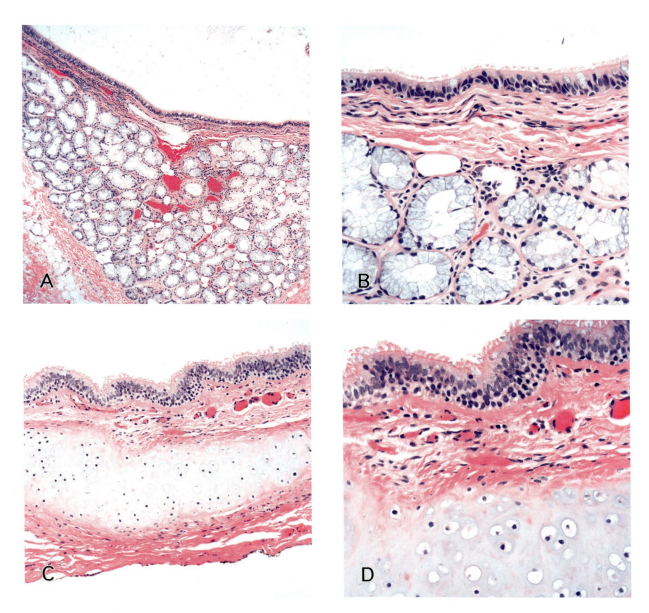

Figure 4-31

BRONCHOGENIC CYST

A,B: A lower neck cystic lesion is lined by ciliated respiratory epithelium with bronchial (mucous) glands in the wall of the cyst.

C,D: The cyst wall also contains cartilage.

cyst. The absence of hair and relative absence of squamous epithelium in bronchogenic cyst differentiates it from a dermoid cyst. Teratomas contain an array of tissue types that are not present in bronchogenic cysts.

Treatment and Prognosis. Excision of the cyst via an external approach generally is curative. Malignant transformation of a mediastinal bronchogenic cyst has not been described, although carcinomas (adenocarcinoma, squamous cell carcinoma, anaplastic carcinoma) have been reported in pulmonary or retrobronchogenic cysts (142–146). Rare examples of congenital anomalies are associated with mediastinal

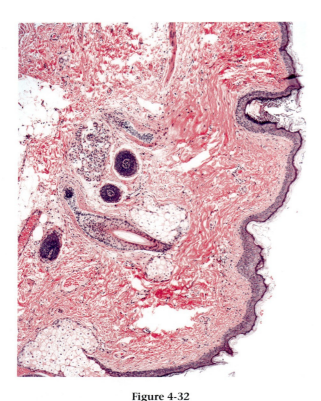

Figure 4-32

DERMOID CYST

The cyst is lined by keratinizing stratified squamous epithelium (right). Cutaneous adnexal structures include sebaceous glands, hair follicles, and eccrine glands in the fibroconnective tissue wall. The adnexal structures are features not found in epidermoid cysts.

bronchogenic cyst but typically these lesions are not associated with developmental anomalies.

Dermoid Cyst

Definition. *Dermoid cyst* is a benign developmental cystic anomaly originating from ectoderm and mesoderm but not endoderm.

Clinical Features. The head and neck area is a fairly common site of occurrence, accounting for approximately 34 percent of all dermoid cysts (147,148). There is an equal gender predilection. Dermoid cysts occur over a wide age range, but are most common in the first decade of life (147,149).

In the head and neck, dermoid cysts are subcutaneous lesions. Common sites of occurrence in the head and neck include orbit, oral cavity, and nasal cavity; less common sites include the mandible, maxilla, middle ear, neck (midline or near midline), upper neck, and near the thyroid cartilage (150,151) or associated with the thyroid gland, suggesting a thyroid nodule (152). Dermoid cysts are slow-growing lesions not associated with pain.

Gross Findings. The lesions are thin-walled cysts containing gray-white friable material. They range in size from a few millimeters to 12 cm in greatest dimension. The internal aspect has a smooth lining.

Microscopic Findings. Dermoid cysts are lined by stratified squamous epithelium with cutaneous adnexal structures (e.g., hair shafts, sebaceous glands, eccrine glands, or apocrine glands) in the fibroconnective tissue wall (fig. 4-32). The cyst content may include keratin or sebaceous material; dermoid cysts may rupture, resulting in a (florid) foreign body giant cell reaction.

Differential Diagnosis. The differential diagnosis includes an epidermal inclusion cyst. Like dermoid cysts, epidermal inclusion cysts are lined by stratified squamous epithelium and are filled with keratin. In contrast to dermoid cysts, however, epidermal inclusion cysts lack adnexal structures in the cyst wall. Teratomas are true neoplasms comprised of tissues from all three germ layers.

Treatment and Prognosis. Simple surgical excision is the treatment of choice and is curative.

INFECTIOUS DISEASES

Mycobacterial Tuberculosis Infection

Definition. *Mycobacterial tuberculosis infection* is an infectious disease caused by *Mycobacterium*, a microorganism classified in the order Actinomycetales and the family Mycobacteriaceae. Mycobacteria include: *Mycobacterium tuberculosis* and nontuberculous ("atypical") mycobacteria.

Mycobacterium tuberculosis is a strictly aerobic bacillus measuring from 1 to 4 μm in length. Identification of the microorganism requires special stains and is based on the capability of forming stable mycolate complexes with certain aryl methane dyes that resist decolorization by acid alcohol; this is referred to as "acid-fastness." The tubercle bacilli that make up the *M. tuberculosis* complex (MTBC) and are the etiologic agents in human tuberculosis include: *M. tuberculosis, M. bovis, M. bovis* Bacille Calmette-Guèrin

[BCG], *M. caprae, M. pinnipedia, M. africanum, M. microtii,* and *M. canetii*.

Nontuberculous mycobacteria are referred to as mycobacteria other than *M. tuberculosis* (MOTT) and represent a group of acid-fast bacilli of which only some are human pathogens. In the immune-competent patient, the nontuberculous mycobacteria do not cause pulmonary disease but often cause localized disease such as lymphadenitis (e.g., scrofula—see below) or a subcutaneous infection. In the immune-compromised patient, these microorganisms cause pneumonia and potentially disseminated (systemic) disease. Some of the nontuberculous mycobacteria include M. *avium-intracellulare, M. scrofulaceum, M. kansasii*, and *M. ulcerans*.

Clinical Features. Mycobacterial infection of the head and neck is uncommon. Overall the incidence of *M. tuberculosis* has decreased over the last five decades, and in a report on extrapulmonary tuberculosis, 12 percent of the patients had mycobacterial infection of the head and neck (153). However, with the advent of the acquired immunodeficiency syndrome (AIDS) associated with immunocompromised conditions, there has been an increased incidence of infection by mycobacteria, especially caused by the nontuberculous mycobacteria (154).

In the head and neck, all sites may be involved but infection primarily involves the cervical lymph nodes, and, much less commonly, tonsils, pharynx, oral cavity, sinonasal region, larynx, salivary glands, external ear, middle ear, and temporal bone (153,155–171). Head and neck involvement may result as a complication of pulmonary involvement (direct infection via expectoration of infected sputum), via hematogenous or lymphatic spread, or as an isolated occurrence as a primary upper aerodigestive tract infection (165,172). *M. tuberculosis* infection may occur in patients with coexisting carcinoma (e.g., squamous cell carcinoma) (170,172,173). Occurrence in association with a Warthin tumor of the parotid gland has also been reported (174).

The symptoms vary according to the site(s) infected. In the cervical lymph nodes, patients present with a neck mass (cervical adenopathy). For mucosal-based disease, patients present with a variety of signs and symptoms that include sore throat, nasal obstruction, mucopurulent rhinorrhea, epistaxis, snoring, hoarseness, dysphagia, odynophagia, serous otitis, hearing loss, tinnitus, and otalgia (171).

The mucocutaneous lesions of secondary tuberculosis, result from hematogenous or lymphatic spread of disease. The nose and cheeks are the most common sites of occurrence. The lesions caused by mycobacteria vary from small papules (e.g., primary inoculation tuberculosis) and warty lesions (e.g., tuberculosis verrucosa cutis) to massive ulcers (e.g., Buruli ulcer) and plaques (e.g., lupus vulgaris) that may be highly deformative/destructive (175). The destructive nature is thought to be due to hypersensitivity to the microorganism in patients with strong immune responses. In approximately 40 percent of patients with lupus vulgaris, there is an association with upper aerodigestive tract lesions and cervical lymphadenitis. Healing may result in scarring and deformity of the involved region.

The clinical workup in suspected cases of tuberculosis includes chest X ray, tuberculin skin test, microbiologic cultures, and molecular diagnostics. The reference ("gold") standard is microbiologic culture for identification on specific media, which allows for testing of drug susceptibility. Depending on the media used, incubation (i.e., growth) takes from 2 to as long as 10 weeks (or longer), potentially resulting in delay in diagnosis and treatment. The media used in the testing for tuberculosis include solid and liquid-based (broth) agents. Solid media include egg-based (Löwenstein-Jensen) and agar-based media (176).

Nonradiometric BACTEC Mycobacteria Growth Indicator Tube 960 (MGIT) has replaced the radiometric BACTEC 460 susceptibility testing system as a liquid-based medium (176). This liquid-based medium is more sensitive and provides more rapid detection of mycobacterial growth (176). In liquid-based media, growth occurs in 1 to 3 weeks, as compared to 3 to 8 weeks for solid media.

The most rapid method for the diagnosis of tuberculosis is the nucleic acid amplification test for the direct detection of MTBC in clinical specimens (e.g., sputum, fluids, and tissue [formalin-fixed paraffin-embedded]). Nucleic acid amplification testing is as sensitive as cultures but requires significantly less time to perform and results take only 4 to 5 hours. It allows for more rapid diagnosis but does not differentiate species in MTBC; however, it can detect as few as 10 organisms in a clinical specimen as compared to the more than 10,000 organisms required for positive identification on smears (176). The available nuclei acid amplification tests include Amplified Mycobacterium Tuberculosis Direct Test (Gen-Probe Inc.) and AMPLICOR Mycobacterium Tuberculosis Test (Roche Diagnostics). The sensitivity of nuclei acid amplification tests generally is slightly lower for nonrespiratory specimens but is useful in the diagnosis of extrapulmonary tuberculosis (176).

Once an isolate is available, drug susceptibility testing is performed. Agar proportion is the standard method of testing susceptibility of MTBC to antituberculosis agents. A liquid-based system allows for quicker turnaround time for results as compared to agar and is recommended. With currently available liquid-based systems, results are available 5 to 7 days after inoculation with the MTBC isolate (176). Molecular methods, including PCR, are developed for the rapid detection of mutations known to be associated with drug resistance including multidrug resistant organisms (MDR-TB) and extensively drug-resistant tuberculosis (XDR-TB) (176).

Microscopic Findings. In the presence of a normal immune status, the main histologic change is caseating (necrotizing) granulomatous inflammation (fig. 4-33). The granulomas are well-formed, surrounded by histiocytes and multinucleated giant cells, and have central areas of necrosis. In up to 25 percent of cases of nontuberculous mycobacterial infections, a caseating granulomatous inflammatory response is not present.

The histochemical identification of microorganisms is often extremely difficult and may defy detection despite an extensive and diligent effort. The identification of microorganisms requires special stains and is based on the capability of forming stable mycolate complexes with certain aryl methane dyes (acid-fastness). Depending on the stain (Acid Fast Bacilli [AFB], Ziehl-Neelsen), the microorganisms appear beaded, red or purple, and are located in necrotic foci and/or within giant cells (fig. 4-33).

In the immune-compromised patient, the typical caseating granulomatous inflammatory response may not be present (fig. 4-34). Rather, diffuse sheets of foamy histiocytes are seen within which numerous AFB-positive microorganisms are identified (fig. 4-34).

Differential Diagnosis. The differential diagnosis includes sarcoidosis (see below) and other infectious necrotizing granulomatous diseases. The latter are rare in head and neck sites and caused by organisms other than *Mycobacterium*. Granulomatosis with polyangiitis (GPA), formerly referred to as Wegener granulomatosis, is characterized by scattered multinucleated giant cells, and while the term "granulomatosis" is applied to this vasculitic-related disease, there is an absence of well-formed granulomas as seen in association with *Mycobacterium* infection.

Treatment and Prognosis. The cornerstone for treatment is multidrug (antituberculous) therapy. First-line drugs include isoniazid, rifampicin, ethambutol, and pyrazinamide (177). The duration of treatment is 6 months, including 2-month intensive therapy with the four drugs and 4-month continued therapy with isoniazid and rifampicin. Second-line drugs include streptomycin, ethionamide, kanamycin, capreomycin, ofloxacin, and rifabutin. Among new cases of tuberculosis, approximately 5 percent worldwide are due to multidrug resistant organisms (MDR-TB), defined as tubercle bacilli resistant to isoniazid and rifampin (177). Mismanagement of drugs used to treat MDR-TB can result in extensive drug-resistant tuberculosis (XDR-TB), defined as MDR-TB plus resistance to any fluoroquinolone and any second-line injectable antituberculosis agent.

Patients with human immunodeficiency (HIV) infection, who have either drug-susceptible or drug-resistant tuberculosis, should receive antiretroviral therapy (ART) while they are receiving treatment for tuberculosis (177). In AIDS patients, therapy for tuberculosis is lifelong. Patients receiving ART and tuberculosis treatment are at high risk for the *immune reconstitution inflammatory syndrome* (IRIS), a sudden systemic inflammation and cytokine storm syndrome resulting from activation of the recovering CD4-positive T cells, often from an unrecognized opportunistic infection (177).

Scrofula

Definition. *Scrofula* is cervical lymph node involvement by mycobacteria. It is also known as *scrofulous gumma*.

Clinical Features. Scrofula is more common in women than men, and may occur over a wide

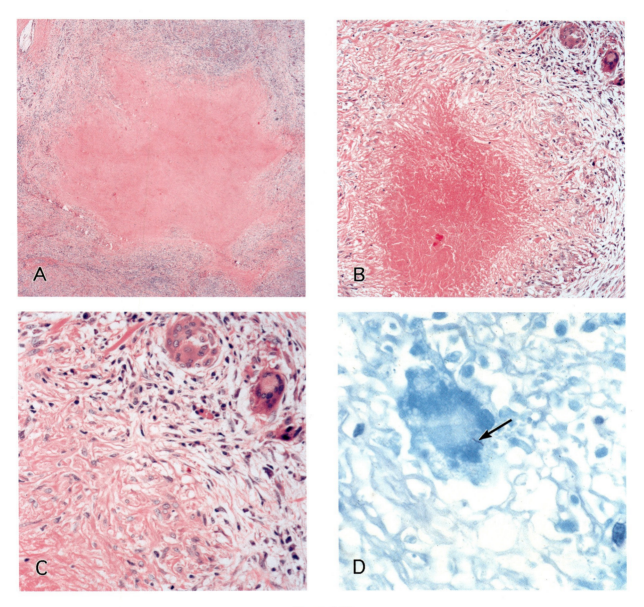

Figure 4-33

MYCOBACTERIAL TUBERCULOSIS INFECTION

A–C: The histologic hallmark of mycobacterial disease in an immune-competent individual includes the presence of (well-formed) caseating (necrotizing) granulomatous inflammation characterized by (central) areas of necrosis surrounded by histiocytes and multinucleated giant cells.

D: Acid-fast bacilli (AFB) staining highlights the microorganism, which appears as a red linear and beaded structure within a multinucleated giant cell (arrow). The microorganisms often are difficult to identify by histochemical staining and may require cultures or molecular analysis for confirmation.

age range but primarily affects children. The high cervical lymph nodes in the region of the submandibular gland are most often affected (fig. 4-35); periparotid, periauricular, and submental lymph nodes may be involved but less often (178).

Scrofula usually presents as a unilateral single or multiple painless lump, mostly located in the posterior cervical or supraclavicular region (179–181); bilateral involvement generally is related to systemic involvement caused by

Non-Neoplastic Diseases of the Head and Neck

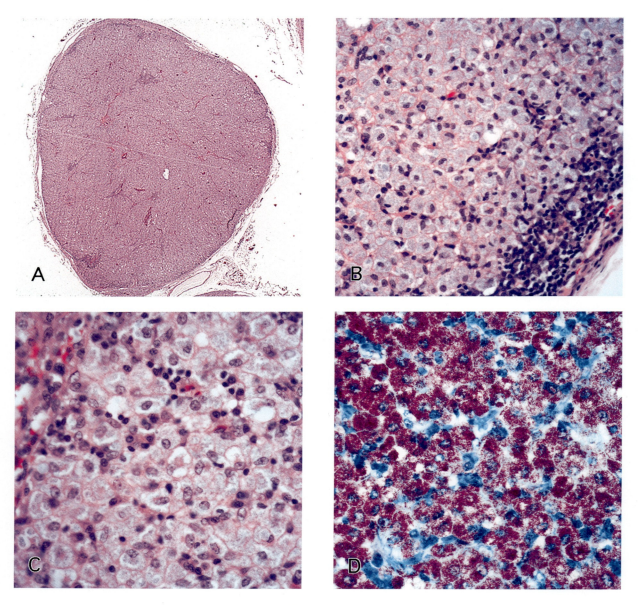

Figure 4-34

ATYPICAL MYCOBACTERIAL INFECTION BY *MYCOBACTERIUM AVIUM-INTRACELLULARE* (MAI) IN CERVICAL NECK LYMPH NODE

A–C: In the immune-compromised patient, well-formed granulomas may not be seen. Instead, the lymph node parenchyma is effaced and replaced by a diffuse proliferation of foamy histiocytes within which numerous.

D: AFB-positive microorganisms are identified

dissemination of *M. tuberculosis*. Patients are afebrile. Scrofula may occur in patients with immune reconstitution inflammatory syndrome (IRIS) (see above) (182). IRIS represents a cohort of HIV-infected patients receiving combined antiretroviral therapy (cART) (177,182).

Radiologic imaging of scrofula of the head and neck is often nonspecific and may be mistaken for carcinoma (183). Tuberculous lymphadenitis is often characterized by areas of low attenuation or low signal intensity, with rim enhancement or calcification (fig. 4-36).

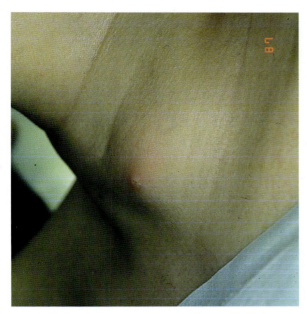

Figure 4-35

MYCOBACTERIAL INVOLVEMENT OF CERVICAL LYMPH NODES (SCROFULA)

Unilateral, firm, red neck mass with focal ulceration of the skin.

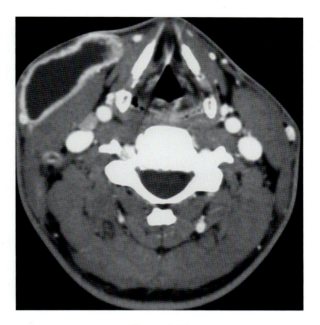

Figure 4-36

SCROFULA

Postcontrast axial image of the neck demonstrates centrally lucent, thick rim-enhancing right-sided lymph nodes showing scattered calcification along the periphery.

Pathogenesis. While the causative microorganism may be *M. tuberculosis*, scrofula is most commonly caused by nontuberculous mycobacteria (*M. scrofulaceum, M. avium-intracellulare, M. kansasii*). Scrofula may be an isolated infection, but it may also be the initial presentation in patients with pulmonary disease. PCR plays a significant role in the identification of the causative infectious agent (i.e., nontuberculous mycobacteria) and in differentiating it from *M. tuberculosis* (184).

Gross Findings. Involved lymph nodes are enlarged and firm. Mucosal involvement appears as granular exudates, with or without associated ulceration; cutaneous ulceration may occur.

Microscopic Findings. Fine-needle aspiration provides a high level of diagnostic accuracy and is reliable as an initial evaluating procedure for the diagnosis of tuberculous lymphadenitis (185,186). Irrespective of the causative microorganism, the histologic picture of mycobacterial infection is the same (i.e., caseating granulomas; see Mycobacterial Tuberculosis Infection).

Differential Diagnosis. The differential diagnosis includes sarcoidosis and cat scratch disease (see later in chapter).

Treatment and Prognosis. Treatment for scrofula caused by nontuberculous mycobacteria is surgical excision, which is considered curative (187). Nontuberculous mycobacteria are nonresponsive to antimycobacterial tuberculosis medications. For infection caused by *M. tuberculosis*, treatment consists of antituberculous chemotherapy.

Mycobacterial Spindle Cell Pseudotumor

Definition. *Mycobacterial spindle cell pseudotumor* is a pseudoneoplastic spindle cell proliferation that almost exclusively occurs in HIV-infected patients. Synonyms include *mycobacterial pseudotumor, M. avium-intracellulare pseudotumor, spindled nontuberculous mycobacteriosis,* and *histioid mycobacteriosis*.

Clinical Features. Mycobacterial spindle cell pseudotumor is an uncommon lesion. There is no gender predilection and it occurs over a wide age range. It is almost always found in immune-compromised individuals due to AIDS/HIV infection or in patients receiving immunosuppressive therapy, including steroids (188–194). Rare occurrence following BCG vaccination has been reported (195). The sites of involvement include the lymph nodes (fig. 4-37), as well as extranodal sites such as skin, spleen, brain, and bone marrow. Rarely, mucosal sites of the upper aerodigestive tract are involved (196–198). The presentation usually includes lymphadenopathy or a subcutaneous firm nodule.

Pathogenesis. The causative microorganism is *M. avium-intracellulare*.

Microscopic Findings. There is a cellular proliferation composed of bland-appearing spindle-shaped cells in a storiform pattern (fig. 4-37). Multinucleated giant cells and foamy histiocytes are not present. Nodal involvement includes partial or complete effacement of the nodal architecture.

Special stains for mycobacteria, including AFB and Ziehl-Neelsen, show the presence of numerous AFB-positive organisms within the cytoplasm of the spindle cells (fig. 4-37). By immunohistochemistry, the spindle cells are CD68, lysozyme, α-antichymotrypsin, and vimentin positive. Based on the CD68 reactivity, the spindle cells represent macrophages. S-100 protein, desmin, and muscle-specific actin may be positive. CD31 and CD34 are negative. PCR assists in identifying the mycobacteria.

Differential Diagnosis. The differential diagnosis includes Kaposi sarcoma, which may occur concomitantly (in same lymph node) as mycobacterial spindle cell tumor (190). Morphologic features that favor Kaposi sarcoma over mycobacterial spindle cell tumor include a prominent fascicular arrangement of spindle cells and slit-like spaces, absence of granular acidophilic cytoplasm, and presence of hyaline globules and mitoses. Further, immunohistochemical features seen in the spindle cells of Kaposi sarcoma include reactivity for human herpesvirus 8 (HHV8), also referred to as Kaposi sarcoma-associated herpesvirus (KSHV), as well as reactivity for CD31 and CD34, and absence of CD68 and S-100 protein. In addition to Kaposi sarcoma, the differential diagnosis may include fibrohistiocytic tumor(s) and Hodgkin disease (nodular sclerosing).

Treatment and Prognosis. Treatment guidelines are based on the species of mycobacteria and susceptibility testing of the isolate that, in some cases, is modified because of the immune status of the patient or other concurrent therapy. If no isolate is obtained, the recommendation is to treat for tuberculosis. The specific drugs chosen depend on the likelihood of drug-resistance based on demographic/epidemiologic factors.

Actinomycosis

Definition. *Actinomycosis* is a chronic granulomatous and suppurative disease caused by Gram-positive, microaerophilic and anaerobic bacteria, the most common isolate being *Actinomyces israelii*. Actinomyces are endogenous saprophytic organisms in the oral cavity and tonsil. They are often seen within the tonsillar crypts as saprophytes, unaccompanied by an inflammatory response.

The disease is classified according to the anatomic site involved and includes cervicofacial, abdominal, and pulmonary sites. The following discussion is limited to cervicofacial actinomycosis.

Clinical Features. *Cervicofacial actinomycosis* is the most common form of disease and is thought to arise secondary to dental manipulation or trauma (199,200). There is no gender predilection and it occurs in all age groups. The neck and area around the angle of the mandible are the most common sites of occurrence; however, clinical infection can occur anywhere in the head and neck (201).

The most common symptom is a painless, slowly enlarging, indurated mass, with or without suppuration (fig. 4-38). The skin overlying the lesion has a characteristic purple color from which a draining sinus may be seen; fistualization is common. A definitive diagnosis is made bacteriologically; the organisms, however, are difficult to culture.

Microscopic Findings. The histology of actinomycotic infection includes a granulomatous reaction with central accumulation of polymorphonuclear leukocytes (abscess formation) and necrosis (fig. 4-39). Within the abscess and enveloped by the neutrophils, microorganism colonies are seen. The microorganisms form a characteristic appearance, referred to as "sulfur granules." Granules are lobular, deep purple, and

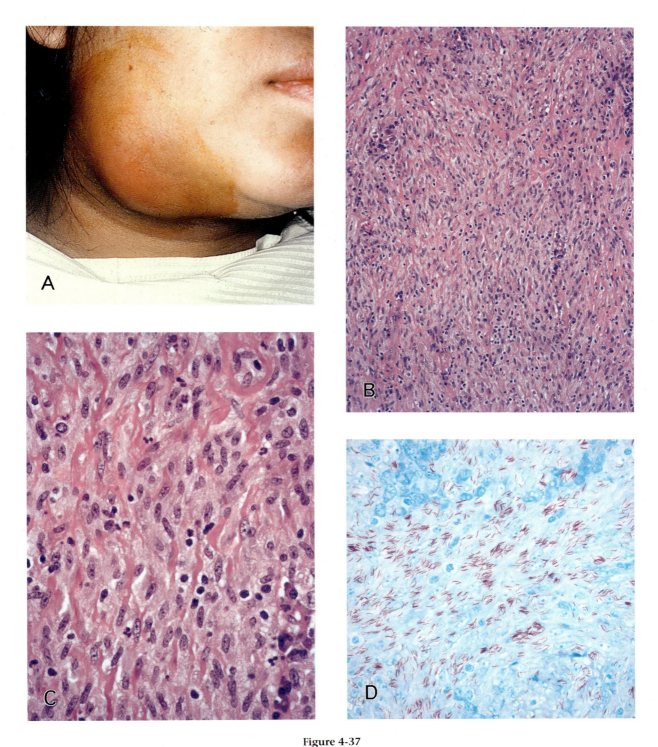

Figure 4-37

MYCOBACTERIAL SPINDLE CELL PSEUDOTUMOR

A: An immunocompromised patient presents with a subcutaneous firm nodule.

B,C: The cellular proliferation is composed of bland-appearing spindle-shaped cells with a storiform pattern; multinucleated giant cells and foamy histiocytes are not present.

D: The AFB stain for mycobacteria shows numerous AFB-positive microorganisms within the cytoplasm of the spindle cells.

Non-Neoplastic Diseases of the Head and Neck

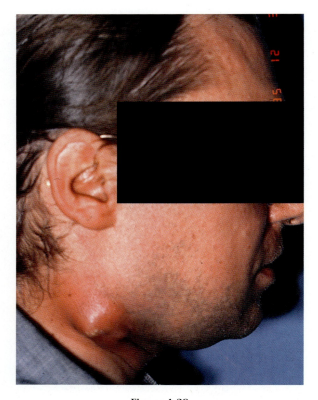

Figure 4-38

CERVICOFACIAL ACTINOMYCOSIS

An indurated, suppurative neck mass is at the angle of the mandible. The skin overlying the lesion is purple.

composed of a central meshwork of filaments that typically have eosinophilic club-shaped ends. Protein often precipitates on the filaments, resulting in thick eosinophilic radiations referred to as the Splendore-Hoeppli phenomenon. The sulfur granules are identified in pus.

A diagnosis of actinomycosis can be made by fine-needle aspiration biopsy (202,203). Smears and cell blocks of the aspirate show the characteristic colonies (sulfur granules) of Actinomyces. The microorganisms stain with Gomori methenamine silver (GMS) and Gram stains (fig. 4-39) and occasionally stain with periodic acid–Schiff (PAS).

Differential Diagnosis. The differential diagnosis includes various infections, including *Nocardia* infection

Treatment and Prognosis. Intravenous penicillin G followed by oral penicillin is the treatment of choice. Patients allergic to penicillin are given tetracycline. In conjunction with antibiotic therapy, surgical excision is advocated, with favorable results (204,205). The prognosis is good if treated early. Acute osteomyelitis of the jaw is the most common complication (fig. 4-40). Once infection reaches bone, tissue destruction may be extensive and involvement of the cranium, meninges, and brain may occur with lethal implications.

Cat Scratch Disease

Definition. *Cat scratch disease* (CSD) is a necrotizing granulomatous lymphadenitis caused by a pleomorphic, Gram-negative bacterium, *Bartonella henselae*, resulting in lymphadenopathy.

Clinical Features. There is no gender predilection and CSD occurs at all ages. The mode of transmission is by direct contact from a cat scratch, bite, or lick through a skin break (206). There is no evidence to support transmission from man to man. The infected cat is not ill and appears to be infectious for only a limited time. In the majority of cases, a history of exposure to a cat can be obtained and the primary inoculation site identified, typically from 7 to 12 days following contact. CSD primarily occurs in immunocompetent individuals but may occur as localized disease in solid organ transplant recipients (207).

The symptoms include enlarged and often tender lymph nodes, with potential involvement of the submental, submandibular, cervical, occipital, and supraclavicular lymph nodes as well as cervical lymph nodes in both the anterior and posterior triangles of the neck (fig. 4-41) (208,209). Obstruction and inflammation may be seen in salivary glands with involved lymph nodes. Atypical head and neck manifestations of CSD including conjunctivitis (Parinaud oculoglandular syndrome), swelling of the parotid gland, and erythema nodosum (209). Constitutional symptoms include low-grade fever, malaise, myalgias, headaches, and weight loss/anorexia (210); less common manifestations/complications include thrombocytopenic purpura, encephalitis/encephalopathy, convulsions, osteomyelitis, retinitis, arthritis, hepatosplenomegaly, pulmonary nodules, and pleurisy (211). A positive skin test confirms the diagnosis (208). Cutaneous lesions appear as a red papule which may become crusted or pustular.

Microscopic Findings. Changes in the affected lymph node vary with time. In early

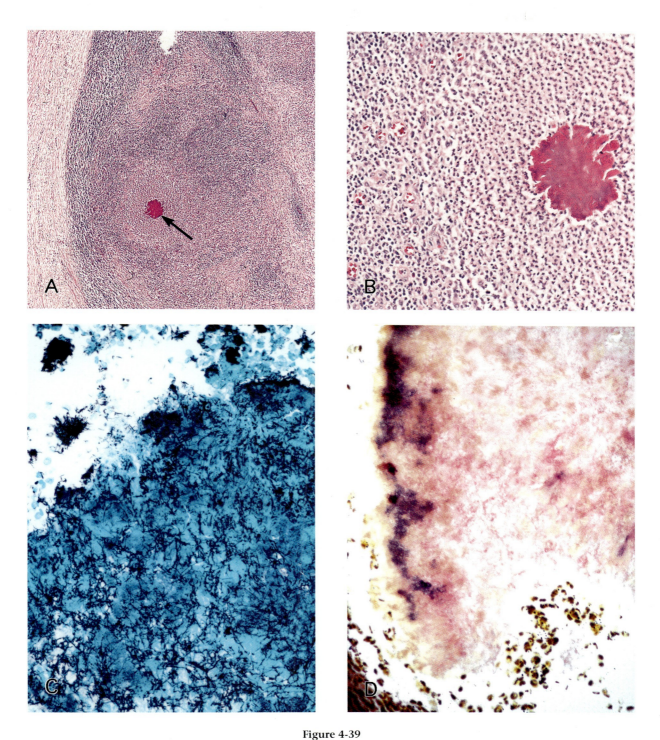

Figure 4-39

CERVICOFACIAL ACTINOMYCOSIS

A: A cervical lymph node has focal abscess formation, within which is the actinomycotic organism (arrow).

B: At higher magnification, the actinomycotic colony has a characteristic appearance, referred to as "sulfur granules"; the granules are lobular, deep purple and composed of a central meshwork of filaments, which typically have thick eosinophilic radiations or club-shaped ends (Splendore-Hoeppli phenomenon).

C,D: The microorganisms stain with the Gomori methenamine silver (GMS) (C) and Gram (D) stains.

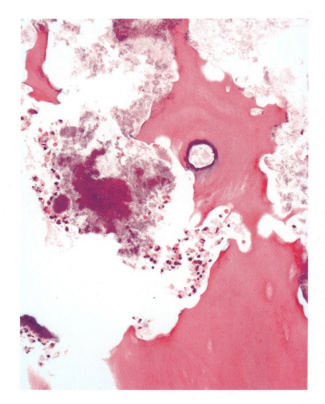

Figure 4-40

CERVICOFACIAL ACTINOMYCOSIS

Acute osteomyelitis is a potential and unfortunately common complication of actinomycotic infection of the jaw.

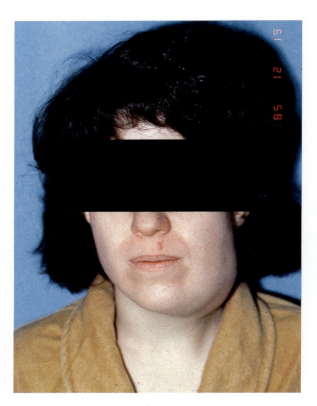

Figure 4-41

CAT SCRATCH DISEASE

This woman presents with enlarged (and tender) left cervical neck lymph nodes.

lesions, follicular hyperplasia and histiocytic proliferations are identified. Intermediate-stage lesions show granulomatous inflammation. In late lesions, abscess formation is present. The appearance of the abscess includes a central area of necrosis with a stellate pattern and an admixture of polymorphonuclear leukocytes surrounded by palisading of histiocytes (fig. 4-42). This pattern is consistently seen and is characteristic of the diagnosis but is not pathognomonic. Nodal sinuses are packed with monocytoid B cells. Skin lesions show necrotic areas within the dermis surrounded by histiocytes.

Cat scratch bacilli can be identified by the Warthin-Starry stain and appear as extracellular pleomorphic coccobacilli (fig. 4-42) (206,212). Staining and culturing for acid-fast microorganisms are negative.

Differential Diagnosis. The primary differential diagnoses include toxoplasmosis and lymphogranuloma venereum.

Treatment and Prognosis. The treatment is supportive and includes analgesics and warm compresses. CSD is usually self-limiting and typically runs its course within a few months. In cases with suppuration, needle aspiration may relieve pain; incision and drainage may produce sinus tract inflammation. Antibiotic therapy appears to be of little benefit (213).

Bacillary Angiomatosis

Definition. *Bacillary angiomatosis* (BA) is a pseudoneoplastic capillary proliferative lesion that occurs as a complication of HIV infection and usually presents as a cutaneous vascular lesion. It is an opportunistic bacterial infection caused by *Rochalimaea* species (*R. henselae*) as well as by *Bartonella quintana*. Synonyms include *epithelioid angiomatosis* and *epithelioid hemangioma-like vascular proliferation*.

Clinical Features. There is no gender predilection. BA occurs over a wide age range. It usually

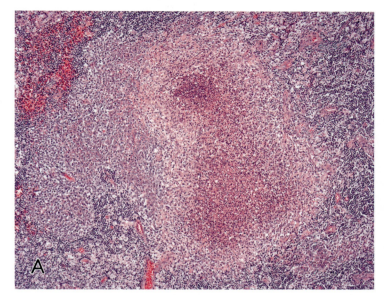

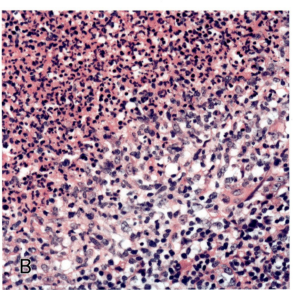
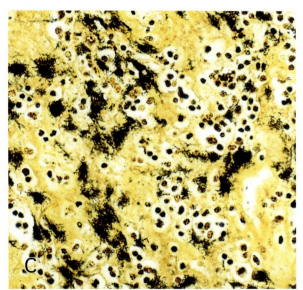

Figure 4-42

NECROTIZING GRANULOMATOUS LYMPHADENITIS

A,B: A central area of necrosis with a stellate pattern and an admixture of polymorphonuclear leukocytes is surrounded by palisading histiocytes. This pattern is consistently seen and is characteristic of the diagnosis but is not pathognomonic.

C: The causative bacterium (*Bartonella henselae*), appearing as extracellular pleomorphic coccobacilli, is identified by the Warthin-Starry stain.

presents as a cutaneous lesion commonly associated with systemic symptoms, including fever, chills, weight loss, and night sweats (214–217). Clinically, the lesions are similar in appearance to lobular capillary hemangioma (pyogenic granuloma) and Kaposi sarcoma, characterized by the presence of multiple erythematous papules with or without crusting. BA may involve other organs sites including lymph nodes, spleen, and liver, as well as mucosal sites of the upper respiratory tract and conjunctiva (218–221).

In addition to its association with HIV and AIDS patients, BA occurs in solid organ transplant recipients (222–224), patients on systemic steroid therapy (225), and patients with Kaposi sarcoma (226–228). In immune-compromised patients coinfection with other opportunistic infections may occur (229). Despite is association with immune-compromised patients, BA has also been reported in (adult and pediatric) immune-competent patients (230–234).

Laboratory studies include conventional microbiologic culturing and molecular techniques, such as PCR (221,235,236). Serologic demonstration of antibodies by direct immunofluorescence and enzyme immunoassay is diagnostic (235).

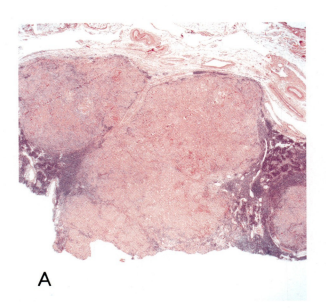 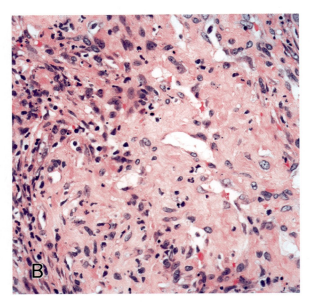

Figure 4-43

BACILLARY ANGIOMATOSIS

A: The lymph node is replaced by circumscribed lobular proliferations.
B: Small capillaries are arranged around ectatic vessels which are lined by prominent endothelial cells.

Proteomic analysis, with identification of immunoreactive antigens, is useful for an improved *Bartonella*-specific serodiagnosis (237).

Gross Findings. The gross features vary widely from cutaneous erythematous papules, to mushroom-shaped papules, and nodules to deep-seated rounded lesions without change in skin color. Exceptionally, BA appears as a mucosal-based, erythematous nodular proliferation.

Microscopic Findings. Regardless of its clinical presentation, the histologic features are the same and include circumscribed nodules of a lobular capillary proliferation with overall features similar to those seen in lobular capillary hemangioma (fig. 4-43). Small capillaries are arranged around ectatic vessels, which are lined by prominent endothelial cells. Cytologic atypia, mitotic figures and necrosis are not usually present but occasionally may be seen. Solid areas may be present and may obscure the vascular proliferation (fig. 4-43). A variable edematous, mucinous, or fibrotic stroma separates the lobular proliferation. An important histologic feature in BA is the presence of neutrophils and neutrophilic debris adjacent to the capillary proliferation, with associated granular clumps (fig. 4-43). In contrast to findings seen in Kaposi sarcoma, BA typically lacks spindled cells, interconnecting vascular channels, or hyaline globules. The overlying epithelium may be ulcerated, thinned, or show pseudoepitheliomatous hyperplasia.

The Warthin-Starry stain shows that the granular material contains bacteria; bacteria are interstitially located (fig. 4-42). No immunoreactivity is present for HHV8 (238–240).

Differential Diagnosis. The differential diagnosis of BA includes a variety of vascular neoplasms, including lobular capillary hemangioma, epithelioid hemangioma, angiosarcoma, and Kaposi sarcoma. The presence of granular material, neutrophils, and neutrophilic debris and the absence of cytologic atypia, ramifying and interconnecting vascular channels, necrosis, mitotic activity, and hyaline globules assist in differentiating BA from these other vascular lesions.

Verruga peruana is another vascular proliferation process caused by an infectious agent (*Bartonella bacilliformis*); it is endemic to Peru (241). The presence of characteristic inclusions, referred to as Rocha-Lima inclusions, allows for differentiation.

Treatment and Prognosis. The treatment for BA is directed at the causative microorganism. Full-dose erythromycin is effective, often

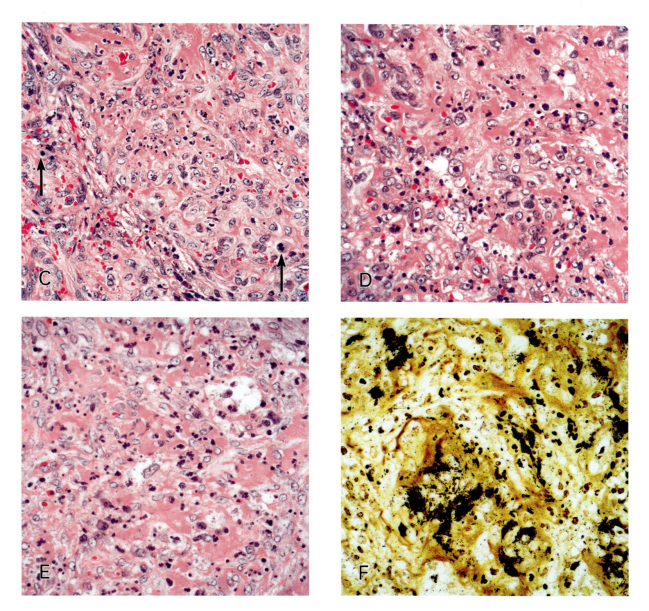

Figure 4-43, continued

C,D: Solid areas may obscure the vascular proliferation and may include the presence of mitotic figures (arrows) and nuclear pleomorphism (D).

E: An important histologic feature is the presence of neutrophils and neutrophilic debris adjacent to the capillary proliferation, with associated granular clumps.

F: Warthin-Starry staining shows that the granular material contains bacteria; the bacteria are interstitially located.

resulting in the resolution of the lesions. If left untreated, BA is progressive and potentially life-threatening (213).

Other Infectious Diseases

Infectious diseases of the lymph nodes in the neck region encompass viral, fungal, protozoan and other infectious diseases. These infections are rare and with some exceptions (e.g., HIV-related infection), cervical nodal involvement typically occurs as part of systemic disease rather than localized disease. HIV related infection is discussed in the section on the pharynx; the histologic alterations occurring in lymph nodes are histologically similar to those seen in association with the extranodal lymphoid structures of the pharynx and nasopharynx (i.e., tonsils, and adenoids). HPV-associated and Epstein-Barr virus (EBV)-associated carcinomas originating from the oropharynx (tonsil, base of tongue) and nasopharynx, respectively, may metastasize to cervical neck lymph nodes. The scope of this text does not allow for discussion of all infectious diseases or viral-associated head and neck carcinomas occurring in association with the neck/cervical lymph nodes. The reader is referred to other texts that deal with these infections.

INFLAMMATORY AND TUMOR-LIKE LESIONS

Sarcoidosis

Definition. *Sarcoidosis* is a multisystem, chronic (noncaseating) granulomatous disease of unknown etiology.

Clinical Features. There is no gender predilection and it occurs in all age groups, but is most commonly seen in young adults. In the United States, sarcoidosis is ten times more common in African Americans, with a female predominance. Any organ system may be involved, with the most common including the lung, skin, and lymph nodes. The usual clinical presentation is fever, weight loss, and hilar adenopathy.

In the head and neck, the most common sites of involvement are the cervical neck lymph nodes (anterior and posterior cervical lymph nodes). Other than cervical lymph node involvement, isolated extranodal (mucosal-based) head and neck involvement only occurs in a small percentage of cases (242). Head and neck mucosal sites of involvement include the pharynx and tonsils, ear and temporal bones, sinonasal region, salivary glands, oral cavity (fig. 4-44), larynx, and eye (242–247). Site-specific involvement may occur as an isolated phenomenon or may coexist with systemic disease, including pulmonary disease. Sarcoidosis and sarcoid-like reactions may rarely occur in association with head and neck cancer (synchronously and metachronously) and may also occur after chemotherapy (248).

Symptoms vary according to site. Cervical lymph node involvement typically presents with cervical adenopathy. Tonsillar and pharyn-

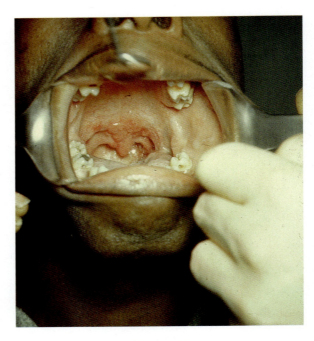

Figure 4-44

ORAL CAVITY (SOFT PALATE) SARCOIDOSIS

Multiple, irregular nodules with a cobblestone appearance are present.

geal involvement presents as pharyngotonsillitis with tonsillar enlargement, airway obstruction, nasal discharge, and epistaxis. Sinonasal involvement may be associated with nasal obstruction, crusting, and epistaxis (249). Sarcoidosis of the salivary glands may clinically simulate Sjögren syndrome, with salivary gland enlargement (fig. 4-45), xerostomia, and xerophthalmia. Involvement of the parotid gland and uveal tract, referred to as uveoparotid fever, or Heerfordt syndrome, may present with facial nerve paralysis.

There are no laboratory findings specific for or diagnostic of sarcoidosis. Cutaneous anergy to skin test ("sarcoid") antigens, referred to as the Kveim test, occurs in most patients with recently diagnosed (subacute) sarcoidosis. The Kveim test reaction may be low or absent in patients with inactive or chronic sarcoidosis. Elevated serum levels of angiotensin-converting enzyme (ACE) are found in patients with active pulmonary sarcoidosis and is considered a marker of sarcoidosis activity (250). ACE levels, however, are elevated in other (nonsarcoid) diseases including liver disease and leprosy.

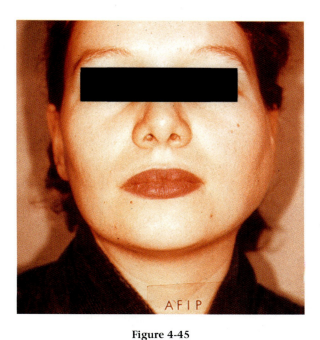

Figure 4-45

SARCOIDOSIS OF SALIVARY GLANDS

This clinically simulates Sjögren syndrome, with salivary gland enlargement as well as xerostomia and xerophthalmia. Sarcoid involvement of the parotid gland is referred to as Heerfordt syndrome.

Although ACE is sensitive to active sarcoidosis, the presence of false-positive findings limits its diagnostic usefulness to an adjunctive role and the assay should be combined with medical evaluation and tissue biopsy (251). ACE inhibitors are used with varying success in the treatment of patients with sarcoidosis. The only confirmatory test is biopsy, showing classic noncaseating granulomas.

Pathogenesis. The etiology of sarcoidosis remains unknown, but there is increasing evidence of finding mycobacterial DNA by PCR in sarcoid granulomas (252–260).

Microscopic Findings. Histologically, sarcoidosis is typically characterized by the presence of multiple, well-formed, noncaseating granulomas consisting of nodules of epithelioid histiocytes surrounded by a mixed inflammatory infiltrate (fig. 4-46). Langhans-type giant cells may be present. Necrosis (caseation) is absent but some examples, especially at extranodal sites, have a small central foci of necrosis. Intracytoplasmic inclusions, including star-shaped and calcified laminated bodies, called asteroid and Schaumann bodies, respectively, may be seen. Calcium oxylate crystals may be present in the cytoplasm of giant cells. All special stains for microorganisms are negative.

Cytogenetics and molecular genetics of sarcoidosis include the presence of major histocompatibility complex (*MHC*) genes and non-*MHC* genes located on short arm of chromosome 6 and implicated as genetic risk factors (261). Genome wide association studies have identified a strong genetic association between sarcoidosis and *ANXA11* (annexin A11) gene on chromosome 10q22.3, representing a new susceptibility locus for sarcoidosis (262). Functional polymorphism within the butyrophilin-like 2 (*BTNL2*) gene has been described as a potential risk factor for sarcoidosis (263).

Differential Diagnosis. A diagnosis of sarcoidosis is generally one of exclusion and is made by correlating the clinical, radiologic, and pathologic findings. While the pathologic features are characteristic, they are not specific for sarcoidosis and the diagnosis can only be rendered in the absence of identifying an infectious agent. The differential diagnosis primarily includes other granulomatous diseases. Noncaseating granulomatous inflammation is seen in tuberculosis (typical and atypical), fungal diseases, leprosy, cat scratch disease, and many other infectious diseases. Noninfectious diseases of the upper aerodigestive tract (e.g., Crohn disease) may also be associated with noncaseating granulomatous inflammation.

Treatment and Prognosis. The treatment for symptomatic sarcoidosis is corticosteroid therapy. The prognosis is generally good, with up to 70 percent of patients improving or remaining stable following therapy. Advanced multisystem disease, leading to extensive pulmonary involvement and respiratory failure, may occur but is seen in only a small percentage of patients.

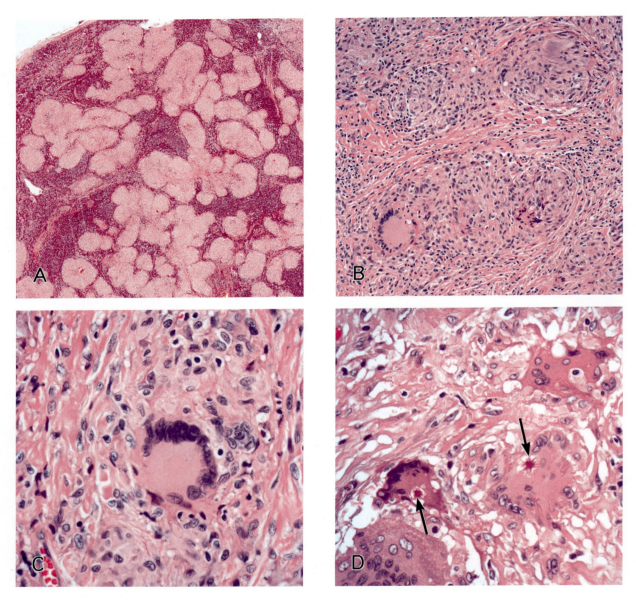

Figure 4-46

SARCOIDOSIS

The histology of sarcoidosis is the same irrespective of location.

A: A cervical neck lymph node is almost completely replaced by multiple well-formed granulomas.

B,C: The granulomas are noncaseating and consist of epithelioid histiocytes and multinucleated Langhans type giant cells.

D: Intracytoplasmic star-shaped inclusions, referred to as asteroid bodies (arrows), are identified. A diagnosis of sarcoidosis is suggested/established only after excluding a possible infectious etiology; to this end, special stains for microorganisms are negative in sarcoidosis.

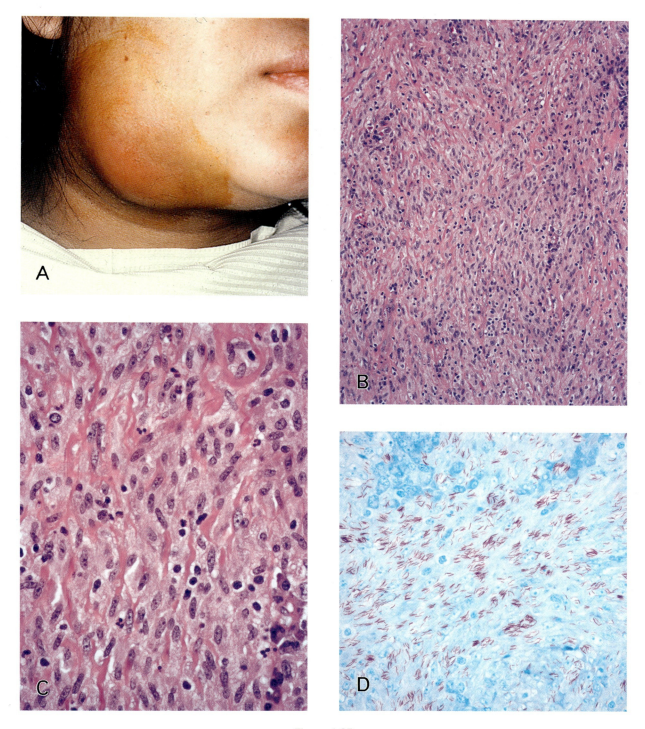

Figure 4-37

MYCOBACTERIAL SPINDLE CELL PSEUDOTUMOR

A: An immunocompromised patient presents with a subcutaneous firm nodule.

B,C: The cellular proliferation is composed of bland-appearing spindle-shaped cells with a storiform pattern; multinucleated giant cells and foamy histiocytes are not present.

D: The AFB stain for mycobacteria shows numerous AFB-positive microorganisms within the cytoplasm of the spindle cells.

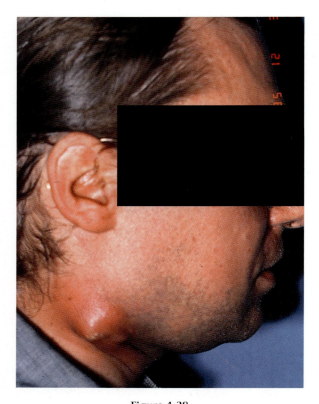

Figure 4-38

CERVICOFACIAL ACTINOMYCOSIS

An indurated, suppurative neck mass is at the angle of the mandible. The skin overlying the lesion is purple.

composed of a central meshwork of filaments that typically have eosinophilic club-shaped ends. Protein often precipitates on the filaments, resulting in thick eosinophilic radiations referred to as the Splendore-Hoeppli phenomenon. The sulfur granules are identified in pus.

A diagnosis of actinomycosis can be made by fine-needle aspiration biopsy (202,203). Smears and cell blocks of the aspirate show the characteristic colonies (sulfur granules) of Actinomyces. The microorganisms stain with Gomori methenamine silver (GMS) and Gram stains (fig. 4-39) and occasionally stain with periodic acid–Schiff (PAS).

Differential Diagnosis. The differential diagnosis includes various infections, including *Nocardia* infection

Treatment and Prognosis. Intravenous penicillin G followed by oral penicillin is the treatment of choice. Patients allergic to penicillin are given tetracycline. In conjunction with antibiotic therapy, surgical excision is advocated, with favorable results (204,205). The prognosis is good if treated early. Acute osteomyelitis of the jaw is the most common complication (fig. 4-40). Once infection reaches bone, tissue destruction may be extensive and involvement of the cranium, meninges, and brain may occur with lethal implications.

Cat Scratch Disease

Definition. *Cat scratch disease* (CSD) is a necrotizing granulomatous lymphadenitis caused by a pleomorphic, Gram-negative bacterium, *Bartonella henselae*, resulting in lymphadenopathy.

Clinical Features. There is no gender predilection and CSD occurs at all ages. The mode of transmission is by direct contact from a cat scratch, bite, or lick through a skin break (206). There is no evidence to support transmission from man to man. The infected cat is not ill and appears to be infectious for only a limited time. In the majority of cases, a history of exposure to a cat can be obtained and the primary inoculation site identified, typically from 7 to 12 days following contact. CSD primarily occurs in immunocompetent individuals but may occur as localized disease in solid organ transplant recipients (207).

The symptoms include enlarged and often tender lymph nodes, with potential involvement of the submental, submandibular, cervical, occipital, and supraclavicular lymph nodes as well as cervical lymph nodes in both the anterior and posterior triangles of the neck (fig. 4-41) (208,209). Obstruction and inflammation may be seen in salivary glands with involved lymph nodes. Atypical head and neck manifestations of CSD including conjunctivitis (Parinaud oculoglandular syndrome), swelling of the parotid gland, and erythema nodosum (209). Constitutional symptoms include low-grade fever, malaise, myalgias, headaches, and weight loss/anorexia (210); less common manifestations/complications include thrombocytopenic purpura, encephalitis/encephalopathy, convulsions, osteomyelitis, retinitis, arthritis, hepatosplenomegaly, pulmonary nodules, and pleurisy (211). A positive skin test confirms the diagnosis (208). Cutaneous lesions appear as a red papule which may become crusted or pustular.

Microscopic Findings. Changes in the affected lymph node vary with time. In early

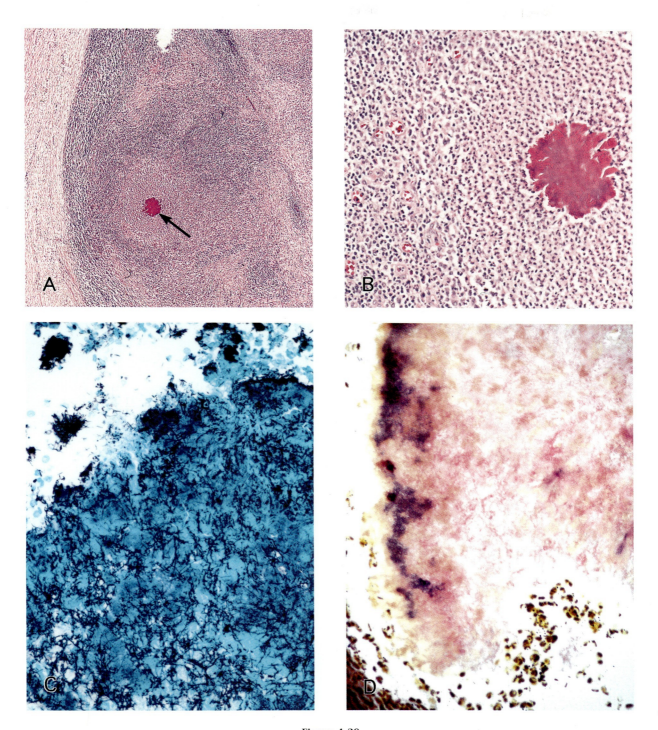

Figure 4-39

CERVICOFACIAL ACTINOMYCOSIS

A: A cervical lymph node has focal abscess formation, within which is the actinomycotic organism (arrow).

B: At higher magnification, the actinomycotic colony has a characteristic appearance, referred to as "sulfur granules"; the granules are lobular, deep purple and composed of a central meshwork of filaments, which typically have thick eosinophilic radiations or club-shaped ends (Splendore-Hoeppli phenomenon).

C,D: The microorganisms stain with the Gomori methenamine silver (GMS) (C) and Gram (D) stains.

Non-Neoplastic Diseases of the Head and Neck

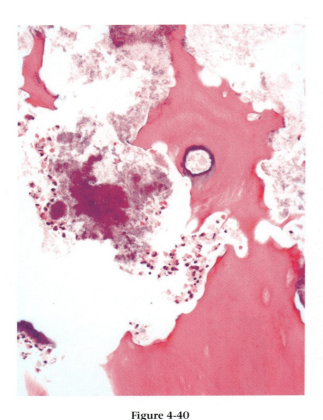

Figure 4-40

CERVICOFACIAL ACTINOMYCOSIS

Acute osteomyelitis is a potential and unfortunately common complication of actinomycotic infection of the jaw.

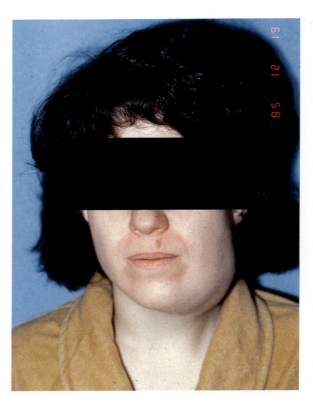

Figure 4-41

CAT SCRATCH DISEASE

This woman presents with enlarged (and tender) left cervical neck lymph nodes.

lesions, follicular hyperplasia and histiocytic proliferations are identified. Intermediate-stage lesions show granulomatous inflammation. In late lesions, abscess formation is present. The appearance of the abscess includes a central area of necrosis with a stellate pattern and an admixture of polymorphonuclear leukocytes surrounded by palisading of histiocytes (fig. 4-42). This pattern is consistently seen and is characteristic of the diagnosis but is not pathognomonic. Nodal sinuses are packed with monocytoid B cells. Skin lesions show necrotic areas within the dermis surrounded by histiocytes.

Cat scratch bacilli can be identified by the Warthin-Starry stain and appear as extracellular pleomorphic coccobacilli (fig. 4-42) (206,212). Staining and culturing for acid-fast microorganisms are negative.

Differential Diagnosis. The primary differential diagnoses include toxoplasmosis and lymphogranuloma venereum.

Treatment and Prognosis. The treatment is supportive and includes analgesics and warm compresses. CSD is usually self-limiting and typically runs its course within a few months. In cases with suppuration, needle aspiration may relieve pain; incision and drainage may produce sinus tract inflammation. Antibiotic therapy appears to be of little benefit (213).

Bacillary Angiomatosis

Definition. *Bacillary angiomatosis* (BA) is a pseudoneoplastic capillary proliferative lesion that occurs as a complication of HIV infection and usually presents as a cutaneous vascular lesion. It is an opportunistic bacterial infection caused by *Rochalimaea* species (*R. henselae*) as well as by *Bartonella quintana*. Synonyms include *epithelioid angiomatosis* and *epithelioid hemangioma-like vascular proliferation*.

Clinical Features. There is no gender predilection. BA occurs over a wide age range. It usually

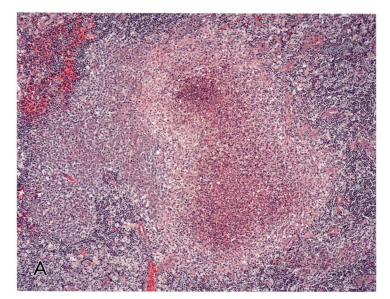
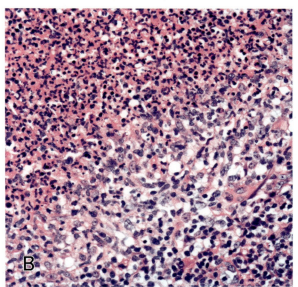
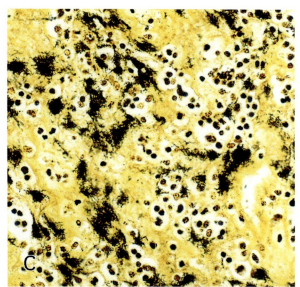

Figure 4-42

NECROTIZING GRANULOMATOUS LYMPHADENITIS

A,B: A central area of necrosis with a stellate pattern and an admixture of polymorphonuclear leukocytes is surrounded by palisading histiocytes. This pattern is consistently seen and is characteristic of the diagnosis but is not pathognomonic.

C: The causative bacterium (*Bartonella henselae*), appearing as extracellular pleomorphic coccobacilli, is identified by the Warthin-Starry stain.

presents as a cutaneous lesion commonly associated with systemic symptoms, including fever, chills, weight loss, and night sweats (214–217). Clinically, the lesions are similar in appearance to lobular capillary hemangioma (pyogenic granuloma) and Kaposi sarcoma, characterized by the presence of multiple erythematous papules with or without crusting. BA may involve other organs sites including lymph nodes, spleen, and liver, as well as mucosal sites of the upper respiratory tract and conjunctiva (218–221).

In addition to its association with HIV and AIDS patients, BA occurs in solid organ transplant recipients (222–224), patients on systemic steroid therapy (225), and patients with Kaposi sarcoma (226–228). In immune-compromised patients coinfection with other opportunistic infections may occur (229). Despite is association with immune-compromised patients, BA has also been reported in (adult and pediatric) immune-competent patients (230–234).

Laboratory studies include conventional microbiologic culturing and molecular techniques, such as PCR (221,235,236). Serologic demonstration of antibodies by direct immunofluorescence and enzyme immunoassay is diagnostic (235).

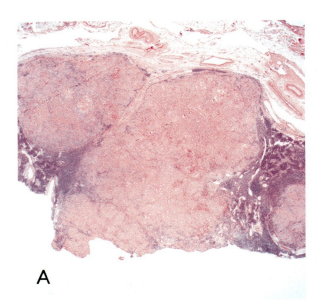
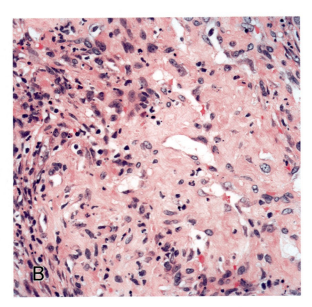

Figure 4-43

BACILLARY ANGIOMATOSIS

A: The lymph node is replaced by circumscribed lobular proliferations.
B: Small capillaries are arranged around ectatic vessels which are lined by prominent endothelial cells.

Proteomic analysis, with identification of immunoreactive antigens, is useful for an improved *Bartonella*-specific serodiagnosis (237).

Gross Findings. The gross features vary widely from cutaneous erythematous papules, to mushroom-shaped papules, and nodules to deep-seated rounded lesions without change in skin color. Exceptionally, BA appears as a mucosal-based, erythematous nodular proliferation.

Microscopic Findings. Regardless of its clinical presentation, the histologic features are the same and include circumscribed nodules of a lobular capillary proliferation with overall features similar to those seen in lobular capillary hemangioma (fig. 4-43). Small capillaries are arranged around ectatic vessels, which are lined by prominent endothelial cells. Cytologic atypia, mitotic figures and necrosis are not usually present but occasionally may be seen. Solid areas may be present and may obscure the vascular proliferation (fig. 4-43). A variable edematous, mucinous, or fibrotic stroma separates the lobular proliferation. An important histologic feature in BA is the presence of neutrophils and neutrophilic debris adjacent to the capillary proliferation, with associated granular clumps (fig. 4-43). In contrast to findings seen in Kaposi sarcoma, BA typically lacks spindled cells, interconnecting vascular channels, or hyaline globules. The overlying epithelium may be ulcerated, thinned, or show pseudoepitheliomatous hyperplasia.

The Warthin-Starry stain shows that the granular material contains bacteria; bacteria are interstitially located (fig. 4-42). No immunoreactivity is present for HHV8 (238–240).

Differential Diagnosis. The differential diagnosis of BA includes a variety of vascular neoplasms, including lobular capillary hemangioma, epithelioid hemangioma, angiosarcoma, and Kaposi sarcoma. The presence of granular material, neutrophils, and neutrophilic debris and the absence of cytologic atypia, ramifying and interconnecting vascular channels, necrosis, mitotic activity, and hyaline globules assist in differentiating BA from these other vascular lesions.

Verruga peruana is another vascular proliferation process caused by an infectious agent (*Bartonella bacilliformis*); it is endemic to Peru (241). The presence of characteristic inclusions, referred to as Rocha-Lima inclusions, allows for differentiation.

Treatment and Prognosis. The treatment for BA is directed at the causative microorganism. Full-dose erythromycin is effective, often

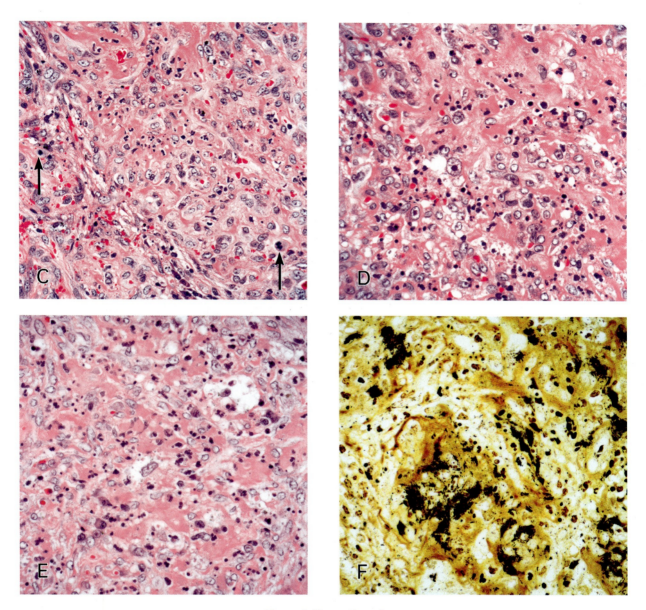

Figure 4-43, continued

C,D: Solid areas may obscure the vascular proliferation and may include the presence of mitotic figures (arrows) and nuclear pleomorphism (D).

E: An important histologic feature is the presence of neutrophils and neutrophilic debris adjacent to the capillary proliferation, with associated granular clumps.

F: Warthin-Starry staining shows that the granular material contains bacteria; the bacteria are interstitially located.

resulting in the resolution of the lesions. If left untreated, BA is progressive and potentially life-threatening (213).

Other Infectious Diseases

Infectious diseases of the lymph nodes in the neck region encompass viral, fungal, protozoan and other infectious diseases. These infections are rare and with some exceptions (e.g., HIV-related infection), cervical nodal involvement typically occurs as part of systemic disease rather than localized disease. HIV related infection is discussed in the section on the pharynx; the histologic alterations occurring in lymph nodes are histologically similar to those seen in association with the extranodal lymphoid structures of the pharynx and nasopharynx (i.e., tonsils, and adenoids). HPV-associated and Epstein-Barr virus (EBV)-associated carcinomas originating from the oropharynx (tonsil, base of tongue) and nasopharynx, respectively, may metastasize to cervical neck lymph nodes. The scope of this text does not allow for discussion of all infectious diseases or viral-associated head and neck carcinomas occurring in association with the neck/cervical lymph nodes. The reader is referred to other texts that deal with these infections.

INFLAMMATORY AND TUMOR-LIKE LESIONS

Sarcoidosis

Definition. *Sarcoidosis* is a multisystem, chronic (noncaseating) granulomatous disease of unknown etiology.

Clinical Features. There is no gender predilection and it occurs in all age groups, but is most commonly seen in young adults. In the United States, sarcoidosis is ten times more common in African Americans, with a female predominance. Any organ system may be involved, with the most common including the lung, skin, and lymph nodes. The usual clinical presentation is fever, weight loss, and hilar adenopathy.

In the head and neck, the most common sites of involvement are the cervical neck lymph nodes (anterior and posterior cervical lymph nodes). Other than cervical lymph node involvement, isolated extranodal (mucosal-based) head and neck involvement only occurs in a small percentage of cases (242). Head and neck mucosal sites of involvement include the pharynx and tonsils, ear and temporal bones, sinonasal region, salivary glands, oral cavity (fig. 4-44), larynx, and eye (242–247). Site-specific involvement may occur as an isolated phenomenon or may coexist with systemic disease, including pulmonary disease. Sarcoidosis and sarcoid-like reactions may rarely occur in association with head and neck cancer (synchronously and metachronously) and may also occur after chemotherapy (248).

Symptoms vary according to site. Cervical lymph node involvement typically presents with cervical adenopathy. Tonsillar and pharyn-

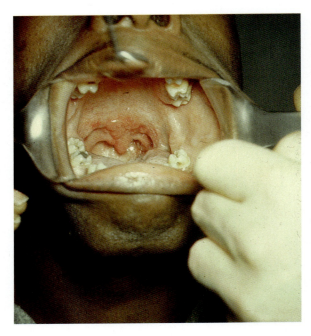

Figure 4-44

ORAL CAVITY (SOFT PALATE) SARCOIDOSIS

Multiple, irregular nodules with a cobblestone appearance are present.

geal involvement presents as pharyngotonsillitis with tonsillar enlargement, airway obstruction, nasal discharge, and epistaxis. Sinonasal involvement may be associated with nasal obstruction, crusting, and epistaxis (249). Sarcoidosis of the salivary glands may clinically simulate Sjögren syndrome, with salivary gland enlargement (fig. 4-45), xerostomia, and xerophthalmia. Involvement of the parotid gland and uveal tract, referred to as uveoparotid fever, or Heerfordt syndrome, may present with facial nerve paralysis.

There are no laboratory findings specific for or diagnostic of sarcoidosis. Cutaneous anergy to skin test ("sarcoid") antigens, referred to as the Kveim test, occurs in most patients with recently diagnosed (subacute) sarcoidosis. The Kveim test reaction may be low or absent in patients with inactive or chronic sarcoidosis. Elevated serum levels of angiotensin-converting enzyme (ACE) are found in patients with active pulmonary sarcoidosis and is considered a marker of sarcoidosis activity (250). ACE levels, however, are elevated in other (nonsarcoid) diseases including liver disease and leprosy.

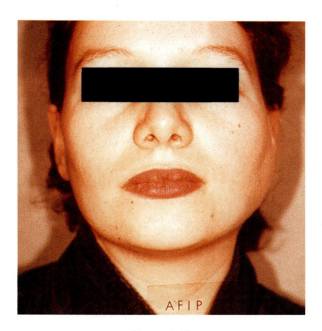

Figure 4-45

SARCOIDOSIS OF SALIVARY GLANDS

This clinically simulates Sjögren syndrome, with salivary gland enlargement as well as xerostomia and xerophthalmia. Sarcoid involvement of the parotid gland is referred to as Heerfordt syndrome.

Although ACE is sensitive to active sarcoidosis, the presence of false-positive findings limits its diagnostic usefulness to an adjunctive role and the assay should be combined with medical evaluation and tissue biopsy (251). ACE inhibitors are used with varying success in the treatment of patients with sarcoidosis. The only confirmatory test is biopsy, showing classic noncaseating granulomas.

Pathogenesis. The etiology of sarcoidosis remains unknown, but there is increasing evidence of finding mycobacterial DNA by PCR in sarcoid granulomas (252–260).

Microscopic Findings. Histologically, sarcoidosis is typically characterized by the presence of multiple, well-formed, noncaseating granulomas consisting of nodules of epithelioid histiocytes surrounded by a mixed inflammatory infiltrate (fig. 4-46). Langhans-type giant cells may be present. Necrosis (caseation) is absent but some examples, especially at extranodal sites, have a small central foci of necrosis. Intracytoplasmic inclusions, including star-shaped and calcified laminated bodies, called asteroid and Schaumann bodies, respectively, may be seen. Calcium oxylate crystals may be present in the cytoplasm of giant cells. All special stains for microorganisms are negative.

Cytogenetics and molecular genetics of sarcoidosis include the presence of major histocompatibility complex (*MHC*) genes and non-*MHC* genes located on short arm of chromosome 6 and implicated as genetic risk factors (261). Genome wide association studies have identified a strong genetic association between sarcoidosis and *ANXA11* (annexin A11) gene on chromosome 10q22.3, representing a new susceptibility locus for sarcoidosis (262). Functional polymorphism within the butyrophilin-like 2 (*BTNL2*) gene has been described as a potential risk factor for sarcoidosis (263).

Differential Diagnosis. A diagnosis of sarcoidosis is generally one of exclusion and is made by correlating the clinical, radiologic, and pathologic findings. While the pathologic features are characteristic, they are not specific for sarcoidosis and the diagnosis can only be rendered in the absence of identifying an infectious agent. The differential diagnosis primarily includes other granulomatous diseases. Noncaseating granulomatous inflammation is seen in tuberculosis (typical and atypical), fungal diseases, leprosy, cat scratch disease, and many other infectious diseases. Noninfectious diseases of the upper aerodigestive tract (e.g., Crohn disease) may also be associated with noncaseating granulomatous inflammation.

Treatment and Prognosis. The treatment for symptomatic sarcoidosis is corticosteroid therapy. The prognosis is generally good, with up to 70 percent of patients improving or remaining stable following therapy. Advanced multisystem disease, leading to extensive pulmonary involvement and respiratory failure, may occur but is seen in only a small percentage of patients.

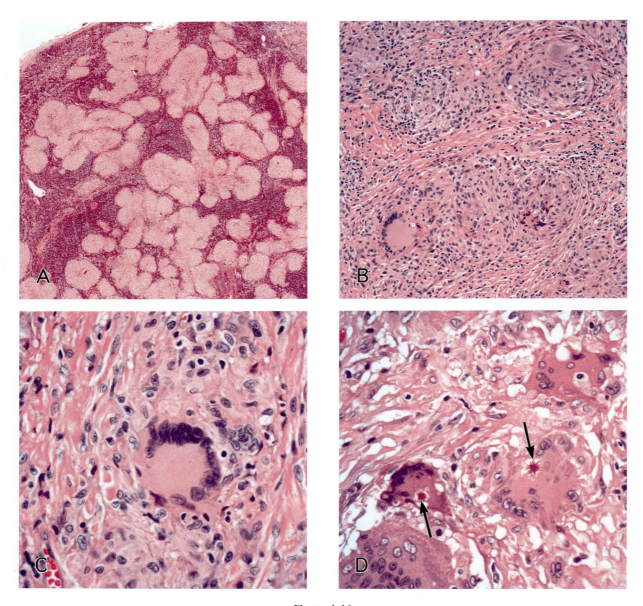

Figure 4-46

SARCOIDOSIS

The histology of sarcoidosis is the same irrespective of location.

A: A cervical neck lymph node is almost completely replaced by multiple well-formed granulomas.

B,C: The granulomas are noncaseating and consist of epithelioid histiocytes and multinucleated Langhans type giant cells.

D: Intracytoplasmic star-shaped inclusions, referred to as asteroid bodies (arrows), are identified. A diagnosis of sarcoidosis is suggested/established only after excluding a possible infectious etiology; to this end, special stains for microorganisms are negative in sarcoidosis.

REFERENCES

Anatomy

1. Hollinshead WH. The neck. In: Hollinshead WH, ed. Anatomy for surgeons, vol. 1, 3rd ed. Philadelphia: Harper & Row; 1982:443-531.
2. Standring S. The neck. In: Standring S, ed. Gray's anatomy, 40th ed. Edinburgh: Elsevier Churchill Livingstone; 2008:435-466.
3. Medina JE, Houck JR Jr. Surgical management of cervical lymph nodes. In: Harrison LB, Sessions RB, Hong WK. Head and neck cancer. A multidisciplinary approach, 2nd ed. Philadelphia; Lippincott Williams & Wilkins; 2004:203-227.

Branchial Cleft Anomalies

4. Moore KL, Persaud TV. The pharyngeal apparatus. In: Moore KL, Persaud TV, eds. The developing human: clinically oriented embryology, 7th ed. Philadelphia: Saunders; 2003:201-240.
5. Hunter AG. Inheritence of branchial sinuses and preauricular fistulas. Teratology 1974;9:225-228.
6. Proctor B, Proctor C. Congenital lesions of the head and neck. Otolaryngol Clin North Am 1970;3:221-248.
7. Alshaiji JM, Handler MZ, Huo R, Freedman A, Schachner LA. HATS syndrome: hemimaxillary enlargement, asymmetry of the face, tooth abnormalities, and skin findings. Cutis 2014;94: E18-21.
8. Welsch MJ, Stein SL. A syndrome of hemimaxillary enlargement, asymmetry of the face, tooth abnormalities, and skin findings (HATS). Pediatr Dermatol 2004;21:448-451.
9. Agaton-Bonilla FC, Gay-Escoda C. Diagnosis and treatment of branchial cleft cysts and fistulae. A retrospective study of 183 patients. Int J Oral Maxillofac Surg 1996;25:449-452.
10. Choi SS, Zalzal GH. Branchial anomalies: a review of 52 cases. Laryngoscope 1995;105(Pt 1):909-13.
11. Mandell DL. Head and neck anomalies related to the branchial apparatus. Otolaryngol Clin North Am 2000;33:1309-1332.
12. Golledge J, Ellis H. The aetiology of lateral cervical (branchial) cysts: past and present theories. J Laryngol Otol 1994;108:653-659.
13. Bhaskar SN, Bernier JL. Histogenesis of branchial cysts: a report of 468 cases. Am J Pathol 1959;35:407-423.

First Branchial Anomalies

14. Aronsohn RS, Batsakis JG, Rice DH, Work WP. Anomalies of the first branchial cleft. Arch Otolaryngol 1976;102:737-740.
15. D'Souza AR, Uppal HS, De R, Zeitoun H. Updating concepts of first branchial defects: a literature review. Int J Pediatr Otorhinolaryngol 2002;62:103-109.
16. Leu YS, Chang KC. First branchial cleft anomalies: report of 12 cases. Ear Nose Throat J 1998; 77:832-823, 837-838.
17. Olsen KD, Maragos NE, Weiland LH. First branchial cleft anomalies. Laryngoscope 1980;90:423-436.
18. Triglia JM, Nicollas R, Ducroz V, Koltai PJ, Garabedian EN. First branchial cleft anomalies: a study of 39 cases and a review of the literature. Arch Otolaryngol Head Neck Surg 1998;124:291-295.
19. Spinelli C, Rossi L, Strambi S, et al. Branchial cleft and pouch anomalies in childhood: a report of 50 surgical cases. J Endocrinol Invest 2016;39:529-535.
20. Nofsinger YC, Tom LW, LaRossa D, Wetmore RF, Handler SD. Periauricular cysts and sinuses. Laryngoscope 1997;107:883-887.
21. Shinn JR, Purcell PL, Horn DL, Sie KC, Manning SC. First branchial cleft anomalies: otologic manifestations and treatment outcomes. Otolaryngol Head Neck Surg 2015;152:506-512.
22. Krishnamurthy A, Ramshanker V. A Type I first branchial cleft cyst masquerading as a parotid tumor. Natl J Maxillofac Surg 2014;5:84-85.
23. Mukherji SK, Tart RP, Slattery WH, Stringer SP, Benson MT, Mancuso AA. Evaluation of first branchial anomalies by CT and MR. J Comput Assist Tomogr 1993;17:576-581.
24. Greenway RE, Hurst L, Fenton NA. An unusual first branchial cleft cyst. J Laryngol 1981;10:219-225.
25. Work WP. Newer concepts of first branchial cleft defects. Laryngoscope 1972;82:1581-1593.

Second Branchial Anomalies

26. Verbin RS, Barnes L. Branchial cysts, sinuses, and fistulas. In: Barnes L, ed. Surgical pathology of the head and neck. Second edition, revised and expanded. New York: Marcel Dekker; 2001:1486-1498.
27. Prasad SC, Azeez A, Thada ND, Rao P, Bacciu A, Prasad KC. Branchial anomalies: diagnosis and management. Int J Otolaryngol 2014;2014: 237015.
28. Chen PS, Lin YC, Lin YS. Nasopharyngeal branchial cleft cyst. J Chin Med Assoc 2012;75:660-662.
29. Papay FA, Kalucis C, Eliachar I, Tucker HM. Nasopharyngeal presentation of second branchial cleft cyst. Otolaryngol Head Neck Surg 1994;110:232-234.
30. Shidara K, Uruma T, Yasuoka Y, Kamei T. Two cases of nasopharyngeal branchial cyst. J Laryngol Otol 1993;107:453-435.
31. Harnsberger HR, Mancuso AA, Muraki AS, et al. Branchial cleft anomalies and their mimics: computed tomographic evaluation. Radiology 1984;152:739-748.

32. Layfield L. Fine needle aspiration biopsy. In: Fu, Y-S, Wenig BM, Abemayor E, Wenig BL, eds. Head and neck pathology with clinical correlations. New York: Churchill Livingstone; 2001:81-109.
33. Elsheikh TM, Singh HK, Saad RS, Silverman JF. Fine needle aspiration of the head and neck. In: Barnes L, ed. Surgical pathology of the head and neck, 3rd ed. New York: Informa Healthcare; 2009:1-94.
34. Pai RK, Erickson J, Pourmand N, Kong CS. p16(INK4A) immunohistochemical staining may be helpful in distinguishing branchial cleft cysts from cystic squamous cell carcinomas originating in the oropharynx. Cancer 2009;117:108-119.
35. Begum S, Gillison ML, Nicol TL, Westra WH. Detection of human papillomavirus-16 in fine-needle aspirates to determine tumor origin in patients with metastatic squamous cell carcinoma of the head and neck. Clin Cancer Res 2007;13:1186-1191.
36. Martin H, Morfit HM, Ehrlich H. The case for branchiogenic cancer (malignant branchioma). Ann Surg 1950;132:867-887.
37. Thompson LDR, Heffner DK. The clinical import of cystic squamous cell carcinomas in the neck: A study of 136 cases. Cancer 1998;82:944-956.
38. Zaifullah S, Yunus MR, See GB. Diagnosis and treatment of branchial cleft anomalies in UKMMC: a 10-year retrospective study. Eur Arch Otorhinolaryngol 2013;270:1501-1506.
39. Blackwell KE, Calcaterra TC. Functional neck dissection for treatment of recurrent branchial remnants. Arch Otolaryngol Head Neck Surg 1994;120:417-421.

Third Branchial Anomalies

40. Cunningham MJ. The management of congenital neck masses. Am J Otolaryngol 1992;13:78-92.
41. Har-el G, Sasaki CT, Prager D, Krespi YP. Acute suppurative thyroiditis and the branchial apparatus. Am J Otolaryngol 1991;12:6-11.
42. Huang RY, Damrose EJ, Alavi S, Maceri DR, Shapiro NL. Third branchial cleft anomaly presenting as a retropharyngeal abscess. Int J Pediatr Otorhinolaryngol 2000;54:167-172.
43. James A, Stewart C, Warrick P, Tzifa C, Forte V. Branchial sinus of the piriform fossa: reappraisal of third and fourth branchial anomalies. Laryngoscope 2007;117:1920-1924.
44. Madana J, Yolmo D, Gopalakrishnan S, Saxena SK. Complete congenital third branchial fistula with left-sided, recurrent, suppurative thyroiditis. J Laryngol Otol 2010;124:1025-1029.
45. Ostfeld EJ, Wiesel JM, Rabinson S, Auslander L. Parapharyngeal (retrostyloid)—third branchial cleft cyst. J Laryngol Otol 1991;105:790-792.
46. Rea PA, Hartley BE, Bailey CM. Third and fourth branchial pouch anomalies. J Laryngol Otol 2004;118:19-24.
47. Sai Prasad TR, Chong CL, Mani A, et al. Acute suppurative thyroiditis in children secondary to pyriform sinus fistula. Pediatr Surg Int 2007;23:779-783.
48. Yolmo D, Madana J, Kalaiarasi R, et al. Retrospective case review of pyriform sinus fistulae of third branchial arch origin commonly presenting as acute suppurative thyroiditis in children. J Laryngol Otol 2012;126:737-742.
49. Cain RB, Kasznica P, Brundage WJ. Right-sided pyriform sinus fistula: a case report and review of the literature. Case Rep Otolaryngol 2012;2012:934968.
50. Harnsberger HR, Wiggins RH III, Hugkins PA, et al. 3rd branchial cleft cyst. In: Harnsberger HR, ed. Diagnostic imaging head and neck. Salt Lake: Amirsys; 2004: IV;1:14-17.
51. Edmonds JL, Girod DA, Woodroof JM, Bruegger DE. Third branchial anomalies. Avoiding recurrences. Arch Otolaryngol Head Neck Surg 1997;123:438-441.
52. Nicoucar K, Giger R, Jaecklin T, Pope HG Jr, Dulguerov P. Management of congenital third branchial arch anomalies: a systematic review. Otolaryngol Head Neck Surg 2010;142:21-28.
53. Pereira KD, Losh GG, Oliver D, Poole MD. Management of anomalies of the third and fourth branchial pouches. Int J Pediatr Otorhinolaryngol 2004;68:43-50.

Fourth Branchial Anomalies

54. Cases JA, Wenig BM, Silver CE, Surks MI. Recurrent acute suppurative thyroiditis in an adult due to a fourth branchial pouch fistula. J Clin Endocrinol Metab 2000;85:953-956.
55. Johnson IJ, Soames JV, Birchall JP. Fourth branchial arch fistula. J Laryngol Otol 1996;110:391-393.
56. Lee FP. Occult congenital pyriform sinus fistula causing recurrent left lower neck abscess. Head Neck 1999;21:671-676.
57. Lin JN, Wang KL. Persistent third branchial apparatus. J Pediatr Surg 1991;26:663-665.
58. Minhas SS, Watkinson JC, Franklyn J. Fourth branchial arch fistula and suppurative thyroiditis: a life-threatening infection. J Laryngol Otol 2001;115:1029-1031.
59. Nicollas R, Ducroz V, Garabedian EN, Triglia JM. Fourth branchial pouch anomalies: a study of six cases and review of the literature. Int J Pediatr Otorhinolaryngol 1998;44:5-10.
60. Ostfeld E, Segal J, Auslander L, Rabinson S. Fourth pharyngeal pouch sinus. Laryngoscope 1985;95:1114-1117.
61. Sharma HS, Razif A, Hamzah M, et al. Fourth branchial pouch cyst: an unusual cause of neonatal stridor. Int J Pediatr Otorhinolaryngol 1996;38:155-161.

62. Nicoucar K, Giger R, Jaecklin T, Pope HG Jr, Dulguerov P. Management of congenital third branchial arch anomalies: a systematic review. Otolaryngol Head Neck Surg 2010;142:21-28.

Thyroglossal Duct Cyst

63. Moore KL, Persaud TV. The pharyngeal apparatus. In: Moore KL, Persaud TVN, eds. The developing human: clinically oriented embryology, 7th ed. Philadelphia: Saunders; 2003:201-240.
64. Ellis PD, van Nostrand AW. The applied anatomy of thyroglossal duct remnants. Laryngoscope 1977;87:765-770.
65. Carcangiu ML. Thyroid. In: Mills, SE, ed. Histology for patholo0gists, 4th ed. Philadelphia: Wolters Kluwer/Lippincott Williams & Wilkins; 2012:1185-1207.
66. de Tristan J, Zenk J, Künzel J, Psychogios G, Iro H. Thyroglossal duct cysts: 20 years' experience (1992-2011). Eur Arch Otorhinolaryngol 2015; 272:2513-2519.
67. Hirshoren N, Neuman T, Udassin R, Elidan J, Weinberger JM. The imperative of the Sistrunk operation: review of 160 thyroglossal tract remnant operations. Otolaryngol Head Neck Surg 2009;140:338-342.
68. Yaman H, Durmaz A, Arslan HH, Ozcan A, Karahatay S, Gerek M. Thyroglossal duct cysts: evaluation and treatment of 49 cases. B-ENT 2011;7:267-271.
69. Allard RH. The thyroglossal cyst. Head Neck Surg 1982;5:134-146.
70. Ward PH, Strahan RW, Acquarelli M, Harris PF. The many faces of cysts of the thyroglossal duct. Trans Am Acad Ophthalmol Otolaryngol 1970;7;310-318.
71. Soni S, Poorey VK, Chouksey S. Thyroglossal duct cyst, variantion in presentation, our experience. Indian J Otolaryngol Head Neck Surg 2014;66:398-400.
72. Aubin A, Lescanne E, Pondaven S, Merieau-Bakhos E, Bakhos D. Stridor and lingual throglossal duct cyst in a newborn. Eur Ann Otorhinolaryngol Head Neck Dis 2011;128:321-323.
73. Fu J, Xue X, Chen L, Fan G, Pan L, Mao J. Lingual thyroglossal duct cyst in newborns: previously diagnosed as laryngomalacia. Int J Pediatr Otorhinolaryngol 2008;72:327-332.
74. Bist SS, Bisht M, Varshney S, Gupta N, Bhatia R. Thyroglossal duct cyst in hyoid bone: unusual location. Indian J Otolaryngol Head Neck Surg 2007;59:366-368.
75. Tas A, Karasalihoglu AR, Yagiz R, Doganay L, Guven S. Thyroglossal duct cyst in hyoid bone: unusual location. J Laryngol Otol 2003;117:656-657.
76. Diaz MC, Stormorken A, Christopher NC. A thyroglossal duct cyst causing apnea and cyanosis in a neonate. Pediatr Emerg Care 2005;21:35-37.
77. Ren W, Zhi K, Zhao L, Gao L. Presentations and management of thyroglossal duct cyst in children versus adults: a review of 106 cases. Oral Surg Oral Med Oral Pathol Oral Radiol Endod 2011;111: e1-6.
78. Branstetter BF, Weissman JL, Kennedy TL, Whitaker M. The CT appearance of thyroglossal duct carcinoma. AJNR Am J Neuroradiol 2000;21:1547-1550.
79. Ayala C, Healy GB, Robson CD, Vargas SO. Psammomatous calcification in association with a benign thyroglossal duct cyst. Arch Otolaryngol Head Neck Surg 2003;129:241-243.
80. Tovi F, Barki Y, Maor E. Cartilage within a thyroglossal duct anomaly. Int J Pediatr Otorhinolaryngol 1988;15:205-210.
81. Davis JP, Toma AG, Robinson PJ, Friedmann I. Ossified thyroglossal cyst—is it of embryological significance? J Laryngol Otol 1994;108:168-170.
82. Shaffer MM, Oertel YC, Oertel JE. Thyroglossal duct cysts: diagnostic criteria by fine-needle aspiration. Arch Pathol Lab Med 1996;120:1039-1043.
83. Gomi K, Kitagawa N, Usui Y, et al. Papillary carcinoma with extensive squamous metaplasia arising from thyroglossal duct cyst in an 11-year-old girl: significance of differentiation from squamous cell carcinoma: a case report. J Pediatr Surg 2011;46:e1-4.
84. Dedivitis RA, Camargo DL, Peixoto GL, Weissman L, Guimaraes AV. Thyroglossal duct: a review of 55 cases. J Am Coll Surg 2002;194:274-277.
85. Geller KA, Cohen D, Koempel JA. Thyroglossal duct cyst and sinuses: a 20-year Los Angeles experience and lessons learned. Int J Pediatr Otorhinolaryngol 2014;78:264-267.
86. Koempel JA. Thyroglossal duct remnant surgery: a reliable, reproducible approach to the suprahyoid region. Int J Pediatr Otorhinolaryngol. 2014;78:1877-1882.
87. Rohof D, Honings J, Theunisse HJ, et al. Recurrences after thyroglossal duct cyst surgery: results in 207 consecutive cases and review of the literature. Head Neck 2015;37:1699-1704.
88. Turkyilmaz Z, Sonmez K, Karabulut R, et al. Management of thyroglossal duct cysts in children. Pediatr Int 2004;46:77-80.
89. Patel NN, Hartley BE, Howard DJ. Management of thyroglossal tract disease after failed Sistrunk's procedure. J Laryngol Otol 2003;117:710-712.
90. Pastore V, Bartoli F. "Extended" Sistrunk procedure in the treatment of recurrent thyroglossal duct cysts: a 10-year experience. Int J Pediatr Otorhinolaryngol 2014;78:1534-1536.
91. Bennett KG, Organ CH Jr, Wiliams GR. Is the treatment for thyroglossal duct cysts too extensive? Am J Surg 1986;152:602-605.
92. Maddalozzo J, Venkatesan TK, Gupta P. Complications associated with the Sistrunk procedure. Laryngoscope. 2001;111:119-123.

93. Cignarelli M, Ambrosi A, Marino A, Lamacchia O, Cincione R, Neri V. Three cases of papillary carcinoma and three of adenoma in thyroglossal duct cysts: clinical-diagnostic comparison with benign thyroglossal duct cysts. J Endocrinol Invest 2002;25:947-954.
94. Astl J, Duskova J, Kraus J, et al. Coincidence of thyroid tumor and thyroglossal duct remnants. Review of the literature and presentation of three cases. Tumori 2003;89:314-320.
95. Chrisoulidou A, Iliadou P, Doumala E, et al. Thyroglossal duct cyst carcinomas: is there a need for thyroidectomy? Hormones (Athens) 2013;12(4):522-528.
96. Doshi SV, Cruz RM, Hilsinger RL Jr. Thyroglossal duct carcinoma: a large case series. Ann Otol Rhinol Laryngol 2001;110:734-738.
97. Forest VI, Murali R, Clark JR. Thyroglossal duct cyst carcinoma: case series. J Otolaryngol Head Neck Surg 2011;40:151-156.
98. Patel SG, Escrig M, Shaha AR, Singh B, Shah JP. Management of well-differentiated thyroid carcinoma presenting within a thyroglossal duct cyst. J Surg Oncol 2002;79:134-139.
99. Ferrer C, Ferrandez A, Dualde D, et al. Squamous cell carcinoma of the thyroglossal duct cyst: report of a new case and literature review. J Otolaryngol 2000;29:311-314.
100. Jaques DA, Chambers RG, Oertel JE. Thyroglossal tract carcinoma. A review of the literature and addition of eighteen cases. Am J Surg 1970;120:439-446.
101. Köybasioglu F, Simsek GG, Onal BU. Tall cell variant of papillary carcinoma arising from a thyroglossal cyst: report of a case with diagnosis by fine needle aspiration cytology. Acta Cytol 2006;50:221-224.
102. LiVolsi VA, Perzin KH, Savetsky L. Carcinoma arising in median ectopic thyroid (including thyroglossal duct tissue). Cancer 1974;34:1303-1315.
103. Renard TH, Choucair RJ, Stevenson WD, Brooks WC, Poulos E. Carcinoma of the thyroglossal duct. Surg Gynecol Obstet 1990;171:305-308.
104. Shah S, Kadakia S, Khorsandi A, Andersen A, Iacob C, Shin E. Squamous cell carcinoma in a thyroglossal duct cyst: A case report with review of the literature. Am J Otolaryngol 2015;36:460-462.
105. Warner E, Ofo E, Connor S, Odell E, Jeannon JP. Mucoepidermoid carcinoma in a thyroglossal duct remnant. Int J Surg Case Rep 2015;13:43-47.
106. Weiss SD, Orlich CC. Primary papillary carcinoma of a thyroglossal duct cyst: report of a case and review of the literature. Br J Surg 1991;78:87-89.
107. Woods RH, Saunders JR, Pearlman S, Hirata RM, Jaques DA. Anaplastic carcinoma arising in a thyroglossal duct tract. Otolaryngol Head Neck Surg 1993;109:945-949.
108. Yanagisawa K, Eisen RN, Sasaki CT. Squamous cell carcinoma arising in a thyroglossal duct cyst. Arch Otolaryngol Head Neck Surg 1992;118:538-541.
109. Agarwal K, Puri V, Singh S. Critical appraisal of FNAC in the diagnosis of primary papillary carcinoma arising in thyroglossal cyst: a case report with review of the literature on FNAC and its diagnostic pitfalls. J Cytol 2010;27:22-25.
110. Miccoli P, Minuto MN, Galleri D, Puccini M, Berti P. Extent of surgery in thyroglossal duct carcinoma: reflections on a series of eighteen cases. Thyroid 2004;14:121-123.
111. Ozturk O, Demirci L, Egeli E, Cukur S, Belenli O. Papillary carcinoma of the thyroglossal duct cyst in childhood. Eur Arch Otorhinolaryngol. 2003;260:541-543.
112. Choi YM, Kim TY, Song DE, et al. Papillary thyroid carcinoma arising from a thyroglossal duct cyst: a single institution experience. Endocr J 2013;60:665-670.

Cervical Thymic Cyst

113. Zarbo RJ, McClatchey KD, Arcen RG, Baker SB. Thymopharyngeal duct cyst: a form of cervical thymoma. Ann Otol Rhinol Laryngol 1983;92:284-289.
114. Barat M, Sciubba JJ, Abramson AL. Cervical thymic cyst: case report and review of literature. Laryngoscope 1985;95:89-91.
115. De Caluwe D, Ahmed M, Puri P. Cervical thymic cysts. Pediatr Surg Int 2002;18:477-479.
116. Fahmy S. Cervical thymic cysts: their pathogenesis and relationship to branchail cysts. J Laryngol Otol 1974;88:47-60.
117. Sturm-O'Brien AK, Salazar JD, Byrd RH, et al. Cervical thymic anomalies—the Texas Children's Hospital experience. Laryngoscope 2009;119:1988-1993.
118. Ridder GJ, Boedeker CC, Kersten AC. Multilocular cervical thymic cysts in adults. A report of two cases and review of the literature. Eur Arch Otorhinolaryngol 2003;260:261-265.
119. Ibrahim M, Hammoud K, Maheshwari M, Pandya A. Congenital cystic lesions of the head and neck. Neuroimaging Clin N Am 2011;21:621-639.
120. Burton EM, Mercado-Deane MG, Howell CG, et al. Cervical thymic cysts: CT appearance of two cases including a persistent thymopharyngeal duct cyst. Pediatr Radiol 1995;25:363-365.

Bronchogenic Cysts

121. Verbin RS, Barnes L. Bronchogenic cysts. In: Barnes L, ed. Surgical Pathology of the head and neck, 2nd ed, revised and expanded. New York: Marcel Dekker; 2001:1501-1504.
122. Abell MR. Mediastinal cysts. AMA Arch Pathol 1956;61:360-379.

123. Eraklis AJ, Griscom NT, McGovern JB. Bronchogenic cysts of the mediastinum in infancy. N Engl J Med 1969;281:1150-1155.
124. Travis WD, Colby TV, Koss MN, Rosado-de-Christenson ML, Müller NL, King TE Jr. Nonneoplastic disorders of the lower respiratory tract. AFIP Atlas of Nontumor Pathology, 1st Series, Fascicle 2. Washington, DC: American Registry of Pathology; 2002:478-481.
125. Fraga S, Helwig EB, Rosen SH. Bronchogenic cysts in the skin and subcutaneous tissue. Am J Clin Pathol 1971;56:230-238.
126. Newkirk KA, Tassler AB, Krowiak EJ, Deeb ZE. Bronchogenic cysts of the neck in adults. Ann Otol Rhinol Laryngol 2004;113:691-695.
127. Teissier N, Elmaleh-Bergès M, Ferkdadji L, François M, Van den Abbeele T. Cervical bronchogenic cysts: usual and unusual clinical presentations. Arch Otolaryngol Head Neck Surg 2008;134:1165-1169.
128. Ustundag E, Iseri M, Keskin G, Yayla B, Muezzinoglu B. Cervical bronchogenic cysts in head and neck region. J Laryngol Otol 2005;119:419-423.
129. Sarper A, Ayten A, Golbasi I, Demircan A, Isin E. Bronchogenic cyst. Tex Heart Inst J 2003;30:105-108.
130. Goswamy J, de Kruijf S, Humphrey G, Rothera MP, Bruce IA. Bronchogenic cysts as a cause of infantile stridor: case report and literature review. J Laryngol Otol 2011;125:1094-1097.
131. Lazar RH, Younis RT, Bassila MN. Bronchogenic cysts: a cause of stridor in the neonate. Am J Otolaryngol 1991;12:117-121.
132. Yerman HM, Holinger LD. Bronchogenic cyst with tracheal involvement. Ann Otol Rhinol Laryngol 1990;99:89-93.
133. Niño-Hernández LM, Arteta-Acosta C, Redondo-de Oro K, Alcalá-Cerra L, Redondo-Bermúdez C, Marrugo-Grace O. Cervical bronchogenic cyst mimicking thyroglossal cyst: case report and literature review. Cir Cir 2011;79:330-333.
134. Tripp HF, Reames MK. Resection of a bronchogenic cyst involving the wall of the mainstem bronchus and repair utilizing a pedicled pericardial flap. Am Surg 1997;63:785-787.
135. Wenig BL, Abramson AL. Tracheal bronchogenic cyst: a new clinical entity? Ann Otol Rhinol Laryngol 1987;96:58-60.
136. Briganti V, Molle P, Miele V, Vallasciani S, Calisti A. [Intramural esophageal bronchogenic cyst: an unusual cause of dysphagia in pediatric patients. Report of a case.] Cir Pediatr 2003;16:99-101. [Spanish]
137. Kawase Y, Takahashi M, Takemura H, Tomita S, Watanabe G. Surgical treatment of a bronchogenic cyst in the interatrial septum. Ann Thorac Surg 2002;74:1695-1697.
138. Prates PR, Lovato L, Homsi-Neto A, et al. Right ventricular bronchogenic cyst. Tex Heart Inst J 2003;30:71-73.
139. Sedwick JD, Giannoni C. Bronchogenic cyst of the oropharynx and hypopharynx in a neonate. Otolaryngol Head Neck Surg 2001l;125:105-106.
140. Hadi UM, Jammal HN, Hamdan AL, Saad AM, Zaatari GS. Lateral cervical bronchogenic cyst: an unusual cause of a lump in the neck. Head Neck 2001;23:590-593.
141. Rapado F, Bennett JD, Stringfellow JM. Bronchogenic cyst: an unusual cause of lump in the neck. J Laryngol Otol 1998;112:893-4.
142. Ashizawa K, Okimoto T, Shirafuji T, Kusano H, Ayabe H, Hayashi K. Anterior mediastinal bronchogenic cyst: demonstration of complicating malignancy by CT and MRI. Br J Radiol 2001;74:959-961.
143. de Perrot M, Pache JC, Spiliopoulos A. Carcinoma arising in congenital lung cysts. Thorac Cardiovasc Surg 2001;49:184-185.
144. Endo C, Imai T, Nakagawa H, Ebina A, Kaimori M. Bronchioloalveolar carcinoma arising in a bronchogenic cyst. Ann Thorac Surg 2000;69:933-935.
145. Miralles Lozano F, Gonzalez-Martinez B, Luna More S, Valencia Rodriguez A. Carcinoma arising in a calcified bronchogenic cyst. Respiration 1981;42:135-137.
146. Sullivan SM, Okada S, Kudo M, Ebihara Y. A retroperitoneal bronchogenic cyst with malignant change. Pathol Int 1999;49:338-341.

Dermoid Cyst

147. McAvoy JM, Zuckerbraun L. Dermoid cysts of the head and neck in children. Arch Otolaryngol. 1976;102:529-531.
148. Taylor BW, Erich JB, Dockerty MD. Dermoids of the head and neck. Minn Med 1966;49:1535-1540.
149. Coppit GL 3rd, Perkins JA, Manning SC. Nasopharyngeal teratomas and dermoids: a review of the literature and case series. Int J Pediatr Otorhinolaryngol 2000;52:219-227.
150. Rosen D, Wirtschafter A, Rao VM, Wilcox TO Jr. Dermoid cyst of the lateral neck: a case report and literature review. Ear Nose Throat J 1998;77:129-132.
151. Smirniotopoulos JG, Chiechi MV. Teratomas, dermoids, and epidermoids of the head and neck. Radiographics 1995;15:1437-1455.
152. Diercks GR, Iannuzzi RA, McCowen K, Sadow PM. Dermoid cyst of the lateral neck associated with the thyroid gland: a case report and review of the literature. Endocr Pathol 2013;24:45-48.

Mycobacterial Infections

153. Alvarez S, McCabe E. Extrapulmonary tuberculosis revisited: a review of experience at Boston City and other hospitals. Medicine (Baltimore) 1984;63:25-55.
154. Srirompotong S, Yimtae K, Srirompotong S. Tuberculosis in the upper aerodigestive tract and human immunodeficiency virus coinfections. J Otolaryngol 2003;32:230-233.
155. Basal Y, Ermisler B, Eryilmaz A, Ertugrul B. Two rare cases of head and neck tuberculosis. BMJ Case Rep 2015;23;2015.
156. Bruzgielewicz A, Rzepakowska A, Osuch-Wójcikewicz E, Niemczyk K, Chmielewski R. Tuberculosis of the head and neck—epidemiological and clinical presentation. Arch Med Sci 2014;10:1160-1166.
157. Chopra RK, Kerner MM, Calcaterra TC. Primary nasopharyngeal tuberculosis: a case report and review of this rare entity. Otolaryngol Head Neck Surg 1994;111:820-823.
158. Cleary KR, Batsakis JG. Mycobacterial disease of the head and neck: current perspective. Ann Otol Rhinol Laryngol 1995;104:830-833.
159. Hajioff D, Snow MH, Thaker H, Wilson JA. Primary tuberculosis of the posterior oropharyngeal wall. J Laryngol Otol 1999;113:1029-1030.
160. Hale RG, Tucker DI. Head and neck manifestations of tuberculosis. Oral Maxillofac Surg Clin North Am 2008;20:635-642.
161. Harrison NK, Knight RK. Tuberculosis of the nasopharynx misdiagnosed as Wegener's granulomatosis. Thorax 1986;41:219-220.
162. Kim YH, Jeong WJ, Jung KY, Sung MW, Kim KH, Kim CS. Diagnosis of major salivary gland tuberculosis: experience of eight cases and review of the literature. Acta Otolaryngol 2005;125:1318-1322.
163. Kim KY, Bae JH, Park JS, Lee SS. Primary sinonasal tuberculosis confeind to the unilateral maxillary sinus. Int J Clin Exp Pathol 2014 15;7:815-818.
164. Khuzwayo ZB, Naidu TK. Head and neck tuberculosis in KwaZulu-Natal, South Africa. J Laryngol Otol 2014;128:86-90.
165. Kurokawa M, Nibu K, Ichimura K, Nishino H. Laryngeal tuberculosis: A report of 17 cases. Auris Nasus Larynx 2015;42:305-310.
166. Nalini B, Vinayak S. Tuberculosis in ear, nose, and throat practice: its presentation and diagnosis. Am J Otolaryngol 2006;27:39-45.
167. Selimoglu E, Sutbeyaz Y, Ciftcioglu MA, Parlak M, Esrefoglu M, Ozturk A. Primary tonsillar tuberculosis: a case report. J Laryngol Otol 1995;109:880-882.
168. Srirompotong S, Yimtae K, Srirompotong S. Clinical aspects of tonsillar tuberculosis. Southeast Asian J Trop Med Public Health. 2002;33:147-150.
169. Waldron J, Van Hasselt CA, Skinner DW, Arnold M. Tuberculosis of the nasopharynx: clinicopathological features. Clin Otolaryngol 1992;17:57-59.
170. Wang WC, Chen JY, Chen YK, Lin LM. Tuberculosis of the head and neck: a review of 20 cases. Oral Surg Oral Med Oral Pathol Oral Radiol Endod 2009;107:381-386.
171. Wang SY, Zhu JX. [Primary mucosal tuberculosis of head and neck region: a clinicopathologic analysis of 47 cases.] Zhonghua Bing Li Xue Za Zhi 2013;42:683-686. [Chinese]
172. Oishi M, Okamoto S, Teranishi Y, Yokota C, Takano S, Iguchi H. Clinical study of extrapulmonary head and neck tuberculosis: a single-instiute 10-year experience. Int Arch Otorhinolaryngol 2016;20:30-33.
173. Caroppo D, Russo D, Merolla F, et al. A rare case of coexistence of metastasis from head and neck squamous cell carcinoma and tuberculosis within a neck lymph node. Diagn Pathol 2015;10:197.
174. Wu KC, Chen BN. Mycobacterial tuberculosis superimposed on a Warthin tumor. Ear Nose Throat J 2012;91:E4-E6.
175. van Zyl L, du Plessis J, Viljoen J. Cutaneous tuberculosis overview and current treatment regimens. Tuberculosis (Edinb) 2015;95:629-638.
176. Woods GL. Mycobacteria. In: McPherson RA, Pincus MR, eds. Henry's clinical diagnosis and management by laboratory methods, 22nd ed. Philadelphia: Elsevier Saunders; 2011:1145-1154.
177. Horsburgh CR Jr, Barry CE 3rd, Lange C. Treatment of tuberculosis. N Engl J Med 2015;373:2149-2160.

Scrofula

178. Saitz EW. Cervical lymphadenitis caused by atypical mycobacteria. Pediatr Clin North Am 1981;28:823-839.
179. Albright JT, Pransky SM. Nontuberculous mycobacterial infections of the head and neck. Pediatr Clin North Am 2003;50:503-514.
180. Bayazit YA, Bayazit N, Namiduru M. Mycobacterial cervical lymphadenitis. ORL J Otorhinolaryngol Relat Spec 2004;66:275-80.
181. Munck K, Mandpe AH. Mycobacterial infections of the head and neck. Otolaryngol Clin North Am 2003;36:569-576.
182. Ablanedo-Terrazas Y, Alvarado-de la Barrera C, Ormsby CE, Reyes-Terán G. Head and neck manifestations of the immune reconstitution syndrome in HIV-infected patients: a cohort study. Otolaryngol Head Neck Surg 2012;147:52-56.
183. Moon WK, Han MH, Chang KH, et al. CT and MR imaging of head and neck tuberculosis. Radiographics 1997;17:391-402.

184. Shrestha NK, Tuohy MJ, Hall GS, Reischl U, Gordon SM, Procop GW. Detection and differentiation of Mycobacterium tuberculosis and nontuberculous mycobacterial isolates by real-time PCR. J Clin Microbiol 2003;41:5121-5126.
185. Bezabih M, Mariam DW, Selassie SG. Fine needle aspiration cytology of suspected tuberculous lymphadenitis. Cytopathology 2002;13:284-290.
186. Handa U, Palta A, Mohan H, Punia RP. Fine needle aspiration diagnosis of tuberculous lymphadenitis. Trop Doct 2002;32:147-149.
187. Esteban J, García-Pedrazuela M, Muñoz-Egea MC, Alcaide F. Current treatment of nontuberculous mycobacteriosis: an update. Expert Opin Pharmacother 2012;13:967-986.

Mycobacterial Spindle Cell Pseudotumor

188. Brandwein M, Choi HS, Strauchen J, Stoler M, Jagirdar J. Spindle cell reaction to nontuberculous mycobacteriosis in AIDS mimicking a spindle cell neoplasia. Evidence for dual histiocytic and fibroblastic-like characteristics of spindle cells. Virchows Arch A Pathol Anal Histopathol 1990;416;281-286.
189. Chen KT. Mycobacterial spindle cell pseudotumor of lymph nodes. Am J Surg Pathol 1992;16:276-281.
190. Logani S, Lucas DR, Cheng JD, Ioachim HL, Adsay NV. Spindle cell tumors associated with mycobacteria in lymph nodes of HIV-positive patients: 'Kaposi sarcoma with mycobacteria' and 'mycobacterial pseudotumor'. Am J Surg Pathol 1999;23:656-661.
191. Umlas J, Federman M, Crawford C, O'Hara CJ, Fitzgibbon JS, Modeste A. Spindle cell pseudotumor due to Mycobacterium avium-intracellulare in patients with acquired immunodeficiency syndrome (AIDS). Positive staining of mycobacteria for cytoskeleton filaments. Am J Surg Pathol 1991;15:1181-1187.
192. Rahmani M, Alroy J, Zoukhri D, Wein RO, Tischler AS. Mycobacterial pseudotumor of the skin. Virchows Arch 2013;463:843-846.
193. Wolf DA, Wu CD, Medeiros LJ. Mycobacterial pseudotumors of lymph node. A report of two cases diagnosed at the time of intraoperative consultation using touch imprint preparations. Arch Pathol Lab Med 1995;119:811-814.
194. Wood C, Nickoloff BJ, Todes-Taylor NR. Pseudotumor resulting from atypical mycobacterial infection: a "histoid" variety of Mycobacterium avium-intracellulare complex infection. Am J Clin Pathol 1985;83:524-527.
195. Yin HL, Zhou XJ, Wu JP, Meng K, Sun YM. Mycobacterial spindle cell pseudotumor of lymph nodes after receiving Bacille Calmette-Guerin (BCG) vaccination. Chin Med J (Engl) 2004;117:308-310.
196. Gunia S, Behrens MH, Stosiek P. Mycobacterial spindle cell pseudotumor (MSP) of the nasal septum clinically mimicking Kaposi's sarcoma: case report. Rhinology 2005;43:70-71.
197. Ilyas S, Youssef D, Chaudhary H, Al-Abbadi MA. Myocbacterium-avium intracellulare associated inflammatory pseudotumor of the anterior nasal cavity. Head Neck Pathol 2011;5:296-301.
198. Ohara K, Kimura T, Sakamoto K, Okada Y. Non-tuberculous mycobacteria-associated spindle cell pseudotumor of the nasal cavity: a case report. Pathol Int 2013;63:266-271.

Actinomycosis

199. Bennhoff DF. Actinomycosis: diagnostic and therapeutic considerations and a review of 32 cases. Laryngoscope 1984;94:1198-1217.
200. Valour F, Sénéchal A, Dupieux C, et al. Actinomycosis: etiology, clinical features, diagnosis, treatment, and management. Infect Drug Resist 2014;7:183-197.
201. Nielsen PM, Novak A. Acute cervico-facial actinomycosis. Int J Oral Maxillofac Surg 1987;16:440-444.
202. Custal-Teixidor M, Tull-Gimbernat JM, Garijo-Lopez G, Valldosera-Rosello M. Fine-needle aspiration cytology in the diagnosis of cervicofacial actinomycosis: report of 15 cases. Med Oral Patol Oral Cir Bucal 2004;9:464-470.
203. Das DK. Actinomycosis in fine needle aspiration cytology. Cytopathology 1994;5:243-250.
204. Boyanova L, Kolarov R, Mateva L, Markovska R, Mitov I. Actinomycoiss: a frequently forgotten disease. Future Microbiol 2015;10:613-628.
205. Moghimi M, Salentijn E, Debets-Ossenkop Y, Karagozoglu KH, Forouzanfar T. Treatment of Cervicofacial actinomycosis: a report of 19 cases and review of literature. Med Oral Patol Oral Cir Bucal 2013;18:e627-632.

Cat Scratch Disease

206. Wear DJ, Margileth AW, Hadfield TL, Fisher GW, Schlagel CJ, King FM. Cat scratch disease: a bacterial infection. Science 1983;221:1403-1405.
207. Rostad CA, McElroy AK, Hilinski JA, et al. Bartonella henselae-mediated disease in solid organ transplant recipients: two pediatric cases and a literature review. Transpl Infect Dis 2012;14:E71-E81.
208. Carithers HA. Cat-scratch disease: an overview based on a study of 1200 patients. Am J Dis Child 1985;139:1124-33.
209. Ridder GJ, Boedeker CC, Technau-Ihlking K, Sander A. Cat-scratch disease: Otolaryngologic manifestations and management. Otolaryngol Head Neck Surg 2005;132:353-358.

210. Margileth AW, Wear DJ, English CK. Systemic cat scratch disease: report of 23 patients with prolonged or recurrent severe bacterial infection. J Infect Dis 1987;155:390-402.
211. Maguiña C, Guerra H, Ventosilla P. Bartonellosis. Clin Dermatol 2009;27:271-280.
212. Miller-Catchpole R, Variakojis D, Vardiman JW, Loew JM, Carter J. Cat scratch disease: identification of bacteria in seven cases of lymphadenitis. Am J Surg Pathol 1986;10:276-281.
213. Prutsky G, Domecq JP, Mori L, et al. Treatment outcomes of human bartonellosis: a systematic review and meta-analysis. Int J Infect Dis 2013;17:e811-e819.

Bacillary Angiomatosis

214. LeBoit PE, Berger TG, Egbert BM, Beckstead JH, Yen TS, Stoler MH. Bacillary angiomatosis. The histopathology and differential diagnosis of a pseudoneoplastic infection in patients with human immunodeficiency virus disease. Am J Surg Pathol 1989;13:909-920.
215. LeBoit PE. Bacillary angiomatosis: a systemic opportunistic infection with prominent cutaneous manifestations. Semin Dermatol 1991;10:194-198.
216. Spach DH, Koehler JE. Bartonella-associated infections. Infect Dis Clin North Am 1998;12:137-155.
217. Tsang WY, Chan JK. Bacillary angiomatosis. A "new" disease with a broadening clinicopathologic spectrum. Histol Histopathol 1992;7:143-152.
218. Batsakis JG, Ro JY, Frauenhoffer EE. Bacillary angiomatosis. Ann Otol Rhinol Laryngol 1995; 104:668-672.
219. Greenspan D, Greenspan JS. Oral manifestations of HIV infection. AIDS Clin Care 1997;9: 29-33.
220. Lopez de Blanc S, Sambuelli R, Femopase F, et al. Bacillary angiomatosis affecting the oral cavity. Report of two cases and review. J Oral Pathol Med 2000;29:91-96.
221. Matar GM, Koehler JE, Malcolm G, et al. Identification of Bartonella species directly in clinical specimens by PCR-restriction fragment length polymorphism analysis of a 16S rRNA gene fragment. J Clin Microbiol 1999;37:4045-4047.
222. Cline MS, Cummings OW, Goldman M, Filo RS, Pescovitz MD. Bacillary angiomatosis in a renal transplant recipient. Transplantation 1999;67:296-298.
223. Juskevicius R, Vnencak-Jones C. Pathologic quiz case: a 17-year-old renal transplant patient with persistent fever, pancytopenia, and axillary lymphadenopathy. Bacillary angiomatosis of the lymph node in the renal transplant recipient. Arch Pathol Lab Med 2004;128:e12-14.
224. Psarros G, Riddell J 4th, Gandhi T, Kauffman CA, Cinti SK. Bartonella henselae infections in solid organ transplant recipients: report of 5 cases and review of the literature. Medicine (Baltimore) 2012;91:111-121.
225. Schwartz RA, Gallardo MA, Kapila R, et al. Bacillary angiomatosis in an HIV seronegative patient on systemic steroid therapy. Br J Dermatol 1996;135:982-987.
226. Berger TG, Tappero JW, Kaymen A, LeBoit PE. Bacillary (epithelioid) angiomatosis and concurrent Kaposi's sarcoma in acquired immunodeficiency syndrome. Arch Dermatol 1989;125:1543-1547.
227. Rosales CM, McLaughlin MD, Sata T, et al. AIDS presenting with cutaneous Kaposi's sarcoma and bacillary angiomatosis in the bone marrow mimicking Kaposi's sarcoma. AIDS Patient Care STDS 2002;16:573-577.
228. Steeper TA, Rosenstein H, Weiser J, Inampudi S, Snover DC. Bacillary epithelioid angiomatosis involving the liver, spleen, and skin in an AIDS patient with concurrent Kaposi's sarcoma. Am J Clin Pathol 1992;97:713-718.
229. Edmonson BC, Morris WR, Osborn FD. Bacillary angiomatosis with cytomegaloviral and mycobacterial infections of the palpebral conjunctiva in a patient with AIDS. Ophthal Plast Reconstr Surg 2004;20:168-170.
230. Bernabeu-Wittel J, Luque R, Corbi R, et al. Bacillary angiomatosis with atypical clinical presentation in an immunocompetent patient. Indian J Dermatol Venereol Leprol 2010;76:682-685.
231. Cockerell CJ, Bergstresser PR, Myrie-Williams C, Tierno PM. Bacillary epithelioid angiomatosis occurring in an immunocompetent individual. Arch Dermatol 1990;126:787-790.
232. Kayaselcuk F, Ceken I, Bircan S, Tuncer I. Bacillary angiomatosis of the scalp in a human immunodeficiency virus-negative patient. J Eur Acad Dermatol Venereol 2002;16:612-614.
233. Smith KJ, Skelton HG, Tuur S, Larson PL, Angritt P. Bacillary angiomatosis in an immunocompetent child. Am J Dermatopathol 1996;18:597-600.
234. Zarraga M, Rosen L, Herschthal D. Bacillary angiomatosis in an immunocompetent child: a case report and review of the literature. Am J Dermatopathol. 2011;33:513-515.
235. Agan BK, Dolan MJ. Laboratory diagnosis of Bartonella infections. Clin Lab Med 2002;22:937-962.
236. Koehler JE, Sanchez MA, Garrido CS, et al. Molecular epidemiology of bartonella infections in patients with bacillary angiomatosis-peliosis. N Engl J Med 1997;337:1876-1883.
237. Eberhardt C, Engelmann S, Kusch H, et al. Proteomic analysis of the bacterial pathogen Bartonella henselae and identification of immunogenic proteins for serodiagnosis. Proteomics 2009;9:1967-1681.

238. Cheuk W, Wong KO, Wong CS, Dinkel JE, Ben-Dor D, Chan JK. Immunostaining for human herpesvirus 8 latent nuclear antigen-1 helps distinguish Kaposi sarcoma from its mimickers. Am J Clin Pathol 2004;121:335-342.
239. Nayler SJ, Allard U, Taylor L, Cooper K. HHV-8 (KSHV) is not associated with bacillary angiomatosis. Mol Pathol 1999;52:345-348.
240. Relman DA, Fredricks DN, Yoder KE, Mirowski G, Berger T, Koehler JE. Absence of Kaposi's sarcoma-associated herpesvirus DNA in bacillary angiomatosis-peliosis lesions. J Infect Dis 1999;180:1386-1389.
241. Maguina C, Gotuzzo E. Bartonellosis. New and old. Infect Dis Clin North Am 2000;14:1-22.

Sarcoidosis

242. Wenig BM, Devaney K, Wenig BL. Pseudoneoplastic lesions of the oropharynx and larynx simulating cancer. Pathol Annu 1995;30(Pt 1):143-187.
243. Alawi F. Granulomatous diseases of the oral tissues: differential diagnosis and update. Dent Clin North Am 2005;49:203-221.
244. Badhey AK, Kadakia S, Carrau RL, Iacob C, Khorsandi A. Sarcoidosis of the head and neck. Head Neck Pathol 2015;9:260-268.
245. Cleary KR, Batsakis JG. Orofacial granulomatosis and Crohn's disease. Ann Otol Rhinol Laryngol 1996;105:166-167.
246. Eveson JW. Granulomatous disorders of the oral mucosa. Semin Diagn Pathol 1996;13:118-127.
247. Serrat Soto A, Lobo Valentin L, Redonod Gonzalez LM, Sanz Santa Cruz C, Verrier Hernandez A. Oral sarcoidosis with tongue involvement. Oral Surg Oral Med Oral Pathol Oral Radiol Endod 1997;83:668-671.
248. Abdel-Galiil K, Anand R, Sharma S, Brennan PA, Ramchandani PL, Ilankovan V. Incidence of sarcoidosis in head and neck cancer. Br J Oral Maxillofac Surg 2008;46:59-60.
249. Aloulah M, Manes RP, Ng YH, et al. Sinonasal manifestations of sarcoidosis: a single institution experience with 38 cases. Int Forum Allergy Rhinol 2013;3:567-572.
250. Lieberman J. The specificity and nature of serum-angiotensin-converting enzyme (serum ACE) elevations in sarcoidosis. Ann N Y Acad Sci 1976;278:488-497.
251. Shultz T, Miller WC, Bedrossian CW. Clinical application of measurement of angiotensin-converting enzyme level. JAMA 1979;242:439-441.
252. Brownell I, Ramírez-Valle F, Sanchez M, Prystowsky S. Evidence for mycobacteria in sarcoidosis. Am J Respir Cell Mol Biol. 2011;45:899-905.
253. Du Bois RM, Goh N, McGrath D, Cullinan P. Is there a role for microorganisms in the pathogenesis of sarcoidosis? J Intern Med 2003;253:4-17.
254. Fidler HM. Mycobacteria and sarcoidosis. Recent advances. Sarcoidosis 1994;11:66-68.
255. Gupta D, Agarwal R, Aggarwal AN, Jindal SK. Sarcoidosis and tuberculosis: the same disease with different manifestations or similar manifestations of different disorders. Curr Opin Pulm Med 2012;18:506-516.
256. Hance AJ. The role of mycobacteria in the pathogenesis of sarcoidosis. Semin Respir Infect 1998;13:197-205.
257. Li N, Bajoghli A, Kubba A, Bhawan J. Identification of mycobacterial DNA in cutaneous lesions of sarcoidosis. J Cutan Pathol 1999;26:271-278.
258. Oswald-Richter KA, Drake WP. The etiologic role of infectious antigens in sarcoidosis pathogenesis. Semin Respir Crit Care Med 2010;31:375-379.
259. Popper HH, Klemen H, Hoefler G, Winter E. Presence of mycobacterial DNA in sarcoidosis. Hum Pathol 1997;28:796-800.
260. Wong CF, Yew WW, Wong PC, Lee J. A case of concomitant tuberculosis and sarcoidosis with mycobacterial DNA present in the sarcoid lesion. Chest 1998;114:626-629.
261. Wennerström A, Pietinalho A, Lasota J, et al. Major histocompatibility complex class II and BTNL2 associations in sarcoidosis. Eur Respir J 2013;42:550-553.
262. Hofmann S, Franke A, Fischer A, et al. Genome-wide association study identifies ANXA11 as a new susceptibility locus for sarcoidosis. Nat Genet 2008;40:1103-1106.
263. Morais A, Lima B, Peixoto MJ, Alves H, Marques A, Delgado L. BTNL2 gene polymorphism associations with susceptibility and phenotype expression in sarcoidosis. Respir Med 2012;106:1771-1777.

5 LARYNX AND TRACHEA

By Drs. Raja R. Seethala and Lester D. R. Thompson

EMBRYOLOGY, ANATOMY, AND HISTOLOGY: LARYNX

Embryology

The epithelium and glands of the larynx arise from the endoderm lining the laryngotracheal groove (1,2). The supraglottic larynx arises from the 3rd and 4th branchial arches, while the glottis and subglottic larynx arise from the 6th branchial arch. The cartilage, muscle, and other connective tissue elements develop from the mesenchyme around the foregut. The thyroid, cricoid, arytenoid, corniculate, and cuneiform cartilages derive from the 4th and 6th branchial arches; the greater cornu and inferior part of the body of the hyoid bone derive from the 3rd branchial arch; the lesser cornu and superior part of the body of the hyoid bone derive from the 2nd branchial arch; the intrinsic muscles of the larynx muscles derive from the 4th and 6th branchial arches; and the superior laryngeal and recurrent laryngeal nerves (both branches of the vagus nerve) are derived from the 4th and 6th branchial arches.

Anatomy

Anatomic Borders. The superior border of the larynx is the tip of the epiglottis, the inferior border is the inferior rim of the cricoid cartilage. The anterior border is the lingual surface of the epiglottis (vallecula), thyrohyoid membrane, anterior commissure, thyroid cartilage, cricothyroid membrane, and anterior arch of the cricoid cartilage. The posterior border is the posterior commissure, arytenoid and interarytenoid space, and mucoperichondrium overlying the cricoid cartilage. The lateral border is the aryepiglottic folds (1,3).

Anatomic Compartments. The supraglottic larynx extends from the tip of the epiglottis to a horizontal line passing through the apex of the ventricle. Structures within this compartment are the epiglottis (lingual and laryngeal aspects), aryepiglottic folds, arytenoids, false vocal cords, and ventricle (fig. 5-1).

The glottic portion of the larynx extends from the ventricle to 1 cm below the free level of the true vocal cord and includes the anterior and posterior commissures and the true vocal

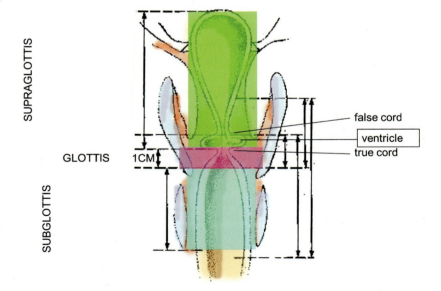

Figure 5-1

ANATOMIC COMPARTMENTS OF THE LARYNX

The supraglottis (green) extends from the tip of the epiglottis to a horizontal line through the apex of the ventricle. The glottis (magenta) extends from this line to 1 cm inferiorly and encompasses the vocal cords. The subglottis (cyan) then extends from this line to the inferior rim of the cricoid cartilage (Adapted from figure 51 from Barnes L. Diseases of the larynx, hypopharynx, and trachea. In: Barnes L, ed. Surgical pathology of the head and neck, 3rd ed. New York: Informa Healthcare; 2009:137.

cord. There is no specific anatomic or histologic structure that forms the inferior boundary of the glottis. The anterior commissure represents a confluence of the vocalis ligament, thyroepiglottic ligament, and perichondrium of the thyroid cartilage to form Broyles ligament (or anterior commissure tendon).

The subglottic larynx extends from 1 cm below the level of the true vocal cord to the inferior rim of the cricoid cartilage. As noted above, the superior border does not have a defining anatomic or histologic structure.

The pre-epiglottic and paraglottic spaces are not actually spaces, but are loose fibroadipose tissues rich in blood vessels. These are of minimal significance in non-neoplastic diseases. Briefly, the pre-epiglottic space is the soft tissue anterior and surrounding the epiglottis, bounded inferiorly to some extent by the thyroepiglottic ligament (4). The paraglottic space is the adipose tissue bounded laterally by the thyroid cartilage and inferomedially by the conus elasticus of the vocal cord. It is beneath but somewhat continuous with the pre-epiglottic space since it is separated by a discontinuous collagen layer (5,6).

Histology

Nonkeratinizing stratified squamous epithelium lines the epiglottis and true vocal cord. Pseudostratified ciliated respiratory epithelium lines the false vocal cord, ventricle, subglottis.

The lining of the supraglottis varies depending on environmental exposure and smoking and drinking status (7–10). The epiglottis, which is more prone to mechanical irritation physiologically, is lined by nonkeratinizing squamous epithelium, while the false cords and ventricle are still lined by respiratory-type epithelium (fig. 5-2). Seromucous glands are present in the supraglottis and prominent in the false cord. Seromucous glands are found in the lower two thirds of the epiglottis and in the ventricular submucosa. The lingual surface of the epiglottis may have varying degrees of lymphoid tonsillar-type stroma extending from the oropharynx.

The true vocal cord is the first structure to squamatize, and is lined by nonkeratinizing stratified squamous epithelium throughout life (fig. 5-2). At birth, the submucosa and vocalis ligament are absent. It is theorized that phonation induces vocal fold stellate cells in the macula flava anterior and posterior cords to produce the extracellular matrix and cytoskeletal alterations required to form the characteristic layered appearance of the adult vocal cord. This consists of submucosa and the vocalis ligament to which the vocalis muscle, a portion of the thyroarytenoid muscle, is tethered (11,12). The specialized submucosa/lamina propria is called the Reinke space and consists of a loose paucicellular myxoid stroma, largely devoid of vessels and lymphatics, and serves as an oncologic barrier to early tumors. It is the compartment involved in vocal cord nodules.

As the matrix is rich in hyaluronic acids, under repeated injury, true chondroid metaplasia may occur. Chondroid metaplasia is usually an incidental finding unassociated with any symptoms, appearing as a single small circumscribed or delineated, nonlobulated cartilaginous nodule (fig. 5-2). It is composed of elastic-type cartilage and typically occurs in the mid and posterior portions of the vocal cord, but may occur in other areas of the larynx (e.g., false cord) and hypopharynx (e.g., piriform sinus). In association with chondroid metaplasia, there may be increased cellularity (as compared to normal cartilage), including binucleated chondrocytes, but no significant cytologic atypia or increased mitotic activity. Associated ossification may be present (fig. 5-2). There is no specific connection between the foci of chondroid metaplasia to the cartilaginous framework, and histologically the nodule merges at the periphery with the surrounding soft tissue (fig. 5-2). The absence of lobulation, absence of connection to the cartilaginous framework, presence of elastic rather than hyaline-type cartilage, and the merging with surrounding soft tissues assist in differentiating chondroid metaplasia from cartilaginous neoplasms (e.g., chondroma and chondrosarcoma).

Posterior to the vocalis muscle (not considered within the paraglottic space) (13) is a bit of the paraglottic space. The perichondrium of the thyroid cartilage is posterior as well.

The subglottis is mainly lined by respiratory-type epithelium and contains seromucinous glands in the submucosa (fig. 5-3). Immature-type epithelium, referred to as intermediate or transitional-type epithelium, may be found

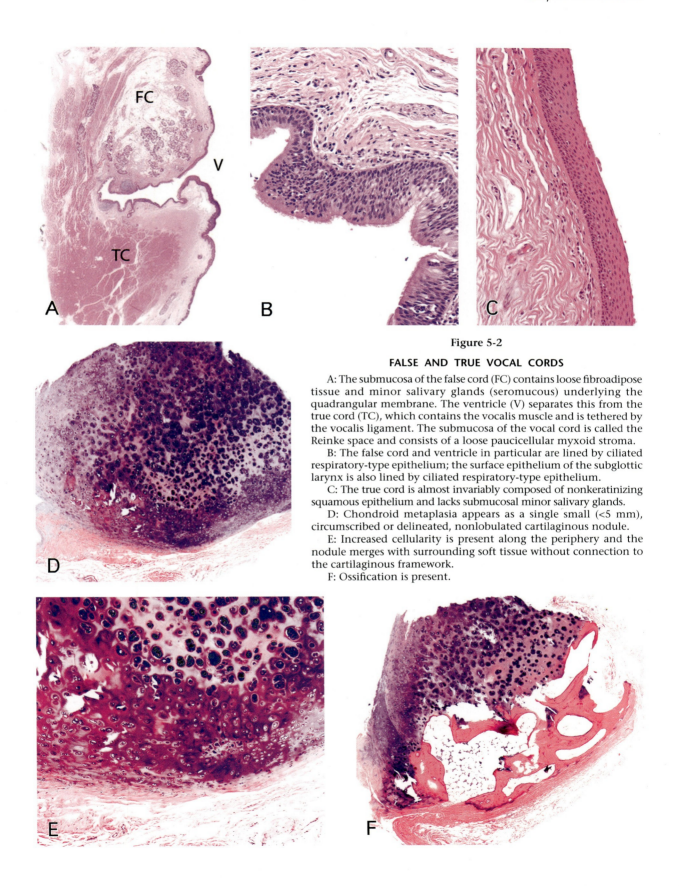

Figure 5-2

FALSE AND TRUE VOCAL CORDS

A: The submucosa of the false cord (FC) contains loose fibroadipose tissue and minor salivary glands (seromucous) underlying the quadrangular membrane. The ventricle (V) separates this from the true cord (TC), which contains the vocalis muscle and is tethered by the vocalis ligament. The submucosa of the vocal cord is called the Reinke space and consists of a loose paucicellular myxoid stroma.

B: The false cord and ventricle in particular are lined by ciliated respiratory-type epithelium; the surface epithelium of the subglottic larynx is also lined by ciliated respiratory-type epithelium.

C: The true cord is almost invariably composed of nonkeratinizing squamous epithelium and lacks submucosal minor salivary glands.

D: Chondroid metaplasia appears as a single small (<5 mm), circumscribed or delineated, nonlobulated cartilaginous nodule.

E: Increased cellularity is present along the periphery and the nodule merges with surrounding soft tissue without connection to the cartilaginous framework.

F: Ossification is present.

Non-Neoplastic Diseases of the Head and Neck

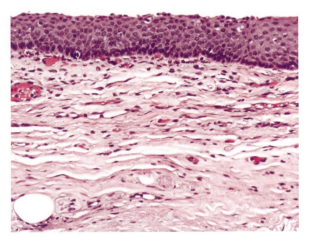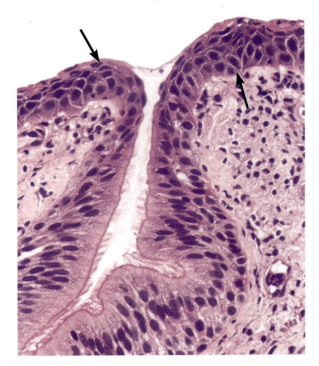

Figure 5-3

SUBGLOTTIC LARYNX

Left: The transitional zone from glottis to subglottis demonstrates more basaloid hyperchromatic epithelium, although still devoid of atypia.

Right: The epithelium (arrows) transitioning to the normal ciliated respiratory-type epithelium shows some disorganization and hyperchromasia, worrisome for dysplasia.

in the transitional zone between the glottis and subglottis. It is identified between the ciliated respiratory epithelium of the supraglottis or subglottis and the squamous epithelium of the true vocal cord. The transitional-type epithelium appears abruptly; is predominantly composed of basaloid or immature squamous cells with hypercellularity, disorganization, absence of maturation, and increased nuclear to cytoplasmic ratio; and may be misdiagnosed on biopsy or by frozen section as severe dysplasia or carcinoma in situ (CIS) (fig. 5-3). In contrast to the latter, the cells are devoid of cytonuclear atypia and mitotic activity.

Deep to the true the vocal cord lies the vocal ligament, thickened elastic tissue lying under the free edge of vocal cord (fig. 5-4). The vocal ligament inserts on the thyroid cartilage anteriorly and the vocal process of arytenoid cartilage posteriorly. Biopsies taken in this anatomic location may include the vocal cord ligament, which if unrecognized, may be misdiagnosed as a cartilaginous neoplasm, myxoma, or peripheral nerve sheath neoplasm.

Laryngeal Cartilages

The epiglottis, and cuneiform and corniculate cartilages are elastic cartilages (14). The epiglottis is fenestrated and perforated by vessels (fig. 5-5). The thyroid and cricoid cartilages are hyaline cartilages. These have a thick perichondrium. The hyaline cartilage components of the larynx may calcify or ossify with age (fig. 5-5). This is a "normal" aging process in the larynx, and if traumatized, may result in a fractured larynx. The articulations between the various laryngeal joints are synovial in type and may be involved by an arthritic process.

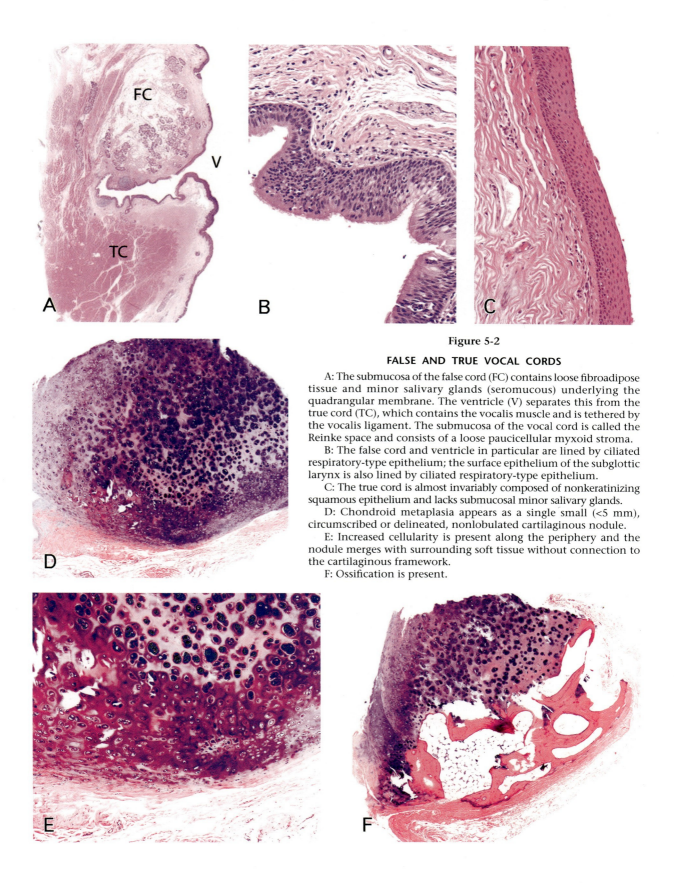

Figure 5-2

FALSE AND TRUE VOCAL CORDS

A: The submucosa of the false cord (FC) contains loose fibroadipose tissue and minor salivary glands (seromucous) underlying the quadrangular membrane. The ventricle (V) separates this from the true cord (TC), which contains the vocalis muscle and is tethered by the vocalis ligament. The submucosa of the vocal cord is called the Reinke space and consists of a loose paucicellular myxoid stroma.

B: The false cord and ventricle in particular are lined by ciliated respiratory-type epithelium; the surface epithelium of the subglottic larynx is also lined by ciliated respiratory-type epithelium.

C: The true cord is almost invariably composed of nonkeratinizing squamous epithelium and lacks submucosal minor salivary glands.

D: Chondroid metaplasia appears as a single small (<5 mm), circumscribed or delineated, nonlobulated cartilaginous nodule.

E: Increased cellularity is present along the periphery and the nodule merges with surrounding soft tissue without connection to the cartilaginous framework.

F: Ossification is present.

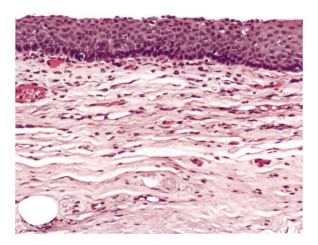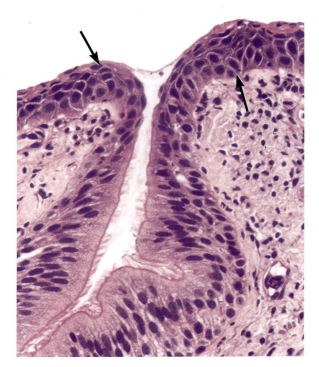

Figure 5-3

SUBGLOTTIC LARYNX

Left: The transitional zone from glottis to subglottis demonstrates more basaloid hyperchromatic epithelium, although still devoid of atypia.

Right: The epithelium (arrows) transitioning to the normal ciliated respiratory-type epithelium shows some disorganization and hyperchromasia, worrisome for dysplasia.

in the transitional zone between the glottis and subglottis. It is identified between the ciliated respiratory epithelium of the supraglottis or subglottis and the squamous epithelium of the true vocal cord. The transitional-type epithelium appears abruptly; is predominantly composed of basaloid or immature squamous cells with hypercellularity, disorganization, absence of maturation, and increased nuclear to cytoplasmic ratio; and may be misdiagnosed on biopsy or by frozen section as severe dysplasia or carcinoma in situ (CIS) (fig. 5-3). In contrast to the latter, the cells are devoid of cytonuclear atypia and mitotic activity.

Deep to the true the vocal cord lies the vocal ligament, thickened elastic tissue lying under the free edge of vocal cord (fig. 5-4). The vocal ligament inserts on the thyroid cartilage anteriorly and the vocal process of arytenoid cartilage posteriorly. Biopsies taken in this anatomic location may include the vocal cord ligament, which if unrecognized, may be misdiagnosed as a cartilaginous neoplasm, myxoma, or peripheral nerve sheath neoplasm.

Laryngeal Cartilages

The epiglottis, and cuneiform and corniculate cartilages are elastic cartilages (14). The epiglottis is fenestrated and perforated by vessels (fig. 5-5). The thyroid and cricoid cartilages are hyaline cartilages. These have a thick perichondrium. The hyaline cartilage components of the larynx may calcify or ossify with age (fig. 5-5). This is a "normal" aging process in the larynx, and if traumatized, may result in a fractured larynx. The articulations between the various laryngeal joints are synovial in type and may be involved by an arthritic process.

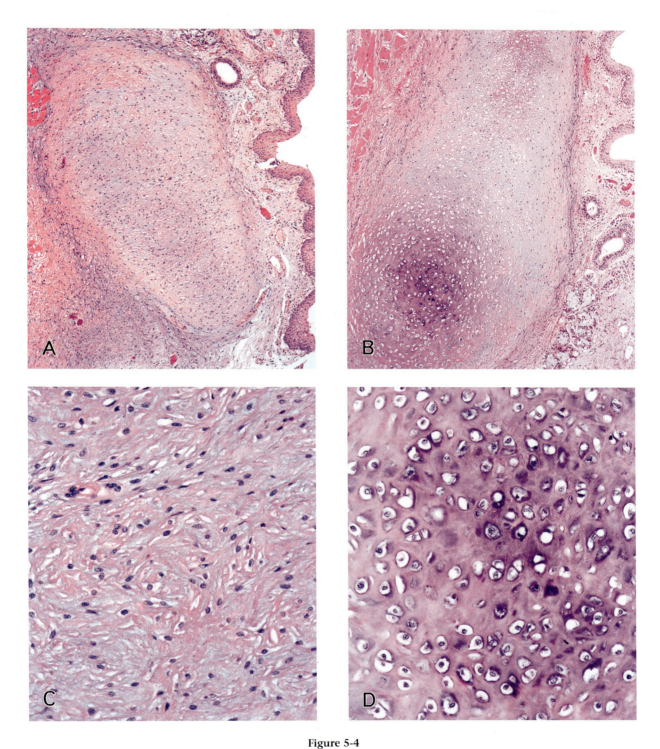

Figure 5-4

VOCAL LIGAMENT

A–D: The vocal ligament is a normal structure located within the submucosa of the true vocal cord. It appears as a circumscribed nodule representing thickened elastic to cartilaginous tissue lying under the free edge of vocal cord. Biopsies taken in this anatomic location may include the vocal ligament, which if unrecognized, may be misdiagnosed as a cartilaginous neoplasm, myxoma, or peripheral nerve sheath neoplasm.

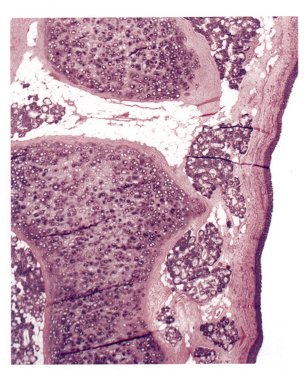 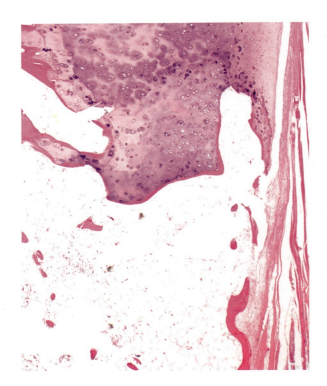

Figure 5-5
LARYNGEAL CARTILAGE
Left: Fenestrated epiglottic cartilage.
Right: Osseous metaplasia in the thyroid cartilage with fatty bone marrow elements.

EMBRYOLOGY, ANATOMY, AND HISTOLOGY: TRACHEA

Embryology

The endodermal lining of the middle segment of the laryngotracheal tube gives rise to the epithelium and glands of the trachea (15). The cartilage, connective tissue, and muscle derive from surrounding splanchnic mesenchyme.

Anatomy

The anatomic borders of the trachea extend from the lower border of the cricoid cartilage to the carina (15). In adults, the trachea averages 11 cm in length and 20 to 27 mm transversally (15). There are a total of 18 to 22 tracheal rings, with approximately 2 tracheal rings per centimeter of trachea. The superior border is continuous with the larynx, the inferior border is continuous with the bronchi, the anterior border is associated with the thyroid gland, and the posterior border is associated with the esophagus.

Histology

The entire lining of the trachea is ciliated respiratory epithelium. Abundant minor salivary glands (seromucous glands) are in the lamina propria. The cartilaginous rings are incomplete and form about two thirds of a circle. The rings are connected to each other by a fibroelastic annular ligament; the posterior (noncartilaginous) membranous part contains smooth muscle.

CLASSIFICATION

The classification of laryngeal and tracheal non-neoplastic lesions is seen in Table 5-1.

DEVELOPMENTAL LESIONS

Laryngomalacia

Definition. *Laryngomalacia (congenital laryngeal stridor, congenital flaccid larynx)* is a developmental anomaly defined by the collapse of supraglottic structures during inspiration with resultant stridor (16-20).

Table 5-1

CLASSIFICATION OF LARYNGEAL/ TRACHEAL NON-NEOPLASTIC LESIONS

Developmental
  Laryngomalacia
  Tracheobronchopathia osteochondroplastica

Hamartomas, Choristomas, Ectopias

Infectious Diseases
  Granulomatous
  Bacterial
  Viral
  Fungal
  Protozoal

Noninfectious Inflammatory Diseases

Autoimmune Diseases
  Granulomatosis with polyangiitis (formerly Wegener granulomatosis)
  Relapsing polychondritis
  Others

Tumor-Like Lesions
  Vocal cord nodules/polyps
  Laryngocele and laryngeal cysts
  Contact ulcer
  Necrotizing sialometaplasia
  Amyloidosis
  Subglottic stenosis
  Rheumatoid nodule
  Teflon granuloma
  Reactive epithelial changes
  Radiation changes

Dermatologic-Related Diseases

Clinical Features. Laryngomalacia is the most common cause of stridor in the pediatric population. The stridor is high pitched and inspiratory (19). Symptoms are usually apparent at several weeks of age, and may worsen over the first 4 to 8 months of life. Up to 20 percent of children have respiratory distress and hypoxemia. Untreated, rare cases progress to pulmonary hypertension. The current theory is that laryngomalacia is a result of abnormal integration or maturation of innervation rather than an anatomic or histologic (i.e., fibroelastic tissue composition) abnormality.

Gross Findings. The gross, or more accurate, the laryngoscopic appearance of laryngomalacia includes shortened aryepiglottic folds, arytenoid collapse into the airway, and a retroflexed epiglottis (19).

Microscopic Findings. Microscopic examination is largely irrelevant with the exception of excluding other causes of stridor (20). The main diagnostic considerations include infectious and inflammatory etiologies. Associated lesions (i.e., reflux esophagitis) may be biopsied as well.

Treatment and Prognosis. Treatment depends on the severity of the disease (19). Mild cases are managed conservatively with positional therapy, formula thickening, and treatment of reflux, if present, to improve feeding. Many cases resolve by 1 year of age and the remainder at 2 years. A small subset require surgical treatment, traditionally tracheotomy, but may now include epiglottoplasty.

Tracheopathia Osteochondroplastica

Definition. *Tracheopathia osteochondroplastica* (TO), also known as *tracheopathia osteoplastica*, is a segmental disorder of the tracheobronchial tree characterized by multiple submucosal cartilaginous and osseous nodules of various sizes narrowing the upper respiratory tract.

Clinical Features. TO usually occurs in persons over 50 years of age, with no gender predilection. Patients frequently present with a chronic cough and variable degrees of dyspnea, either acute or chronic. About 20 percent present with hemoptysis and 10 percent with pneumonia (21,22). Wheezing and ronchi are common, but stridor is rare. The most common extratracheal finding is atrophic rhinitis (over 25 percent of patients). The scalloped, nodular, calcified opacities seen radiologically in the submucosa suggest the diagnosis (fig. 5-6). The diagnosis is confirmed after endoscopic and pathologic examination (23).

Pathogenesis. The etiology is unclear but has been linked to chronic inflammation, since many cases occur in patients with chronic inflammatory conditions. In addition, trauma has been suggested as a possible cause. Half of patients with acute symptomatology have positive bacterial cultures, with *Klebsiella ozaenae* and *Pseudomonas aeruginosa* being the most common organisms (24).

Gross Findings. Nodules typically occur along the proximal tracheobronchial tree of the upper and mid trachea. The posterior wall is usually spared.

Microscopic Findings. Histologically, metaplastic cartilage and bone are found in the submucosa (figs. 5-6, 5-7), often in continuity with the inner surface of the tracheal cartilage.

Non-Neoplastic Diseases of the Head and Neck

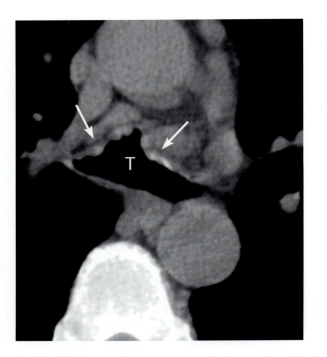
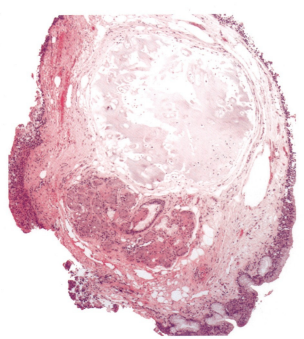

Figure 5-6

TRACHEOPATHIA OSTEOCHONDROPLASTICA

Left: A computerized tomographic (CT) scan demonstrates the nodularity of the anterior trachea (arrows) and sparing of the membranous posterior trachea.

Right: Histologically, submucosal cartilaginous nodules are noted. Ossification may also be seen as implied by the name for this entity.

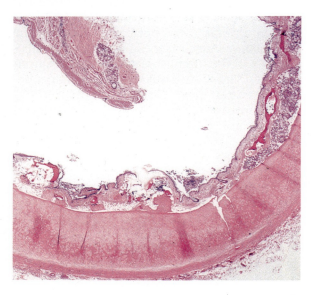
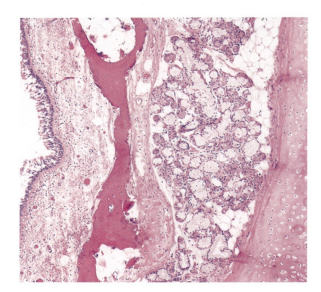

Figure 5-7

TRACHEOPATHIA OSTEOCHONDROPLASTICA

Left: Submucosal bone deposition or metaplasia is found separated from the cartilage. This finding, combined with the clinical presentation, is distinctive for tracheopathia osteoplastica.

Right: A spicule of metaplastic bone is separated from the mucosa and cartilage.

The overlying mucosa is intact and may appear normal or metaplastic. There is an overall rigidity to the trachea. The nodules may become ossified, and heterotopic bone formation is seen in the soft tissue or stroma. The bony lamellae may protrude into the mucosa, giving the characteristic appearance on bronchoscopy. The irregular bony spicules have thin walls surrounding fatty bone marrow. In children, there is often a limited degree of calcification (25). Diagnosis requires clinicoradiologic correlation with the biopsy.

Differential Diagnosis. The primary clinical differential diagnostic considerations are tracheobronchomegaly and tracheomalacia; these are readily distinguished by laryngoscopic examination. Histologically, rare cases of myositis ossificans of the larynx or even some forms of osseous tracheal stenosis are considerations. TO, however, does not have the maturation or zonal pattern/phenomenon seen in myositis ossificans, characterized by a central cellular area, an intermediate zone of osteoid formation, and a peripheral shell of highly organized bone. The posterior sparing distribution helps separate TO from tracheal stenosis (26).

Treatment and Prognosis. Localized disease may not require treatment, but significant narrowing requires laser removal and dilatation. Meticulous tracheobronchial hygiene is imperative in long-term clinical management.

HAMARTOMAS, CHORISTOMAS, AND ECTOPIAS

Definition. *Hamartoma* is a non-neoplastic developmental anomaly caused by excessive and disordered growth of normal cells or tissue indigenous to its site of occurrence. *Choristoma* is a non-neoplastic developmental anomaly of essentially normal tissue but with the tissue elements being foreign to its anatomic location. Choristoma is also referred to as *heterotopia*, *ectopia*, and *aberrant rest*.

Clinical Features. Hamartomas, choristomas, and ectopias are identified in the supraglottic and posterior commissure regions, although no region of the larynx or trachea is excluded. This group of lesions accounts for less than 5 percent of all primary "mass" lesions in the larynx and trachea (27–30). The lesions may have variable clinical manifestations, although hoarseness and obstructive symptoms are most common.

Hamartomas specifically are described in association with other congenital anomalies, such as cleft larynx, and are most frequently congenital disorders presenting in infancy.

The most frequent choristoma is *ectopic thyroid tissue* (ETT) (31–34). Patients with intratracheal ETT usually present with signs of dyspnea or upper airway obstruction, but varying levels of hormone stimulation appear to play a major role, since there is often an associated nodular thyroid disease. Its clinical manifestations often correlate with the surgical resection of the thyroid gland since the removal may induce the quiescent thyroid tissue mass to enlarge, resulting in symptoms. Women between 30 and 50 years of age are most frequently affected by ETT.

Gross Findings. The masses are nodular or polypoid, firm to soft, mobile or fixed, yellow, white, or red, measuring up to 5 cm in greatest dimension. They are often in a submucosal location. Without a characteristic gross appearance, histologic examination of the excised specimen is mandatory to confirm the diagnosis.

Microscopic Findings. Hamartomas of the larynx and trachea have epithelial and mesenchymal components arranged in a haphazard fashion throughout the lesion (fig. 5-8). Squamous or respiratory-type epithelium, glandular elements, adipose connective tissue, skeletal or smooth muscle, cartilage, fibrous connective tissue or collagen, nerves, lymphoid elements, and blood vessels are all present in a variable combination and disorganization. The lesions may not be encapsulated and lack demarcation from the rest of the tissue. Cartilaginous islands are frequently present, but in close approximation with other epithelial or mesenchymal elements (fig. 5-8).

Choristoma may be composed of any tissue type but most frequently are ETT. There is a predilection for the posterolateral subglottic wall, which is postulated to be a result of "in growth" via a path of least resistance in contrast to the conus elasticus and vocalis ligament more anterocranially (34,35). The histologic appearance is that of benign thyroid parenchyma, although, rarely, a papillary thyroid carcinoma develops (36).

Differential Diagnosis. The differential diagnosis includes teratoma, dermoid cyst, and chondroma. An immature teratoma can be included in the differential diagnosis of hamartomas and ectopias, however, three germ layers

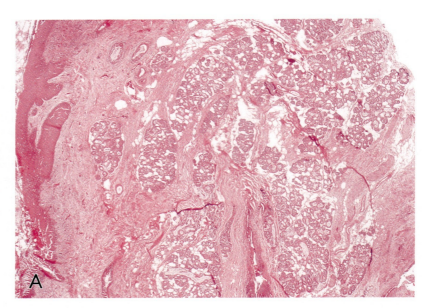

Figure 5-8

LARYNGEAL HAMARTOMA

A,B: This seromucous gland hamartoma consists of increased numbers of submucosal seromucous glands with focal retention of the lobular architecture. The diffuse proliferation of seromucous glands is out of proportion to the normal amount of such glands in the larynx.

C: Chondroid hamartoma is composed of a cartilaginous island close to the normal seromucous glands.

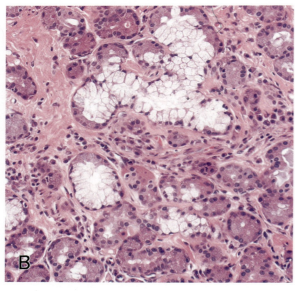

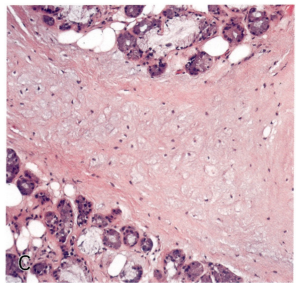

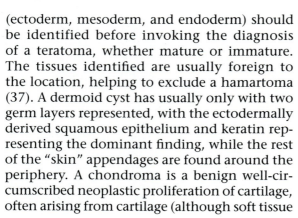

(ectoderm, mesoderm, and endoderm) should be identified before invoking the diagnosis of a teratoma, whether mature or immature. The tissues identified are usually foreign to the location, helping to exclude a hamartoma (37). A dermoid cyst has usually only with two germ layers represented, with the ectodermally derived squamous epithelium and keratin representing the dominant finding, while the rest of the "skin" appendages are found around the periphery. A chondroma is a benign well-circumscribed neoplastic proliferation of cartilage, often arising from cartilage (although soft tissue forms have been noted) in the posterior subglottic region, without nuclear pleomorphism and also without other epithelial or mesenchymal elements.

Treatment and Prognosis. Surgery is the mainstay of treatment and is curative.

INFECTIOUS DISEASES

Infectious diseases of the larynx and trachea are defined for specific groups of microorganisms as listed below. They encompass a spectrum of disease that includes laryngitis, epiglottitis, "croup," and laryngotracheobronchitis.

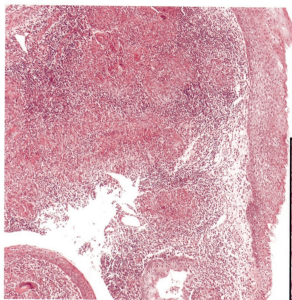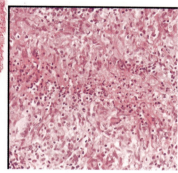

Figure 5-9

GRANULOMATOUS LARYNGITIS

This patient with known tuberculosis has well-formed granulomas within the submucosa. Inset: central necrosis is seen in several of the granulomas.

Often, the clinical disease caused by infection depends on the age of the patient. In general, findings on histologic examination are nonspecific, with edema and an inflammatory infiltrate without a discrete lesion. There may be cord compromise and ulceration. Acute bacterial lesions tend to demonstrate neutrophilic infiltrates; viral infections may show lymphoid and histiocytic elements; fungal and parasitic organisms may show eosinophilia. A wide spectrum of organisms may manifest with granulomatous inflammation. Because the manifestations of laryngopharyngitis are nonspecific, close correlation with the clinical setting, in addition to serology, cytologic preparations, microbiologic cultures or tests, precipitant tests for fungi, and other clinical studies (thyroid function tests, skin tests), are imperative to obtain a complete view of the disease process.

Treatment is determined by the infectious agent identified. Similarly, prognosis for infectious diseases of the larynx is dependent on a number of factors including the agent identified, response to therapy, and clinical scenario in which the infection occurs (e.g., immunocompetent or immunosuppressed condition).

Granulomatous Laryngopharyngitis

Granulomatous laryngopharyngitis is identified in a variety of infections, including bacterial, mycobacterial, and fungal. The nodules are present throughout the respiratory tract, along with the characteristic epithelioid histiocytes, giant cells, chronic inflammation, and variable necrosis or caseation, depending upon the infectious agent (fig. 5-9). The overlying epithelium may be atrophic, to normal, to hyperplastic.

The degree of granulomatous inflammation depends upon the host immune response to the organism; for instance, nonspecific inflammation primarily comprised of foamy histiocytes may be encountered in a mycobacteria tuberculosis infection in an immunocompromised patient rather than the characteristic caseating granulomas. Careful examination is necessary, often under oil immersion, frequently of multiple slides, in order to identify the causative agent. Mycobacterial agents, including *M. tuberculosis*, *M. avium-intracellulare* complex, and *M. leprae* are identified with acid-fast stains (Ziehl-Neelsen) or with fluorochrome dyes (auramine and rhodamine) (38–42). Lupus vulgaris is a secondary form of tuberculosis which can present in the mucosa of the larynx, usually as a result of extension from cervical lymphadenitis.

The laryngeal equivalent of rhinoscleroma is rare but also associated with *Klebsiella rhinoscleromatis*. It consists of a more loosely organized granulomatous inflammation, a rich inflammatory infiltrate, and characteristic histiocytes referred to as Mikulicz cells (43). The organisms fill these cells, and are highlighted by a tissue Warthin-Starry or Gram stain (38,41,44,45).

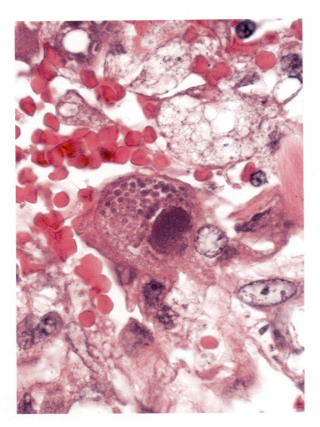

Figure 5-10

CYTOMEGALOVIRUS (CMV) INFECTION OF THE LARYNX

The characteristic eosinophilic, intranuclear, "bull's-eye" type inclusion is present, with a more basophilic cytoplasmic inclusion.

Actinomycosis israelii (usually part of oral flora) may manifest as granulomatous laryngopharyngitis. The organism engenders a granulomatous inflammatory response, but usually with a greater degree of necrosis (abscess formation) and fibrosis, often demonstrating "sulfur granules" (spheres of organisms arranged in a radiating pattern). A Gram stain accentuates the fine filamentous organism, which is not positive with acid-fast stains (41,46,47).

Cat-scratch disease, caused by *Bartonella henslae*, may extend into the larynx from the surrounding lymph nodes, in which a palisaded granuloma with stellate necrosis is characteristic. The Warthin-Starry stain helps identify the Gram-negative bacillus, and now immunohistochemical antibodies are available for easier identification (48).

A modified Dieterle stain documents the presence of spirochetes if syphilis or borreliosis is suspected, although now immunohistochemical antibodies are available for these as well (49). Syphilis presents with primary (mucosal ulceration), secondary, or tertiary manifestations (perichondritis, gumma formation, and fibrosis). Tertiary stage is the more common laryngeal manifestation, with gumma, granuloma, and ulceration. The associated vasculitis, rich plasma cell infiltrate (plasma cell endarteritis), and positive testing by various algorithms (rapid plasma reagin [RPR], venereal disease research laboratory [VDRL], and/or fluorescent treponemal antibody-absorption [FTA-ABS]) confirm the diagnosis (50).

In the setting of granulomatous inflammation, malakoplakia also needs to be excluded. The demonstration of Michaelis-Gutmann bodies, appearing as round, target-like calcified structures, is satisfactory for the diagnosis, although cultures usually grow *Escherichia coli* or another bacterial organism (51).

Viruses

A full spectrum of viral infections can affect the larynx, trachea, and hypopharynx, including but not limited to picornaviridae (rhinovirus and enterovirus), paramyxoviridae (parainfluenza viruses, mumps, measles [morbillivirus], and respiratory syncytial virus [pneumovirus]), orthomyxoviridae (influenza viruses), adenovirus, human papillomavirus, herpesviridae (cytomegalovirus [CMV]) (fig. 5-10), herpes simplex virus (fig. 5-11), varicella-zoster virus, and Epstein-Barr virus (EBV). With some exceptions, the histologic appearance of these is identical, as are the clinical manifestations, which are frequently dependent upon the age, sex, and nutritional and immunologic status of the patient.

An extensive laboratory investigation to document the specific type of virus causing a "common cold" is probably not warranted except in extreme cases. The mucous membranes are erythematous and swollen on gross examination, while the histologic findings consist of nonspecific inflammatory cells and edema fluid, occasionally coupled with specific "viral-type" inclusions.

Frequently, secondary infections by bacterial agents complicate the clinical and histologic appearance. *Fibrinous laryngotracheobronchitis* is

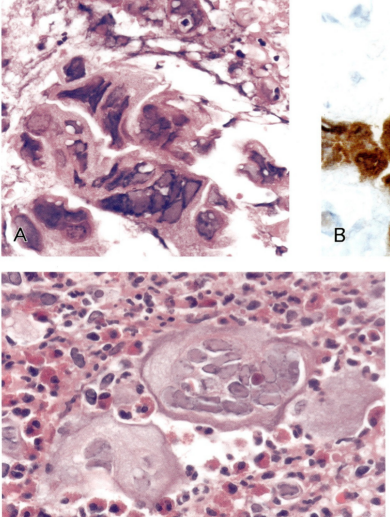
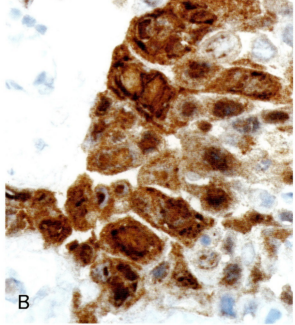

Figure 5-11

HERPETIC LARYNGITIS

A: Sloughed epithelium within a neutrophilic/fibrinous exudate demonstrates the characteristic margination, multinucleation, and moulding of the herpes simplex virus (HSV) cytopathic effect.

B: HSV1 immunostain is positive, confirming the diagnosis.

C: Another example of HSV infection resulting in the characteristic "ground glass" appearance found in a multinucleated giant cell.

thought to be caused by both a virus and secondary bacterial infection, with destruction of the ciliated epithelium. Cultures help identify the superinfecting bacteria in order to provide additional antibiotic therapy, but clinical management prior to laboratory results is imperative (52,53).

Human papillomavirus (HPV) DNA is an oral colonizer in about 7 percent of the general population, although it is increased in patients with adult recurrent respiratory papillomatosis (54,55). Factors that influence the conversion of HPV exposure to active HPV infection resulting in an epithelial proliferation are still unclear.

Bacteria

Bacterial infections include *Haemophilus influenzae* (type B specifically, although all subtypes are involved), pneumococci, hemolytic streptococci or staphylococci (also including scarlet fever sequela), *Neisseria* species, micrococci, *Klebsiella*

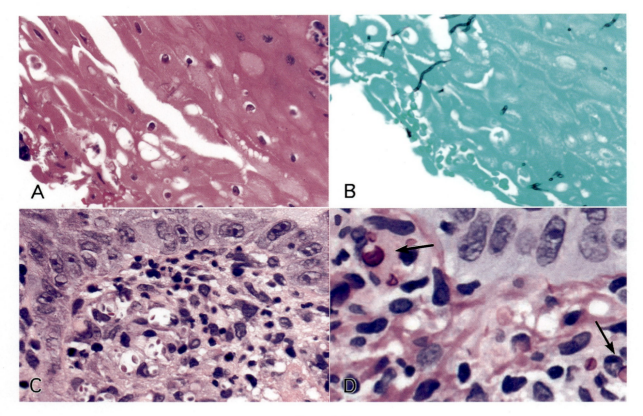

Figure 5-12

FUNGAL LARYNGITIDES

A: *Candida* is often characterized by a hyperplastic/keratotic epithelium with acute mucositis (top right corner).
B: The Gomori methenamine silver (GMS) stain highlights the spores and hyphae of the fungi.
C: Less common organisms, such as *Histoplasma capsulatum,* may manifest as a submucosal granuloma.
D: DPAS staining highlights the budding yeast (arrows).

species, *Bordetella pertussis* (whooping cough), *Corynebacterium diphtheriae* (diphtheria), *Salmonella typhi* (typhoid fever) and *Rickettsia* species (typhus). These bacteria result a spectrum of diseases including acute epiglottitis, acute laryngeotracheobronchitis, and laryngeal diphtheria. They result in diffuse erythema of the laryngeal mucosa, with an exudate that often extends into the subglottis or trachea. Mucopurulent discharge may be seen grossly. Histologic examination demonstrates microabscesses and mixed inflammation, often with surface ulceration.

Clinical management is mandatory, often requiring emergent therapy without laboratory confirmation of the etiologic agent. Once the etiologic agent is determined, appropriate antibiotic therapy can be instituted (38,56–59).

Diphtheria still occurs and antitoxin should be given as clinically indicated, not delayed by a lack of laboratory confirmation or confirmation by a Schick test (intradermal injection of diphtheria toxin: the skin around the injection becomes red and swollen, indicating a positive result). A diphtheritic, dirty-gray membrane can be seen, coupled with a foul odor.

Retropharyngeal abscess, peritonsillar abscess, or laryngeal abscess may result in obstruction of the larynx, usually resulting from a suppurative infection of a retropharyngeal lymph node or the posterior tonsillar pillar, or related to deep penetrating trauma. Prompt surgical intervention and protection of the airway become the primary concern; *H. influenzae* is the most common organism implicated (60,61).

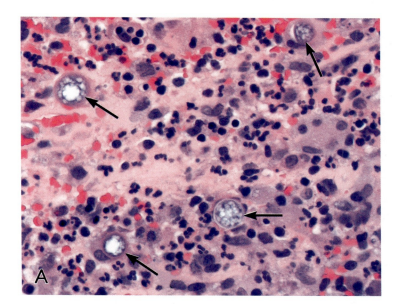
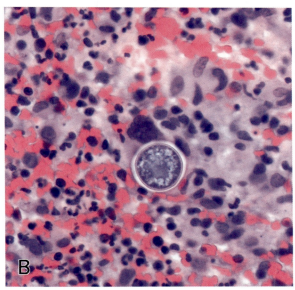
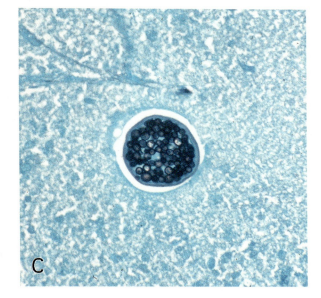

Figure 5-13

COCCIDIOIDES IMMITIS

A: Multiple spherules (arrows) are identified in a background of granulomatous inflammation and acute inflammatory cells.

B: At higher magnification, endospores are identified within the spherule found within a multinucleated giant cell

C: The spherule and endospores of *Coccidioides immitis* are accentuated with GMS stain.

Fungi

A variety of fungi cause laryngitis, all with a similar histologic appearance of inflammation, usually granulomatous in nature, with acute and chronic inflammation. Fungal organisms (either yeast or mold forms) that cause laryngitis include: *Candida albicans,* appearing as oval, budding cells with long, tubular hyphae (fig. 5-12), which can be seen on Gram stain; *Histoplasma capsulatum,* appearing as small, variably shaped, intracytoplasmic organisms often in regions of viable tissues (fig. 5-12); *Coccidioides immitis,* appearing as thick, double-walled spherules with endospores (fig. 5-13); *Cryptococcus neoformans* (polysaccharide encapsulated variable-sized, oval-shaped organisms); *Blastomyces dermatitidis,* appearing as thick, double-contoured, "refractile" organisms with broad-based budding (fig. 5-14); *Paracoccidioides brasiliensis,* appearing as circular organisms with "mariner's wheel" type multiple budding; *Aspergillus* species, appearing as narrow fungi with acute angle branching and septations; and *Mucor* species, appearing as broad, aseptate, "ribbon"-like mold forms) (38,41,47,62–67). Each

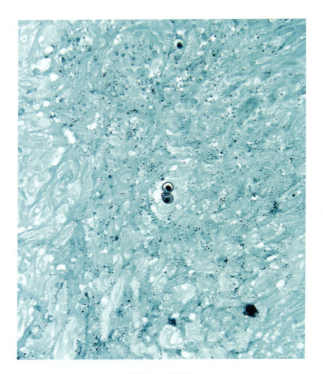

Figure 5-14

LARYNGEAL BLASTOMYCOSIS

Broad-based budding is accentuated with a silver-impregnation preparation.

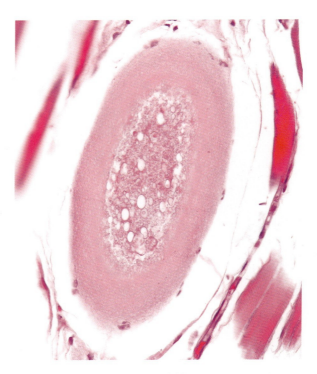

Figure 5-15

TRICHINELLA

A nurse cell within the skeletal musculature of the larynx contains multiple encysted and degenerated larva of the *Trichinella* species.

of these organisms has a characteristic fungal or yeast form in tissue and in culture.

Documentation of the organism in tissue can be facilitated with mucicarmine, periodic acid–Schiff (PAS), calcafluor white, Warthin-Starry, Gomori methenamine silver (GMS), and immunoperoxidase antibodies, as suggested by the histologic appearance, or confirmed with blood cultures or serologic titers (complement fixation, latex agglutination or precipitant test) or cutaneous hypersensitivity testing (less specific). Although isolated disease can occur, fungal infections are more often part of systemic disease, and accentuated in immunocompromised patients. Laryngeal lesions of acquired immunodeficiency syndrome (AIDS) are caused by a variety of infectious agents, most frequently *Candida* species and herpes simplex virus (66).

Protozoa

Only rare case reports document laryngeal involvement by parasitic organisms, which include *Trichinella* (fig. 5-15), *Ascaris lumbricoides*, *Hirudinea* (leeches), *Limnatis maculosa*, and *Leishmania* (68).

NONINFECTIOUS INFLAMMATORY DISEASES

Angioedema/Allergic Laryngitis

Definition. *Angioedema* of the larynx is an allergic immune-mediated reaction to various environmental agents or drugs.

Clinical Features. Usually, the clinical onset is abrupt after environmental exposure, distinctly different from infectious agents, and almost 20 percent of patients require intubation (69,70). Previous allergic sensitivity helps establish the diagnosis. In addition to angiotensin converting enzyme (ACE) inhibitors, other drugs associated with laryngeal angioedema include various antibiotics such as ciprofloxacin (71,72). Hereditary angioedema as a result of C1q esterase deficiency may also affect the larynx although less frequently and with less severity than environmental causes (73).

Gross Findings. Areas affected tend to be boggy and edematous. With glottic involvement, there may be Reinke space edema. But unlike the spectrum of diseases in vocal cord nodules, this edema is not restricted to the Reinke space, and is often supraglottic and occasionally subglottic.

Microscopic Findings. The histologic examination shows only edema fluid and variable inflammation. Chronic nonspecific inflammation with associated squamous metaplasia and epithelial thickening may result from repeated episodes of laryngitis.

Treatment and Prognosis. Treatment is supportive. In acutely obstructive and threatening cases of angioedema, airway preservation is critical, and may require epinephrine.

Sarcoidosis

Definition. *Sarcoidosis* is a multiorgan noncaseating granulomatous disease of unknown etiology that can affect lymph nodes, lung, mucosal sites of the upper aerodigestive tract, salivary glands, skin, spleen, and liver.

Clinical Features. Isolated laryngeal disease has been described, but must be supported by additional clinical, radiographic, or laboratory evidence. Involvement of the larynx as part of systemic disease is a much more likely scenario, and cutaneous manifestations, fever, and adenopathy are usually present (26,74–76).

There are no laboratory findings specific for, or diagnostic of, sarcoidosis. Cutaneous anergy to skin test antigens (Kveim test) occurs in 60 to 85 percent of patients. An elevated ACE level is a marker for sarcoid disease activity but is not unique to sarcoidosis and can be elevated in other diseases including liver disease and leprosy. The etiology remains unknown, but there is increasing evidence that mycobacterial DNA, assessed by polymerase chain reaction, is associated with sarcoid granulomas.

Gross Findings. Macroscopically, there is a diffuse, symmetric, swollen, nodular, exophytic or edematous lesion, most often of the supraglottic structures. A miliary nodular appearance, with small submucosal bumps, has also been described with laryngeal involvement, with associated epithelial hyperplasia or keratosis. Larger, lobulated masses, all submucosal, have also been described (26,74–76).

Microscopic Findings. The microscopic diagnosis of sarcoidosis is generally one of exclusion, with clinical, radiographic, and laboratory correlation needed to confirm the histologic appearance. Small to medium-sized, "tightly" clustered, noncaseating epithelioid granulomas are present in the stroma. The rich inflammatory infiltrate consists of plasma cells and lymphocytes interspersed with occasional Langhans and foreign body-type giant cells (fig. 5-16). The epithelioid histiocytes are polyhedral cells with abundant cytoplasm and vesicular nuclei. Although not specific for sarcoid, asteroid bodies (stellate intracytoplasmic inclusions in giant cells) (fig. 5-16), Schaumann bodies (concentrically laminated calcified bodies), and Hamazaki-Wesenberg bodies (yellow-brown structures similar to fungal organisms) are identified. With progression of the disease, fibrosis and hyalinization of the stroma occur, possibly obscuring the granulomatous inflammation.

Differential Diagnosis. As noted previously, there are numerous infectious causes of granulomatous laryngitis, and it is thus imperative to rule out other infectious and inflammatory or neoplastic conditions before diagnosing sarcoidosis. Bacteria and fungal organisms should be sought through tissue staining or culture. A foreign body reaction can be excluded through polarization. Malakoplakia does not have the tight distribution of epithelioid granulomas that is seen is sarcoidosis, and demonstrates Michaelis-Gutmann bodies as part of the granulomatous inflammation (51). Granulomatous inflammation is also be seen in association with malignant tumors, especially as a reaction to the keratinaceous debris (keratin granuloma) of a squamous cell carcinoma (26,41,74–76). Sarcoidosis and sarcoid-like reactions may occur in association with head and neck cancer (synchronously or metachronously) and may also occur after chemotherapy.

Treatment and Prognosis. Most patients with laryngeal sarcoidosis do not require therapy. In the presence of airway obstruction, however, parenteral steroid therapy is indicated.

AUTOIMMUNE DISEASES

Granulomatosis with Polyangiitis

Definition. *Granulomatosis with polyangiitis* (GPA), formerly referred to as Wegener granulomatosis, is a necrotizing characteristically

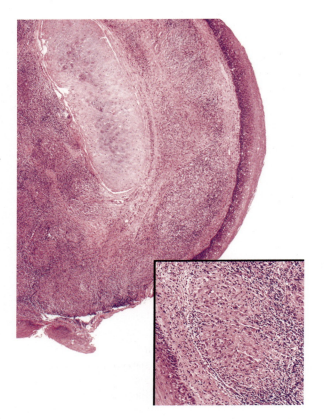
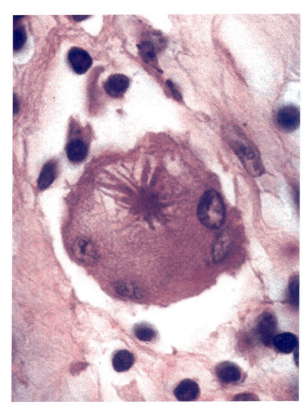

Figure 5-16

SARCOIDOSIS OF THE EPIGLOTTIS

Left and inset: Numerous submucosal, well-formed, noncaseating granulomas are seen.

Right: The asteroid body seen here is a stellate intracytoplasmic inclusion in a giant cell, present in a few conditions, but most frequently in sarcoidosis.

systemic vasculitic disorder that involves multiple organs, although localized involvement of the upper aerodigestive tract, especially the sinonasal tract, but also the larynx occurs. For a more complete discussion of GPA, including additional illustrations, see chapter 1.

Clinical Features. Laryngeal (and tracheal) involvement occurs in approximately 25 percent of patients with GPA (77–79). Primary laryngeal presentation is uncommon since the disease is generally systemic by the time laryngeal involvement is biopsied or suspected (44,77–82). While there is a male predilection for GPA involvement of other head and neck sites, there is a female predilection for laryngeal GPA of the subglottic region. Any portion of the larynx can be affected, but it is usually a subglottic disease with extension into the trachea (the latter especially more frequent in females).

Patients with laryngeal GPA have nonspecific symptoms initially, progressing to total subglottic obstruction in late-stage disease. Antineutrophil cytoplasmic antibody (ANCA) and proteinase 3 (PR3) are now well established as a serologic markers associated with the disease. A significant delay in the diagnosis and in the start of appropriate therapy can adversely affect the disease course and patient outcome. Therefore, occasionally, empiric therapy is initiated while a definitive diagnosis is pending.

Gross Findings. A reddish, friable to ulcerated, circumferential subglottic narrowing or stenosis is the typical gross finding, with pseudotumor formation and ulcerating tracheal lesions identified in a number of patients. These nonspecific findings must be coupled with a histologic examination and additional studies as clinically warranted.

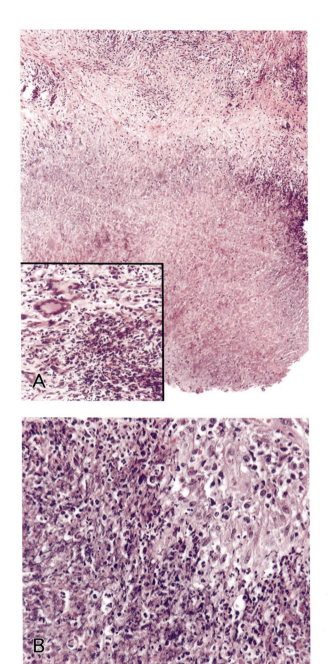
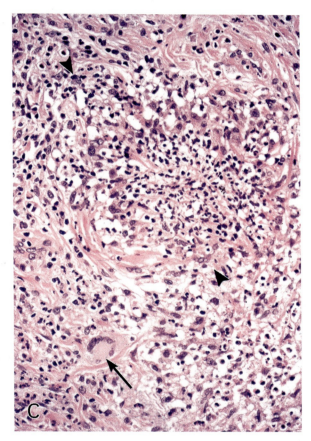

Figure 5-17

LARYNGEAL (SUBGLOTTIC) GRANULOMATOSIS WITH POLYANGIITIS (GPA)

A: Geographic necrobiosis. Inset: Granulomas are not well-formed but consist of scattered giant cells.

B: Necrobiosis with basophilic destruction of the tissues is a hallmark of GPA. A small vessel (upper right) demonstrates vasculitis, with lymphoid cells and acute inflammatory cells identified within the wall.

C: Perivascular inflammation with the ultimate destruction of the vessel (arrowheads), necrobiosis, and a multinucleated giant cell (arrow) are helpful in diagnosing GPA, especially when combined with the clinical findings, including elevated serologic titers of c-ANCA and proteinase 3.

Microscopic Findings. The classic histologic triad of GPA includes granulomas, necrosis, and vasculitis (79). This is considered a misrepresentation, however, since it is actually the hallmark ischemic-type necrobiosis, a severe distortion and basophilic destruction of collagenous and mesenchymal tissues (vascular smooth muscle), that characterizes this entity (fig. 5-17). This necrobiosis has a "geographic" or serpiginous border, and is characterized by finely to coarsely granular blue debris and neutrophilic microabscesses.

Despite being part of the classic triad, vasculitis is considered a secondary process. In fact, Dr. Wegener himself wrote: "The vasculitis that accompanies the disease is a secondary feature that presents at a later stage" (83). When true vasculitis is present, small to medium-sized vessels have fibrinoid necrosis of the media or may have microabscesses within the wall. When a leukocytoclastic vasculitis or fibrosing vasculitis is demonstrated, it is usually associated with a more advanced form or late stage of the disease. The inflammatory cells include lymphocytes, histiocytes, eosinophils, and neutrophils. Similarly, while granulomas are part of this triad, true well-formed palisaded granuloma formation is rare, but instead scattered multinucleated giant cells are more typical (fig. 5-17) (44,77–82,84,85). Outside the sinonasal tract, the histologic presentation may be less classic, occasionally showing more chronicity in the form of perivascular fibrosclerosis (79).

Special Stains. Staining for microorganisms (e.g., GMS, PAS, acid-fast bacillus [AFB]), is invariably negative. Elastic stains help clarify the presence of vasculitis. Immunohistochemical staining shows reactivity for B-cell markers (e.g., CD20) and T-cell markers (CD3) but staining for CD56, TIA1, granzyme B, and perforin, and in situ hybridization for EBV-encoded RNA (EBER) are negative.

Differential Diagnosis. The diagnosis of GPA (see Table 1-4 in chapter 1 for differential diagnosis) is one of both inclusion of the characteristic clinical and serologic findings, and exclusion of a variety of infectious diseases, collagen vascular/autoimmune diseases, and hematolymphoid neoplasms. As noted above, fungal cultures, infectious serologies, and histochemical stains are important for the exclusion of infectious etiologies. Churg-Strauss disease (also referred to as allergic granulomatosis and vasculitis) may show some overlap with GPA histologically, and even serologically, but shows tissue and peripheral eosinophilia, and has a more integral small vessel vasculitic component (86). NK/T-cell lymphoma of larynx is rare, and may be angiocentric and granuloma forming, but on careful examination, shows lymphoid atypia. Stains for EBV and lymphoid markers (e.g., CD 56, TIA1, granzyme, perforin) establish the diagnosis (87).

Treatment and Prognosis. Localized disease is managed by medical therapy (cyclophosphamide and steroids), although surgery may be needed to maintain a patent airway in progressive disease (88–90).

Relapsing Polychondritis

Definition. *Relapsing polychondritis* (RP) also termed *systemic chondromalacia* and *polychondropathy*, is an uncommon systemic, episodic or relapsing disease characterized by progressive degeneration of cartilaginous structures throughout the body. For a more complete discussion of RP, including illustrations, see chapter 7.

Clinical Features. Patients with RP usually present in the fifth decade with one or more of the following progressive degenerative changes in the cartilages of the body: recurrent bilateral auricular chondritis, inflammatory polyarthritis, nasal chondritis, ocular inflammation, tracheal or laryngeal chondritis, and cochlea or vestibular damage. Other immunologically mediated diseases may be associated with RP, including systemic lupus erythematosus, rheumatoid arthritis, and Sjögren syndrome (91,92). There is an association with HLA-DR4.(93,94) Type II and anti-matrilin-1 tests are now sensitive or specific for the diagnosis (95). Laryngotracheal manifestations range from mild, such as hoarseness, to severe airway compromise.

Gross Findings. Although the gross findings are nonspecific, there is an overall thickening of the epiglottis and aryepiglottic folds, with softening and friability of the cricoid and tracheal rings (and tracheal wall). The larynx and trachea decrease in size and frank collapse may occur in the later stages of the disease (91–93,96–99).

Microscopic Findings. At low magnification, RP shows a loss of cartilage basophilia, assuming a more eosinophilic quality, as well as fragmentation of the cartilage with necrosis and lysis of cartilaginous plates. The outer perichondrium is permeated by a spectrum of inflammatory cells, including neutrophils, eosinophils, lymphocytes, and plasma cells, frequently associated with edema or gelatinous cystic degeneration. When there is no well-defined perichondrium, there is an imperceptible blending of the degenerated fibrillar cartilage with the surrounding inflammatory cells. With progression of the disease, the dissolved lacunae are replaced with granulation-type tissue or fibrosis, which can completely replace the cartilage structure. Occasionally, the cartilage has a deranged architecture, perhaps affiliated with regeneration as the disease progresses (91,97,98,100,101).

Differential Diagnosis. The histologic differential diagnosis for RP in the larynx is limited, but may include chondronecrosis, either inflammatory or secondary to radiotherapy, and tracheal stenosis secondary to prolonged intubation (102). These entities do not show the typical zonation of RP, and the clinical history is also useful. Infectious diseases may similarly show alterations of the laryngotracheal cartilage. Obtaining cultures or performing histochemical stains helps to rule out infectious organisms.

Treatment and Prognosis. Anti-inflammatory agents, steroids, antimetabolite drugs, and immunosuppressive medications are used in variable combinations to treat patients, depending upon the severity of the disease. Surgery is used only in severe airway compromise or collapse. Airway compromise is a frequent cause of death in this uncommon disorder (91,92,94,97).

TUMOR-LIKE PROCESSES

Vocal Cord Nodules and Polyps

Definition. *Vocal cord nodule* (VCN) is an edematous fibrovascular response to excessive phonotrauma involving the Reinke space. There is a variable inflammatory component (103,104). Synonyms include *Reinke space edema*, *vocal cord polyp*, *singer nodule*, *preacher nodule*, and *corditis nodosa*.

A nodule and a polyp are not clinically synonymous, although they frequently are interchangeable in the pathology community. Clinicians distinguish between nodules and polyps based on whether the lesions is sessile (nodule) or pedunculated (polyp).

Clinical Features. Nodules are more frequent in young women, are associated with vocal abuse (phonologic disorder), and often are bilateral, involving the anterior or middle third of the vocal cord. A polyp occurs in any age group, is associated with infection and smoking, and tends to be a single lesion arising from the true vocal cord. For nodules and polyps, vocal changes, specifically hoarseness and "breaking" of the voice, are the most frequent presenting symptoms.

Pathogenesis. VCNs occur in patients who subject themselves to phonotrauma, namely singers, teachers, and broadcasters. The phonotrauma may either represent long-term abuse, or in some cases, a highly traumatic acute incident (i.e., yelling at a concert) (104). Other contributory causes include gastroesophageal reflux and smoking, which may lower the threshold for damage from phonotrauma. Infrequently, hypothyroidism causes vocal cord edema which may progress to the formation of a (myxoid) polyp.

Gross Findings. As the many synonyms indicate, this spectrum of disease may manifest as diffuse edema, nodule (fig. 5-18), polyp, or even a cyst, typically in the middle third of the vocal cord, the presumed region of maximal vibration. Polyps and nodules range from edematous to hemorrhagic. VCNs are rarely over 0.5 cm, and by definition, are restricted to the Reinke space. Polyps may be somewhat larger as a result of secondary vascular changes (105–107).

Microscopic Findings. VCNs, specifically polypoid lesions, are divided into four main histologic subtypes: myxoid/edematous, vascular, fibrous, and hyaline (fig. 5-18). Often, all of these change are seen in the same polyp. The dominant histologic pattern determines the type. The types mirror the presumed pathogenesis of VCN. The edematous type is a result of early increased permeability secondary to the phonotrauma and has a loose myxoid paucicellular stroma. The vascular type is a result of hemorrhage and neovascularization (108). The fibrous type shows a fibroproliferative response in longer-standing lesions, and the hyaline type often shows dense acellular fibrinoid deposits and extensive sclerosis indicative of very late changes (103–105,107,109). The surface epithelium may become metaplastic, atrophic, keratotic, and hyperplastic to a degree that may mimic squamous dysplasia, and even demonstrate pseudoepitheliomatous changes (fig. 5-18). Uncommonly, coexisting high-grade intraepithelial dysplasia (i.e., moderate to severe) and/or invasive squamous cell carcinoma may be identified

Differential Diagnosis. The differential diagnosis is based on the predominant morphology. Edematous VCN may mimic myxoma, vascular VCN may mimic hemangioma or other vascular neoplasms, fibrous VCN may mimic neurofibroma, and hyaline VCN may resemble laryngeal amyloid. Key distinguishing features for all VCNs are the small size and restriction to the true vocal cord. In some cases, immunohistochemical stains are useful.

Treatment and Prognosis. Excision of a polyp and treatment of the underlying cause of a nodule is generally sufficient therapy. Treatment of hypothyroidism can also be beneficial. Nodules may recur with repeated phonotrauma.

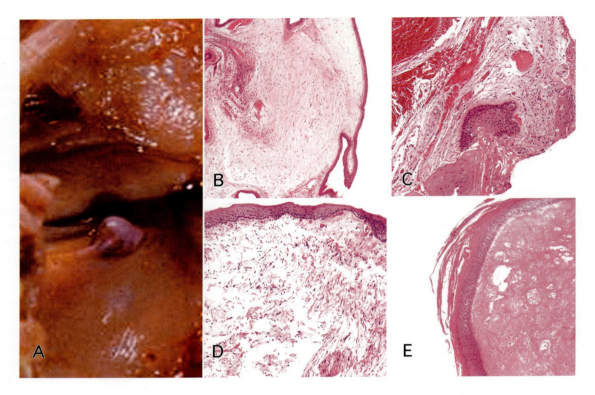

Figure 5-18

VOCAL CORD NODULE/POLYP

A: Vocal cord nodules are exophytic, variably hyperemic, soft nodules or polyps emanating from the free edge of the vocal cord. (Courtesy Dr. E. L. Barnes, Pittsburgh, PA.)

B–E: The histologic types include: myxoid (B), vascular (C), fibrous stage (D), and hyaline (E). In figure C there is tangential sectioning and pseudoepitheliomatous change which may be mistaken for intraepithelial dysplasia or carcinoma. In figure E there is associated keratosis and epithelial hyperplasia.

Laryngocele and Saccular Cyst

Definition. *Laryngocele* is an abnormal dilatation or outpouching from the laryngeal ventricle and saccule that contains air and maintains an open communication with the laryngeal lumen. *Saccular cyst* is a similar outpouching, but is a result of fluid accumulation and dilation of a noncommunicating saccule (110).

Clinical Features. There is no gender predilection and laryngoceles are most common in the fifth to eighth decades of life. Most cases are unilateral, but are bilateral in up to 25 percent of patients. Laryngoceles are congenital or acquired, and divided clinically into internal (expansion into the false vocal fold) and external (extension through the thyrohyoid membrane into the soft tissues of the neck) types, with most presenting as internal unilateral masses (111, 112). Symptoms are variable because the air may decompress spontaneously, removing the airway obstruction or hoarseness. Patients who repeatedly are subjected to increased pressure (e.g., glassblowers, musicians, and weight lifters) are more likely to have laryngoceles. Saccular cysts are divided into anterior and lateral types. Laryngoceles and saccular cysts are seen in conjunction with laryngeal squamous cell carcinoma.

The diagnosis of laryngocele is made by clinical and radiologic correlation. Radiologically, laryngocele is a thin-walled air-filled cystic lesion communicating with the laryngeal ventricle (fig. 5-19). Internal laryngoceles appear as low density masses in the supraglottic space. Mixed laryngoceles appear as low density, thin-walled masses seen in the low submandibular space that can be followed into larynx through the thyrohyoid membrane; the internal component

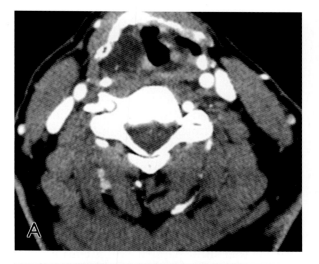
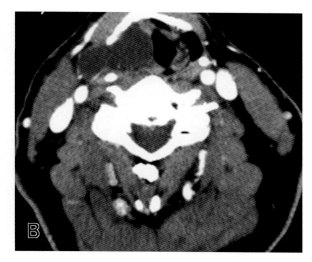
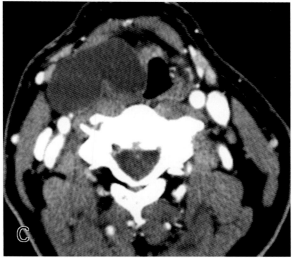

Figure 5-19

LARYNGOCELE

Axial contrast-enhanced images through the soft tissue of the neck show a cystic abnormality in the supraglottic larynx filling the right paraglottic space and extending through the thyrohyoid membrane. (Courtesy of Dr. A. Khorsandi, New York, NY.)

may be collapsed or dilated. Infected laryngoceles (*laryngopyolocele*), by contrast-enhanced computerized tomography (CT) have a thick, enhancing wall surrounding the laryngocele (fig. 5-20). Saccular cysts may show fluid levels.

Gross Findings. The gross appearance recapitulates the radiologic appearance.

Microscopic Findings. The histologic findings are nondescript and recapitulate the appearance of the laryngeal ventricle and saccule (fig. 5-21). Squamous metaplasia may occur (112–114).

Differential Diagnosis. The clinical differential diagnosis for laryngocele includes external jugular phlebectasia (a congenital dilatation of the jugular vein), which frequently presents as a neck mass particularly during straining or crying (Valsalva maneuver), similar to a laryngocele. It does not, however, require surgery, although surgery is often performed for cosmetic purposes. The histologic appearance is readily discernible from a saccular cyst because it is a vascular space (115,116). Saccular cysts have a clinical appearance similar to other laryngeal cysts of seromucinous derivation.

Treatment and Prognosis. Treatment is not required for asymptomatic cases; however, surgery (simple excision, marsupialization) may be necessary for large and symptomatic lesions. Surgery is curative. The complications associated with laryngoceles include airway obstruction and infection (laryngopyolocele).

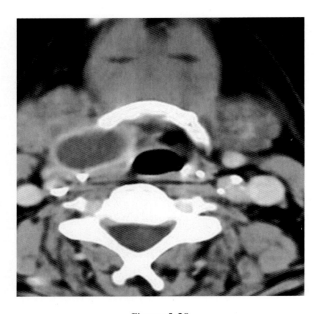

Figure 5-20

LARYNGOPYOCELE

Axial contrast-enhanced images show a rim enhancement of the cystic lesion in the right parapharyngeal space extending through the thyrohyoid membrane. (Courtesy of Dr. A. Khorsandi, New York, NY.)

Other Laryngeal Cysts

Definition. *Retention cysts* result from obstruction of seromucinous ducts and may be present throughout the larynx. *(Papillary) oncocytic cystadenoma* is a salivary-type cyst that occurs in the larynx.

Clinical Features. There is no gender predilection. Laryngeal cysts occur over a wide age range but tend to be most common in individuals older than the sixth decade of life. Most occur in the supraglottic larynx where there are more prominent seromucinous glands; less frequently, glottic and subglottic cysts occur. Many laryngeal cysts are asymptomatic and identified incidentally. The symptoms that are associated with laryngeal cysts include hoarseness, coughing, dyspnea, dysphagia, sensation of foreign body in the throat, neck mass, and pain. Infants may present with feeding problems.

Gross Findings. The gross appearance of cysts in the larynx is often determined by the point of origin in the larynx and the type of cyst. In contrast to laryngoceles, there is no direct communication of the cyst with the lumen or ventricle (117). Eversion and prolapse of the ventricle and saccule have been described, further complicating the classification of cysts of the larynx. The cyst wall may appear shiny and thinned, contains fluctuant to firm contents, and is often streaked with blood vessels. The cysts range in size from 0.5 cm to 8.0 cm. They are variably filled with thin serous fluid to tenacious, thick, mucinous, gelatinous or bloody fluid. They range from colorless to yellow, gray, or red, and frequently are translucent.

Microscopic Findings. The cyst lining determines the cyst subtype. Retention cysts resemble saccular cysts, with a squamous or respiratory-type lining in keeping with excretory duct morphology. Oncocytic cysts range from simple cysts to those that show papillary proliferations and solid areas, and may be referred to as *oncocytic cystadenoma* and *papillary oncocytic cystadenoma*, respectively (fig. 5-22) (118–120).

Differential Diagnosis. The differential diagnosis is limited. Ventricular prolapse may mimic a cyst but can be resituated unlike laryngeal cysts (121). Occasionally, large branchial cleft cysts and thyroglossal duct cysts may push into the larynx, but proper localization will resolve these considerations (122).

Treatment and Prognosis. Simple excision is curative.

Contact Ulcer of the Larynx

Definition. *Contact ulcer of the larynx* (CUL) is a benign, reactive, tumor-like condition etiologically related to gastroesophageal reflux, vocal abuse, or intubation. Synonyms include *pyogenic granuloma of the larynx* and *intubation granuloma*.

Clinical Features. CUL affects men more than women, and occurs over a wide age range. Generally, this is a lesion seen in adult populations and is considered uncommon in children, but is not restricted to any specific age group (123). In the intubation setting, female patients are affected more commonly, especially in an emergency setting when an inappropriately sized endotracheal tube has been selected. The most common site of occurrence is along the posterior aspect of one or both vocal cords, primarily in the area of the vocal cord process of the arytenoid cartilage. The clinical presentation may include hoarseness (most common), sore throat, and pain. Patients often have chronic throat clearing or habitual coughing.

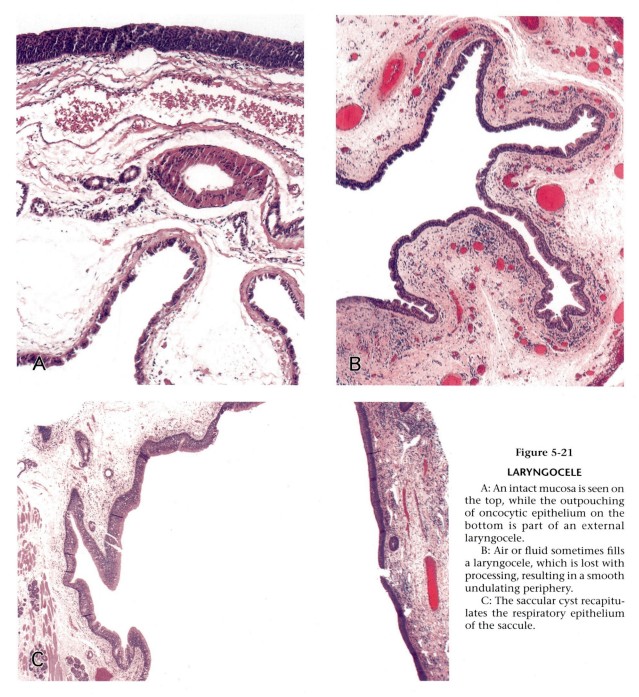

Figure 5-21

LARYNGOCELE

A: An intact mucosa is seen on the top, while the outpouching of oncocytic epithelium on the bottom is part of an external laryngocele.

B: Air or fluid sometimes fills a laryngocele, which is lost with processing, resulting in a smooth undulating periphery.

C: The saccular cyst recapitulates the respiratory epithelium of the saccule.

Pathogenesis. Etiologic factors include gastroesophageal reflux disease (GERD) with acid regurgitation, vocal abuse (excessive shouting, persistent coughing or throat clearing), and postintubational trauma (123,124). Gastric-laryngeal reflux, or GERD is frequently missed as the patient is unaware of the underlying cause, although they may report heartburn and belching. A hiatal hernia, peptic esophagitis, or gastritis will cause acid reflux, usually during sleep, thereby causing a contact ulcer without the patient's knowledge. Pepsin is thought to be the injurious agent and not the hydrochloric acid (123–126). The smaller tracheal lumen in

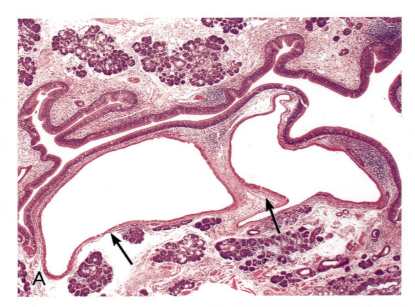

Figure 5-22

ONCOCYTIC CYST/CYSTADENOMA

A: Submucosal cysts (arrows) lined by cells with brightly eosinophilic cytoplasm (oncocytic epithelium) recapitulate the salivary duct. Lesions with proliferative changes are often designated as cystadenomas.

B: Oncocytic cystadenoma of the larynx is composed of enlarged cells with abundant eosinophilic cytoplasm.

C: Papillary oncocytic cystadenoma is composed of polyhedral cells with small, round to elongated nuclei and abundant granular eosinophilic (oncocytic) cytoplasm.

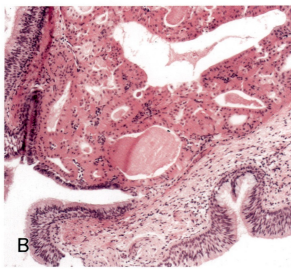
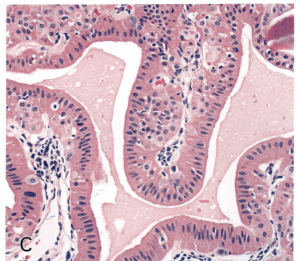

women results in a greater frequency of postintubational CUL than in men. The lesion may not become manifest until weeks to months following intubation injury.

Gross Findings. CUL usually presents as an ulcerated, polypoid or nodular mass, most frequently involving the posterior vocal cord. The lesion is red to tan-white and up to 3 cm in size. The frequent bilateral involvement of the cords results in a "kissing ulcer" on the opposite side of the vocal cord lesion. Involvement of the cartilage may be seen on generous biopsy specimens.

Microscopic Findings. The surface is ulcerated, covered by fibrin or fibrinoid necrosis overlying exuberant granulation tissue (fig. 5-23). The vessels in the granulation tissue are lined by plump, reactive endothelial cells, and surrounded by acute and chronic inflammatory cells and histiocytes. The vascular spaces are haphazard in configuration, and richly invested by lymphocytes, plasma cells, neutrophils, and histiocytes (including giant cell forms). Surface bacterial or fungal colonization is frequently identified.

In the early stages, surface ulceration without granulation tissue may be seen. With the progression of time, the chronic phase of the disease may demonstrate an irregular hyperplastic epithelium resulting from the regenerative

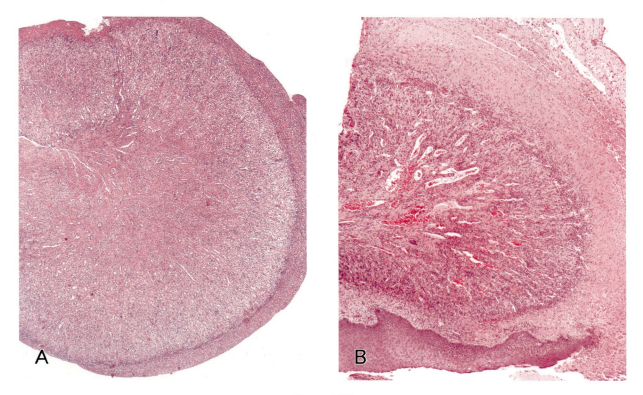

Figure 5-23

CONTACT ULCER OF THE LARYNX

A: The polypoid mass has surface ulceration and associated fibrinoid necrosis and granulation tissue.

B: Most of the surface epithelium has been denuded and replaced by fibrinoid necrosis. The vasculature in the granulation tissue is arranged perpendicular to the surface and is surrounded by rich granulation-type tissue.

surface re-epithelialization, but a residuum of fibrinoid necrosis is often identified below the surface. Prominent fibrosis may also be present in the stroma with progression of disease (123).

Differential Diagnosis. The differential diagnosis of CUL is broad given the nonspecific histologic appearance and includes previously mentioned infectious and inflammatory conditions, as well as vascular lesions such as hemangioma, and even epithelial lesions, ranging from papilloma to even carcinoma variants such as spindle cell squamous carcinoma or verrucous carcinoma. As such, clinicopathologic correlation with site and antecedent trauma, and the use of histochemical stains for microorganisms, and in some cases immunohistochemical stains, help resolve the diagnosis. Aggressive vascular lesions such as Kaposi sarcoma and epithelial neoplasms such as spindle cell squamous carcinoma and verrucous carcinoma often "declare" themselves by demonstrating greater depth of extension than the changes of CUL. Kaposi sarcoma expresses vascular markers and human herpesvirus (HHV)-8. Spindle cells squamous carcinomas are often immunoreactive for keratins and p63.

Treatment and Prognosis. The correct diagnosis allows for the identification of CUL with directed treatment of the underlying cause, including medical therapy for GERD and voice therapy for voice abuse.

Necrotizing Sialometaplasia

Definition. *Necrotizing sialometaplasia* (NSM) is a benign self-limiting process that mimics malignancy. For a more complete discussion, including illustrations, see chapter 6.

Clinical Features. While the development of (necrotizing) sialometaplasia following radiotherapy for squamous cell carcinoma is fairly common and underreported, primary NSM of the larynx is rare (127). Cases are associated with pain, numbness or a burning sensation, and

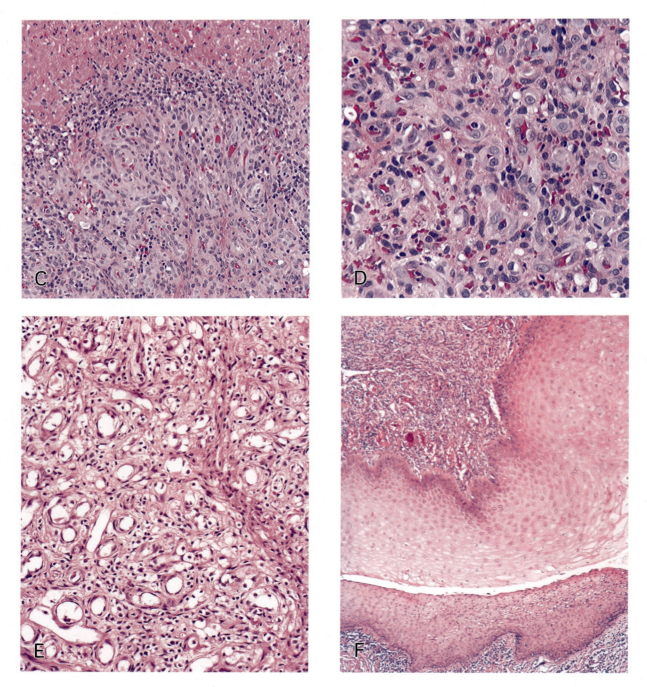

Figure 5-23, continued

C: The granulation tissue is exuberant with acute and chronic inflammatory cells and fibrinoid necrosis, which has a homogenized eosinophilic quality.

D: Plump, reactive endothelial cells almost completely obscure the vascular lumens. Mitotic figures are abundant, but cytologic atypia or pleomorphism is absent. Extravasated erythrocytes are common.

E: A haphazard arrangement of vessels can be seen in this area of granulation tissue deep in the center of a contact ulcer and may suggest the presence of a vascular neoplasm.

F: Because of the absence of a definitive diagnosis, and the chronic nature of the disease, re-epithelialization of the surface squamous epithelium over the defect, but with granulation-type tissue within the submucosa, may be seen in conjunction with active disease in the form of ulceration (not shown).

dysphagia. NSM may appear as a uninodular ulcerated lesion or as a nodular swelling. As in the palate, NSM is thought to be an ischemic event, possibly related to intubation trauma, radiotherapy, and in rare cases, atheromatous embolization (128). Even in the absence of antecedent radiotherapy, NSM may be seen in association with other lesions, including carcinoma (129,130).

Gross Findings. A submucosal nodular swelling will, after sloughing, give way to an ulcerative, crater-like lesion, usually less than 3 cm in greatest dimension. In the larynx, glottic sites are less likely to be involved since it is the supraglottic and subglottic larynx that contain seromucinous glands. In the trachea, NSM often appears over the tracheal rings first, resulting in stratified squamous epithelium replacing pseudostratified respiratory epithelium (127,131).

Microscopic Findings. NSM of the larynx has a similar appearance to that seen in the palate, and consists of ulceration with pseudoepitheliomatous hyperplasia of the adjacent mucosa, infarction of the salivary lobule, mucus extravasation, varying degrees of fibrosis, and squamous metaplasia of the ductoacinar units. Although frequent in other sites of NSM, pseudoepitheliomatous hyperplasia is not seen in the laryngeal cases, although the proximity to carcinoma in some reported cases adds to the challenge (127,130).

Differential Diagnosis. The differential diagnosis for NSM is summarized in Table 6-5 of chapter 6 and specifically includes squamous cell carcinoma, adenosquamous carcinoma, and mucoepidermoid carcinoma. While the key feature that distinguishes NSM from these considerations is the retention of the lobular architecture, this may not be apparent on a small biopsy or frozen section specimen, in which case it is appropriate to defer diagnosis. The presence of surface dysplasia also helps distinguish squamous cell carcinoma and adenosquamous carcinoma from NSM.

Treatment and Prognosis. NSM is self-limiting in the palate, and the same likely holds true for the larynx and trachea, although in some cases this is an incidental finding adjacent to a more significant lesion that would precipitate surgery anyway. Alone, it is reasonable to expect a favorable outcome without intervention.

Laryngeal Amyloidosis

Definition. *Laryngeal amyloidosis* encompasses a family of different types of benign accumulations of extracellular, fibrillar, insoluble protein deposits with a characteristic structure. The deposition of amyloid may be either localized or systemic, and primary or secondary.

Clinical Features. Laryngeal amyloidosis occurs over a wide patient age range but most patients present in the fifth to seventh decades of life, although children can rarely be affected (132–136). Almost all patients experience hoarseness or voice changes, usually caused by mechanical factors, and conditioned by the size and location of the amyloid; other symptoms include dyspnea and cough. There is no gender predilection.

Laryngeal amyloidosis can affect any portion of the larynx, but most frequently is seen along the true vocal cords, false vocal cords, and ventricle. It may be nodular or diffuse, single or multiple, and may be associated with a laryngocele.

Laryngeal amyloidosis is commonly localized and primary, although rare, accounting for less than 1 percent of benign laryngeal tumors. Multifocal disease is present in up to 15 percent of patients (132–136). There have been a variety of classifications of amyloidosis, according to its distribution (localization), clinical type, presence or absence of underlying disease, and by its precursor protein and patterns of extracellular deposition (132–136). The three forms of systemic amyloidosis include the primary form, the reactive form, and the familial form. The localized form is rare, with the larynx affected more frequently than any other single site and, conversely, most laryngeal cases are primary and focal, only occasionally part of systemic disease. Different sources of amyloid are recognized: immunoglobulin light chains (AL), serum amyloid A in reactive amyloidosis (AA), transthyretin type in familial or senile amyloidosis (ATTR), hemodialysis-associated β2 microglobulin amyloid (Aβ2M), and more recently, leukocyte cell-derived chemotaxin 2 amyloid (ALECT2) (137,138).

A diagnosis of laryngeal amyloidosis should prompt clinical evaluation to exclude the presence of primary or secondary amyloidosis. The evaluation includes serum and urine electrophoresis, immunoelectrophoresis, and

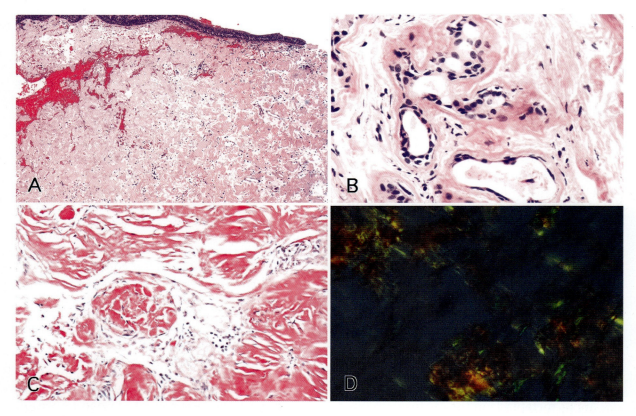

Figure 5-24

LARYNGEAL AMYLOID

A: Typically, there is abundant stromal deposition of waxy, amorphous, pink matrix.
B: Ductal accentuation in seromucous glands is common.
C: As in other sites, amyloid is intensely congophilic.
D: The amyloid demonstrates the typical birefringence that may appear "apple green."

aspiration biopsy of the abdominal fat pad to evaluate for the presence of amyloid, which is positive in up to 95 percent of patients with primary (systemic) amyloidosis and approximately two thirds of patients with secondary (systemic) amyloidosis.

Gross Findings. The lesion has a firm, "starch-like," waxy, translucent cut surface. Lesions range from a few millimeters up to 4 cm in greatest dimension. The disease may be multifocal in the upper aerodigestive tract.

Microscopic Findings. Amyloid consists histologically (irrespective of any associated findings) of a subepithelial, extracellular, acellular, hyaline-like, homogeneous, eosinophilic matrix material dispersed randomly throughout the stroma, although revealing a predilection for vessels or seromucous glands (fig. 5-24). A sparse inflammatory infiltrate composed of lymphocytes and plasma cells, with occasional histiocytes and a few giant cells, is present either at the peripheral margin of, or enclosed within, the amyloid. There is no significant cytologic atypia of the lymphoplasmacytic infiltrate.

Special Stains. Amyloid is confirmed with histochemical techniques including Congo red (fig. 5-24) and methyl violet (metachromatic pink-violet) staining. The appearance of amyloid by cross polarization of light with a polarizer and analyzer, however, is what is most frequently used to establish the diagnosis. The physics of this phenomenon are more complex than conveyed by the simple term "apple green birefringence," (fig. 5-24) (139). While this remains a memorable basic descriptor, the spectrum of color under cross polarization ranges from various shades of green yellow to blue-green, which transitions to red when polarizer and analyzer are uncrossed. Electron microscopy reveals the characteristic interlacing meshwork of nonbranching, 7- to 10-nm fibrils as the protein arranges itself into β-pleated sheets (140).

Although CD20 and CD3 highlight B cells and T cells in the sparse lymphoplasmacytic infiltrate, respectively, T cells tend to predominate, especially at the periphery of the amyloid deposits. Most cases of laryngeal amyloidosis are of the AL type; immunoreactivity with amyloid P and light chains (κ and λ) is more variable, although light chain restriction of the plasma cells can be seen. The mucosal presentation of laryngeal amyloidosis, the recurrence and multifocal presentation in other mucosal sites, the monoclonal nature of the associated lymphoplasmacytic infiltrate in some cases, and a possible systemic plasma cell dyscrasia imply that at least a few laryngeal amyloid cases are the result of an immunocyte dyscrasia or lymphoproliferative disorder with an origin from mucosa-associated lymphoid tissue (MALT).

Differential Diagnosis. The differential diagnosis includes hyalinized vocal cord polyps (usually lacks an associated lymphoplasmacytic infiltrate), ligneous conjunctivitis (a hereditary or familial disease associated with plasminogen mutations/deficiency that presents as pseudomembranous-covered, fibrous, woody, plaque-like deposits in the larynx or trachea consisting of accumulated acid mucopolysaccharides and hyaluronic acid and surrounded by inflammatory cells and vessels) (141,142), and lipoid proteinosis (a disease characterized by *ECM1* mutations, with systemic cutaneous and mucosal amorphous hyaline deposits) (143). These are all negative for amyloid stains.

Treatment and Prognosis. Localized laryngeal amyloidosis has a favorable prognosis, and is cured by local endoscopic resection. Persistent or recurrent local disease may rarely occur, usually within 5 years of the initial treatment. Systemic amyloidosis involving the larynx, on the other hand, requires an appropriate workup as noted above.

Subglottic Stenosis

Definition. *Subglottic stenosis* (SS) is acquired or congenital narrowing (partial or complete) of the larynx (subglottis) due to excessive growth of fibrous tissue. Synonyms include *laryngotracheal stenosis* and *tracheal stenosis*.

Clinical Features. SS is a rare condition, with acquired stenosis being more common than congenital stenosis. There is no gender predilection although idiopathic SS is more common in women than in men. SS affects all age groups.

Symptoms relate to airway obstruction and include progressive respiratory difficulty, biphasic stridor, dyspnea, and air hunger. Other symptoms include hoarseness, abnormal cry, aphonia, dysphagia, and feeding abnormalities. In congenital stenosis, symptoms appear at or shortly after birth. In acquired stenosis, usually there is a history of trauma followed by a latent period of 1 month or longer prior to the manifestation of symptoms.

Pathogenesis. For acquired SS, various etiologic factors come into play, with postintubation injury, smoke inhalation, and burn injury the most frequent. The airway obstruction is further classified as extrinsic, intrinsic, or intraluminal, and segmental or circumferential. While there are a host of clinical staging systems for children and adults, the degree of stenosis (length and percent of luminal narrowing/compromise) is the most important single factor. Patients come to clinical attention because of increasing dyspnea upon exertion or wheezing with exercise. Laryngoscopic examination reveals webs, synechia, strictures, bridging, and circumferential narrowing.

Gross Findings. SS involves the region from the insertion of the conus elasticus into the vocal cords to the inferior margin of the cricoid cartilage, not including the upper trachea. Most cases are either cartilaginous or soft tissue stenosis, "hard" or "soft," respectively, clinically, although fibrosis can occur in both categories depending upon maturity. Cricoid cartilage abnormalities (absence, deformity, small for age), trapped first tracheal ring, and fibrosis cause the cartilaginous types (congenital) while granulation tissue, mucinous gland hyperplasia (usually on the posterior wall), and associated fibrosis cause the soft tissue types (including acquired or idiopathic). A large anterior or posterior lamina, and generalized thickening resulting in circumferential narrowing, elliptical shape,

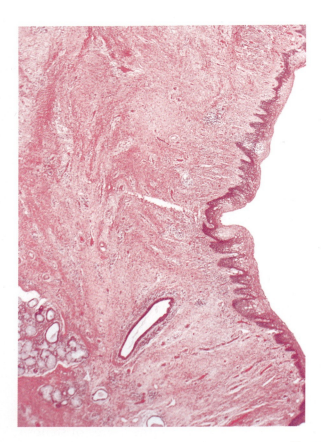 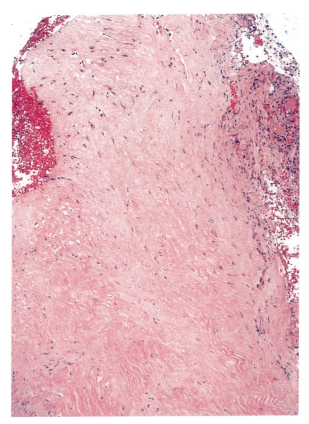

Figure 5-25

SUBGLOTTIC STENOSIS

Left: The stenosis is characterized by a dense, almost keloid-like scar.
Right: At higher magnification, the dense fibrosis is fairly hypocellular, and consists of bland fibroblasts without significant atypia. The histologic findings are nonspecific and require clinical correlation to render a diagnosis of subglottic stenosis.

or a submucous cleft are the most frequent abnormalities of the cricoid cartilage, but the cartilage may also be too small for the size of the larynx. Absence of the cricoid is associated with laryngeotracheoesophageal cleft or atresia. It is uncommon to find only a single abnormality, but instead, there are degrees of involvement of both the "hard" and "soft" types in the same specimen (144–149).

Microscopic Findings. Although the histologic findings are nonspecific, careful documentation of the abnormalities of the gross specimen allows appropriate clinical management. The idiopathic form of SS is histologically characterized by the presence of submucosal fibrosis, with dense eosinophilic collagen deposition (keloid-like) associated with a sparse population of fibroblasts (fig. 5-25). The fibroblasts are composed of uniform spindled-shaped cells with oval nuclei, inconspicuous nucleoli, and a variable amount of cytoplasm. Nuclear pleomorphism, mitotic figures, and necrosis are not identified. A mixed inflammatory cell infiltrate is variably present, and may be scant or large. The overlying surface epithelium is benign, may show metaplastic changes (e.g., squamous), or may be ulcerated with replacement by granulation tissue. The subjacent cartilage is generally unremarkable.

Differential Diagnosis. While there are a number of causes of subglottic stenosis, the histopathologic differential diagnosis is usually limited, once a variety of infectious and inflammatory conditions are excluded by the clinical features. Occasionally, mesenchymal lesions, such as benign peripheral nerve sheath tumor (e.g., schwannoma) or fibromatosis are considered, but if there is adequate material for immunohistochemical stains such as S-100 protein (positive in benign peripheral nerve sheath tumors) and nuclear beta-catenin (positive in fibromatosis), the diagnosis is clear.

In congenital SS, laryngomalacia enters the differential but is distinguished clinically since the obstruction is secondary to the collapse of the larynx into the lumen rather than true stenosis. Congenital SS, in contrast to acquired SS, tends to have the associated lesions such as webs, synechia, and atresias.

Treatment and Prognosis. The treatment is predicated on the underlying cause of the stenosis, and in establishing a patent airway. Airway maintenance may require excision (endoscopic, laser) tracheotomy or segmental resection. Local recurrences are common. The prognosis is usually good, although re-stenosis can develop, especially in patients with circumferential stenosis associated with cartilaginous abnormalities.

Rheumatoid Nodule

Definition. *Rheumatoid nodule* is a nodular necrobiotic granulomatous process seen in patients with rheumatoid arthritis.

Clinical Features. Laryngeal involvement by rheumatoid arthritis is uncommon (150–157). The cricoarytenoid or cricothyroid joint may be involved, with the former more frequently involved. Cricoarytenoid arthritis is usually bilateral. Rheumatoid nodules develop in approximately one quarter of patients with rheumatoid arthritis, but laryngeal involvement is rare, typically involving the true vocal cord, and thus presenting with hoarseness, dysphonia, and dysphagia. Other sites of involvement include the false vocal cords, epiglottis, and soft tissues around the cricoarytenoid joint. Rarely, laryngeal amyloidosis is associated with rheumatoid arthritis (154).

Gross Findings. The lesions at laryngoscopy are nonspecific and may present as erythematous vocal cords with submucosal nodules or as ulcerated granulation tissue, often bilateral. The nodules are soft and often yellow. Joint destruction and ankylosis develop with the passage of time. The manifestations within the cricoarytenoid or thyroid joint in the acute phase include inflammation, joint effusion, and a synovial proliferation.

Microscopic Findings. Rheumatoid nodules have the same histologic appearance as seen in other sites, with subepithelial areas of fibrinoid necrosis of the collagen surrounded by palisading histiocytes, with associated fibrosis and inflammatory cells (fig. 5-26). There can be more extensive inflammation with fibroblasts, edema, and endothelial proliferation in the fibrous connective tissue (150–157). Laryngeal amyloidosis has been rarely described as a finding in rheumatoid arthritis (154).

Differential Diagnosis. The differential diagnosis includes other causes of arthritis in the laryngeal joints (systemic lupus erythematosus, gout, Reiter disease) and other granulomatous diseases (infectious and autoimmune). The clinical setting of the disease helps define the sometimes nonspecific inflammatory findings. Gout can involve the larynx and gouty tophi may have a similar appearance to rheumatoid nodules. Tophi usually show urate crystals, or clefts within the tissue if the crystals do not survive processing (158–160). Infectious granulomas and granulomatosis with polyangiitis often have a different character of necrosis that is "bluer," with more karyorrhectic debris, and inflammatory infiltrates. Correlation with clinical, culture, and serologic findings is a requisite.

Treatment and Prognosis. Treatment for laryngeal arthritis includes high doses of prednisone and, in some cases, injection into the joint space. Ankylosis of the joint is a feared complication that may result in airway compromise necessitating surgical intervention (e.g., tracheotomy) (151).

Teflon Granuloma

Definition. *Teflon granuloma* (*teflonoma*) is a foreign body granulomatous tissue response to the extravasation of Teflon® injected for the treatment of vocal cord paralysis.

Clinical Features. Teflon® (fluorocarbon, polytetrafluoroethylene) is among the most viscous substances used in injection medialization laryngoplasties to treat unilateral vocal fold paralysis (UFVP) (161). Historically the most popular substance for injection, Teflon has now fallen out of favor because of the tendency for a granulomatous response, and the performance superiority of more flexible, less viscous agents. A Teflon granuloma is a submucosal, polypoid,

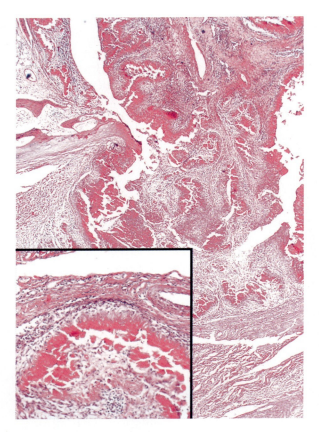 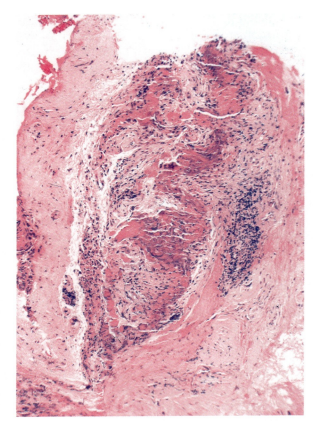

Figure 5-26

CRICOARYTENOID RHEUMATOID ARTHRITIS

Left: The rheumatoid nodules disrupt the thyroid cartilage. The necrobiotic nodules show fragmentation. Inset: Palisading histiocytes are located at the periphery of the nodule.

Right: In another example, the circumscribed nodule is associated with necrobiosis.

tumor-like accumulation of Teflon paste. The use of Teflon to correct UFVP was generally limited to the adult population, making Teflon granuloma mainly a lesion of adulthood, although they have been reported in children (162). Teflon granulomas produce persistent dysphonia, but may also present with obstruction (163).

Gross Findings. Macroscopically, the vocal cord is usually stiff and nonpliable, erythematous and hard. "Tumors" may appear as polypoid lesions within the submucosal compartment of the vocal cord area or may be well-delineated, firm masses when identified in the soft tissues of the neck. The lesions vary from a few millimeters to 2 cm (164).

Microscopic Findings. The granulomatous or foreign body giant cell reaction is more frequently identified in the arytenoid region than the mid-vocal cord; it occurs in the submucosa and extends into the underlying muscle and cartilage (fig. 5-27) (165). Depending upon the exact chronologic point at which the biopsy is taken, the initial findings may only consist of edema, inflammation, and a marked mononuclear histiocytic response. The irregular brown to black, birefringent (under polarized light) fibers of Teflon appear as glassy crystals within the giant cells or loose within the extensive fibrous connective tissue. Occasionally, they appear as black fibers if carbon coated. There is only a limited inflammatory reaction, with dense fibrous connective tissue "encapsulating" the lesion, especially when it has been present for some time. Giant cells are only seen occasionally at this late stage of the disorder.

Electron microscopy, infrared absorption spectrophotometry (IAS), and energy dispersive

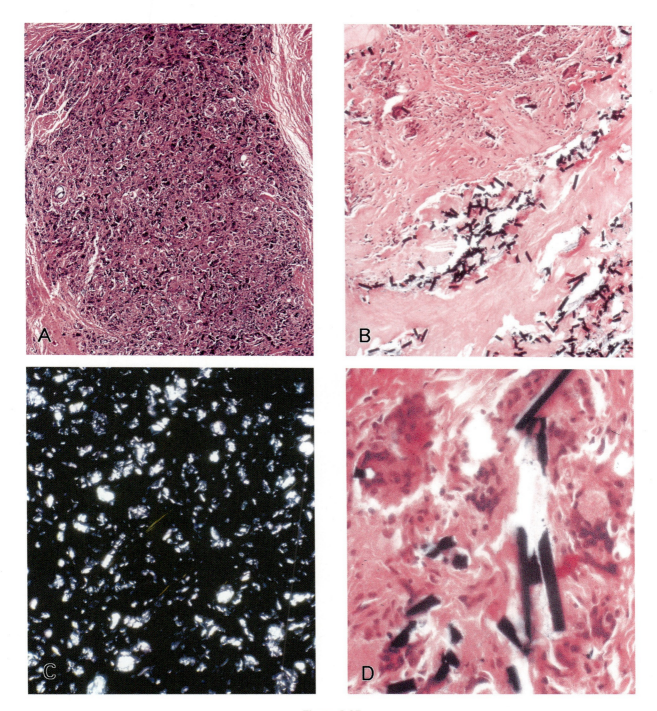

Figure 5-27

TEFLON GRANULOMA

A: The particles of Teflon are aggregated as a circumscribed stromal nodule. A significant inflammatory or foreign body giant cell reaction is lacking.

B: The brown-black fibers of Teflon are in close association with foreign body giant cells.

C: Polarization of the specimen shows the highly refractile (Teflon) particles.

D: Carbon coating is used on Teflon in some instances, yielding black rod-shaped particles, often identified within foreign body giant cell macrophages.

X-ray analysis (EDXA) are more conclusive methodologies to confirm the presence of Teflon (165), but are mainly of historical interest, as the clinical history is confirmatory.

Differential Diagnosis. Aside from the other necrobiotic and infectious granulomatous lesions noted above, other substances used for injection laryngoplasty may enter the differential diagnosis for Teflon granuloma but are distinguished by their distinctive appearance. Injectable substances are divided broadly into hyaluronic acid–derived and nonhyaluronic acid–derived substances, including collagen, Teflon, calcium hydroxyapatite (Coaptite®) in gel carrier, as well as autologous elements such as adipose tissue or bone marrow (161). Some materials, such as calcium hydroxyapatite gel, have histologic documentation, mainly in animal models (166,167), but most do not, which is itself telling in that these other materials are less problematic than Teflon and thus less likely to result in a biopsy specimen in humans. Autologous fat does not generally elicit a strong granulomatous response (168).

Treatment and Prognosis. Correct placement and appropriate amount of the injection help to decrease the possible negative effects of the therapy. Since Teflon is a permanent implant that is not absorbed, surgical resection remains the only way to remove the Teflon-induced granulomatous reaction. After debulking of the Teflon particles, an improvement in vocal function can be expected, although the poor voice quality is often permanent.

Reactive Epithelial Changes

Definition. *Reactive epithelial changes* (i.e., keratosis without dysplasia, hyperplasia) are potentially reversible, reactive or reparative, benign processes reflecting the epithelial response to a stimulus or to injury. There is still no uniformity and consistency in the terminology used to classify reactive epithelial changes in relation to precancerous epithelial lesions (i.e., dysplasia). A fundamental problem here is both the histologic and biologic overlap with such lesions. In some classification systems, basal layer hyperplasia actually equates with dysplasia (169).

Clinical Features. Distinctive reactive lesions with a known etiology have been described in detail above. The remainder of such lesions also occur in patients with the same epidemiologic and risk factors for squamous dysplasia and carcinoma: mainly those over the fifth decade of life, with a male predilection and history of tobacco and alcohol exposure. Patients typically present with sore throat; those with glottic lesions have hoarseness or changes in phonation.

Gross Findings. Most of these lesions involve the true vocal cords, frequently bilaterally, rarely involving the commissures. The lesions range from a circumscribed thickening of the mucosa to an ill-defined plaque, often exhibiting a rough surface. Unfortunately, no clinical appearance is consistently correlated to the underlying histology since the same appearance can be attributed to dysplastic and even early carcinomatous lesions. The changes may be localized to a small area of the vocal cord or may be diffuse, involving virtually the entire larynx (*pachyderma laryngis*) (170).

Microscopic Findings. As there is overlap with early precancerous or dysplastic lesions, restricting the spectrum of changes in reactive epithelial hyperplasia is challenging, and may vary depending on location. For instance, a metaplastic or immature basaloid appearance is more acceptable in transitional areas of supraglottic and subglottic regions, but is more alarming on the true vocal cords (171). Perhaps the most consistent model to help define changes is the free edge of the true vocal fold. Reactive lesions include *simple hyperplasia*, *basal layer hyperplasia*, and *keratosis without dysplasia* (fig. 5-28). Some lesions are more exophytic, including *pseudoepitheliomatous hyperplasia* (fig. 5-28) and *verrucous hyperplasia* (fig. 5-29).

Keratosis is present in a wide variety of alterations, including reactive and hyperplastic lesions, premalignant changes, and carcinomas. Keratosis is the abnormal production and accumulation of keratin at the surface of the (laryngeal) mucosa, in which is it normally absent. The keratin is often present in an exophytic or stalactitic pattern. The term hyperkeratosis is not used in the larynx since keratin is not a normal constituent of the epithelium, making this term redundant (the term keratosis suffices). Nuclear atypia or pleomorphism is not implied by "keratosis" although keratosis can have atypia present (atypia is not synonymous with pleomorphism.). Parakeratosis refers to the presence of nuclei within the keratotic layer.

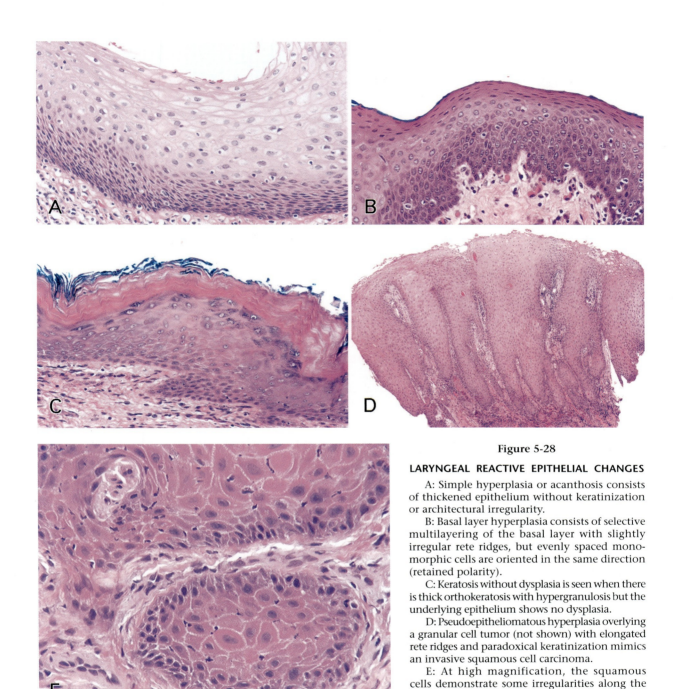

Figure 5-28

LARYNGEAL REACTIVE EPITHELIAL CHANGES

A: Simple hyperplasia or acanthosis consists of thickened epithelium without keratinization or architectural irregularity.

B: Basal layer hyperplasia consists of selective multilayering of the basal layer with slightly irregular rete ridges, but evenly spaced monomorphic cells are oriented in the same direction (retained polarity).

C: Keratosis without dysplasia is seen when there is thick orthokeratosis with hypergranulosis but the underlying epithelium shows no dysplasia.

D: Pseudoepitheliomatous hyperplasia overlying a granular cell tumor (not shown) with elongated rete ridges and paradoxical keratinization mimics an invasive squamous cell carcinoma.

E: At high magnification, the squamous cells demonstrate some irregularities along the periphery, but no cytologic atypia.

Keratosis in laryngeal mucosa by itself does not have any prognostic significance and is only a part of the complex response seen in the laryngeal mucosa. There is an approximately 4 percent risk of subsequently identifying carcinoma in patients with an initial diagnosis of keratosis (172,173). A *keratoma* is a flat to warty or villous mass about the anterior to middle third of the vocal cord, although involvement of the entire length has been described.

Epithelial hyperplasia may produce verrucous or papillary growth with surface keratinization, lacking loss of polarity and nuclear atypia (174). *Verrucous hyperplasia*, or *proliferative verrucous*

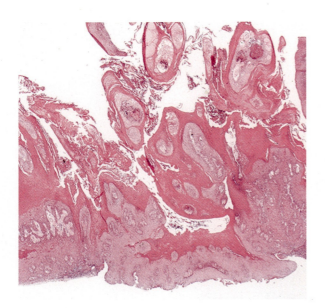 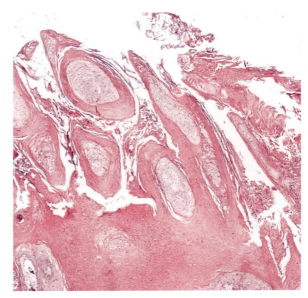

Figure 5-29

VERRUCOUS HYPERPLASIA

Left, right: Verrucous hyperplasia is characterized by papillary fronds of squamous epithelium covered with tiered-appearing keratin and lacking the architectural and cytologic features of malignancy. Differentiating verrucous hyperplasia from verrucous carcinoma is challenging.

leukoplakia (PVL), similarly is considered a preinvasive form of verrucous carcinoma based on oral cavity data (175). The terminology should thus fit the regional and cultural norm to ensure that the appropriate connotation and biology is conveyed. Realistically, many cases of reactive epithelial change cannot be reliably separated from preneoplastic lesions.

Special Stains. Immunohistochemical staining for various keratins (CK13) has been proposed as a means of distinguishing between reactive epithelial changes and carcinoma. CK13 is expressed in reactive conditions but decreased or absent in dysplasia and carcinoma (176). Differential keratin staining, however, has not proved reliable in differentiating reactive processes from dysplasia or carcinoma. Ki-67 (MIB1) and known biomarkers of carcinogenesis, such as p53 and other tumor suppressor gene losses (177), have limited value in the diagnosis and differential diagnosis.

Differential Diagnosis. The differential diagnosis encompasses different lesions within the reactive and hyperplastic category as well as separation from dysplasia and carcinoma. It is well accepted that dysplasia (squamous intraepithelial lesion, squamous intraepithelial neoplasia) is a precancerous lesion, but the issue of how much "atypia" makes a lesion dysplastic is not well established and poorly reproducible between practitioners. Since there is a sequential continuum or arc of development, it is nearly impossible to rigidly divide a particular lesion categorically into reactive versus neoplastic, as no combination of features consistently or accurately separates the two. Therefore, degrees of atypia and subtle changes often portend impending carcinoma transformation but may at that time not represent a true "carcinoma."

A listing of the maturation and cellular alterations associated with dysplasia is detailed in Table 5-2 and prove useful in separating dysplasia from reactive processes. Markers of dysplasia not seen in benign reactive conditions include: dyskeratosis, a lack of maturity or irregular epithelial stratification toward the surface ("basal zone"-type cells identified above the basal zone), anisonucleosis (abnormal nuclear size), anisocytosis (abnormal cell size), pleomorphism (nuclear shape irregularities, chromatin distribution disturbance, nuclear hyperchromasia), changes in the nuclear to cytoplasmic ratio, atypical

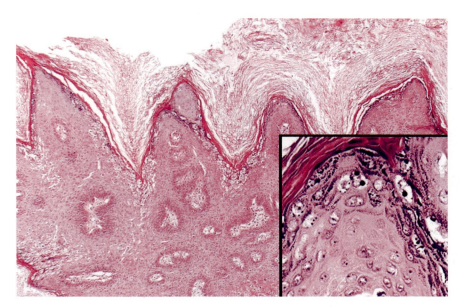

Figure 5-30

VERRUCA VULGARIS

Verrucoid keratosis is associated with orthokeratosis and hypergranulosis. Inset: Dense keratohyaline granules. (Courtesy Dr. E. L. Barnes, Pittsburgh, PA.)

Table 5-2
HISTOMORPHOLOGIC CHANGES ASSOCIATED WITH DYSPLASIA[a]
Architectural Abnormalities
Irregular epithelial stratification with elongated rete ridges extending in a downward fashion into submucosa
Loss of maturation with increased cellularity in the superficial epithelium
Crowding of cells with loss of polarity especially in the basal zone
Increased mitotic activity, especially away from the basal zone involving the mid- and upper (superficial) portions of the surface epithelium (may include atypical forms)
Abnormal keratosis (dyskeratosis)
Cellular Abnormalities
Abnormal variation in the nuclear size (anisonucleosis)
Abnormal variation in the nuclear shape (i.e., nuclear pleomorphism)
Nuclear hyperchromasia with irregularities in the nuclear contour
Prominent nucleoli (not unique to dysplasia, may be seen in reactive or reparative processes)

[a]Adapted from Table 16-2 from Wenig BM. Neoplasms of the larynx and trachea. In Wenig BM, ed. Atlas of head and neck pathology, 3rd ed. Philadelphia: Elsevier; 2016:719.

mitotic figures, premature keratinization lower in the proliferating epithelium (toward the basal zone), and increased mitotic figures. Nutritional deficiencies of vitamin B12 and folate can imitate dysplasia, but the clinical history and other laboratory data help to make this separation.

For verrucoid lesions, verruca vulgaris is a rare consideration in the larynx but it does occur. Features include marked acanthosis, papillomatosis, orthokeratosis, prominent granular cell layer, irregular coarsely aggregated keratohyaline granules, koilocytes, and thin, penetrating rete ridges (fig. 5-30) (178).

Treatment and Prognosis. Technically, true hyperplasia and reactive epithelial lesions are self-limiting and reversible. But because of the morphologic overlap with early preneoplastic lesions, even a keratosis without dysplasia has a small (2 to 4 percent) risk of progression to carcinoma. Thus limited surveillance may be appropriate.

Radiation-Associated Changes

Definition. *Radiation-associated changes* are distinctive epithelial and stromal changes associated with radiation therapy.

Clinical Features. The gender and demographics typically follow those associated with laryngeal squamous cell carcinoma, which more often affects men than women and occurs over a wide range of adult ages. Radiation injury to mucosal sites results in alterations in the surface epithelium, minor salivary glands, fibroblasts, skeletal muscle, and endothelial cells. Radiation-induced changes may be acute or chronic. Acute changes occur from days to weeks (usually 6 weeks) following treatment; chronic changes are seen from 6 to 7 weeks following therapy to years later (179,180). Biopsies are

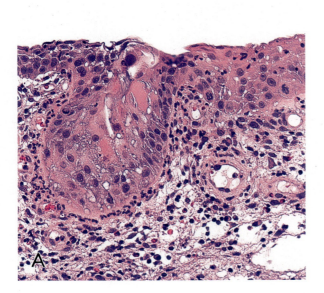 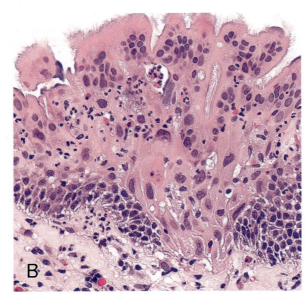

Figure 5-31

RADIATION-ASSOCIATED CHANGES

Epithelial alterations may include the following:
A: Nuclear enlargement with prominent eosinophilic nucleoli, although the cells still maintain their polarity with a low nuclear to cytoplasmic ratio. In the submucosa there is marked inflammation and vascular proliferation with associated enlarged endothelial cells.
B: Papillary-like growth is composed of markedly enlarged cells with nuclear hyperchromasia and irregularity but with a low nuclear to cytoplasmic ratio. Associated acute inflammation is present.

taken following radiation therapy to primarily exclude the possibility of recurrent carcinoma.

Gross Findings. Early changes, when present, include an edematous to erythematous, erosive appearance, while late changes are grossly characterized by fibrosis. The vocal folds may be attenuated, showing scarring and loss of pliability.

Microscopic Findings. During the acute postirradiation phase (days to weeks), biopsies are seldom obtained. These early changes include stromal edema, vascular congestion, and mucosal erosion (179). Biopsies taken in the later (chronic) postirradiation period show variable histologic changes including: 1) thinner than normal surface epithelium, surface ulceration, and squamous epithelial atypia (fig. 5-31); 2) atrophy of minor salivary gland acini (fig. 5-31) and sialometaplasia, which may include atypical squamous epithelium; 3) mesenchymal or stromal alterations that may include submucosal fibrosis, vascular alterations characterized by telangiectatic capillaries often with prominent (plump) endothelial cells, myointimal proliferation, foamy histiocytes within the intima and thrombosis, atypical (bizarre) (myo)fibroblasts, and bizarre striated muscle degeneration (fig. 5-31) (177).

Differential Diagnosis. The differential diagnosis for radiation atypia primarily but not exclusively includes differentiating radiation-related epithelial atypia from dysplasia or carcinoma involving the surface epithelium, minor salivary glands, or submucosa. Despite the bizarre atypia of the surface epithelium occasionally seen following radiotherapy, the constellation of nuclear changes seen in association with dysplasia is absent. Relative to sialometaplasia, there is retention of the lobular configuration of the minor salivary glands following radiation while such glands tend to be effaced in the presence of carcinoma. Stromal changes (i.e., atypical fibroblasts) may mimic a postirradiation sarcoma or squamous cell carcinoma. While both processes may have atypical hyperchromatic cells, post-irradiation change tends to show "smudgy" rather than coarse chromatin characteristics. Further, the atypical fibroblasts tend to be isolated in contrast to the cohesive cell

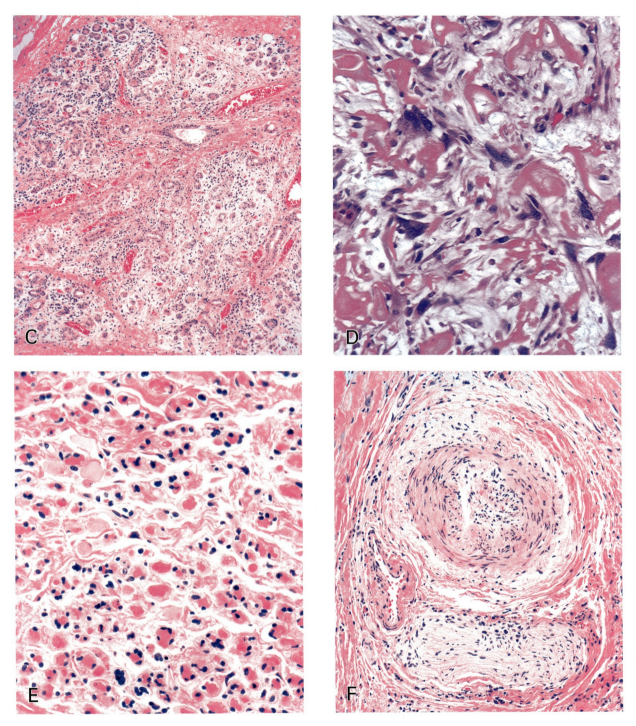

Figure 5-31, continued
C: There is atrophy of minor salivary glands, although lobular growth is retained.
D: Atypical stromal cells that represent myofibroblastic cells are characterized by smudged nuclei, low nuclear to cytoplasmic ratio, and in some cells "axonal"-like cytoplasmic extensions.
E: Degenerative changes of skeletal muscle are seen.
F: Blood vessel myointimal proliferation is seen.

clusters seen in carcinoma. In some cases immunohistochemical staining may be required to exclude a carcinoma (keratin positive) and differentiate it from fibroblasts (keratin negative).

Occasionally, the fibrovascular response in radiation change may also mimic an angiosarcoma. However, the architecture of the vessels is maintained and the anastomosing channels seen in angiosarcoma are absent.

Treatment and Prognosis. Radiation atypia eventually resolves to some extent although the fibrosis and intimal hyperplasia remain. Postirradiation sarcomas of the larynx can occur, although they are rare (181,182).

LARYNGEAL MANIFESTATIONS OF DERMATOLOGIC DISORDERS

Many dermatologic disorders have systemic manifestations that include involvement of the mucous membranes of the larynx. An exhaustive recitation of these clinical conditions is beyond the scope of this volume, and only a few key entities are described.

Epidermolysis Bullosa

Epidermolysis bullosa (EB) is an inherited group of diseases that include *junctional EB, EB simplex* or *dystrophic EB*, and *Kindler syndrome*, depending on the level of blistering and thus the molecular component affected (183). *EB acquisita* is an acquired autoimmunity to type VII collagen, and rarely involves the larynx (184). Junctional EB most frequently involves the larynx (185).

The symptoms of laryngotracheal EB range from hoarseness to obstruction. Findings range from bullae, with or without ulceration and superinfection, to laryngeal stenosis in dystrophic EB (186).

Histologically, there is a blister or disruption of the basal cell layer, although this depends upon the duration of the lesion. There may be regeneration of the epithelium, and so the blister location within the epithelium may vary. A PAS stain to accentuate the basement membrane demonstrates the bullae on the luminal side of the basement membrane. In the chronic forms, granulation tissue with scaring may be seen, along with cystic dilatation of the submucosal glands. A skin biopsy with direct immunofluorescence or electron microscopy to confirm the location of the bullae and the type of antibody deposit is ideal, but if the larynx is the only site of involvement, the biopsy should be taken from an uninvolved region or the edge of a blister to reveal the best changes.

EB of the larynx tends to be a marker of aggressive behavior and poor prognosis (184). An association with an increased risk of carcinoma development is postulated, but not validated (187).

Pemphigus

Pemphigus is classified as pemphigus vulgaris (PV), *pemphigus foliaceus, paraneoplastic pemphigus* (PNP), *drug-induced pemphigus*, and *IgA pemphigus* (188), but laryngeal involvement is mainly associated with PV, an autoimmune disease with antibodies targeting desmoglein-3 (PV antigen). PV involvement of the laryngopharynx is likely underreported, as symptomatology is noted in about a quarter of patients and is even more frequent in patients with exacerbations (189,190). Patients present with findings ranging from tenderness to odynophagia and hoarseness. Endoscopic findings include erosions and blisters as are typical at other sites. Pemphigus is defined by suprabasal acantholysis with inflammatory changes, although dyskeratosis is not as prominent as seen in Darier disease. Immunofluorescence is generally useful to delineate PV and PNP.

Mucous Membrane Pemphigoid

Mucous membrane pemphigoid (MMP) is a subepithelial immune-mediated bullous disease predominantly affecting the mucous membranes, unlike bullous pemphigoid. About half of patients have pharyngeal symptoms, while one fourth have laryngeal symptoms. Similar to other bullous diseases, MMP shows a spectrum of blister morphology. The blister is formed subepithelially, with the basement membrane noted on the roof of the blister. MMP is characterized by linear IgG along the basement membrane, often with C3 and even IgA (191). Laryngeal involvement correlates with ocular involvement and is thus considered an ominous feature.

REFERENCES

Embryology, Anatomy and Histology

1. Standring S, Larynx. In: Standring S, ed. Gray's Anatomy. The anatomical basis of clinical practice, 40th ed. Edinburgh: Elsevier Churchill Livingstone; 2008:577-594.
2. Moore KL, Persaud DV. The respiratory system. In: Moore ML, Persaud DV, eds. The developing human: clinically oriented embryology. Philadelphia: Saunders; 2003:241-253.
3. Hollinshead WH. The pharynx and larynx. In: Hollinshead, WD, ed. Anatomy for surgeons. Philadelphia: Harper & Row; 1982:389-441.
4. Reidenbach MM. The periepiglottic space: topographic relations and histological organisation. J Anat, 1996;188(Pt 1):173-182.
5. Reidenbach MM. Borders and topographic relationships of the paraglottic space. Eur Arch Otorhinolaryngol 1997;254:193-195.
6. Sato K, Kurita S, Hirano M. Location of the preepiglottic space and its relationship to the paraglottic space. Ann Otol Rhinol Laryngol 1993;102:930-934.
7. Fawcett DW. The Larynx. In: Fawcett B, ed. A textbook of histology. Philadelphia: WB Saunders; 1986:734-735.
8. Mills SE. Larynx and Pharynx. In: Mills SE, ed. Histology for pathologists. Philadelphia: Lippincott-Williams & Wilkins; 2012:461-475.
9. Stiblar-Martincic D. Histology of laryngeal mucosa. Acta Otolaryngol Suppl 1997;527:138-141.
10. Hirabayashi H, Koshii K, Uno K, et al., Laryngeal epithelial changes on effects of smoking and drinking. Auris Nasus Larynx 1990;17:105-114.
11. Sato K, Hirano M, Nakashima T. 3D structure of the macula flava in the human vocal fold. Acta Otolaryngol 2003;123:269-273.
12. Sato K, Kurita T, Chitose S, Umeno H, Nakashima T. Cytoskeleton of newborn vocal fold stellate cells. Laryngoscope 2014;124:2551-2554.
13. Rucci L, Gammarota L, Simonetti L, Cirri MB. TNM glottic: role of the vocal muscle, arytenoid cartilage, and inferior paraglottic space in impaired vocal cord mobility (T2). An embryological and clinical study. Ann Otol Rhinol Laryngol 1998;107:1038-1045.
14. Claassen H, Schicht M, Sel S, Paulsen F. Special pattern of endochondral ossification in human laryngeal cartilages: X-ray and light-microscopic studies on thyroid cartilage. Clin Anat 2014;27:423-430.
15. Standring S. Pleura, lungs, trachea and bronchi. In: Standring S, ed. Gray's Anatomy. The anatomical basis of clinical practice, 40th ed. Edinburg: Elsevier Churchill Livingstone; 2008:968-1006.

Developmental Lesions
Laryngomalacia

16. McGill T. Congenital diseases of the larynx. Otolaryngol Clin North Am 1984;17:57-62.
17. Belmont JR, Grundfast K. Congenital laryngeal stridor (laryngomalacia): etiologic factors and associated disorders. Ann Otol Rhinol Laryngol 1984;93(Pt 1):430-437.
18. Ferguson CF. Treatment of airway problems in the newborn. Ann Otol Rhinol Laryngol 1967;76:762-73.
19. Thorne MC, Garetz SL. Laryngomalacia: Review and summary of current clinical practice in 2015. Paediatr Respir Rev 2016;17:3-8.
20. Templer J, Hast M, Thomas JR, Davis WE. Congenital laryngeal stridor secondary to flaccid epiglottis, anomalous accessory cartilages and redundant aryepiglottic folds. Laryngoscope 1981;91:394-397.

Tracheopathia Osteochondroplastica

21. Leske V, Lazor R, Coetmeur D, et al. Tracheobronchopathia osteochondroplastica: a study of 41 patients. Medicine (Baltimore) 2001;80:378-90.
22. Harma RA, Suurkari S. Tracheopathia chondro-osteoplastica. A clinical study of thirty cases. Acta Otolaryngol 1977;84:118-123.
23. Birzgalis AR, Farrington WT, O'Keefe L, Shaw J. Localized tracheopathia osteoplastica of the subglottis. J Laryngol Otol 1993;107:352-353.
24. Liétin B, Vellin JF, Bivahagumye L, et al. Tracheopathia osteoplastica. Ann Otolaryngol Chir Cervicofac 2008;125:208-212.
25. Marchal G, Baert AL, van der Hauwaert L. Calcification of larynx and trachea in infancy. Br J Radiol, 1974;47:896-897.
26. Wenig BM, Devaney K, Wenig BL. Pseudoneoplastic lesions of the oropharynx and larynx simulating cancer. Pathol Annu 1995;30(Pt 1):143-187.

Hamartomas, Choristomas, and Ectopias

27. Archer SM, Crockett DM, McGill TJ. Hamartoma of the larynx: report of two cases and review of the literature. Int J Pediatr Otorhinolaryngol 1988;16:237-243.
28. Cohen SR. Posterior cleft larynx associated with hamartoma. Ann Otol Rhinol Laryngol 1984;93(Pt 1):443-446.
29. Weinberger J, Kassim O, Birt BD. Hamartoma of the larynx. J Otolaryngol 1985;14:305-308.

30. Lyons TJ, Variend S. Posterior cleft larynx associated with hamartoma: a case report and literature review. J Laryngol Otol 1988;102:471-472.
31. Donegan JO, Wood MD. Intratracheal thyroid—familial occurrence. Laryngoscope 1985;95:6-8.
32. Byrd MC, Thompson LD, Wieneke JA. Intratracheal ectopic thyroid tissue: a case report and literature review. Ear Nose Throat J 2003;82:514-518.
33. See AC, Patel SG, Montgomery PQ, Rhys Evans PH, Fisher C. Intralaryngotracheal thyroid--ectopic thyroid or invasive carcinoma? J Laryngol Otol 1998;112:673-676.
34. Dossing H, Jørgensen KE, Oster-Jørgensen E, Krogdahl A, Hegedüs L. Recurrent pregnancy-related upper airway obstruction caused by intratracheal ectopic thyroid tissue. Thyroid 1999;9:955-958.
35. Dowling EA, Johnson IM, Collier FC, Dillard RA. Intratracheal goiter: a clinico-pathologic review. Ann Surg 1962;156:258-267.
36. Hari CK, Brown MJ, Thompson I. Tall cell variant of papillary carcinoma arising from ectopic thyroid tissue in the trachea. J Laryngol Otol 1999;113:183-185.
37. Cannon CR, Johns ME, Fechner RE. Immature teratoma of the larynx. Otolaryngol Head Neck Surg 1987;96:366-368.

Infectious Diseases

38. Lederer FJ, Soboroff BJ. Medical problems related to diseases of the larynx. Otolaryngol Clin North Am 1970;3:599-608.
39. Khan I. Tuberculous granuloma of the epiglottis. J Laryngol Otol 1983;97:969-971.
40. Klimala KJ. [Tuberculosis of the larynx in material from the ORL ward of the District General Hospital in Czestochowa in the years 1980-1992]. Pneumonol Alergol Pol 1996;64:68-70. [Polish]
41. Pillsbury HC 3rd, Sasaki CT. Granulomatous diseases of the larynx. Otolaryngol Clin North Am 1982;15:539-551.
42. Couldery AD. Tuberculosis of the upper respiratory tract misdiagnosed as Wegener's granulomatosis—an important distinction. J Laryngol Otol 1990;104:255-258.
43. Miller RH, Shulman JB, Canalis RF, Ward PH. Klebsiella rhinoscleromatis: a clinical and pathogenic enigma. Otolaryngol Head Neck Surg 1979;87:212-221.
44. Lerner DM, Deeb Z. Acute upper airway obstruction resulting from systemic diseases. South Med J 1993;86:623-627.
45. Amoils CP, Shindo ML. Laryngotracheal manifestations of rhinoscleroma. Ann Otol Rhinol Laryngol 1996;105:336-340.
46. Bartels LJ, Vrabec DP. Cervicofacial actinomycosis. Arch Otolaryngol 1978;104:705-708.
47. Vrabec DP. Fungal infections of the larynx. Otolaryngol Clin North Am 1993;26:1091-1114.
48. Huang J, Dai L, Lei S, et al. [Application of Warthin-Starry stain, immunohistochemistry and transmission electron microscopy in diagnosis of cat scratch disease.] Zhonghua Bing Li Xue Za Zhi 2010;39:225-229. [Chinese]
49. Martin-Ezquerra G, Fernandez-Casado A, Barco D, et al. Treponema pallidum distribution patterns in mucocutaneous lesions of primary and secondary syphilis: an immunohistochemical and ultrastructural study. Hum Pathol 2009;40:624-630.
50. Morshed MG. Current trend on syphilis diagnosis: issues and challenges. Adv Exp Med Biol 2014;808:51-64.
51. Mollo JL, Groussard O, Baldeyrou P, Molas G, Fournier M, Pariente R. Tracheal malacoplakia. Chest 1994;105:608-610.
52. Nash G, Foley FD. Herpetic infection of the middle and lower respiratory tract. Am J Clin Pathol 1970;54:857-863.
53. Yeh V, Hopp ML, Goldstein NS, Meyer RD. Herpes simplex chronic laryngitis and vocal cord lesions in a patient with acquired immunodeficiency syndrome. Ann Otol Rhinol Laryngol 1994;103:726-731.
54. Kaya H, Kotiloglu E, Inanli S, et al. Prevalence of human papillomavirus (HPV) DNA in larynx and lung carcinomas. Pathologica 2001;93:531-534.
55. Born H, Ruiz R, Verma A, et al. Concurrent oral human papilloma virus infection in patients with recurrent respiratory papillomatosis: a preliminary study. Laryngoscope 2014;124:2785-2790.
56. Hawkins DB, Miller AH, Sachs GB, Benz RT. Acute epiglottitis in adults. Laryngoscope 1973;83:1211-1220.
57. Johnson GK, Sullivan JL, Bishop LA. Acute epiglottitis. Review of 55 cases and suggested protocol. Arch Otolaryngol 1974;100:333-337.
58. Katori H, Tsukuda M. Acute epiglottitis: analysis of factors associated with airway intervention. J Laryngol Otol 2005;119:967-972.
59. Liston SL, Gehrz RC, Jarvis CW. Bacterial tracheitis. Arch Otolaryngol 1981;107:561-564.
60. Heeneman H, Ward KM. Epiglottic abscess: its occurrence and management. J Otolaryngol 1977;6:31-36.
61. Hsieh JK, Phelan MP, Wu G, Bricker A, Anne S. Epiglottic abscess. Am J Emerg Med 2015;33:734 e5-7.
62. Benson-Mitchell R, Tolley N, Croft CB, Gallimore A. Aspergillosis of the larynx. J Laryngol Otol 1994;108:883-835.
63. Boyle JO, Coulthard SW, Mandel RM. Laryngeal involvement in disseminated coccidioidomycosis. Arch Otolaryngol Head Neck Surg 1991;117:433-438.

64. Donegan JO, Wood MD. Histoplasmosis of the larynx. Laryngoscope 1984;94(Pt 1):206-209.
65. Isaacson JE, Frable MA. Cryptococcosis of the larynx. Otolaryngol Head Neck Surg 1996;114:106-109.
66. Marcusen DC, Sooy CD. Otolaryngologic and head and neck manifestations of acquired immunodeficiency syndrome (AIDS). Laryngoscope 1985;95:401-405.
67. Ward PH, Berci G, Morledge D, Schwartz H. Coccidioidomycosis of the larynx in infants and adults. Ann Otol Rhinol Laryngol 1977;86(Pt 1):655-660.
68. Lewy RB. Carcinoma of larynx and trichinosis. Arch Otolaryngol 1964;80:320-321.

Non-infectious Inflammatory Diseases

69. Williams RI. Allergic laryngitis. Ann Otol Rhinol Laryngol 1972;81:558-565.
70. Brook CD, Devaiah AK, Davis EM. Angioedema of the upper aerodigestive tract: risk factors associated with airway intervention and management algorithm. Int Forum Allergy Rhinol 2014;4:239-245.
71. Chiu AG, Newkirk KA, Davidson BJ, Burningham AR, Krowiak EJ, Deeb ZE. Angiotensin-converting enzyme inhibitor-induced angioedema: a multicenter review and an algorithm for airway management. Ann Otol Rhinol Laryngol 2001;110:834-840.
72. Vidal C, Suarez J, Martinez M, Gonzalez-Quintela A. Ciprofloxacin-induced glottic angioedema. Postgrad Med J 1995;71:318.
73. Javaud N, Charpentier S, Lapostolle F, et al. Angiotensin-converting enzyme inhibitor-induced angioedema and hereditary angioedema: a comparison study of attack severity. Intern Med 2015;54:2583-2588.
74. Benjamin B, Dalton C, Croxson G. Laryngoscopic diagnosis of laryngeal sarcoid. Ann Otol Rhinol Laryngol 1995;104:529-531.
75. Devine KD. Sarcoidosis and sarcoidosis of the larynx. Laryngoscope 1965;75:533-569.
76. Neel HB 3rd, McDonald TJ. Laryngeal sarcoidosis: report of 13 patients. Ann Otol Rhinol Laryngol 1982;91(Pt 1):359-362.

Autoimmune Diseases

77. Arauz JC, Fonseca R. Wegener's granulomatosis appearing initially in the trachea. Ann Otol Rhinol Laryngol 1982;91(Pt 1):593-596.
78. Daum TE, Specks U, Colby TV, et al. Tracheobronchial involvement in Wegener's granulomatosis. Am J Respir Crit Care Med 1995;151(Pt 1):522-526.
79. Devaney KO, Travis WD, Hoffman G, Leavitt R, Lebovics R, Fauci AS. Interpretation of head and neck biopsies in Wegener's granulomatosis. A pathologic study of 126 biopsies in 70 patients. Am J Surg Pathol 1990;14:555-564.
80. Hoare TJ, Jayne D, Rhys Evans P, Croft CB, Howard DJ. Wegener's granulomatosis, subglottic stenosis and antineutrophil cytoplasm antibodies. J Laryngol Otol 1989;103:1187-1191.
81. McDonald TJ, Neel HB 3rd, DeRemee RA. Wegener's granulomatosis of the subglottis and the upper portion of the trachea. Ann Otol Rhinol Laryngol 1982;91(Pt 1):588-592.
82. McDonald TJ, DeRemee RA. Wegener's granulomatosis. Laryngoscope 1983;93:220-31.
83. Wegener F. Wegener's granulomatosis. Thoughts and observations of a pathologist. Eur Arch Otorhinolaryngol 1990;247:133-142.
84. Matsubara O, Yoshimura N, Doi Y, Tamura A, Mark EJ. Nasal biopsy in the early diagnosis of Wegener's (pathergic) granulomatosis. Significance of palisading granuloma and leukocytoclastic vasculitis. Virchows Arch 1996;428:13-19.
85. Heffner DK. Wegener's granulomatosis is not a granulomatous disease. Ann Diagn Pathol 2002;6:329-333.
86. Greco A, Rizzo MI, De Virgilio A, et al. Churg-Strauss syndrome. Autoimmun Rev 2015;14:341-348.
87. Monobe H, Nakashima M, Tominaga K. Primary laryngeal natural killer/T-cell lymphoma—report of a rare case. Head Neck 2008;30:1527-1530.
88. Rao JK, Weinberger M, Oddone EZ, Allen NB, Landsman P, Feussner JR. The role of antineutrophil cytoplasmic antibody (c-ANCA) testing in the diagnosis of Wegener granulomatosis. A literature review and meta-analysis. Ann Intern Med 1995;123:925-932.
89. Talerman A, Wright D. Laryngeal obstruction due to Wegener's granulomatosis. Arch Otolaryngol 1972;96:376-379.
90. Langford CA, Sneller MC, Hallahan CW, et al. Clinical features and therapeutic management of subglottic stenosis in patients with Wegener's granulomatosis. Arthritis Rheum 1996;39:1754-1760.
91. McAdam LP, O'Hanlan MA, Bluestone R, Pearson CM. Relapsing polychondritis: prospective study of 23 patients and a review of the literature. Medicine (Baltimore) 1976;55:193-215.
92. McCaffrey TV, McDonald TJ, McCaffrey LA. Head and neck manifestations of relapsing polychondritis: review of 29 cases. Otolaryngology 1978;86(Pt 1):ORL473-478.
93. Lang B, Rothenfusser A, Lanchbury JS, et al. Susceptibility to relapsing polychondritis is associated with HLA-DR4. Arthritis Rheum 1993;36:660-664.
94. Longo L, Greco A, Rea A, Lo Vasco VR, De Virgilio A, De Vincentiis M. Relapsing polychondritis: a clinical update. Autoimmun Rev 2016;15:539-543.

95. Puechal X, Terrier B, Mouthon L, Costedoat-Chalumeau N, Guillevin L, Le Jeunne C. Relapsing polychondritis. Joint Bone Spine 2014;81:118-124.
96. Bhalla M, Grillo HC, McLoud TC, Shepard JO, Weber AL, Mark EJ. Idiopathic laryngotracheal stenosis: radiologic findings. AJR Am J Roentgenol 1993;161:515-517.
97. Damiani JM, Levine HL. Relapsing polychondritis—report of ten cases. Laryngoscope 1979;89(Pt 1):929-946.
98. Purcelli FM, Nahum A, Monell C. Relapsing polychondritis with tracheal collapse. Ann Otol Rhinol Laryngol 1962;71:1120-119.
99. Hussain SS. Relapsing polychondritis presenting with stridor from bilateral vocal cord palsy. J Laryngol Otol 1991;105:961-963.
100. Dolan DL, Lemmon GB Jr, Teitelbaum SL. Relapsing polychondritis. Analytical literature review and studies on pathogenesis. Am J Med 1966;41:285-299.
101. Kaye RL, Sones DA. Relapsing polychondritis. Clinical and pathologic features in fourteen cases. Ann Intern Med 1964;60:653-664.
102. Kashima HK, Holliday MJ, Hyams VJ. Laryngeal chondronecrosis: clinical variations and comments on recognition and management. Trans Sect Otolaryngol Am Acad Ophthalmol Otolaryngol 1977;84:ORL878-881.

Tumor-like Processes: Vocal Cord Nodules/Polyps

103. Strong MS, Vaughan CW. Vocal cord nodules and polyps—the role of surgical treatment. Laryngoscope 1971;81:911-923.
104. Kleinsasser O. Pathogenesis of vocal cord polyps. Ann Otol Rhinol Laryngol 1982;91(Pt 1):378-381.
105. Yanagisawa E, Hausfeld JN, Pensak ML. Sudden airway obstruction due to pedunculated laryngeal polyps. Ann Otol Rhinol Laryngol 1983;92(Pt 1):340-343.
106. Sataloff RT, Spiegel JR, Emerich KA, Rosen D. Post-hemorrhagic vocal fold polyps. Ear Nose Throat J 1994;73:883.
107. Sataloff RT, Hawkshaw M, Rosen DC. Vocal fold polyp and varicosity. Ear Nose Throat J 1993;72:780.
108. Werner JA, Schünke M, Rudert H, Tillmann B. Description and clinical importance of the lymphatics of the vocal fold. Otolaryngol Head Neck Surg 1990;102:13-19.
109. Kambic V, Radsel Z, Zargi M, Acko M. Vocal cord polyps: incidence, histology and pathogenesis. J Laryngol Otol 1981;95:609-618.

Laryngocele and Saccular Cyst

110. Sniezek JC, Johnson RE, Ramirez SG, Hayes DK. Laryngoceles and saccular cysts. South Med J 1996;89:427-430.
111. Matino Soler E, Martínez Vecina V, León Vintró X, Quer Agustí M, Burgues Vila J, de Juan M. [Laryngocele: clinical and therapeutic study of 60 cases.] Acta Otorrinolaringol Esp 1995;46:279-286. [Spanish]
112. Griffin JL, Ramadan HH, Wetmore SJ. Laryngocele: a cause of stridor and airway obstruction. Otolaryngol Head Neck Surg 1993;108:760-762.
113. Luzzago F, Nicolai P, Tomenzoli D, Maroldi R, Antonelli AR. [Laryngocele: analysis of 18 cases and review of the literature.] Acta Otorhinolaryngol Ital 1990;10:399-412. [Italian]
114. Chu L, Gussack GS, Orr JB, Hood D. Neonatal laryngoceles. A cause for airway obstruction. Arch Otolaryngol Head Neck Surg 1994;120:454-458.
115. Balik E, Erdener A, Taneli C, Mevsim A, Sayan A, Yüce G. Jugular phlebectasia in children. Eur J Pediatr Surg 1993;3:46-47.
116. Pul N, Pul M. External jugular phlebectasia in children. Eur J Pediatr 1995;154:275-276.
117. Arens C, Glanz H, Kleinsasser O. Clinical and morphological aspects of laryngeal cysts. Eur Arch Otorhinolaryngol 1997;254:430-436.
118. Gallagher JC, Puzon BQ. Oncocytic lesions of the larynx. Ann Otol Rhinol Laryngol 1969;78:307-318.
119. Lundgren J, Olofsson J, Hellquist H. Oncocytic lesions of the larynx. Acta Otolaryngol 1982;94:335-344.
120. Oliveira CA, Roth JA, Adams GL. Oncocytic lesions of the larynx. Laryngoscope 1977;87(Pt 1):1718-1725.
121. Civantos FJ, Holinger LD. Laryngoceles and saccular cysts in infants and children. Arch Otolaryngol Head Neck Surg 1992;118:296-300.
122. Shaari CM, Ho BT, Som PM, Urken ML. Large thyroglossal duct cyst with laryngeal extension. Head Neck 1994;16:586-588.

Contact Ulcer of the Larynx

123. Wenig BM, Heffner DK. Contact ulcers of the larynx. A reacquaintance with the pathology of an often underdiagnosed entity. Arch Pathol Lab Med 1990;114:825-828.
124. Koufman JA. The otolaryngologic manifestations of gastroesophageal reflux disease (GERD): a clinical investigation of 225 patients using ambulatory 24-hour pH monitoring and an experimental investigation of the role of acid and pepsin in the development of laryngeal injury. Laryngoscope 1991;101(Pt 2 Suppl 53):1-78.
125. Keane WM, Denneny JC, Rowe LD, Atkins JP Jr. Complications of intubation. Ann Otol Rhinol Laryngol 1982;91(Pt 1):584-587.

126. Ward PH, Zwitman D, Hanson D, Berci G. Contact ulcers and granulomas of the larynx: new insights into their etiology as a basis for more rational treatment. Otolaryngol Head Neck Surg 1980;88:262-269.

Necrotizing Sialometaplasia

127. Wenig BM. Necrotizing sialometaplasia of the larynx. A report of two cases and a review of the literature. Am J Clin Pathol 1995;103:609-613.
128. Walker GK, Fechner RE, Johns ME, Teja K. Necrotizing sialometaplasia of the larynx secondary to atheromatous embolization. Am J Clin Pathol 1982;77:221-223.
129. Ben-Izhak O, Ben-Arieh Y. Necrotizing sialometaplasia of the larynx. Am J Clin Pathol 1996;105:251-253.
130. Ravn T, Trolle W, Kiss K, Balle VH. Adenosquamous carcinoma of the larynx associated with necrotizing sialometaplasia—a diagnostic challenge. Auris Nasus Larynx 2009;36:721-724.
131. Romagosa V, Bella MR, Truchero C, Moya J. Necrotizing sialometaplasia (adenometaplasia) of the trachea. Histopathology 1992;21:280-282.

Laryngeal Amyloidosis

132. Thompson LD, Derringer GA, Wenig BM, Amyloidosis of the larynx: a clinicopathologic study of 11 cases. Mod Pathol 2000;13:528-535.
133. Lewis JE, Olsen KD, Kurtin PJ, Kyle RA. Laryngeal amyloidosis: a clinicopathologic and immunohistochemical review. Otolaryngol Head Neck Surg 1992;106:372-377.
134. Hellquist H, Olofsson J, Sökjer H, Odkvist LM. Amyloidosis of the larynx. Acta Otolaryngol 1979;88:443-450.
135. Godbersen GS, Leh JF, Hansmann ML, Rudert H, Linke RP. Organ-limited laryngeal amyloid deposits: clinical, morphological, and immunohistochemical results of five cases. Ann Otol Rhinol Laryngol 1992;101:770-775.
136. Wierzbicka M, Budzynski D, Piwowarczyk K, Bartochowska A, Marszalek A, Szyfter W. How to deal with laryngeal amyloidosis? Experience based on 16 cases. Amyloid 2012;19:177-181.
137. Naiki H, Okoshi T, Ozawa D, Yamaguchi I, Hasegawa K. Molecular pathogenesis of human amyloidosis: lessons from β2-microglobulin-related amyloidosis. Pathol Int 2016;66:193-201.
138. Comenzo RL. LECT2 makes the amyloid list. Blood 2014;123:1436-1437.
139. Howie AJ, Brewer DB, Howell D, Jones AP. Physical basis of colors seen in Congo red-stained amyloid in polarized light. Lab Invest 2008;88:232-242.
140. Eliachar I, Lichtig C. Local amyloid deposits of the larynx. Electron microscopic studies of three cases. Arch Otolaryngol 1970;92:163-166.
141. Hidayat AA, Riddle PJ. Ligneous conjunctivitis. A clinicopathologic study of 17 cases. Ophthalmology 1987;94:949-959.
142. Schuster V, Mingers AM, Seidenspinner S, Nüssgens Z, Pukrop T, Kreth HW. Homozygous mutations in the plasminogen gene of two unrelated girls with ligneous conjunctivitis. Blood 1997;90:958-966.
143. Xu W, Wang L, Zhang L, Han D, Zhang L. Otolaryngological manifestations and genetic characteristics of lipoid proteinosis. Ann Otol Rhinol Laryngol 2010;119:767-771.

Subglottis Stenosis

144. Schroeder JW Jr, Holinger LD. Congenital laryngeal stenosis. Otolaryngol Clin North Am 2008;41:865-875, viii.
145. Morita K, Yokoi A, Bitoh Y, et al. Severe acquired subglottic stenosis in children: analysis of clinical features and surgical outcomes based on the range of stenosis. Pediatr Surg Int 2015;31:943-947.
146. Manickavasagam J, Yapa S, Bateman ND, Thevasagayam MS. Congenital familial subglottic stenosis: a case series and review of literature. Int J Pediatr Otorhinolaryngol 2014;78:359-362.
147. Harpman JA. Cricoid cartilage abnormalities. Arch Otolaryngol 1969;90:634-635.
148. Tucker GF, Ossoff RH, Newman AN, Holinger LD. Histopathology of congenital subglottic stenosis. Laryngoscope 1979;89(Pt 1):866-877.
149. Holinger LD. Histopathology of congenital subglottic stenosis. Ann Otol Rhinol Laryngol 1999;108:101-111.

Rheumatoid Nodule

150. Abdou AG, Asaad NY. Rheumatoid nodule of the vocal cord. Int J Surg Pathol 2012;20:481-482.
151. Voulgari PV, Papazisi D, Bai M, Zagorianakou P, Assimakopoulos D, Drosos AA. Laryngeal involvement in rheumatoid arthritis. Rheumatol Int 2005;25:321-325.
152. Sorensen WT, Moller-Andersen K, Behrendt N. Rheumatoid nodules of the larynx. J Laryngol Otol 1998;112:573-574.
153. Woo P, Mendelsohn J, Humphrey D. Rheumatoid nodules of the larynx. Otolaryngol Head Neck Surg 1995;113:147-150.
154. Brooker DS. Rheumatoid arthritis: otorhinolaryngological manifestations. Clin Otolaryngol Allied Sci 1988;13:239-246.
155. Schwartz IS, Grishman E. Rheumatoid nodules of the vocal cords as the initial manifestation of systemic lupus erythematosus. JAMA 1980;244:2751-2752.

156. Friedman BA. Rheumatoid nodules of the larynx. Arch Otolaryngol 1975;101:361-363.
157. Abadir WF, Forster PM. Rheumatoid vocal cord nodules. J Laryngol Otol 1974;88:473-478.
158. Habermann W, Kiesler K, Eherer A, Beham A, Friedrich G. Laryngeal manifestation of gout: a case report of a subglottic gout tophus. Auris Nasus Larynx 2001;28:265-267.
159. Guttenplan MD, Hendrix RA, Townsend MJ, Balsara G. Laryngeal manifestations of gout. Ann Otol Rhinol Laryngol 1991;100:899-902.
160. Marion RB, Alperin JE, Maloney WH. Gouty tophus of the true vocal cord. Arch Otolaryngol 1972;96:161-162.

Teflon Granuloma

161. Lisi C, Hawkshaw MJ, Sataloff RT. Viscosity of materials for laryngeal injection: a review of current knowledge and clinical implications. J Voice 2013;27:119-123.
162. Butskiy O, Mistry B, Chadha NK. Surgical interventions for pediatric unilateral vocal cord paralysis: a systematic review. JAMA Otolaryngol Head Neck Surg 2015;141:654-660.
163. Costello D. Change to earlier surgical interventions: contemporary management of unilateral vocal fold paralysis. Curr Opin Otolaryngol Head Neck Surg 2015;23:181-184.
164. Varvares MA, Montgomery WW, Hillman RE. Teflon granuloma of the larynx: etiology, pathophysiology, and management. Ann Otol Rhinol Laryngol 1995;104:511-515.
165. Wenig BM, Heffner DK, Oertel YC, Johnson FB. Teflonomas of the larynx and neck. Hum Pathol 1990;21:617-623.
166. Chhetri DK, Jahan-Parwar B, Hart SD, Bhuta SM, Berke GS. Injection laryngoplasty with calcium hydroxylapatite gel implant in an in vivo canine model. Ann Otol Rhinol Laryngol 2004;113:259-264.
167. Ozudogru E, Cakli H, Asan E, et al. The neocartilaginous formation with hydroxyl-apatite in injection laryngoplasty: an experimental study on rabbit model. Eur Arch Otorhinolaryngol 2008;265:199-202.
168. Sasai H, Watanabe Y, Muta H, et al. Long-term histological outcomes of injected autologous fat into human vocal folds after secondary laryngectomy. Otolaryngol Head Neck Surg 2005;132:685-688.

Reactive Epithelial Changes

169. Gale N, Gnepp DR, Poljak M, et al. Laryngeal squamous intraepithelial lesions: an updated review on etiology, Classification, molecular changes, and treatment. Adv Anat Pathol 2016;23:84-91.
170. Hellquist H, Lundgren J, Olofsson J. Hyperplasia, keratosis, dysplasia and carcinoma in situ of the vocal cords—a follow-up study. Clin Otolaryngol Allied Sci 1982;7:11-27.
171. Koren R, Kristt D, Shvero J, Yaniv E, Dekel Y, Gal R. The spectrum of laryngeal neoplasia: the pathologist's view. Pathol Res Pract 2002;198:709-715.
172. Crissman JD. Laryngeal keratosis and subsequent carcinoma. Head Neck Surg 1979;1:386-391.
173. Gale N, Kambic V, Michaels L, et al. The Ljubljana classification: a practical strategy for the diagnosis of laryngeal precancerous lesions. Adv Anat Pathol 2000;7:240-251.
174. Kimmich T, Kleinsasser O. Benign keratoma of the vocal cords. Eur Arch Otorhinolaryngol 1993;250:143-147.
175. Poh CF, Zhang L, Lam WL, et al. A high frequency of allelic loss in oral verrucous lesions may explain malignant risk. Lab Invest 2001;81:629-634.
176. Klijanienko J, Micheau C, Carlu C, Caillaud JM. Significance of keratin 13 and 6 expression in normal, dysplasic and malignant squamous epithelium of pyriform fossa. Virchows Arch A Pathol Anat Histopathol 1989;416:121-124.
177. Califano J, van der Riet P, Westra W, et al. Genetic progression model for head and neck cancer: implications for field cancerization. Cancer Res 1996;56:2488-2492.
178. Barnes L, Yunis EJ, Krebs FJ 3rd, Sonmez-Alpan E. Verruca vulgaris of the larynx. Demonstration of human papillomavirus types 6/11 by in situ hybridization. Arch Pathol Lab Med 1991;115:895-899.

Radiation-Associated Changes

179. Fajardo LF, Berthrong M. Radiation injury in surgical pathology. Part I. Am J Surg Pathol 1978;2:159-199.
180. Weidner N, Askin FB, Berthrong M, Hopkins MB, Kute TE, McGuirt FW. Bizarre (pseudomalignant) granulation-tissue reactions following ionizing-radiation exposure. A microscopic, immunohistochemical, and flow-cytometric study. Cancer 1987;59:1509-514.
181. Mudaliar KM, Borrowdale R, Mehrotra S. Post-radiation atypical vascular lesion/angiosarcoma arising in the larynx. Head Neck Pathol 2014;8:359-363.
182. Bonetta A, Gelli MC, Zini G, et al. Postradiation sarcoma of head and neck: report of two cases. Tumori 1996;82:270-272.

**Laryngeal Manifestations
of Dermatologic Disorders**

183. Intong LR, Murrell DF. Inherited epidermolysis bullosa: new diagnostic criteria and classification. Clin Dermatol 2012;30:70-77.
184. Hester JE, Arnstein DP, Woodley D. Laryngeal manifestations of epidermolysis bullosa acquisita. Arch Otolaryngol Head Neck Surg 1995;121:1042-1044.
185. Liu RM, Papsin BC, de Jong AL. Epidermolysis bullosa of the head and neck: a case report of laryngotracheal involvement and 10-year review of cases at the Hospital for Sick Children. J Otolaryngol 1999;28:76-82.
186. Haruyama T, Furukawa M, Matsumoto F, Kawano K, Ikeda K. Laryngeal stenosis in epidermolysis bullosa dystrophica. Auris Nasus Larynx 2009;36:106-109.
187. Mizutani H, Masuda K, Nakamura N, Takenaka H, Tsuruta D, Katoh N. Cutaneous and laryngeal squamous cell carcinoma in mixed epidermolysis bullosa, kindler syndrome. Case Rep Dermatol 2012;4:133-138.
188. Santoro FA, Stoopler ET, Werth VP. Pemphigus. Dent Clin North Am 2013;57:597-610.
189. Hale EK, Bystryn JC. Laryngeal and nasal involvement in pemphigus vulgaris. J Am Acad Dermatol 2001;44:609-611.
190. Kavala M, Altintas S, Kocatürk E, et al. Ear, nose and throat involvement in patients with pemphigus vulgaris: correlation with severity, phenotype and disease activity. J Eur Acad Dermatol Venereol 2011;25:1324-1327.
191. Alexandre M, Brette MD, Pascal F, et al. A prospective study of upper aerodigestive tract manifestations of mucous membrane pemphigoid. Medicine (Baltimore) 2006;85:239-252.

6 SALIVARY GLANDS

By Drs. Raja R. Seethala and Bruce M. Wenig

EMBRYOLOGY, ANATOMY, AND HISTOLOGY

Embryology

All salivary glands develop as solid proliferations or buds from the epithelium of the stomodeum. The parotid anlage is recognized as early as the 5th to 6th week of embryologic life, and consists of a mixed ectodermal and endodermal derivation, which may explain the frequent finding of intraparotid sebaceous glands. The parotid gland is followed, in sequence, by the submandibular gland and sublingual gland, each about 1 week apart (1,2). The minor salivary glands of the oral cavity, the seromucous glands of the sinonasal tract, and the remainder of the aerodigestive tract evolve at around 12 weeks (3).

The major salivary glands are encapsulated by mesodermal fibroconnective tissue, which forms various fasciae in the neck. Despite being the first gland to form, the parotid gland is the last to become encapsulated, which thus allows the lymphoid tissue to intermingle with the parotid gland, resulting in intraparotid lymph nodes as well as salivary inclusions in the neck lymph nodes (3).

Anatomy

Parotid Gland. The parotid gland is the largest salivary gland, with an average total weight of 25 g. The parotid gland is divided into the larger superficial and smaller deep lobes by the traversing facial nerve and its branches. The superficial lobe is pyramidal or wedge shaped, situated between the mandibular ramus and mastoid process (fig. 6-1). The tail of the parotid forms the "apex" of the pyramid and extends into the neck level II (4). The parotid gland is encapsulated, although the composition of the superficial parotid fascia is complex: the upper two thirds of the superficial parotid lobe are dense and closely opposed to the superficial cervical fascia while the remainder is fairly thin (5–7). The deep lobe is situated in the parapharyngeal space.

The anatomic borders of the parotid gland are as follows: the anterior border overlies the superficial surface of the masseter muscle; the posterior border overlaps the sternocleidomastoid muscle and wraps around the lower ear; the lateral or superficial border is the skin and dermis of the face; the medial or deep border is buttressed by the styloid process and its associated muscles (styloglossus, stylohyoid, stylopharyngeal) and by the carotid sheath and

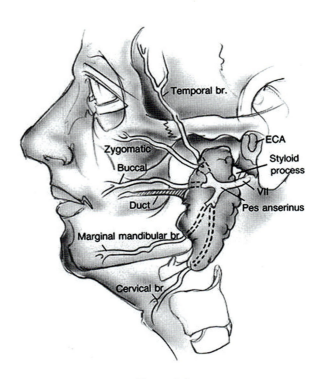

Figure 6-1

ANATOMY OF PAROTID GLAND

Anatomic localization of the parotid gland with respect to the facial nerve and its branches. (From fig. 47.2 from Walvekar RR, Loehn BC, Wilson MN. Anatomy and physiology of the salivary glands. In: Johnson JT, Rosen CA, eds. Bailey's head and neck surgery–otolaryngology, 5th ed. Philadelphia: Lippincott Williams & Wilkins; 2013:692.)

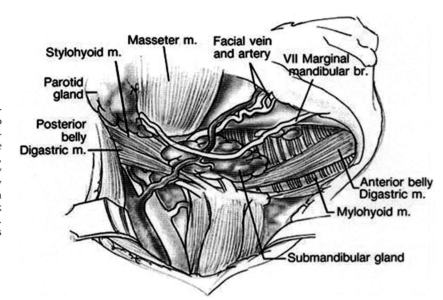

Figure 6-2

ANATOMY OF SUBMANDIBULAR GLAND

Anatomic localization of the submandibular gland with respect to the musculature and marginal mandibular branch of the facial nerve (From fig. 47.7 from Walvekar RR, Loehn BC, Wilson MN. Anatomy and physiology of the salivary glands. In: Johnson JT, Rosen CA, eds. Bailey's head and neck surgery–otolaryngology, 5th ed. Philadelphia: Lippincott Williams & Wilkins; 2013:695.)

its contents (internal carotid artery, internal jugular vein, and cranial nerves IX, X, XII); the superior border is the zygomatic arch; and the inferior border is the sternocleidomastoid muscle (oblique anterior border).

The main parotid duct, or Stensen duct, is approximately 4 to 7 mm in length and originates from the anterior portion of the gland, coursing forward over the masseter muscle, where it enters the buccal fat pad. It pierces the buccinator muscle, opening in the oral cavity opposite the second maxillary molar (parotid papilla) (8). In about 20 percent of the population, accessory parotid tissue is found along the anterior portion of the gland and the Stensen duct.

Submandibular Gland. The submandibular (submaxillary) glands are encapsulated and "walnut-shaped," located in the submandibular triangle situated below the angle of the mandible (fig. 6-2). Each submandibular gland weighs 10 to 15 g. The submandibular glands technically also consist of a superficial and deep lobe, although the latter is a minor component and can only be palpated in the floor of the mouth.

The anatomic borders of the submandibular glands are as follows: the anterior border is the anterior belly of the digastric muscle; the posterior border is the stylomandibular ligament which separates it from the lower part of the parotid gland; the lateral border is found in relation to the submandibular fossa on the inner surface of the body of the mandible; the medial border is bounded by several muscles (mylohyoid, styloglossus, hyoglossus, stylohyoid, and posterior belly of the digastric) and nerves (hypoglossal, glossopharyngeal, and lingual); the superior border is the inferior border of the body of the mandible; and the inferior border is the skin, platysma, and deep fascia.

The submandibular duct, or Wharton duct, runs forward along the inner surface of the mandible, in parallel with the lingual nerve. It passes medial to the lower border of the sublingual gland, at which point the duct may receive the major sublingual duct (Bartholin duct) prior to opening in the oral cavity at the sublingual caruncle or papilla lateral to the frenulum.

Sublingual Gland. The sublingual glands are the smallest of the major salivary glands, each weighing between 2 and 4 g. They are ovoid or almond-shaped and located submucosally in the floor of the mouth (fig. 6-3).

The anatomic borders of the sublingual gland are as follows: the anterior border is the opposite sublingual gland; the posterior border is the deep part of the submandibular gland; the lateral border is the internal aspect of the body of the mandible; the medial border is the genioglossus muscle; the superior border is the mucosa of the floor of the mouth which it raises to form the sublingual fold; and the inferior border is the mylohyoid muscle. The sublingual gland's large duct system is different from the other major salivary glands in that there is a

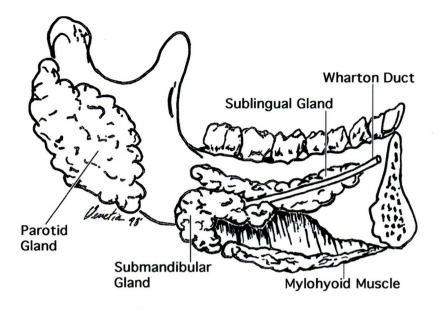

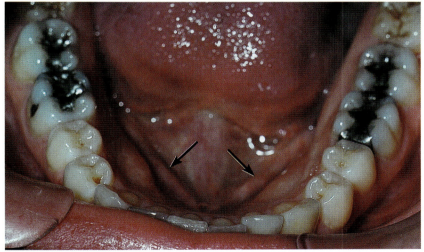

Figure 6-3

ANATOMY OF SUBLINGUAL GLAND

Top: The medial surface of the mandible and mylohyoid muscle shows the relationship of the submandibular, sublingual, and parotid glands. The submandibular duct (Wharton duct) runs anteriorly to the anterior floor of the mouth.

Bottom: The right and left submandibular ducts (arrows) course anteromedially in the floor of the mouth to openings at the lingual carunculae, which are only a few millimeters apart.

common sublingual (Bartholin) duct, which merges as noted with the Wharton duct, as well as numerous smaller Rivinus ducts, which open into the oral cavity proper (fig. 6-3).

Minor Salivary Glands and Seromucous Glands. The minor salivary glands or seromucous glands are located throughout the submucosa of the entire upper aerodigestive tract. They are not generally encapsulated and do not generally have distinctive anatomic landmarks.

Histology

All salivary and seromucous glands consist of an arborizing epithelial ductal system, which is responsible for the production of saliva via distal luminal secretory cells and the delivery of the secretions via the branching structures to the oral cavity. Most of this system is arranged in a bilayer of luminal cells with secretory function and a delimiting abluminal basal/myoepithelial cell layer (fig. 6-4). The latter layer consists mainly of myoepithelial cells, which are situated distally relative to the acini, and intercalated ducts where contractile properties are required for saliva delivery. More proximally to the striated and excretory ducts are strictly "basal cells" with a proliferative capacity.

The microanatomic organization from distal to proximal for the major salivary ducts follows (fig. 6-5). *Acini* represent the most distal

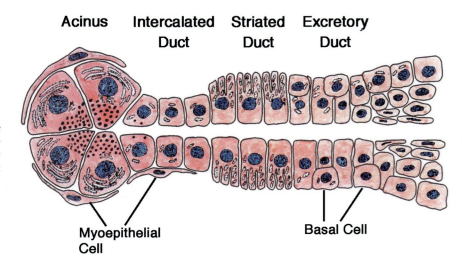

Figure 6-4

SCHEMATIC OF BASIC SALIVARY GLAND UNIT

Cytomorphologic features of various portions of the salivary system from the distal secretory end (left) to the proximal duct end (right).

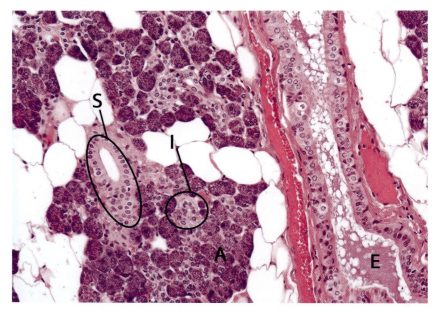

Figure 6-5

MICROANATOMY OF PAROTID GLAND

Lobules of acini (A, all serous with granular basophilic cytoplasm) transition to intercalated ducts (I), which are compressed and interspersed between acini and consist of small cuboidal cells with slightly eosinophilic, but scant cytoplasm. These components are lined by attenuated myoepithelial cells that are difficult to note on light microscopy. Striated ducts (S) transition from intercalated ducts and consist of columnar cells with granular eosinophilic cytoplasm. Rather than myoepithelial cells, the attenuated outer cell layer transitions to a purely basal cell type. Striated ducts then empty into excretory ducts (E).

terminal secretory cells and include serous or mucous cells which produce the saliva. They are lined by attenuated myoepithelial cells.

Serous acinar cells are triangular to pyramidal-shaped cells with a narrow apex toward the luminal aspect, round nuclei near the basal one third of the cell, and abundant cytoplasm containing numerous basophilic zymogen granules situated at the apical portion. Zymogen granules are diastase-resistant, periodic acid–Schiff (PAS) positive, and mucicarmine negative.

Mucous acinar cells are pyramidal-shaped cells with basally located flattened nuclei and clear to faintly basophilic, finely granular cytoplasm. Mucicarmine, alcian blue, and diastase-resistant PAS are positive.

Myoepithelial cells are flat, elongated to stellate cells with cytoplasmic processes extending and surrounding the acinar cells. They are in the space between the basement membrane and the basal plasma membrane of the luminal acinar cells. Myoepithelial cells are difficult to appreciate by light microscopy, but can be highlighted by immunohistochemistry; immunohistochemical stains that are positive in myoepithelial cells include cytokeratins (low- and high-molecular weight), p63, S-100 protein, calponin, and smooth muscle actin.

Basal cells differ from myoepithelial cells by the absence of myoid markers by immunohistochemistry and myofilaments by electron microscopy. They are difficult to appreciate by light microscopy, but can be highlighted by immunohistochemistry; cytokeratins (low- and high-molecular weight) and p63 are positive.

Intercalated ducts transition from acini and tend to be more prominent in the parotid and submandibular glands than the sublingual glands. These are analogous to the terminal ducts of the minor salivary glands.

Striated ducts transition from the intercalated ducts. They are columnar, with abundant oncocytic granular cytoplasm. The surrounding cell layers here are no longer myoepithelial but are basal cells that still appear attenuated. Only the major salivary glands have striated ducts.

Excretory ducts transition from the striated ducts. Their appearance ranges from striated duct-like to more multilayered, with squamoid, mucous, and ciliated components. In the major salivary glands, these continuously converge into progressively larger ducts, ultimately into the named duct(s) for the corresponding gland.

In the major salivary glands, the ductoacinar units coalesce to form lobules that are divided by fibrous tissue septa. The ducts then converge into larger named duct branches and eventually the named duct itself. Interstitial fat composition varies, and is more pronounced in the parotid gland.

The minor salivary glands are arranged more like a lobule of a major salivary gland, with their excretory duct emptying into an excretory duct that connects directly with the mucosa. As noted above, the equivalent of intercalated ducts in these glands is the terminal duct, and there are technically no striated ducts in the minor salivary and in sinonasal seromucous glands.

There are considerable differences in the composition of the acini in the various salivary glands. The *parotid gland* (fig. 6-6) is entirely serous, although rare mucous acini are identified. Sebaceous glands or scattered sebocytes are heavily vacuolated and lipid-laden, as seen in the skin. They are positive for fat stains (oil red O on frozen tissue) but negative for mucin stains. Immunohistochemical stains for epithelial membrane antigen (EMA) and lipoproteins are positive.

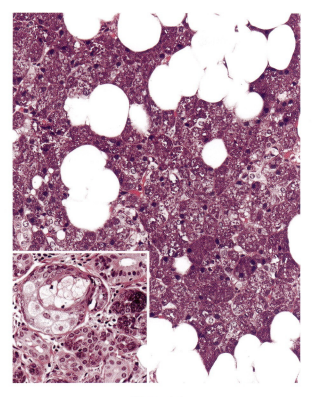

Figure 6-6

PAROTID GLAND

Acini are entirely serous, as seen here. Inset: sebaceous elements may be noted.

The *intraparotid lymph nodes* are common. They often contain normal parotid parenchymal structures, including ducts and acini, which may give rise to intraparotid salivary gland lesions or neoplasms (benign and malignant).

The *submandibular gland* (fig. 6-7) has predominantly serous (about 75 percent) acini with a significant mucous acinar component. The serous cells typically are arranged as crescent-shaped caps, or so-called demilunes (of Gianucci), along the periphery of the mucous acinar cells.

The *sublingual gland* (fig. 6-8) has mostly mucous acini, with rare seromucinous demilunes. Serous cells, even when present, are less basophilic, with lower zymogen granule density.

The *minor salivary glands* and *sinonasal seromucous glands* (fig. 6-9) have a mixture of serous and mucous acinar cells in most of the oral cavity, sinonasal tract, pharynx, and larynx. Serous cells, even when present, are less basophilic, with lower zymogen granule density. The

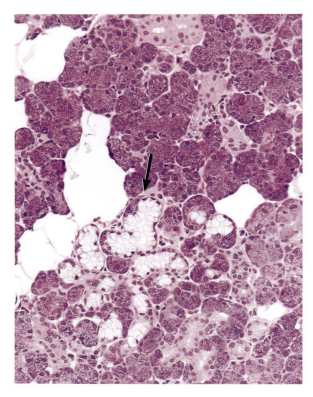

Figure 6-7

SUBMANDIBULAR GLAND

Acini are a mixture of serous and mucous cells. Serous cells are arranged in a crescent (or demilune) surrounding mucous acini (arrow).

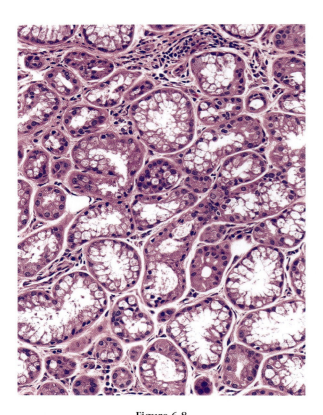

Figure 6-8

SUBLINGUAL GLAND

This gland consists mainly of mucous acini.

Figure 6-9

SINONASAL SEROMUCOUS GLANDS

A mixture of serous and mucous acini is seen. Serous acini are more eosinophilic, with less granularity, in contrast to those of the major salivary glands. The excretory duct empties onto the surface respiratory mucosa (left).

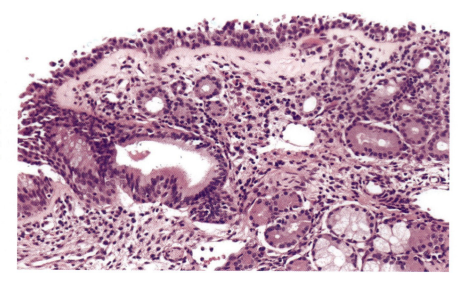

Table 6-1
NON-NEOPLASTIC LESIONS OF SALIVARY GLANDS

Developmental Lesions
  Accessory parotid gland
  Heterotopias (ectopias, choristomas)
  Hamartomas; adenomatoid hyperplasia of mucous
    salivary glands

Salivary Cysts
  Salivary duct cyst and mucous retention cyst
  Mucous extravasation phenomenon (extravasation
    mucocele)
  Ranula
  Lymphoepithelial cyst
  Polycystic (dysgenetic) disease

Metaplasia and Hyperplasia
  Oncocytic metaplasia and oncocytosis
  Sialadenosis

Infectious, Inflammatory, and Reactive Diseases
  Acute sialadenitis and viral parotitis (mumps)
  Chronic nonautoimmune sialadenitis
  HIV[a]-salivary gland disease
  Lymphoepithelial sialadenitis (benign lymphoepi-
    thelial lesion and Sjögren syndrome)
  Chronic sclerosing sialadenitis (IgG4 related)
  Sarcoidosis

Tumor-Like Lesions
  Necrotizing sialometaplasia
  Subacute sclerosing sialadenitis
  Extranodal sinus histiocytosis with massive lymph-
    adenopathy (Rosai-Dorfman disease)
  Others

[a]HIV = human immunodeficiency virus.

palate and anterior lingual salivary glands (of Blandin or Nuhn) are composed almost purely of mucous acini. The posterior lingual salivary glands, near the circumvallate papillae (von Ebner glands), contain mainly serous acini.

CLASSIFICATION

The classification of non-neoplastic salivary gland lesions is seen in Table 6-1.

DEVELOPMENTAL LESIONS

Accessory Parotid Glands

Definition. *Accessory parotid glands* are lobules of parotid gland parenchyma separated from the main body of the gland, and usually situated along a major salivary duct (9).

Clinical Features. Accessory parotid glands are common and have been reported in up to 56 percent in patients in an autopsy series (10). They usually lie on the masseter, situated on the buccal fat pad. The accessory tissue is normally connected to the Stensen duct by one or more accessory ducts (11). Even without a neoplasm, accessory parotid glands may present as buccal space masses. Computerized tomographic (CT) and magnetic resonance imaging (MRI) modalities are useful in establishing this, as well as identifying lesions that arise in the accessory gland.

Gross Findings. Accessory parotid tissue is ovoid and delicate "rice-like," without a complete fascial covering. The size ranges from 0.5 to 3.0 cm (12).

Microscopic Findings. Accessory parotid glands are histologically identical to the main parotid gland. However, unlike the main parotid gland in which mucous acini are rare, up to 25 percent of accessory parotid tissue shows mucous acinar components (12) Usually, diffuse or systemic processes are similar in accessory and main parotid glands. Various tumor types may arise from accessory parotid glands (9,10,13–19).

Treatment and Prognosis. An accessory parotid gland without disease does not require treatment, although it may be excised as a result of presenting as a mass lesion in the buccal space. Accessory parotid glands are usually excised in tandem with a superficial parotidectomy, particularly for neoplasms (20). The prognosis is based on the type of neoplasm identified.

Salivary Gland Heterotopia (Ectopias, Choristomas)

Definition. *Salivary gland heterotopia* is salivary gland tissue located in sites other than those appropriate for the normal anatomic distribution of salivary glands. Strict criteria defining true heterotopic salivary glands exclude salivary tissue of accessory glands and that associated with branchial cleft anomalies, although this distinction is somewhat debatable since one of the proposed developmental hypotheses for salivary gland heterotopia is a branchial cleft derivation (21).

Clinical Features. Most heterotopic salivary gland tissue occurs in head and neck sites. The most common locations are the periparotid lymph nodes, the middle ear, and the lower neck (9). Less frequent sites of occurrence include the upper neck, external auditory canal,

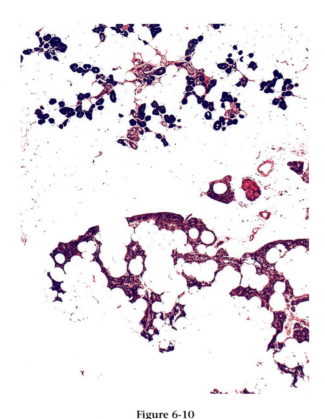

Figure 6-10

HETEROTOPIC SALIVARY TISSUE

Serous acini (left) are associated with a parathyroid gland (right).

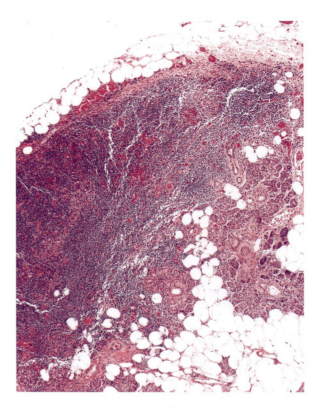

Figure 6-11

INTRANODAL PAROTID TISSUE

The parotid tissue is present toward the hilum of this level II lymph node.

intraosseous sites (e.g., mandible), cerebellopontine angle, and pituitary gland. In addition, salivary gland tissue has been reported in thyroglossal duct, capsules of the thyroid gland and parathyroid glands (fig. 6-10), mediastinum, tonsils, and gingiva, as well as more distant sites including the prostate gland, vulva, and rectum (22).

Heterotopic Salivary Gland Tissue in the Lower Neck. Most reported cases of salivary gland heterotopia are in the lower anterolateral neck, along the medial border of the sternocleidomastoid muscle. The most common presenting symptom is a draining sinus on the anterior aspect of the neck along the medial border of the sternocleidomastoid muscle near the sternoclavicular joint (9,21). Patients present typically with localized, nontender swelling associated with the sinus. These sinuses may drain small quantities of saliva-type secretions that may fluctuate with meals.

Intranodal Periparotid Salivary Gland Tissue. Salivary inclusions are fairly common in periparotid and neck level II lymph nodes and may not be true heterotopias, strictly speaking, since the prevailing hypothesis is entrapment during embryologic development in areas that are expected to have parotid tissue (23). Histologically, the salivary gland tissue is predominantly serous with ducts (fig. 6-11); mucous acini are exceptional.

Heterotopic Salivary Gland Tissue in the Middle Ear. Heterotopic salivary gland tissue in the middle ear, often labeled salivary choristoma, is rare, with under 40 cases reported in the literature (24). It typically occurs in the first and second decades (range, 9 months to 52 years), and is associated with conductive hearing loss and ossicular chain abnormalities. This association implicates first and second branchial arch abnormalities since the malleus and incus are derived from the first arch, and the stapes from the second arch (25). Heterotopic salivary gland tissue is associated with anomalies that suggest the branchio-otorenal (BOR) syndrome (26,27). A provisional syndrome of heterotopia, preauricular pits, and facial nerve abnormalities has been proposed as well (28).

Intraosseous Heterotopic Salivary Gland Tissue. Intraosseous salivary gland tissue is rare and incidental, comprising less than 1 percent of bone marrow samples of the maxillofacial bones in one study (29). It occurs in the posterior mandible near the angle beneath the mandibular canal, and less frequently, in the anterior mandible. This tissue must be distinguished from Stafne defects, which are bone cavities into which normal salivary tissue presumably invaginates (30). Rare cases are sellar, without association with pituitary or Rathke cleft cyst, although they too are presumed Rathke cleft abnormalities (31).

Gross Findings. When visible grossly, heterotopic salivary tissue is lobular, tan-yellow with a similar appearance to normal salivary gland elsewhere.

Microscopic Findings. Most heterotopias consist of either serous or seromucinous acini surrounding an excretory duct that may be ectatic or cystic. In lower neck salivary heterotopias, this duct connects with a sinus (9).

Treatment and Prognosis. Salivary heterotopias are often incidental findings that require no further treatment beyond conservative excision. A subset, however, come to attention because they have developed into a tumor (32). Intranodal salivary inclusions, in particular, may be involved by a spectrum of salivary gland lesions including cyst formation, oncocytic metaplasia, oncocytic adenomatous hyperplasia, and neoplasia (33). In fact, one of the hypotheses for some tumors with prominent lymphoid stroma, like Warthin tumor and lymphadenoma, is evolution from salivary inclusions in an intraparotid/periparotid stroma (34). Heterotopic salivary gland tumors are treated in a similar fashion to their orthotopic counterparts.

Salivary Gland Hamartomas and Adenomatoid Hyperplasia

Definition. *Salivary gland hamartoma* is a malformation or disorganized tumor-like proliferation of salivary tissue at a site where salivary gland parenchyma is normally located. *Adenomatoid hyperplasia* is a nodular proliferation of mucous acini of salivary glands.

Clinical Features. Salivary tissue is often a component of head and neck hamartomas consisting of mesenchymal and occasionally cutaneous/melanocytic elements (35,36). Seromucinous hamartomas can arguably fit into this category and are discussed in chapter 1.

Adenomatoid hyperplasia is "minimally" hamartomatous and is likely more common than reported. It typically presents as a painless mass of the palate, uvula, or retromolar trigone, usually in the fourth decade of life (37–40). Rarely, patients have obstructive sleep apnea from uvular involvement (34).

Gross Findings. The lesions are firm and sessile and range from 0.5 to 3.0 cm.

Microscopic Findings. Histologically, salivary tissue in hamartomas is mixed seromucinous and interspersed haphazardly within adipose tissue, imparting a sialolipoma-like appearance. Adenomatous hyperplasia is composed of hypertrophied and hyperplastic lobules of mucous acini (fig. 6-12). Slight mucus extravasation may be noted, albeit with little if any reaction. The overlying mucosa is unremarkable.

Differential Diagnosis. The main diagnostic considerations are mucin-rich tumors such as mucoepidermoid carcinoma. The retention of the lobular acinar architecture is a key feature in recognizing adenomatous hyperplasia.

Treatment and Prognosis. Surgical excision is curative.

SALIVARY CYSTS

Salivary Duct Cyst and Mucous Retention Cyst

Definition. *Salivary duct cysts* and *mucous retention cysts* (also known as *sialocysts*, *simple cysts*, and *retention mucoceles*) are true cysts of the salivary duct with an epithelial lining (41). Etiologic differences (i.e., developmental versus postobstructive) are difficult to use to define these categories. Generally, the term salivary duct cyst is used to describe cysts in the major salivary glands. Mucous retention cysts are histologically similar but the term is used for minor salivary glands cysts. These represent the minority (5 to 20 percent) subset of lesions collectively labeled mucocele (42).

Non-Neoplastic Diseases of the Head and Neck

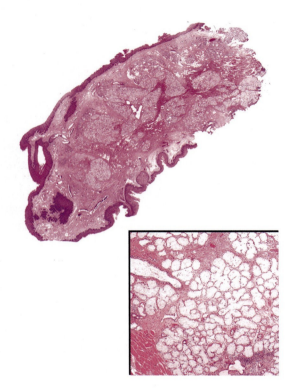

Figure 6-12

ADENOMATOUS HYPERPLASIA OF THE SALIVARY TISSUE

The hyperplasia in an enlarged uvula presents as a mass. Mucous acini retain the lobular architecture but are enlarged and the ducts are somewhat ectatic (inset).

Clinical Features. While most salivary "cysts" excised are cystic neoplasms, salivary duct cysts are the most common non-neoplastic salivary cysts, comprising about 1.5 percent of all salivary gland diseases in one study (43). Over 80 percent of salivary duct cysts occur in the parotid gland. Mucous retention cysts are typically located in on the palatoglossal fold (44) and even occur in gingiva. These typically present as painless masses and occur across all age groups. Mucus retention cysts have a female predilection and occur in the elderly (fifth to eighth decades) (45,46).

Gross Findings. These cysts are unilocular and filled with serous to mucoid material. Sialoliths can develop in longstanding major gland salivary duct cysts. Superficial mucus retention cysts are raised, fluctuant, bluish submucosal nodules.

Microscopic Findings. Salivary duct and mucous retention cysts are well demarcated and tend to recapitulate the excretory duct. They are lined by cuboidal, columnar, or squamous epithelium with interspersed goblet cells (fig. 6-13). Oncocytic metaplasia may be seen in older individuals. The cyst wall is usually collagenized and may show inflammatory changes secondary to rupture, ranging from sparse lymphocytic inflammation to a granulomatous reaction (47).

Figure 6-13

SALIVARY DUCT CYSTS (SIALOCYSTS)

Left: This simple cyst has a thin fibrous wall and is lined by cuboidal to columnar eosinophilic cytoplasm (inset), recapitulating the appearance of an excretory duct.

Right: This cyst demonstrates rupture-related inflammatory changes, a thicker wall, and is lined by squamous epithelium (inset).

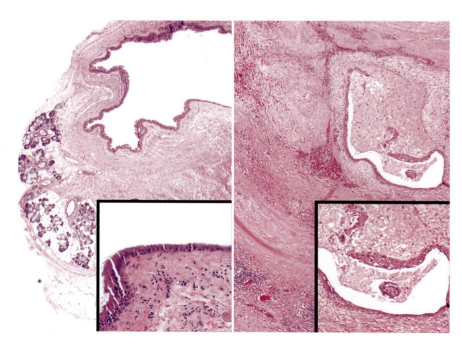

Differential Diagnosis. The main differential diagnostic considerations are true cystic neoplasms and lymphoepithelial cysts. True cystic neoplasms include cystadenomas, cystadenocarcinomas, low-grade mucoepidermoid carcinoma, acinic cell adenocarcinoma, and mammary analogue secretory carcinoma, among others. Salivary gland cystic tumors are distinguished by their greater architectural complexity, ranging from solid to cribriform/tubular to papillary, and prominent (increased) cellularity including defining cell populations (e.g., epidermoid cells, mucocytes, and intermediate cell types in mucoepidermoid carcinoma). In contrast, the salivary duct cyst recapitulates the normal epithelium seen in a salivary duct cyst. Occasionally, immunohistochemical staining may be required and helps define specific tumor types including discovered on Gist 1 (DOG1) for acinic cell adenocarcinoma and S-100 protein and mammaglobin in mammary analogue secretory carcinoma.

Treatment and Prognosis. Rare complications include superimposed infections. Recurrences are exceptional and result from incomplete excision.

Mucus Extravasation Phenomenon (Extravasation Mucocele)

Definition. *Mucous extravasation phenomenon (extravasation mucocele)* is a pseudocystic proliferation lined by resulting from the escape of saliva as a result of injury to the duct of a minor salivary gland.

Clinical Features. Mucous extravasation phenomenon comprises the majority (80 to 95 percent) of what is designated as a mucocele in the oral cavity. The lip is the most common site (80 percent), and occurrence is in the second to third decade (48–51). Like mucous retention cysts, these often present as fluctuant submucosal bluish nodules.

Gross Findings. Mucous extravasation phenomenon ranges from 0.1 to 4.0 cm (48,49).

Microscopic Findings. The characteristic appearance of mucous extravasation phenomenon is the extravasation of mucus with intermixed, mucus-laden foamy to vacuolated macrophages or "muciphages" (fig. 6-14). Pseudocysts lined by these muciphages may be present. The mucus is typically mucicarmine and PAS positive. The

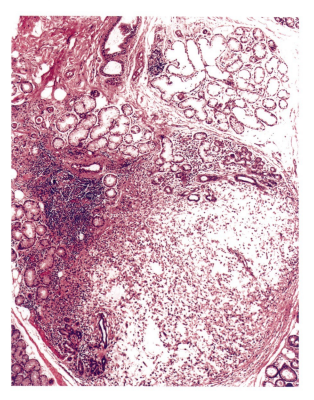

Figure 6-14

LIP MINOR SALIVARY TISSUE WITH MUCOUS EXTRAVASATION PHENOMENON

The mucus is extravasated and bounded by lobular septa. Muciphages are interspersed within. There is a small lymphoid cuff surrounding the extravasation.

adjacent salivary tissue may show associated secondary inflammatory postobstructive changes. Less than 1 percent are intraepithelial, and less than 1 percent show unusual lamellated, inspissated, mucin-rich fibroinflammatory spheres, designated as myxoglobulosis (48).

Differential Diagnosis. The differential diagnosis is mainly that of a mucin-rich salivary neoplasm, and the absence of an epithelial neoplastic component essentially excludes this. Occasionally, the muciphages resemble signet ring cell carcinoma, primary or metastatic (fig. 6-15), but expression of histiocyte lineage markers (e.g., CD68, others) and absence of keratin(s) eliminate this diagnostic consideration.

Treatment and Prognosis. Treatment generally consists of excision of the cyst along with the associated salivary gland lobule to minimize recurrence.

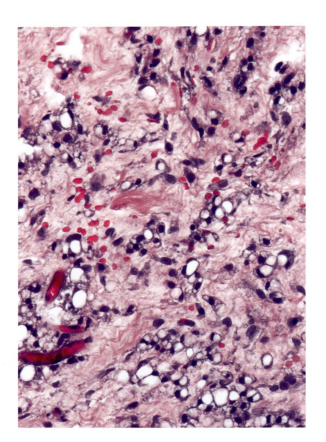 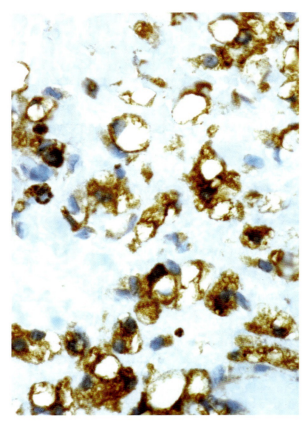

Figure 6-15

MUCUS EXTRAVASATION PHENOMENON WITH SIGNET RING CELLS

Left: Signet ring-like muciphages mimic a signet ring cell carcinoma.
Right: Positive immunoreactivity for CD68 demonstrates the histiocyte lineage and allows for differentiation from signet ring carcinoma cells.

Ranula

Definition. *Ranula* is a term derived from the Latin phrase for frog belly, and defines a distinctive mucocele (either extravasation or retention type) involving the floor of the mouth and arising from the sublingual gland (52,53). Ranulas are divided as follows: *simple (submandibular, oral) ranulae* present with intraoral swelling only; *plunging ranulae* extend into the neck, herniating through the mylohyoid muscle; and *mixed ranulae* show both intraoral and neck swelling.

Clinical Features. Ranulae predominate in the second decade, with a wide age range. Simple ranulae present as lateral floor fluctuant masses that may cause tongue deviation, snoring, or even obstructive sleep apnea. Plunging ranulae present as painless neck masses in the submental or submandibular triangle. Mixed ranulae may show features of both (53).

Gross Findings. Ranulae range from fluctuant to solid, with a cystic gelatinous cut surface. In one literature review, over half of simple ranulae were less than 2 cm, while almost all plunging ranulae were greater than 2 cm (52).

Microscopic Findings. Ranulae microscopically have an appearance similar to that of mucous retention cyst and mucous extravasation phenomenon. Simple ranulae are more likely to show retention cyst morphology, namely, an attenuated ductal epithelial lining, while plunging ranulae are invariably an exaggerated form of mucous extravasation with varying degrees of fibrosis, chronic inflammation, and muciphages. After histologic examination, the diagnosis is straightforward.

Differential Diagnosis. The clinical and gross differential diagnoses include myxoid or mucinous lesions such as pleomorphic adenoma, lipoma with myxoid change, and mucoepidermoid carcinoma. Cystic lesions of the neck, such as thyroglossal duct cyst, epidermoid cyst, branchial cleft cyst, and lymphangioma are additional diagnostic considerations for plunging ranula.

Treatment and Prognosis. The overall recurrence rate is about 20 percent (54) but varies greatly based on treatment. Aspiration and marsupialization result in higher recurrence rates than resection with sublingual gland excision (52). Some patients develop secondary submandibular mucus extravasation from leakage of the Wharton duct near the orifice of the Bartholin duct of the excised sublingual gland if the latter is not ligated (55).

Lymphoepithelial Cysts

Definition. *Lymphoepithelial cysts* (LECs) are salivary duct cysts with associated lymphoid stroma. LECs do not include first branchial cleft anomalies secondarily involving the parotid gland, human immunodeficiency virus (HIV)-associated cystic lymphoid hyperplasia, and cystic change in lymphoepithelial sialadenitis (LESA) of Sjögren syndrome.

Clinical Features. LECs predominate in the parotid gland, and like salivary duct cysts, occur over a wide age range, although on average they occur in the fifth decade (56). LECs typically present as solitary painless masses, although superinfection may result in tenderness. Bilateral cysts not related to HIV infection have been described. While some contend that these are branchial cleft related, the histologic features and high amylase content in the cyst fluid suggest a salivary duct derivation. An origin from intranodal salivary inclusions is also postulated (57,58).

Gross Findings. The cysts are usually unilocular and range from 0.5 to 6.0 cm. The fluid contents are more caseous and debris laden than salivary duct cysts, and their inner lining may show nodularity reflecting lymphoid hyperplasia (59).

Microscopic Findings. LECs are well delineated from the surrounding gland by fibrous tissue and recapitulate the lining of the salivary excretory duct: they are lined by a mixture of cuboidal,

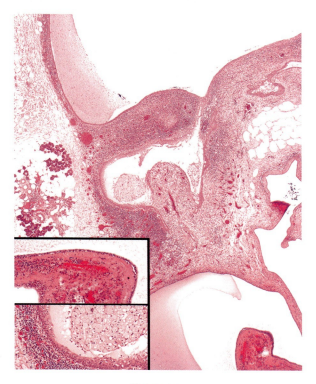

Figure 6-16

LYMPHOEPITHELIAL CYST OF THE PAROTID GLAND

Multilocular cyst shows a lymphoid cuff with germinal centers. The cyst epithelial lining is similar to that of a salivary cyst and ranges from cuboidal/columnar (inset top) to squamous (inset bottom).

columnar ductal, and squamous cells. Oncocytic and goblet cell components may be noted. The cyst wall is characterized by a prominent lymphoid stroma with germinal centers (fig. 6-16).

Differential Diagnosis. LEC must be distinguished from lymphoid stroma-rich (also referred to as tumor-associated lymphoid proliferation, or TALP) (60) cystic neoplasms such as Warthin tumor, mucoepidermoid carcinoma, and acinic cell adenocarcinoma. The architectural complexity and defining cell types help resolve this differential diagnosis. LEC may show considerable overlap with HIV-related cystic lymphoid hyperplasia and cystic change in LESA of Sjögren syndrome. The surrounding salivary tissue in solitary LEC is minimally altered in contrast to these other considerations. LESA with cystic change (and to a lesser extent HIV-related cystic lymphoid hyperplasia) show lymphocytic infiltration of the epithelial lining as well as lymphoepithelial lesions (i.e., epimyoepithelial islands). HIV-associated cystic lymphoid hyperplasia may show isolated giant cells (61,62) and a relative abundance of CD8-positive lymphocytes (given the decrease in CD4-positive T cells) (63,64). See later in this chapter for a more complete discussion of HIV-related salivary gland disease and Sjögren syndrome.

Treatment and Prognosis. Like salivary duct cysts, lymphoepithelial cysts are essentially cured by complete excision.

Polycystic (Dysgenetic) Disease

Definition. *Polycystic (dysgenetic) disease* is extremely rare cystopathy that diffusely involves the salivary gland (65–71).

Clinical Features. Polycystic disease occurs in a wide age range, but almost exclusively in the parotid glands of females (65–71). The one case reported in a male was actually documented in the submandibular gland (68). Typically, this disease is bilateral, presenting as nontender masses or swellings (65–71). One case was reported to fluctuate in size with pregnancy, implicating hormonal-related growth (72). At least three cases have a familial association, although the responsible genetic alteration has not yet been identified (67,71,73).

Gross Findings. These lesions present as diffuse spongy masses with multiple cysts of various sizes, similar to polycystic disease at other organ sites (i.e., liver, kidney).

Microscopic Findings. The epithelium is attenuated and cuboidal, and the cyst wall is delicate with minimal fibrosis or inflammation (fig. 6-17). Tufting, vacuolated cytoplasm, and apocrine snouts may be seen. The lumens may contain concentric eosinophilic secretions. These concretions are PAS positive and diastase resistant, but may also be congophilic (65–71).

Differential Diagnosis. The main entity in the differential diagnosis is sclerosing polycystic adenosis, which is now considered a neoplasm (74). Unlike sclerosing polycystic adenosis, which is often a well-demarcated or multinodular process, polycystic dysgenetic disease is diffuse and does not demonstrate the same degree of sclerosis or proliferative ductal or acinar changes.

Treatment and Prognosis. To date, recurrence has been only occasionally described (73).

METAPLASIA AND HYPERPLASIA

Oncocytic Metaplasia and Oncocytosis

Definition. *Oncocytic metaplasia* is non-neoplastic transformation of salivary parenchyma into oncocytes, which are cells engorged by abundant, often ultrastructurally abnormal, mitochondria imparting a granular eosinophilic appearance to cells by light microscopy. *Oncocytosis* (also referred to as *oncocytic (adenomatous) hyperplasia*) is a non-neoplastic mass-forming proliferation of oncocytic cells within the salivary gland encompassing diffuse and nodular oncocytic hyperplasia. Usually there are nodular foci, referred to as *nodular oncocytic hyperplasia* or *nodular oncocytosis*. Less commonly, there is a diffuse alteration in the affected salivary gland, referred to as *diffuse oncocytosis*.

Clinical Features. Oncocytic metaplasia is a senescent phenomenon typically occurring after the fifth decade of life. It is an incidental finding, often in the minor salivary gland tissue of the larynx and hypopharynx. Oncocytosis presents as unilateral or bilateral parotid gland enlargement (75).

Gross Findings. Oncocytic metaplasia is not grossly detectable. Similar to oncocytic lesions at other sites, oncocytosis presents with a tan to dark, "mahogany," brown cut surface. Multinodular growth is more common than diffuse growth. Cystic change may be evident. The nodules are often well demarcated. In either the nodular or diffuse form, presentation is as a clinically detectable mass lesion, causing difficulties in differentiation from oncocytoma.

Microscopic Findings. In contrast to oncocytoma (and oncocytosis), oncocytic metaplasia is a nonmass-forming focal or limited change in one or more areas within the salivary gland. Oncocytic metaplastic foci appear as isolated clusters of oncocytic cells within otherwise normal-appearing parenchyma (fig. 6-18) and usually represent an incidental histologic finding in salivary glands excised for other reasons. The oncocytic cells are characterized by abundant granular eosinophilic cytoplasm.

Nodular oncocytic hyperplasia consists of multiple (often two or more) separate solid unencapsulated nodules of oncocytes with a compressed tubulotrabecular growth pattern and delicate vasculature (fig. 6-18). The nodules

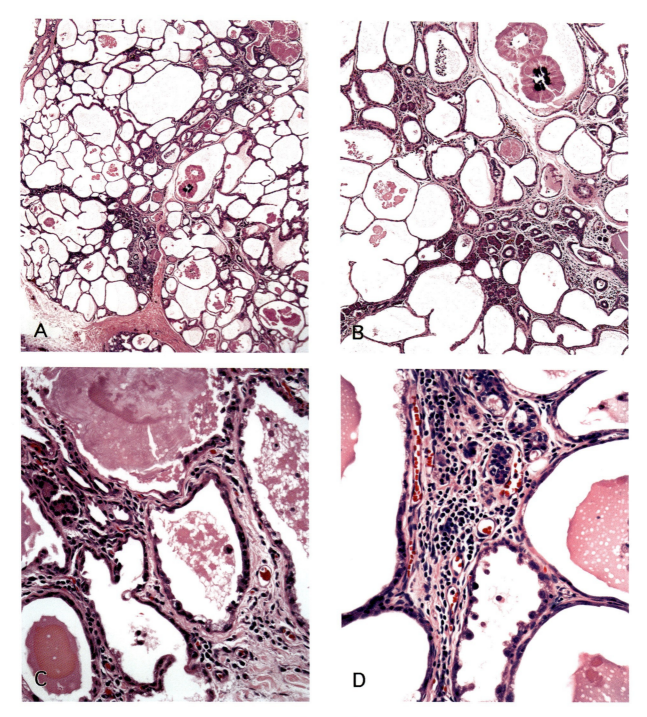

Figure 6-17

POLYCYSTIC (DYSGENETIC) DISEASE

A,B: The involved gland is diffusely replaced by multiple variably sized epithelial-lined cysts creating a honeycomb or lattice-like appearance.

C: Cysts are lined by flattened to cuboidal to columnar-appearing epithelium; intraluminal proteinaceous and eosinophilic concretions with concentric laminations resembling microliths are present.

D: Apocrine-like snouting may be present; entrapped salivary gland acini and ducts can be seen between the cysts.

Non-Neoplastic Diseases of the Head and Neck

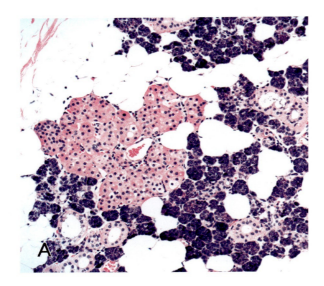

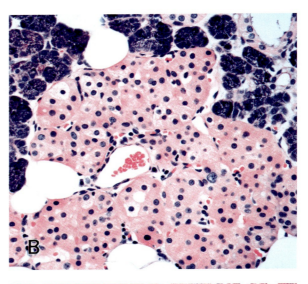

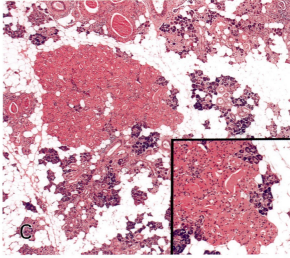

Figure 6-18

ONCOCYTIC METAPLASIA AND ONCOCYTOSIS

A: Incidentally identified focus of oncocytic metaplasia in a parotid gland from an older individual.

B: At higher magnification, the oncocytic cells show the characteristic granular eosinophilic cytoplasm.

C: Nodular oncocytic hyperplasia consists of an unencapsulated nodule of oncocytes interspersed within the parotid gland and merging with (nononcocytic) salivary gland parenchyma. Inset: These nodules consist of compressed tubules and trabeculae of cuboidal to columnar oncocytes with granular eosinophilic cytoplasm.

D: Mass-forming oncocytic nodule that appears circumscribed but not encapsulated gradually merging with and incorporating residual salivary gland parenchyma.

E: Higher magnification shows oncocytic cells with granular eosinophilic cytoplasm and acini characterized by intracytoplasmic basophilic (zymogen) granules.

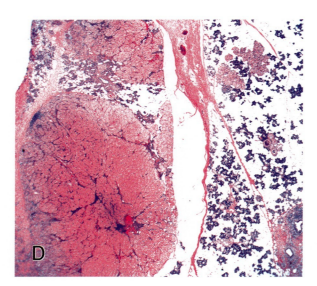

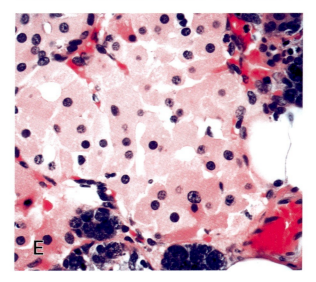

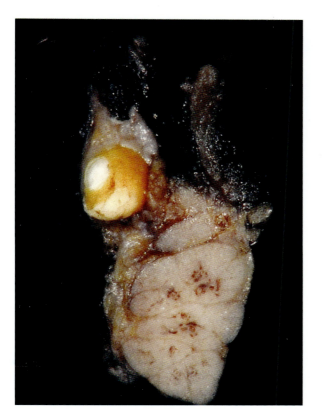 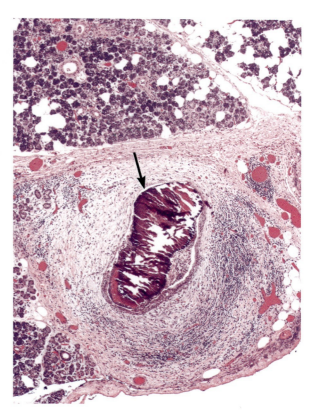

Figure 6-20

SIALOLITHIASIS

Left: Gross sialolith (top) within the Wharton duct.
Right: Microscopic sialoliths are present in the excretory duct (arrow), surrounded by a fibroinflammatory reaction.

interlobular fibrosis and atrophy of lobules. Sialolithiasis typically results in duct ectasia with stones that may be identifiable grossly (fig. 6-20), if not previously removed (96).

Microscopic Findings. Chronic sialadenitis demonstrates excretory duct ectasia, periductal fibrosis, and a mixture of lymphocytic, histiocytic, and plasmacytic infiltrates. Ducts may undergo squamous or mucinous metaplasia. Microliths may be seen in some cases, even when there is no gross sialolithiasis (fig. 6-20). Advanced cases show acinar atrophy with an abundance of intercalated duct cells. Radiation may induce stromal and ductal atypia (fig. 6-21). In chronic granulomatous sialadenitis, infectious etiologies are highlighted by Grocott methenamine silver (GMS) stains for fungi and acid-fast (AFB) stains for mycobacteria.

Treatment and Prognosis. The prognosis depends on the underlying etiology. Complications include superinfection with fistula or sinus tract formation (97) and xerostomia. Surgical treatment may prevent superinfection but xerostomia, particularly in the radiation setting, does not resolve (98,99).

Human Immunodeficiency Virus Salivary Gland Disease

Definition. *Human immunodeficiency virus salivary gland disease* (HIV-SGD) is defined as xerostomia in HIV-infected individuals, with enlargement of one or more major salivary glands (100–102). HIV-SGD is characterized by cystic lymphoid hyperplasia. It is also known as *acquired immunodeficiency syndrome (AIDS)-related parotid cyst.*

Clinical Features. The prevalence of HIV-SGD is about 3 to 6 percent in adults and 10 to 30 percent in children (100–102), although this may have decreased with the advent of highly active antiretroviral treatment (HAART); the type of

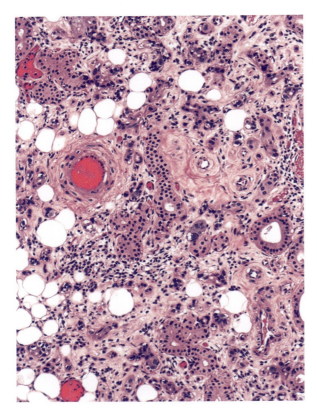

Figure 6-21

RADIATION-RELATED CHANGES IN THE SUBMANDIBULAR GLAND

There is acinar atrophy with residual prominent intercalated ducts surrounded by a fibromyxoid stroma. The nuclei in the ductal cell vary in size and amount of cytoplasm.

HAART may influence prevalence (103). The most common presentation is salivary gland swelling, and 60 percent of cases are bilateral. Over 95 percent of cases occur in the parotid gland. In adults, there is a male predilection, although gender distribution is equal in the pediatric population.

The typical presentation is painless swelling, xerostomia, dry eyes, and arthralgias. Salivary gland disease may present throughout the disease course and its prevalence does not correlate well with the CD4-positive count, with perhaps the exception of submandibular gland involvement (104).

Rarely, HIV-SGD is attributable to the syndrome of *diffuse infiltrating lymphocytosis* (DILS). Criteria for DILS include (105): 1) HIV infection, 2) bilateral salivary gland enlargement or xerostomia, 3) 6-month persistence of signs/symptoms, and 4) histologic confirmation of salivary or lacrimal gland lymphocytic infiltrates unrelated to granulomas or neoplasm. This subtype occurs in 3 to 7 percent of patients, there is an African-American preponderance, and the presentation mimics that of Sjögren syndrome (106). Unlike Sjögren syndrome, however, DILS (and all HIV-SGD types) does not generally manifest with autoantibodies such as anti-SSA, anti-SSB, antinuclear antibody (ANA), or rheumatoid factor (RF) (107). The salivary gland enlargement and extrasalivary manifestations are more extreme in DLS, including pulmonary, renal, gastrointestinal, and neuromuscular involvement (108). Median CD4-positive counts are over $350/mm^2$ in association with DILS (105,109), but about 25 percent of cases demonstrate opportunistic infection (thus fulfilling the criteria for AIDS). Unlike the usual HIV-SGD, DILS is associated with more systemic findings.

Gross Findings. Grossly, HIV-SGD is classically characterized by cysts that range from single to multiple. The parenchymal lobular septation may be attenuated or effaced, showing a firmer tan appearance rather than the typical lobular yellow color.

Microscopic Findings. HIV-SGD is typically a cystic lymphoid hyperplasia. The epithelial lining of the cyst resembles that of a lymphoepithelial cyst, ranging from cuboidal to columnar with varying degrees of oncocytic change and squamous metaplasia (fig. 6-22). The initial assumption was that these are cystic dilatations of salivary inclusions in hyperplastic intraparotid/periparotid lymph nodes, similar to other non-HIV lymphoepithelial cysts (110). While this is likely accurate to some extent, three-dimensional reconstruction studies suggest that a large component of HIV-SGD is a cystic dilatation of the native ductal system in the setting of lymphoid hyperplasia (111). The lymphoid hyperplasia resembles that seen the lymph nodes of HIV patients and includes florid follicular hyperplasia, thinning (attenuation) to loss of the mantle zone lymphocytes, follicle lysis, and multinucleated giant cells that may be isolated or clustered in interfollicular areas or approximating or within the cystic epithelial lining (fig. 6-22). Lymphoepithelial sialadenitis (LESA)-like change, similar to that seen in Sjögren syndrome (fig. 6-22), is common.

Salivary Glands

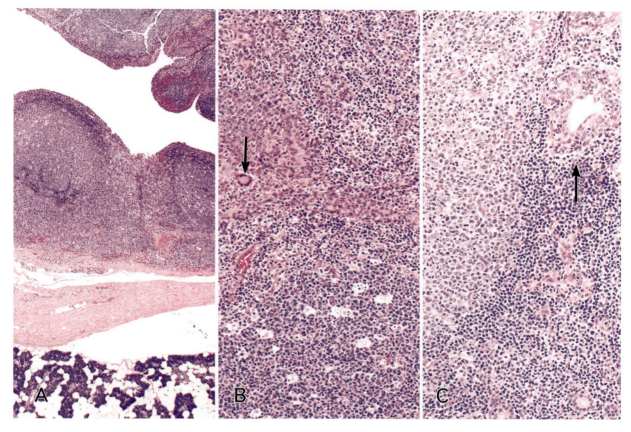

Figure 6-22

HUMAN IMMUNODEFICIENCY VIRUS SALIVARY GLAND DISEASE (HIV-SGD)

A: A cystic epithelial lesion is characterized by lymphoid follicular hyperplasia and attenuation and an absence of mantle lymphocytes.

B: Scattered giant cells (arrow) are noted in the lymphoid stroma; at the lower portion of the image, there is a follicle permeated by lymphocytes resulting in follicle lysis.

C: Lymphoepithelial lesions resembling those seen in lymphoepithelial sialadenitis may be present (arrow).

The histologic manifestations are similar in DILS, but the lymphoid component may be more extensive. Evidence for DILS is provided by minor salivary gland biopsy which shows lymphocytic sialadenitis similar to that seen in Sjögren syndrome, but with ductal atypia (109). See chapter 3 for additional images of HIV-associated diseases.

The diagnosis by fine-needle aspiration biopsy of HIV-SGD is feasible, simple, and cost-effective in cystic parotid gland lesions (112,113). The key cytologic findings include a heterogeneous lymphoid population, scattered single or clustered foamy macrophages, numerous multinucleated giant cells, and superficial or anucleated squamous cells (114–116).

Ancillary studies are not usually necessary for the diagnosis. Immunohistochemical assessment of the lymphoid population may show a preponderance of CD8-positive lymphocytes, which may help delineate HIV-SGD from LESA (117,118). Clonality by T-cell receptor gene rearrangement is common in patients with DILS/CD8-positive lymphocytosis, but progression to lymphoma has not been seen (119). HIV p24 antigen is detected in the germinal center (follicular dendritic cells), scattered lymphoid cells, and multinucleated giant cells (fig. 6-23) (100,101,116,120,121). Given the occasional S-100 protein, CD21, and CD35 reactivity, some of these giant cells may actually be dendritic cells phenotypically (122,123). Further evidence of dendritic

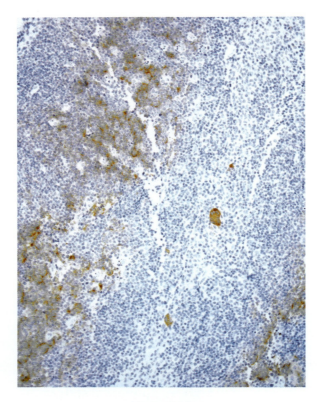

Figure 6-23

HUMAN IMMUNODEFICIENCY VIRUS SALIVARY GLAND DISEASE

HIV infection is confirmed by immunohistochemical reactivity with HIV p24 core antigen. p24 expression is present in a germinal center (bottom and top right) and in scattered interfollicular multinucleated giant cells.

cell derivation is the p55 dendritic cell markers in the multinucleated giant cells (124).

Treatment and Prognosis. HAART is a mainstay of "treatment" as the prevalence of HIV-SGD, especially DILS, has decreased as a result. Other therapeutic options include surgery, surveillance, and radiation (125–127). Recent evidence supports the value of radiotherapy (104). Malignant transformation of the lymphoid component is rare (102,128–130). Post-transplant lymphoproliferative disorder-like lesions in the setting of HIV-SGD rarely have been described, typically of the polymorphous type consisting of lymphoplasmacytic infiltrates and an association with EBV (103). While carcinomas arising in the setting of HIV have been described, this appears coincidental (131).

Table 6-2

LYMPHOEPITHELIAL SIALADENITIS: ASSOCIATION WITH SALIVARY GLAND DISEASES

Sialolithiasis

Sialadenitis (infectious and noninfectious)

Sjögren syndrome and other connective tissue disorders

Human immunodeficiency virus salivary gland disease (HIV-SGD)

Lymphomas

Peritumoral response

Lymphoepithelial Sialadenitis

Lymphoepithelial sialadenitis (LESA) is a non-neoplastic enlargement of the salivary glands characterized by a distinctive pattern of lymphocytic infiltrates. Synonyms include *benign lymphoepithelial lesion, myoepithelial sialadenitis, immunosialadenitis, Godwin lesion*, and *punctate parotitis*. As the synonyms indicate, this lesion has a rich evolutionary history since its original description (132), with the current favored term being lymphoepithelial sialadenitis (133).

LESA is classically viewed as an autoimmune sialadenitis, specifically associated with Sjögren syndrome (SS). As a pure pathologic diagnosis, however, it represents a pattern of sialadenitis that while distinctive, is not specific for SS (134). Table 6-2 summarizes the spectrum of salivary lesions that may manifest histologically as LESA.

Sjögren Syndrome

Definition. Salivary and lacrimal gland enlargement were first described by Jan Mikulicz-Radecki in 1888. In 1925, Gougerot recognized a generalized condition consisting of dryness of the eyes, upper aerodigestive tract, and genitourinary tract. Henrik Sjögren expanded on this constellation after observing that polyarthritis and an elevated erythrocyte sedimentation rate were also disease manifestations, and this disease eventually bore his name, *Sjögren syndrome* (135).

Despite the characterization over the ensuing decades, there is no single standard test for the diagnosis. The general definition of SS is 1) a systemic autoimmune disease, 2) chronic and progressive in nature, and 3) characterized by secretory dysfunction (136).

Clinical Features. SS is divided into primary and secondary SS. *Primary SS* occurs in the absence of another connective tissue disease, and comprises the majority of cases. Secondary SS occurs in the setting of other autoimmune diseases (i.e., polyautoimmunopathy). The most common of these secondary diseases are autoimmune thyroiditis, rheumatoid arthritis, and systemic lupus erythematosus (137). Primary SS has a prevalence of 0.1 to 3.0 percent in the general population, with a striking female predominance (about 9 to 1). It typically occurs in the fourth to sixth decades, and is rare in children.

The typical presentation is one of dryness, xerophthalmia, or xerostomia (138). When salivary or lacrimal gland swelling occurs, parotid involvement predominates in over 80 percent of cases. Pediatric SS is more likely to present with parotitis (139). The oral sequelae of xerostomia include primary or recurrent dental carries, angular cheilitis, and patchy or generalized oral mucosal erythema with dorsal tongue fissuring and papillary atrophy (140). Extrasalivary manifestations include Raynaud phenomenon, primary biliary cirrhosis, diffuse interstitial lung disease, interstitial nephritis, atrophic gastritis, hepatobiliary diseases, neuropathies, and inflammatory vascular disease (141–146).

Laboratory Findings. While the pathogenesis is complex and not fully understood, the hallmark of SS is the presence of autoantibodies to ribonucleoproteins Ro/SSA and La/SSB, which are the main serologies used clinically. Autoantibodies to fodrin, alpha-amylase, and carbonic anhydrase have been demonstrated as well (147). Antinuclear antibodies (ANA) and rheumatoid factor (RF) are also elevated in SS (148–150). Antineutrophil cytoplasmic antibody (ANCA) positivity is less common but may be associated with vascular manifestations (151).

More general laboratory findings include hypergammaglobulinemia, mild anemia, leukopenia, eosinophilia, and elevated erythrocyte sedimentation rates. High resolution salivary proteomic analysis is investigational but may be useful in delineating primary SS from secondary SS (152).

Diagnostic Criteria. Recent American College of Rheumatology (ACR) guidelines using evidence-based statistical validation of a large cohort of patients have simplified the criteria for diagnosis (summarized in Table 6-3) (136). These correlate with criteria of the prior American-European Consensus Group (AECG), although the latter shows more subjectivity (153).

Table 6-3

AMERICAN COLLEGE OF RHEUMATOLOGY CLASSIFICATION CRITERIA FOR SJÖGREN SYNDROME[a]

Two of the following three are required:
1. Positive serum anti-SSA and/or anti-SSB or positive rheumatoid factor and ANA ≥1:320
2. Ocular staining score ≥3
3. Presence of focal lymphocytic sialadenitis with focus score ≥1 focus/4 mm² in labial salivary gland biopsies

The following are exclusionary criteria:
   hepatitis C, human immunodeficiency virus (HIV), sarcoidosis, amyloidosis, active tuberculosis, graft versus host disease, autoimmune connective tissue diseases other than rheumatoid arthritis or lupus erythematosus, past head and neck radiation treatment, current treatment with daily eye drops for glaucoma, corneal surgery in the last 5 years to correct vision, cosmetic eyelid surgery in the last 5 years.

[a]Table 7 from reference 136.

Pathogenesis. The pathogenesis is likely multifactorial, with both environmental and genetic causes. The exact antigenic stimulus remains elusive but has been postulated to be viral. Key components that summarize the cascade of autocrine pathways include B-cell hyperactivity and an interferon (IFN) signature. Genome-wide association studies have shown that traditional human leukocyte antigen (HLA) associations are associated with SS risk: HLADQA1*0501, HLA-DQB1*0201, and HLA-DRB*0301; non-HLA factors (IRF5, STAT4, BLK, and CXCR5) are also implicated (154).

Gross Findings. The salivary glands show diffuse or nodular involvement with SS. Cystic change may occur, and the cut surface may show varying degrees of fibrosis and a firm tan appearance.

Microscopic Findings. LESA is almost invariably associated with SS. LESA consists of periductal lymphocytic infiltrates with germinal center formation and infiltration of duct epithelium, which results in solid, vaguely spindled, epithelial nests formerly designated as epimyoepithelial islands but now referred to as lymphoepithelial lesions (fig. 6-24). It is now suggested that these are not truly myoepithelial, although still metaplastic (155,156). In early disease, there

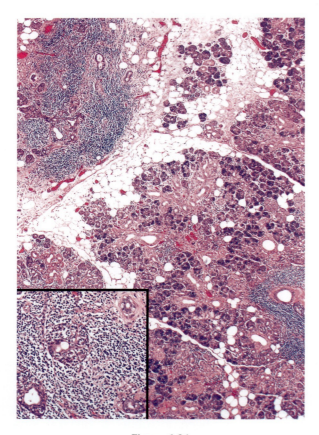

Figure 6-24

LYMPHOEPITHELIAL SIALADENITIS (LESA) IN SJÖGREN SYNDROME

Periductal lymphoid infiltrates and germinal centers are present. Inset: Classic lymphoepithelial lesions consist of metaplastic solid to spindled ducts infiltrated by lymphocytes.

are only periductal lymphoid aggregates with little epitheliotropism. Late-stage disease, on the other hand, shows a prominent lymphoid stroma with loss of salivary acinar parenchyma (134). Plasma cells may be present in longstanding SS. The lymphocytes and plasma cells have a limited heavy chain V gene (VH) repertoire even among different patients, suggesting antigenic stimulation from a common epitope, and adding further support to possible viral stimulation (157).

Immunohistochemically, the lymphoid component in LESA shows polyclonality including reactivity for B-cell and T-cell markers, with the B-cell population being greater than the T-cell population. Lymphoepithelial lesions are cytokeratin positive.

By molecular evaluation, the lymphoid infiltrates may reveal heavy and light chain *Ig* gene rearrangements. The presence of molecular evidence of B-cell clonality may be seen in the absence of histologic features diagnostic of a lymphoma; the meaning and importance of this finding remain controversial. Most cases with monoclonal populations have an uneventful course. The significance of clonality in LESA without morphologic evidence of lymphoma remains controversial. Detecting oligoclonality or monoclonality in this context is not diagnostic of lymphoma, which requires effacement of the architecture by a nodular expansion of monocytoid lymphocytes.

Lip Biopsy. While the clinical and gross manifestations of SS are most vividly reflected in the major salivary glands, lip biopsy results are commonly used as an indication of the objective criteria that qualify a patient for the diagnosis. The basis of lip biopsy evaluation revolves around the focus score. Foci are then counted by specific area (see below).

Recently, the Sjögren International Collaborative Clinical Alliance (SICCA) registry established fairly reproducible guidelines that correlate with symptomatology and serologic findings. Adequacy is defined by area of foci rather than lobules and at minimum should be 4 mm^2, although optimally 10 mm^2 is desired. Focal lymphocytic sialadenitis, a diagnostic category in this registry, is used to support the diagnosis of SS (Table 6-4) (154). Focal lymphocytic sialadenitis consists of periductal or perivascular foci as defined above (fig. 6-25). Germinal centers and lymphoepithelial lesions are less common in lip biopsies but are highly correlated with other SS findings, when present. In contrast, nonspecific chronic sialadenitis consists of plasma cells, duct ectasia, and atrophy, and chronic sclerosing sialadenitis shows more prominent sclerosis (158). IgG4 disease is exceptionally rare in lip biopsies but would fall under this category (159). Rarely, granulomatous inflammation, other diseases, and lymphomas are detected by lip biopsy and are categorized as such. The registry is simplistic in the approach to the latter (158), and a standard evaluation for these diseases (i.e., microbial histochemical stains for granulomas and immunophenotypic workup of a potential lymphoma) is appropriate.

Table 6-4
SJÖGREN INTERNATIONAL COLLABORATIVE CLINICAL ALLIANCE (SICCA) REGISTRY DIAGNOSTIC CATEGORIES OF SJÖGREN SYNDROME

1. *Within Normal Limits* or *Unremarkable* or *No Significant Abnormalities*: normal architecture, densely arranged normal acini and scattered plasma cells with no or few lymphocytes
2. *Nonspecific Chronic Sialadenitis*: the presence of scattered or focal infiltrates of lymphocytes that are not immediately adjacent to normal-appearing acini and located in gland lobules, lobes, or entire glands that exhibit some combination of mild to moderate acinar atrophy, interstitial fibrosis, and duct dilation, often filled with inspissated mucus
    not enough lymphocytes to make a lymphoid focus
    even if there is what qualifies as a focus, adjacent acini are atrophic or ectatic
3. *Focal Lymphocytic Sialadenitis*: the presence of one or more foci containing dense aggregates of 50 or more lymphocytes that are usually located in perivascular or periductal locations
    these foci are adjacent to normal mucous acini, in lobes or lobules that lack duct dilation and contain no more than a minority proportion of plasma cells
    this diagnosis is assigned when these foci are the only inflammation present in a specimen, or the most prominent feature
    should mention germinal centers when present
    should mention lymphoepithelial lesion ("epimyoepithelial islands") when present (rare)
4. *Chronic Sclerosing Sialadenitis*: generally considered an advanced stage of nonspecific chronic sialadenitis with interstitial fibrosis, chronic inflammation; IgG4 disease falls into this group but very rare
5. *Granulomatous Inflammation*: self-explanatory
6. *Lymphoma*: self-explanatory

Typically, foci are confluent and difficult to quantitate in lymphomas.

Differential Diagnosis. The main entity in the differential diagnosis, as well as sequela of SS, is small B-cell lymphoma, usually marginal zone or mucosa-associated lymphoid tissue (MALT) type. The earliest histologic changes of MALT lymphoma are the presence of "halos" of monocytoid or centrocyte-like B cells that are slightly pale on low-power magnification (160). These coalesce into sheets and eventually form mass lesions. Involvement of intraparotid and periparotid lymph nodes is common. Immunohistochemical and flow cytometric analysis show a population of B cells that are CD19 positive, CD20 positive, CD5 negative, CD10 negative, and CD23 negative. CD43, typically seen in T cells, is aberrantly expressed. MALT lymphomas often, but not always, show light chain restriction (161). In the salivary gland, the most common translocation is t(14;18)(q32;q21), which is the fusion of *IGH/MALT1*, while trisomy 3 is the most common alteration overall. The significance of these alterations is unclear at this point (162)

Treatment and Prognosis. SS is characterized by a long disease course and may be punctuated by activity, which is assessed with a quantitative and qualitative index (163). About two thirds of

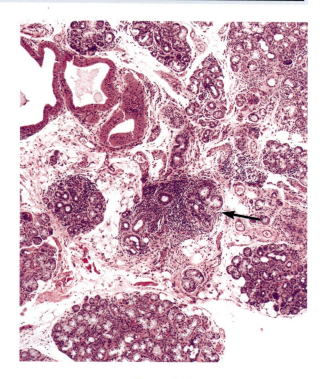

Figure 6-25
FOCAL LYMPHOCYTIC SIALADENITIS IN SJÖGREN SYNDROME
The lip biopsy shows a periductal lymphoid focus (arrow) showing an early lymphoepithelial lesion.

patients have or will manifest systemic disease. Patients with SS have a 40-fold increased risk for the development of MALT lymphoma in comparison to the general population, and 6 to 9 percent eventually progress to lymphoma (133,161,164–166). Patients with so-called SSA-, SSB-negative SS have a lower risk for lymphoma progression (167).

In rare instances, the epithelial component of LESA in SS may transform into a malignancy, usually undifferentiated nonkeratinizing nasopharyngeal carcinoma, although keratinizing squamous cell carcinomas have been described (168–170). Lymphoepithelial carcinomas of the parotid gland, similar to their nasopharyngeal counterparts, are often associated with EBV infection. Wu et al. (171) showed the presence of EBV small RNA-1 (EBV-encoded RNA [EBER-1]) in benign lymphoepithelial lesions, with carcinomatous transformation in both the benign and malignant areas, while typical LESA was negative for EBER-1 (171).

IgG4-Related Sialadenitis

Definition. *IgG4-related sialadenitis* is a chronic fibroinflammatory salivary gland disease with characteristic morphology within the spectrum of the systemic IgG4-related diseases that include autoimmune pancreatitis and involvement of extrapancreatic organs (e.g., kidney, lung, retroperitoneum, liver, gallbladder, lymph nodes, breast, salivary glands, lacrimal glands, aorta).

IgG4-related sialadenitis includes *chronic sclerosing sialadenitis* (CSS) (also called *Küttner tumor* and *punctate parotitis*) and *Mikulicz disease* (MD), which was considered to be a subtype of SS based on histopathologic similarities, but recently has been shown to be an IgG4-related disease because of the high serum IgG4 concentration (172). CSS was categorized originally as nonspecific localized chronic sialadenitis. While this remains true for some cases, a subset or possibly most cases are autoimmune in etiology, have elevated serum IgG4 levels, and often have multiple fibrosclerosing exocrinopathies, including multigland involvement and extrasalivary disease such as primary sclerosing cholangitis, idiopathic retroperitoneal fibrosis, and lymphoplasmacytic sclerosing pancreatitis. This was initially characterized in Japanese cohorts (173,174) but confirmed in western populations as well (172,175).

In order to establish a definitive diagnosis of IgG4-related sialadenitis in the clinical and pathologic settings that correlate to CSS and MD, immunohistochemical staining is necessary to determine the number and fraction of plasma cells with IgG4 (see below). Not all cases of CSS and MD show the requisite increase in the number of IgG4 to IgG plasma cells to establish a definitive diagnosis of IgG4-related sialadenitis, and in such a scenario a diagnosis of nonspecific (idiopathic) CSS is rendered.

Clinical Features. IgG4-sialadenitis shows a slight male predilection and typically involves the submandibular gland of middle-aged adults. About a quarter of cases are bilateral. Systemic manifestations occur in 30 to 40 percent of patients. The finding of a fibrosclerotic disease spectrum in association with IgG4 implicates an unusual pathogenesis, since this is the least common subclass of IgG (3 to 6 percent of total IgG) (176). While the clinicopathologic findings are well characterized, the etiology of this disease is elusive and no potential self-antigen or microbial agent has been implicated. It is not even clear whether the IgG4 is responsible for the pathologic findings, or is merely a marker of a dysregulation of T- and B-cell populations (177).

Laboratory Findings. Patients with IgG4-related sialadenitis have elevated serum levels of IgG4, IgG, and IgG4/IgG. Antibodies associated with SS (e.g., anti-SSA, anti-SSB) are absent in IgG4-associated sialadenitis. Serum ANCA and proteinase 3 levels are not elevated. Eosinophilia, hypergammaglobulinemia, and ANA may be present in systemic disease but are not typically elevated in localized disease.

Gross Findings. Grossly, IgG4-related sialadenitis/CSS is characterized by a firm, nodular, tan-white cut surface with retention of normal lobularity (fig. 6-26). In some cases, the fibrosis surrounds the parenchymal lobules, simulating a "cirrhotic" appearance.

Microscopic Findings. IgG4-related sialadenitis is characterized by dense fibrosclerosis with retention of the lobular architecture but with acinar atrophy. A dense lymphoplasmacytic inflammatory cell infiltrate is present within the lobules and extends into the fibrosis (fig. 6-27). Enlarged and irregular lymphoid follicles, with

Salivary Glands

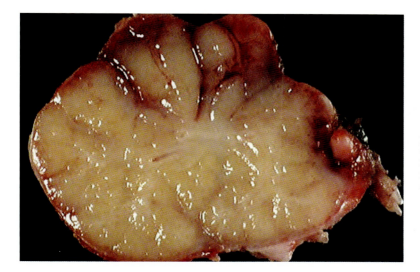

Figure 6-26

IgG4-RELATED SIALADENITIS

A submandibular gland was firm to palpation, with near complete effacement of the gland parenchyma. The parenchyma is tan-yellow, with foci of white (center) irregular fibrosis (sclerosis) but retention of the lobular architecture.

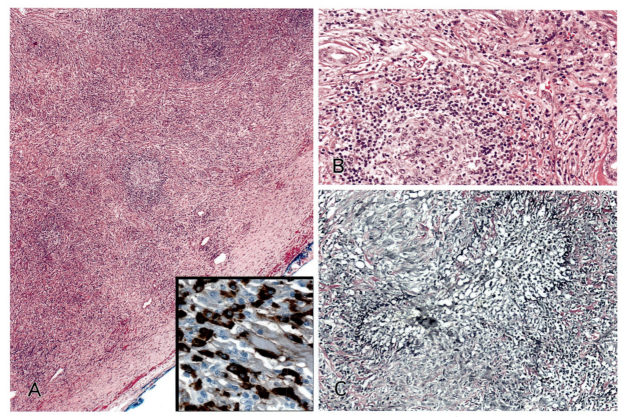

Figure 6-27

IgG4-RELATED SIALADENITIS

A: A dense fibrosclerosing proliferation is present with acinar atrophy and an associated mixed inflammatory cell infiltrate with identifiable germinal centers. Inset: Immunohistochemical staining shows the plasma cell to IgG4 subpopulation of plasma cell ratio is pronounced.

B: The fibrosclerosis has a storiform appearance, with "cracking" artifact and a mixed chronic inflammatory cell infiltrate dominated by mature plasma cells.

C: Elastic stain demonstrates an obliterated vein (obliterative phlebitis), characteristic of IgG4-related diseases.

or without (expanded) germinal centers, may be present (fig. 6-27).

The fibrosclerosis of IgG4-related sialadenitis, like IgG4 diseases at other sites, is often "storiform" with cracking of collagen (fig. 6-27), but the typical storiform-type fibrosis seen in other organs (e.g., pancreas) may not be as frequently present in the salivary glands. Other cases show a more "pseudolymphomatous" lymphoplasmacytic infiltrate overlying the fibrosclerosis (176). The inflammatory cell infiltrate is dominated by mature plasma cells, which may appear in sheets and, of course, as the association would imply, an increased IgG4-positive plasma cell fraction defines this disease.

While organ sites vary in terms of the threshold IgG4-positive cell count for establishing the diagnosis, general guidelines suggest that it should be greater than 50 per high-power field or the fraction to total IgG should be greater than 0.4 (176). Occasional neoplastic and non-neoplastic entities show elevated IgG4 fractions of plasma cells within this range. Without the appropriate clinical and morphologic context, the presence of increased IgG4-positive plasma cells does not equate with a diagnosis of IgG4-related disease (178). In addition to the lymphoplasmacytic cell infiltrate, eosinophils and noncaseating granulomas are occasionally noted, and there may be squamous or mucous cell (ciliated or goblet cells) metaplasia of the ducts. Another hallmark of IgG4-related sialadenitis is the presence of obliterative phlebitis, noted in about three quarters of cases, but may be challenging to identify in any given case; an elastic stain highlights this manifestation (fig. 6-27). The absence of obliterative phlebitis does not exclude the diagnosis of IgG4-related sialadenitis.

IgG4-related sialadenitis is occasionally diagnosed, or at least considered, on fine-needle aspiration biopsy (FNAB), which would then render surgical intervention unnecessary (179). Aspirates are paucicellular but characterized by occasional fibrous fragments, ductal structures surrounded by sclerosis, and a prominent lymphoplasmacytic background. A caveat is that on FNAB, IgG4-related sialadenitis may mimic the findings of a salivary gland neoplasm (180).

The occasional case still labeled CSS, but not associated with IgG4 disease, may be a result of localized obstruction. While the periductal fibrosis, lymphoplasmacytic infiltrate, retention of architecture, and acinar atrophy may be present, the fibrosis is not typically storiform, and there is no obliterative phlebitis.

Differential Diagnosis. The differential diagnosis encompasses neoplastic and non-neoplastic entities. Unlike LESA, there are no lymphoepithelial lesions in IgG4-related sialadenitis/CSS. Additionally, LESA predominates in parotid glands associated with SS, while CSS is usually a submandibular gland disease. Postobstructive sialadenitis, as noted above, may represent the cases of CSS without IgG4 type morphology. Occasionally, the reason for the obstruction (i.e., sialolith) is evident.

The main neoplastic considerations include IgG4-positive lymphomas and sclerosing mucoepidermoid carcinoma. Lymphomas arising in the salivary gland may contain a high IgG4-positive plasma cell fraction. Rare cases reported include B-cell lymphomas of MALT or mantle zone type (181,182). The keys to recognition are the diagnostic immunophenotype and morphology in the lymphoid-rich areas.

While a few carcinoma types have been described in association with IgG4 elevation (183,184), the classic tumor in the differential diagnosis is sclerosing mucoepidermoid carcinoma, also characterized by IgG4-positive plasma cell elevation (185). Biopsies may prove troublesome, but the presence of a multicystic epithelial proliferation with a mixture of mucous, epidermoid, and intermediate-type cells excludes CSS. To date, sclerosing mucoepidermoid carcinoma has not been associated with systemic disease.

Treatment and Prognosis. IgG4-related sialadenitis is often diagnosed when a gland is resected. Regarding the resected gland, no further treatment is needed. IgG4-related sialadenitis, however, may be a manifestation of systemic disease. Systemic disease is treated with steroids or rituximab (177).

Sarcoidosis

Definition. *Sarcoidosis* is a multiorgan, noncaseating granulomatous disease of unknown etiology that affects lymph nodes, lung, mucosal sites of the upper aerodigestive tract, salivary gland, skin, spleen, and liver. It is also known as *Boeck disease*.

Clinical Features. Sarcoidosis involves the salivary glands, mainly the parotid and submandibular glands in to 4 to 30 percent of patients. Most salivary involvement occurs in the second to fourth decades, with a slight female predominance (186). A syndromic variant of sarcoidosis, known as *Heerfordt syndrome*, consists of uveitis, facial nerve palsy, and parotitis, and occurs in less than 1 percent of all cases (187,188).

Involvement is classically bilateral, and extrasalivary involvement is typical. Only rare cases present as isolated unilateral parotitis. Xerostomia is typical, and there is some overlap with the presentation of SS (189).

Pathogenesis. The pathogenesis remains unknown. One of the leading theories is that sarcoidosis represents an immune response to mycobacterial antigens (190), although viruses and even other bacteria have been implicated as well. Other considerations include environmental agents (similar to berylliosis) (191).

There are no specific chemical or serologic tests for sarcoidosis, although angiotensin-converting enzyme (ACE) levels are often elevated with lung involvement. Classically, the Kveim test, which is an epithelial reaction to intradermal injections of sarcoid homogenates, is positive in active or subacute disease. Proteomic analysis using matrix-associated laser desorption/ionization-time of flight mass spectrometry has identified one of the antigens in the Kveim reagent, *Mycobacterium tuberculosis* catalase-peroxidase protein, adding further support to an infectious agent (190). HLA haplotypes may modulate the presenting manifestations of the disease. HLA-DRB1*04 allele is associated with Heerfordt syndrome (187).

Gross Findings. The parotid glands involved by sarcoidosis range from grossly normal to fibrotic.

Microscopic Findings. The defining feature of sarcoidosis is the presence of "tight," well-formed noncaseating granulomas, often in a periductal or perivascular distribution, with varying degrees of fibrosis (fig. 6-28). The granulomas consist of epithelioid histiocytes and Langhans-type giant cells. Intracytoplasmic inclusions, including those that are star-shaped and referred to as asteroid bodies and calcific laminated bodies called Schaumann bodies, are present.

As a requisite, other causes of granulomatous inflammation must be excluded, notably infectious disease (mycobacterial and fungal), and

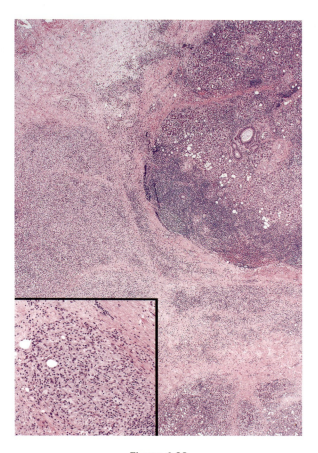

Figure 6-28

SARCOIDOSIS OF THE PAROTID GLAND

There is background sialadenitis and dense fibrosis. Inset: Within the fibrous areas are several noncaseating granulomas. Stains for microorganisms (e.g., acid-fast bacillus [AFB], Gomori methenamine silver [GMS]) were negative.

foreign body giant cell reaction. To this end, acid-fast stains and Gomori methenamine silver are essential. The intraparotid/periparotid lymph nodes often show noncaseating granulomas as well. FNAB may help establish the diagnosis of sarcoidosis when the granulomatous component is present in the aspirate (192,193).

Differential Diagnosis. The differential diagnosis includes other granulomatous processes. While classically tuberculosis demonstrates caseating granulomas, other mycobacterial species have findings that overlap with those of sarcoidosis. Granulomatosis with polyangiitis (GPA, formerly referred to as Wegener granulomatosis) only rarely involves the parotid gland (194). Typically, GPA is not a true granuloma-forming disease but rather consists of scattered multinucleated giant cell granulomas. Further, GPA is characterized by geographic-type or ischemic necrosis, associated vasculitis, and elevated serologic c-ANCA levels (see chapter 1 for a more complete discussion). Occasionally, post-obstructive change and mucus extravasation result in prominent granulomatous inflammation, but the granulomas are localized to these areas (195).

Treatment and Prognosis. Treatment is determined by the severity and extent of disease. Some patients have spontaneous remission. Corticosteroids are the mainstay of therapy, but other agents, such as methotrexate, are used as second-line therapy (196). The overall mortality from sarcoidosis is estimated at 1 to 5 percent in population-based studies. The prognostic features include race, age, persistence of symptomatology, extent of lung involvement, and specific types of extrapulmonary involvement (i.e., cardiac, neurologic, osseous) (197).

TUMOR-LIKE LESIONS

Necrotizing Sialometaplasia

Definition. *Necrotizing sialometaplasia* (NSM) is a benign self-limiting process of the salivary glands that mimics malignancy (198).

Clinical Features. NSM typically occurs in the fourth decade, with a male predilection (male to female ratio, 1.9 to 1.0) (199–202). Although the palate is the most frequently involved site, NSM has been described in seromucous glands throughout the upper and lower respiratory tract (199,203–206). The typical presentation is a single unilateral ulcer at the junction of the hard and soft palate (199–201). The inciting incident (see below) is postulated to precede the development of the NSM by about 2 to 3 weeks. Roughly 10 percent are bilateral, and 15 percent are asymptomatic (199). A burning sensation and nerve symptomatology are rare (207,208).

Pathogenesis. Classic NSM is thought to be the result of spontaneous infarction of the seromucous glands. However, a clinically and histologically identical picture is seen as a result of surgery, radiation, trauma, or vasculitis among other distortive injuries (209,210). The self-limiting nature and histologic features suggest vascular compromise, with ischemic injury and subsequent regeneration as the main pathogenic mechanism (199,202,211).

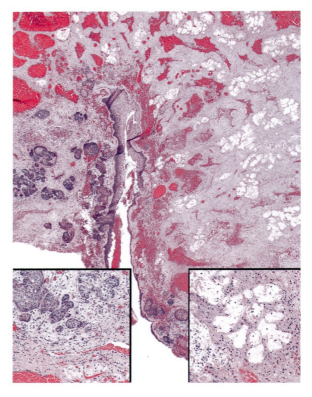

Figure 6-29

NECROTIZING SIALOMETAPLASIA

Palate lesion shows infarcted or ghost-like acini (top of image) as well as squamous metaplasia of the minor salivary glands (bottom). The lobular architecture of the minor salivary glands is retained.

Left inset: Higher magnification of the squamous metaplasia of the minor salivary glands.

Right inset: Higher magnification of the infarcted acini.

The occasional association with repeated emesis seen in bulimia and other disorders suggests chemical injury as a contributing factor (212,213).

Gross Findings. NSM is typically a well-demarcated, raised, erythematous ulcer. The underlying salivary tissue is a soft, friable and gray-tan (202,214). The mean size in one large series was 1.9 cm (range, 0.7 to 5.0 cm) (199).

Microscopic Findings. The defining microscopic criteria include infarction of the salivary lobule with mucus extravasation, varying degrees of fibrosis, and squamous metaplasia of the ducto-acinar units. In early lesions, infarcted "ghosts" of acinar units, with mucus extravasation and mucosal ulceration, may be prominent (fig. 6-29). As a lesion matures, however, fibrosis and squamous

Table 6-5
NECROTIZING SIALOMETAPLASIA: DIFFERENTIAL DIAGNOSIS

	NS[a]	MEC, Low-Grade	SCC
Architecture/growth	Retention of lobular architecture	Haphazard, infiltrative growth	Haphazard, infiltrative growth
Cellular components	Smooth round to oval nests of metaplastic squamous epithelium with bland cytology; may show residual duct lumens with with mucous cells	Admixture of mucous, intermediate ("basaloid") and epidermoid (squamous) cells; bland cytology; irregular cell nests	Nests and cords of squamous cells with irregular outlines and variable amount of cytologic atypia; may entrap residual glands, but the tumor itself contains no mucin
Cyst formation	Absent	Present (prominent component)	Absent
Surface epithelium	May show PEH; usually not connected with NS	Uninvolved; not connected with tumor	Often dysplastic and/or indirect continuity with the carcinoma; may be ulcerated
Extravasated mucin	May be present	Present	Absent
Necrosis	Lobular infarction of salivary gland acini	Absent	May show tumor necrosis
Inflammation	May be prominent	May be prominent with mucin extravasation	May be present; associated desmoplasia

[a]NS = necrotizing sialometaplasia; MEC = mucoepidermoid carcinoma; SCC = squamous cell carcinoma; PEH = pseudoepitheliomatous hyperplasia.

metaplasia of these units ensues, along with surface pseudoepitheliomatous change. Ulceration with pseudoepitheliomatous hyperplasia of the adjacent mucosa may or may not be present in association with NSM. Histochemical stains for epithelial mucin (e.g., mucicarmine, PAS with diastase) may help identify residual mucocytes (goblet cells) of the metaplastic minor salivary gland units.

Differential Diagnosis. The admixture of histologic features of NSM suggests two main differential diagnostic considerations: squamous cell carcinoma and mucoepidermoid carcinoma (Table 6-5). While cytonuclear features are useful, the key to the distinction of NSM from these malignancies is the retention of the lobularity and ductoacinar configuration. Mucoepidermoid carcinoma tends to be more haphazard and multicystic in configuration. Even a well-differentiated squamous cell carcinoma still demonstrates more dyskeratosis and peripheral/basal layer atypia than NSM. Immunostains for p53, Ki-67, and BCL-2 are useful in this distinction although rarely necessary (215).

Treatment and Prognosis. NSM is self-limiting, lasting from a few days to a few months, and does not recur (199). Debridement and saline rinses may be helpful, but surgical resection is not needed.

Subacute Necrotizing Sialadenitis

Definition. *Subacute necrotizing sialadenitis* (SANS) is a rare idiopathic reactive (inflammatory) process of the minor salivary glands (200,216–219). SANS shares several clinical and pathologic features with NSM.

Clinical Features. SANS occurs typically in patients in the second decade, somewhat younger than those with NSM. Similar to NSM, however, SANS typically occurs as a mass of the palate, although nonulcerated in contrast to NSM. The male predominance is reportedly pronounced (about 3 to 1) but may be an artifact of military population bias (200,219).

The etiology of SANS is unclear. Some view it as a variant of NSM (217). The association in a significant number of patients with upper respiratory tract infections, close living quarters, and a winter month incidence raises the possibility of a viral etiology.

Gross Findings. Grossly, these are nonulcerated submucosal masses ranging from 0.3 to 2.5 cm.

Microscopic Findings. The histologic criteria devised by Werning et al. (219) include: acinar cell necrosis and loss, and a mixed inflammatory infiltrate consisting of neutrophils, eosinophils (occasionally prominent), and plasma cells. In contrast to NSM, SANS does not show squamous metaplasia or fibrosis. Ultrastructurally, dense particles have been identified in the acini, which either represent viral particles or lysosomes (200,219).

Treatment and Prognosis. SANS is also a self-limiting disease, with an even more rapid course than NSM: all cases reported resolved within 4 weeks (200,217,218).

Extranodal Sinus Histiocytosis with Massive Lymphadenopathy (Rosai-Dorfman Disease)

Definition. *Extranodal sinus histiocytosis with massive lymphadenopathy* (ESHML) is an idiopathic, histiocytic proliferative disorder that usually resolves spontaneously (220,221). Often a nodal-based proliferation that occurs as part of a generalized process involving the lymph nodes, sinus histiocytosis with massive lymphadenopathy (SHML) may involve extranodal sites independent of the lymph node status. Extranodal sinus histiocytosis with massive lymphadenopathy is technically a misnomer since extranodally there are no sinuses. Synonyms include *Rosai-Dorfman disease* and *Destombes-Rosai-Dorfman syndrome*.

Clinical Features. SHML typically occurs in the cervical lymph nodes, with over three quarters of extranodal cases occurring in the head and neck region; it typically manifests in the second decade, and there is a slight male predominance (225,227,240). Sinonasal disease predominates at extranodal head and neck sites (see chapter 1), but the salivary gland may be involved either in isolation or in conjunction with other sites. The parotid and submandibular glands are the most common glands involved (222–224). The most common presentation in salivary gland is a painless mass. In the salivary gland, there appears to be an equal sex predilection (224).

Pathogenesis. The etiology for SHML is unclear. The lesional cells bear the phenotype of mature macrophage-derived cell types (226). Recently, a *KRAS* K117N missense variant has been detected by next generation sequencing, raising the possibility of a clonal process (227). SHML has been reported in the setting of HIV (228), Langerhans cell histiocytosis (224), and SS (229) There is a debatable association with IgG4-related disease (230–232). Other, even more tenuous associations include EBV, human herpesvirus (HHV)6, and HHV8 (233–236).

Gross Findings. The salivary glands have a tan-white to yellow appearance on cut surface.

Microscopic Findings. SHML is a histiocytic proliferation with a fibroinflammatory background consisting of lymphocytes and plasma cells, which typically form aggregates, although well-formed germinal centers are rare. Histiocytes often percolate through the lymphoid aggregates, imparting a "mottled" appearance. The histiocytes themselves are plump, with abundant granular, pale to eosinophilic cytoplasm. The nuclei are conspicuously round to oval with vesicular nuclei. The hallmark finding is emperipolesis in the histiocytes, which often engulf lymphocytes but may also include other cell types. True granulomas are not typically seen. See chapter 1 for illustrations of ESHML.

The characteristic immunophenotype for SHML is CD68 and S-100 positivity in the histiocytes (225,226), but staining for CD1a and langerin are negative. Plasma cells often show an elevated IgG4 fraction, hence the debate over whether SHML is related to IgG4 fibrosclerosing disease (231).

Differential Diagnosis. The main entities in the differential diagnosis are infectious granulomatous diseases, histiocytic dendritic cell neoplasms, and occasionally, hematolymphoid neoplasms. In addition to the absence of true granulomas, no infectious organisms are noted in SHML. While there is immunohistochemical overlap with histiocytic/dendritic cell lesions and neoplasms (e.g., Langerhans cell histiocytosis), other markers (CD1a, langerin, CD21) are negative. Histiocyte-rich lymphomas do not generally have as prominent a histiocytic component, nor do the histiocytes demonstrate the CD68- and S-100-positive phenotype or emperipolesis. Rarely, SHML progresses to lymphoma (237).

Treatment and Prognosis. There is no standard treatment for SHML. Asymptomatic patients are often only observed. Surgical excision for symptomatic lesions (i.e., salivary gland masses) is considered. Other options, such as corticosteroids, systemic chemotherapy, or radiotherapy, are reserved for more advanced disease. SHML regresses spontaneously in roughly 20 percent of cases, and is stable in the majority. Only about 1 percent progress and actually have lethal complications. Multivisceral involvement predicts aggressive disease (222).

Intercalated Duct Lesion

Definition. *Intercalated duct lesion* (IDL) is a rare lesion that includes hyperplasia, adenoma, or both (hybrid lesions), and may be a precursor lesion of a salivary gland neoplasm (238). It is also known as *adenomatous ductal hyperplasia* (239).

The proposal that IDL may represent a precursor to salivary gland neoplasms is based on the presence of small foci of IDL in cases of basal cell adenoma, epithelial-myoepithelial carcinoma, pleomorphic adenoma, mucoepidermoid carcinoma, basal cell adenocarcinoma, Warthin tumor, acinic cell carcinoma, and others (238–243). The role as a precursor lesion is not definitively proven.

Clinical Features. IDLs are rare lesions. They are more common in females than males, and occur over a wide age range from the second to ninth decades, with a mean in the sixth decade. Most occur in the parotid gland and less often in the oral cavity and submandibular gland. IDLs are typically incidental findings in association with another lesion.

Gross Findings. IDL is usually a small lesion, measuring less than 5 mm in greatest dimension.

Microscopic Findings. *Interelated duct hyperplasia* (IDH) is the most common type of IDL (238). IDH is a unifocal or multifocal and diffuse unencapsulated proliferation of small ducts, with minimal intervening stroma, merging/blending imperceptively with acinar and mucous cells of the surrounding salivary gland parenchyma (fig. 6-30). At low magnification, IDHs appear as irregular pale foci in contrast with the surrounding darker salivary gland parenchyma. Intercalated ducts are lined by a single layer of cuboidal to columnar cells with small round nuclei and eosinophilic to amphophilic cytoplasm. There is an absence of nuclear pleomorphism or increased mitotic activity. Acinic cells may be incorporated within the proliferation or identified at the periphery of most lesions (fig. 6-30). Myoepithelial cells are consistently present around the ducts but are not discernible by light microscopy, thus requiring immunohistochemical staining with p63 or other markers (e.g., calponin, CK14) for identification. Stromal hyalinization that may be periductal is seen. Other less common features include perilesional follicular lymphoid hyperplasia, clear myoepithelial cells, entrapment of nerve within the lesion, presence of focal luminal eosinophilic secretions, cystic change, and basal lamina-like material with a cribriform pattern (242).

The ductal cells are reactive for CK7, S-100 protein, DOG1 (often with apical expression), lysozyme, and estrogen receptor; progesterone receptor is negative (238,239,241–243). The myoepithelial cells are positive for calponin, CK14, smooth muscle actin, and p63 (238,239,241–243). The proliferation rate, as determined by Ki-67 (MIB1) staining, is typically low (less than 5 percent) (242).

Hybrid intercalated duct lesion (HIDL) is the least common IDL. HIDL may have a partially rounded, encapsulated, adenoma-like appearance admixed with irregular hyperplasia-like areas, giving the impression of transition from hyperplastic intercalated ducts to adenomatous areas. Alternatively, HIDL may include a completely encapsulated adenoma with separate discrete, hyperplastic foci immediately adjacent to the capsule. Entrapped irregular ductal structures are identified within the capsule of the adenoma.

Differential Diagnosis. In contrast to IDH, intercalated duct adenoma (IDA) is a discrete, rounded, partially to completely encapsulated nodule with a well-defined contour. The fibrous capsule varies in thickness and may contain entrapped, irregular-appearing ducts. IDAs are composed of intercalated ducts lined by a single layer of cuboidal to columnar cells with small round nuclei and eosinophilic to amphophilic cytoplasm; there is minimal intervening stroma. There is an absence of nuclear pleomorphism. Occasionally, acinic cells are interspersed among the ductular structures.

The differential diagnosis also includes basal cell adenoma (BCA), in particular, the tubular variant, which may coexist with IDL. The difference between the adenoma-like subset of IDL and tubular BCA is the larger number of myoepithelial cells identified in tubular BCA (242,243). In BCA, there are areas with obvious bilayering of the tubules, including outer myoepithelial cells as seen with routine hematoxylin and eosin (H&E) staining, a finding not seen in the

Figure 6-30
INTERCALATED DUCT HYPERPLASIA

A: An intraparotid circumscribed but unencapsulated cellular proliferation is composed of closely packed ducts that incorporate acinar cells.

B,C: At higher magnification there are closely packed ducts and incorporation of acinar cells in more central areas (B) as well as along the periphery of the proliferation (C). The ducts are lined by cuboidal cells with small round nuclei and eosinophilic cytoplasm. There is an absence of nuclear pleomorphism or increased mitotic activity. The acinar cells are characterized by intracytoplasmic basophilic (zymogen) granules. Myoepithelial cells are not readily identified.

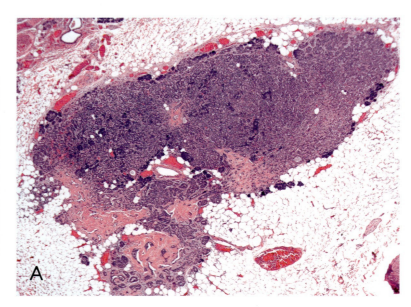

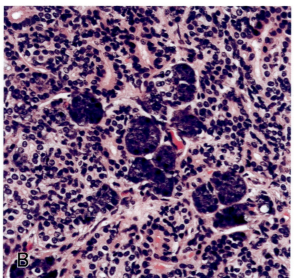

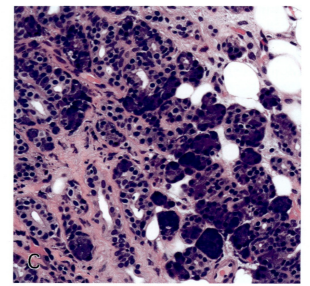

tubular variant of BCA and reflecting a smaller number of myoepithelial cells in IDL (242,243). Further, in BCA there is a significant stromal spindle cell component showing S-100 protein immunoreactivity (242), another feature not found typically in IDL.

The incorporation of acinic cells within the intercalated duct proliferation at the periphery of most IDLs may suggest infiltrative growth and a possible diagnosis of a low-grade carcinoma. Awareness of the existence of IDL, including the full array of pathologic findings, should allow for the correct diagnosis and preclude mistaking these lesions for a carcinoma.

Treatment and Prognosis. No specific treatment required. Given their usual small size, they are typically cured by excision without known untoward biology. More critical issues relative to treatment and prognosis relate to associated neoplasms, some of which include malignant salivary gland neoplasms.

REFERENCES

Embryology, Anatomy, and Histology

1. Moore KL, Persaud TV. The pharyngeal apparatus. In: Moore KL, Persaud TV. The developing human: clinically oriented embryology. Philadelphia: Saunders; 2003:202-240.
2. Peel RL, Seethala RR. Salivary gland pathology. In: Myers EN, Ferris RL. Salivary gland disorders. New York: Springer; 2007:33-105.
3. Hiatt JL, Sauk JJ. Embryology and anatomy of the salivary glands. In: Ellis GL, Auclair PL, Gnepp DR. Surgical pathology of the salivary glands. Philadelphia: W.B. Saunders; 1991:2-9
4. Seethala RR. Current state of neck dissection in the United States. Head Neck Pathol 2009;3:238-245.
5. Hollinshead WH. The head and neck. In: Hollinshead, WH, ed. Anatomy for surgeons. Philadelphia: Harper & Row; 1982;291-323.
6. Martinez-Madrigal F, Bosq J, Casiraghi O. Major salivary glands. In: Mills SE, ed. Histology for pathologists. Philadelphia: Lippincott Williams & Wilkins; 2007:445-470.
7. Ramsaroop L, Singh B, Allopi L, Moodley J, Partab P, Satyapal KS. The surgical anatomy of the parotid fascia. Surg Radiol Anat 2006;28:33-37.
8. Hollinshead WH. The jaws, palate and tongue. In: Hollinshead WH, ed. Anatomy for Surgeons. Philadelphia: Harper & Row; 1982:325-387.

Developmental Lesions

9. Batsakis JG. Heterotopic and accessory salivary tissues. Ann Otol Rhinol Laryngol 1986;95(Pt 1):434-435.
10. Tamiolakis D, Chimona TS, Georgiou G, et al. Accessory parotid gland carcinoma ex pleomorphic adenoma. Case study diagnosed by fine needle aspiration. Stomatologija 2009;11:37-40.
11. Frommer J. The human accessory parotid gland: its incidence, nature, and significance. Oral Surg Oral Med Oral Pathol 1977;43:671-676.
12. Toh H, Kodama J, Fukuda J, Rittman B, Mackenzie I. Incidence and histology of human accessory parotid glands. Anat Rec 1993;236:586-590.
13. Horii A, Honjo Y, Nose M, Ozaki M, Yoshida J. Accessory parotid gland tumor: a case report. Auris Nasus Larynx 1997;24:105-110.
14. Isogai R, Kawada A, Ueno K, Aragane Y, Tezuka T. Myoepithelioma possibly originating from the accessory parotid gland. Dermatology 2004;208:74-78.
15. Johnson FE, Spiro RH. Tumors arising in accessory parotid tissue. Am J Surg 1979;138:576-578.
16. Kawashima Y, Kobayashi D, Ishikawa N, Kishimoto S. A case of myoepithelioma arising in an accessory parotid gland. J Laryngol Otol 2002;116:474-476.
17. Khadaroo RG, Walton JM, Ramsay JA, Hicks MJ, Archibald SD. Mucoepidermoid carcinoma of the parotid gland: a rare presentation in a young child. J Pediatr Surg 1998;33:893-895.
18. Sakurai K, Urade M, Kishmoto H, Takahashi Y, Hozumi S, Yanagisawa T. Primary squamous cell carcinoma of accessory partoid gland duct epithelium: report of a case. Oral Surg Oral Med Oral Pathol Oral Radiol Endod 1998;85:447-451.
19. Tamiolakis D, Thomaidis V, Tsamis I, Jivannakis T, Cheva A, Papadopoulos N. Malignant mucoepidermoid tumor arising in the accessory parotid gland: a case report. Acta Medica (Hradec Kralove) 2003;46:79-83.
20. Rodino W, Shaha AR. Surgical management of accessory parotid tumors. J Surg Oncol 1993;54:153-156.
21. Lassaletta-Atienza L, Lopez-Rios F, Martin G, et al. Salivary gland heterotopia in the lower neck: a report of five cases. Int J Pediatr Otorhinolaryngol 1998;43:153-161.
22. Downs-Kelly E, Hoschar AP, Prayson RA. Salivary gland heterotopia in the rectum. Ann Diagn Pathol 2003;7:124-126.
23. Warnock GR, Jensen JL, Kratochvil FJ. Developmental diseases. In: Ellis GL, Auclair PL, Gnepp DR, eds. Surgical pathology of the salivary glands. Major problems in pathology, Vol 25. Philadelphia: WB Saunders; 1991:10-15.
24. Rinaldo A, Ferlito A, Devaney KO. Salivary gland choristoma of the middle ear. A review. ORL J Otorhinolaryngol Relat Spec 2004;66:141-147.
25. Abadir WF, Pease WS. Salivary gland choristoma of the middle ear. J Laryngol Otol 1978;92:247-252.
26. Amrhein P, Sittel C, Spaich C, et al. [Middle ear salivary gland choristoma related to branchio-oto-renal syndrome diagnosed by array-CGH]. HNO 2014;62:374-377. [German]
27. Joseph MP, Goodman ML, Pilch BZ, Bieber FR, Holmes LB, Reardon E. Heterotopic cervical salivary gland tissue in a family with probable branchio-otorenal syndrome. Head Neck Surg 1986;8:456-462.
28. Buckmiller LM, Brodie HA, Doyle KJ, Nemzek W. Choristoma of the middle ear: a component of a new syndrome? Otol Neurotol 2001;22:363-368.

29. Bouquot JE, Gnepp DR, Dardick I, Hietanen JH. Intraosseous salivary tissue: jawbone examples of choristomas, hamartomas, embryonic rests, and inflammatory entrapment: another histogenetic source for intraosseous adenocarcinoma. Oral Surg Oral Med Oral Pathol Oral Radiol Endod 2000;90:205-217.
30. Assaf AT, Solaty M, Zrnc TA, et al. Prevalence of Stafne's bone cavity—retrospective analysis of 14,005 panoramic views. In Vivo 2014;28:1159-1164.
31. Tatter SB, Edgar MA, Klibanski A, Swearingen B. Symptomatic salivary-rest cyst of the sella turcica. Acta Neurochir (Wien) 1995;135:150-153.
32. Ferlito A, Bertino G, Rinaldo A, Mannara GM, Devaney KO. A review of heterotopia and associated salivary gland neoplasms of the head and neck. J Laryngol Otol 1999;113:299-303.
33. Shinohara M, Harada T, Nakamura S, Oka M, Tashiro H. Heterotopic salivary gland tissue in lymph nodes of the cervical region. Int J Oral Maxillofac Surg 1992;21:166-171.
34. Peel RL, Seethala RR. Salivary gland pathology. In: Myers EN, Ferris RL, eds. Salivary gland disorders. E. New York: Springer: 2007:33-105.
35. Harada H, Morimatsu M, Kusukawa J, Kameyama T. A hamartoma-like mass on the palate? A possible discussion regarding the components of a pigmented naevus and hyperplastic salivary gland. J Laryngol Otol 1997;111:296-299.
36. Wushou A, Liu W, Bai XF, et al. Clinical analysis of 194 cases of head and neck hamartoma. Oral Surg Oral Med Oral Pathol Oral Radiol 2013;115:299-303.
37. Arafat A, Brannon RB, Ellis GL. Adenomatoid hyperplasia of mucous salivary glands. Oral Surg Oral Med Oral Pathol 1981;52:51-55.
38. Barrett AW, Speight PM. Adenomatoid hyperplasia of oral minor salivary glands. Oral Surg Oral Med Oral Pathol Oral Radiol Endod 1995;79:482-487.
39. Brannon RB, Houston GD, Meader CL. Adenomatoid hyperplasia of mucous salivary glands: a case involving the retromolar area. Oral Surg Oral Med Oral Pathol 1985;60:188-190.
40. Buchner A, Merrell PW, Carpenter WM, Leider AS. Adenomatoid hyperplasia of minor salivary glands. Oral Surg Oral Med Oral Pathol 1991;71:583-587.

Salivary Duct Cyst and Mucus Retention Cyst

41. Batsakis JG, Raymond AK. Sialocysts of the parotid glands. Ann Otol Rhinol Laryngol 1989;98:487-489.
42. Oliveira DT, Consolaro A, Freitas FJ. Histopathological spectrum of 112 cases of mucocele. Braz Dent J 1993;4:29-36.
43. Seifert G, Donath K. Classification of the pathohistology of diseases of the salivary glands—review of 2,600 cases in the Salivary Gland Register. Beitr Pathol 1976;159:1-32.
44. Eveson J, Nagao T. Diseases of the salivary glands. In: Barnes EL, ed. Surgical pathology of the head and neck. New York: Informa; 2009;1:474-648.
45. Granholm C, Olsson Bergland K, Walhjalt H, Magnusson B. Oral mucoceles; extravasation cysts and retention cysts. A study of 298 cases. Swed Dent J 2009;33:125-130.
46. Seifert G, Donath K, von Gumberz C. [Mucoceles of the minor salivary glands. Extravasation mucoceles (mucus granulomas) and retention mucoceles (mucus retention cysts) (author's transl).] HNO 1981;29:179-191. [German]
47. Peel RL, Seethala. Salivary gland pathology. In: Myers EN, Ferris RL, eds. Salivary gland disorders. New York: Springer: RR 2007:33-105.

Mucus Extravasation Phenomenon (Extravasation Mucocele) and Ranula

48. Chi AC, Lambert PR 3rd, Richardson MS, Neville BW. Oral mucoceles: a clinicopathologic review of 1,824 cases, including unusual variants. J Oral Maxillofac Surg 2011;69:1086-1093.
49. More CB, Bhavsar K, Varma S, Tailor M. Oral mucocele: A clinical and histopathological study. J Oral Maxillofac Pathol 2014;18(Suppl 1):S72-77.
50. Oliveira DT, Consolaro A, Freitas FJ. Histopathological spectrum of 112 cases of mucocele. Braz Dent J 1993;4:29-36.
51. Seifert G, Donath K, von Gumberz C. [Mucoceles of the minor salivary glands. Extravasation mucoceles (mucus granulomas) and retention mucoceles (mucus retention cysts) (author's transl).] HNO 1981;29:179-191. [German]
52. Patel MR, Deal AM, Shockley WW. Oral and plunging ranulas: What is the most effective treatment? Laryngoscope 2009;119:1501-1509.
53. Zhao YF, Jia Y, Chen XM, Zhang WF. Clinical review of 580 ranulas. Oral Surg Oral Med Oral Pathol Oral Radiol Endod 2004;98:281-287.
54. Harrison JD. Modern management and pathophysiology of ranula: literature review. Head Neck 2010;32:1310-1320.
55. Chen CJ, Guo P, Chen XY. Recurrent sublingual ranula or saliva leakage from the submandibular gland? Anatomical consideration of the ductal system of the sublingual gland. J Oral Maxillofac Surg 2015;73:675.e1-7.

Lymphoepithelial Cysts

56. Jensen JL. Lymphoepithelial cysts. In: Ellis GL, Auclair PL, Gnepp DR, eds. Surgical pathology of the salivary glands. Major problems in pathology, Vol 25. Philadelphia: WB Saunders; 1991:66-69.

57. Fujibayashi T, Itoh H. Lymphoepithelial (so-called branchial) cyst within the parotid gland. Report of a case and review of the literature. Int J Oral Surg 1981;10:283-292.
58. Piattelli A, Tete S. Lymphoepithelial cyst of the parotid gland. Acta Stomatol Belg 1995;92:137-138.
59. Peel RL, Seethala RR. Salivary gland pathology. In: Myers EN, Ferris RL, eds. Salivary gland disorders. New York, Springer; 2007:33-105.
60. Auclair P. Tumor-associated lymphoid proliferation in the parotid gland. A potential diagnostic pitfall. Oral Surg Oral Med Oral Pathol 1994;77:19-26.
61. Elliott JN, Oertel YC. Lymphoepithelial cysts of the salivary glands. Histologic and cytologic features. Am J Clin Pathol 1990;93:39-43.
62. Vicandi B, Jimenez-Heffernan JA, Lopez-Ferrer P, et al. HIV-1 (p24)-positive multinucleated giant cells in HIV-associated lymphoepithelial lesion of the parotid gland. A report of two cases. Acta Cytol 1999;43:247-251.
63. Chetty R. HIV-associated lymphoepithelial cysts and lesions: morphological and immunohistochemical study of the lymphoid cells. Histopathology 1998;33:222-229.
64. Mandel L, Kim D, Uy C. Parotid gland swelling in HIV diffuse infiltrative CD8 lymphocytosis syndrome. Oral Surg Oral Med Oral Pathol Oral Radiol Endod 1998;85:565-568.

Polycystic (Dysgenetic) Disease

65. Batsakis JG, Bruner JM, Luna MA. Polycystic (dysgenetic) disease of the parotid glands. Arch Otolaryngol Head Neck Surg 1988;114:1146-1148.
66. Dobson CM, Ellis HA. Polycystic disease of the parotid glands: case report of a rare entity and review of the literature. Histopathology 1987;11:953-961.
67. Ficarra G, Sapp JP, Christensen RE, Polyakov V. Dysgenetic polycystic disease of the parotid gland: report of case. J Oral Maxillofac Surg 1996;54:1246-1249.
68. Garcia S, Martini F, Caces F, Andrac L, De Micco C, Charpin C. [Polycystic disease of the salivary glands: report of an attack of the submaxillary glands.] Ann Pathol 1998;18:58-60. [French]
69. McFerran DJ, Ingrams DR, Gallimore AP, Grant HR. Polycystic disease of salivary glands. J Laryngol Otol 1995;109:165-167.
70. Ortiz-Hidalgo C, Cervantes J, de la Vega G. Unilateral polycystic (dysgenetic) disease of the parotid gland. South Med J 1995;88:1173-1175.
71. Seifert G, Thomsen S, Donath K. Bilateral dysgenetic polycystic parotid glands. Morphological analysis and differential diagnosis of a rare disease of the salivary glands. Virchows Arch A Pathol Anat Histol 1981;390:273-288.
72. Kumar KA, Mahadesh J, Setty S. Dysgenetic polycystic disease of the parotid gland: Report of a case and review of the literature. J Oral Maxillofac Pathol 2013;17:248-252.
73. Smyth AG, Ward-Booth RP, High AS. Polycystic disease of the parotid glands: two familial cases. Br J Oral Maxillofac Surg 1993;31:38-40.
74. Skalova A, Gnepp DR, Simpson RH, et al Clonal nature of sclerosing polycystic adenosis of salivary glands demonstrated by using the polymorphism of the human androgen receptor locus (HUMARA) as a marker. Am J Surg Pathol 2006;30:939-944.

Metaplasia and Hyperplasia

75. Skalova A, Michal M, Ryska A, et al. Oncocytic myoepithelioma and pleomorphic adenoma of the salivary glands. Virchows Arch 1999;434:537-546.
76. Brandwein MS, Huvos AG. Oncocytic tumors of major salivary glands. A study of 68 cases with follow-up of 44 patients. Am J Surg Pathol 1991;15:514-528.
77. Peel RL, Seethala RR. Salivary gland pathology. In: Myers EN, Ferris RL, eds. Salivary gland disorders. New York: Springer: 2007:33-105.
78. McHugh JB, Hoschar AP, Dvorakova M, Parwani AV, Barnes EL, Seethala RR. p63 immunohistochemistry differentiates salivary gland oncocytoma and oncocytic carcinoma from metastatic renal cell carcinoma. Head Neck Pathol 2007;1:123-131.
79. Mandel L, Carrao V. Bilateral parotid diffuse hyperplastic oncocytosis: case report. J Oral Maxillofac Surg 2005;63:560-562.
80. Chilla R. Sialadenosis of the salivary glands of the head. Studies on the physiology and pathophysiology of parotid secretion. Adv Otorhinolaryngol 1981;26:1-38.
81. Donath K. [Sialadenosis of the parotid gland. Ultrastructural, clinical and experimental findings in disturbances of secretion (author's transl).] Veroff Pathol 1976;(103):1-122. [German]
82. Mignogna MD, Fedele S, Lo Russo L. Anorexia/bulimia-related sialadenosis of palatal minor salivary glands. J Oral Pathol Med 2004;33:441-442.
83. Donath K, Seifert G. Ultrastructural studies of the parotid glands in sialadenosis. Virchows Arch A Pathol Anat Histol 1975;365:119-135.
84. Eversole L. Salivary gland pathology. In: Fu Y, Wenig BM, Abemayor E, Wenig BL, eds. Head and neck pathology: with clinical correlations. Philadelphia: Churchill-Livingstone; 2001:242-291.

Infections, Inflammatory and Reactive Diseases
Acute Sialadenitis and Viral Parotitis (Mumps)

85. McQuone SJ. Acute viral and bacterial infections of the salivary glands. Otolaryngol Clin North Am 1999;32:793-811.
86. Brook I. Acute bacterial suppurative parotitis: microbiology and management. J Craniofac Surg 2003;14:37-40.
87. Raad II, Sabbagh MF, Caranasos GJ. Acute bacterial sialadenitis: a study of 29 cases and review. Rev Infect Dis 1990;12:591-601.
88. Silvers AR, Som PM. Salivary glands. Radiol Clin North Am 1998;36:941-966, vi.
89. Peel RL, Seethala RR. Salivary gland pathology. In: Myers EN, Ferris RL, eds. Salivary gland disorders. New York: Springer; 2007:33-105.

Chronic Nonautoimmune Sialadenitis

90. Eversole L. Salivary gland pathology. In: Fu Y, Wenig BM, Abemayor E, Wenig BL, eds. Head and neck pathology: with clinical correlations. Philadelphia: Churchill-Livingstone; 2001:242-291.
91. Baurmash HD. Chronic recurrent parotitis: a closer look at its origin, diagnosis, and management. J Oral Maxillofac Surg 2004;62:1010-1018.
92. Seifert G. Aetiological and histological classification of sialadenitis. Pathologica 1997;89:7-17.
93. McQuone SJ. Acute viral and bacterial infections of the salivary glands. Otolaryngol Clin North Am 1999;32:793-811.
94. Lee IK, Liu JW. Tuberculous parotitis: case report and literature review. Ann Otol Rhinol Laryngol 2005;114:547-551.
95. Van der Walt JD, Leake J. Granulomatous sialadenitis of the major salivary glands. A clinicopathological study of 57 cases. Histopathology 1987;11:131-144.
96. Peel RL, Seethala RR. Salivary gland pathology. In: Myers EN, Ferris RL, eds. Salivary gland disorders. New York: Springer; 2007:33-105.
97. Arriaga MA, Myers EN. The surgical management of chronic parotitis. Laryngoscope 1990;100:1270-1275.
98. Grotz KA, Wustenberg P, Kohnen R, et al. Prophylaxis of radiogenic sialadenitis and mucositis by coumarin/troxerutine in patients with head and neck cancer—a prospective, randomized, placebo-controlled, double-blind study. Br J Oral Maxillofac Surg 2001;39:34-39.
99. Teymoortash A, Simolka N, Schrader C, Tiemann M, Werner JA. Lymphocyte subsets in irradiation-induced sialadenitis of the submandibular gland. Histopathology 2005;47:493-500.

Human Immunodeficiency Virus Salivary Gland Disease

100. Labouyrie E, Merlio JP, Beylot-Barry M, et al. Human immunodeficiency virus type 1 replication within cystic lymphoepithelial lesion of the salivary gland. Am J Clin Pathol 1993;100:41-46.
101. Marie B, Labouyrie E, Scheid P, et al. Human immunodeficiency virus type 1 in an unusual cystic lymphoepithelial lesion of the lung. Histopathology 1997;31:83-86.
102. Stewart JM, Krishnamurthy S. Fine-needle aspiration cytology of a case of HIV-associated anaplastic myeloma. Diagn Cytopathol 2002;27:218-222.
103. Nador RG, Chadburn A, Gundappa G, Cesarman E, Said JW, Knowles DM. Human immunodeficiency virus (HIV)-associated polymorphic lymphoproliferative disorders. Am J Surg Pathol 2003;27:293-302.
104. Mourad WF, Young R, Kabarriti R, et al. 25-year follow-up of HIV-positive patients with benign lymphoepithelial cysts of the parotid glands: a retrospective review. Anticancer Res 2013;33:4927-4932.
105. Itescu, S, Brancato LJ, Buxbaum J, et al. A diffuse infiltrative CD8 lymphocytosis syndrome in human immunodeficiency virus (HIV) infection: a host immune response associated with HLA-DR5. Ann Intern Med 1990;112:3-10.
106. Ulirsch RC, Jaffe ES. Sjogren's syndrome-like illness associated with the acquired immunodeficiency syndrome-related complex. Hum Pathol 1987;18:1063-1068.
107. Atkinson JC, Schiodt M, Robataille S, Greenspan D, Greenspan JS, Fox PC. Salivary autoantibodies in HIV-associated salivary gland disease. J Oral Pathol Med 1993;22:203-206.
108. Itescu S, Winchester R. Diffuse infiltrative lymphocytosis syndrome: a disorder occurring in human immunodeficiency virus-1 infection that may present as a sicca syndrome. Rheum Dis Clin North Am 1992;18:683-697.
109. Ghrenassia E, Martis N, Boyer J, Burel-Vandenbos F, Mekinian A, Coppo P. The diffuse infiltrative lymphocytosis syndrome (DILS). A comprehensive review. J Autoimmun 2015;59:19-25.
110. Bernier JL, Bhaskar SN. Lymphoepithelial lesions of salivary glands; histogenesis and classification based on 186 cases. Cancer 1958;11:1156-1179.
111. Ihrler S, Zietz C, Riederer A, Diebold J, Lohrs U. HIV-related parotid lymphoepithelial cysts. Immunohistochemistry and 3-D reconstruction of surgical and autopsy material with special reference to formal pathogenesis. Virchows Arch 1996;429:139-147.

112. Casiano RR, Cooper JD, Gould E, Ruiz P, Uttamchandani R. Value of needle biopsy in directing management of parotid lesions in HIV-positive patients. Head Neck 1991;13:411-414.
113. Chhieng DC, Argosino R, McKenna BJ, Cangiarella JF, Cohen JM. Utility of fine-needle aspiration in the diagnosis of salivary gland lesions in patients infected with human immunodeficiency virus. Diagn Cytopathol 1999;21:260-264.
114. Elliott JN, Oertel YC. Lymphoepithelial cysts of the salivary glands. Histologic and cytologic features. Am J Clin Pathol 1990;93:39-43.
115. Finfer MD, Gallo L, Perchick A, Schinella RA, Burstein DE. Fine needle aspiration biopsy of cystic benign lymphoepithelial lesion of the parotid gland in patients at risk for the acquired immune deficiency syndrome. Acta Cytol 1990;34:821-826.
116. Vicandi B, Jimenez-Heffernan JA, Lopez-Ferrer P, et al. HIV-1 (p24)-positive multinucleated giant cells in HIV-associated lymphoepithelial lesion of the parotid gland. A report of two cases. Acta Cytol 1999;43:247-251.
117. Chetty R. HIV-associated lymphoepithelial cysts and lesions: morphological and immunohistochemical study of the lymphoid cells. Histopathology 1998;33:222-229.
118. Mandel L, Kim D, Uy C. Parotid gland swelling in HIV diffuse infiltrative CD8 lymphocytosis syndrome. Oral Surg Oral Med Oral Pathol Oral Radiol Endod 1998;85:565-568.
119. Smith PR, Cavenagh JD, Milne T, et al. Benign monoclonal expansion of CD8+ lymphocytes in HIV infection. J Clin Pathol 2000;53:177-181.
120. Bruner JM, Cleary KR, Smith FB, Batsakis JG. Immunocytochemical identification of HIV (p24) antigen in parotid lymphoid lesions. J Laryngol Otol 1989;103:1063-1066.
121. Uccini S, Riva E, Antonelli G, et al. The benign cystic lymphoepithelial lesion of the parotid gland is a viral reservoir in HIV type 1-infected patients. AIDS Res Hum Retroviruses 1999;15:1339-1344.
122. Said JW, Pinkus JL, Yamashita J, et al. The role of follicular and interdigitating dendritic cells in HIV-related lymphoid hyperplasia: localization of fascin. Mod Pathol 1997;10:421-427.
123. Orenstein JM. The Warthin-Finkeldey-type giant cell in HIV infection, what is it? Ultrastruct Pathol 1998;22:293-303.
124. Frankel SS, Wenig BM, Burke AP, et al. Replication of HIV-1 in dendtritic cell-derived syncytia at the mucosal surface of the adenoid. Science 1996;272:115-117.
125. Beitler JJ, Smith RV, Brook A, et al. Benign parotid hypertrophy on +HIV patients: limited late failures after external radiation. Int J Radiat Oncol Biol Phys 1999;45:451-455.
126. Beitler JJ, Smith RV, Silver CE, et al. Cosmetic control of parotid gland hypertrophy using radiation therapy. AIDS Patient Care 1995;9:271-275.
127. Kooper DP, Leemans CR, Hulshof MC, Claessen FA, Snow GB. Management of benign lymphoepithelial lesions of the parotid gland in human immunodeficiency virus-positive patients. Eur Arch Otorhinolaryngol 1998;255:427-429.
128. Del Bono V, Pretolesi F, Pontali E, et al. Possible malignant transformation of benign lymphoepithelial parotid lesions in human immunodeficiency virus-infected patients: report of three cases. Clin Infect Dis 2000;30:947-949.
129. Ioachim HL, Antonescu C, Giancotti F, Dorsett B. EBV-associated primary lymphomas in salivary glands of HIV-infected patients. Pathol Res Pract 1998;194:87-95.
130. Klassen MK, Lewin-Smith M, Frankel SS, Nelson AM. Pathology of human immunodeficiency virus infection: noninfectious conditions. Ann Diagn Pathol 1997;1:57-64.
131. Goldman, N, Shuja S, Makary R, Griffin RL. Mucoepidermoid carcinoma presenting as a large cyst of the parotid gland in HIV disease. Ear Nose Throat J 2013;92:310-311.

Lymphoepithelial Sialadenitis (Benign Lymphoepithelial Lesion and Sjögren Syndrome)

132. Godwin JT. Benign lymphoepithelial lesion of the parotid gland adenolymphoma, chronic inflammation, lymphoepithelioma, lymphocytic tumor, Mikulicz disease. Cancer 1952;5:1089-1103.
133. Harris NL. Lymphoid proliferations of the salivary glands. Am J Clin Pathol 1999;111(Suppl 1):S94-103.
134. Batsakis JG. Lymphoepithelial lesion and Sjögren's syndrome. Ann Otol Rhinol Laryngol 1987;96(Pt 1):354-355.
135. Daniels TE. Benign lymphoepithelial lesion and Sjögren's syndrome. In: Ellis GL, Auclair PL, Gnepp DR. Surgical pathology of the salivary glands. Philadelphia: WB Saunders; 1991:83-106.
136. Shiboski SC, Shiboski CH, Criswell L, et al. American College of Rheumatology classification criteria for Sjögren's syndrome: a data-driven, expert consensus approach in the Sjogren's International Collaborative Clinical Alliance cohort. Arthritis Care Res (Hoboken) 2012;64:475-487.
137. Aggarwal R, Anaya JM, Koelsch KA, Kurien BT, Scofield RH. Association between secondary and primary Sjögren's syndrome in a large collection of lupus families. Autoimmune Dis 2015;2015:298506.

138. Maslinska M, Przygodzka M, Kwiatkowska B, Sikorska-Siudek K. Sjögren's syndrome: still not fully understood disease. Rheumatol Int 2015;35:233-241.
139. Saad Magalhaes C, de Souza Medeiros PB, Oliveira-Sato J, Custodio-Domingues MA. Clinical presentation and salivary gland histopathology of paediatric primary Sjögren's syndrome. Clin Exp Rheumatol 2011;29:589-593.
140. Daniels TE, Fox PC. Salivary and oral components of Sjögren's syndrome. Rheum Dis Clin North Am 1992;18:571-589.
141. Fox RI, Howell FV, Bone RC, Michelson P. Primary Sjögren syndrome: clinical and immunopathologic features. Semin Arthritis Rheum 1984;14:77-105.
142. Hietaharju A, Yli-Kerttula U, Hakkinen V, Frey H. Nervous system manifestations in Sjögren's syndrome. Acta Neurol Scand 1990;81:144-152.
143. Moutsopoulos HM. Sjögren's syndrome: autoimmune epithelitis. Clin Immunol Immunopathol 1994;72:162-165.
144. Pokorny G, Karacsony G, Lonovics J, Hudak J, Nemeth J, Varro V. Types of atrophic gastritis in patients with primary Sjögren's syndrome. Ann Rheum Dis 1991;50:97-100.
145. Provost TT, Vasily D, Alexander E. Sjögren's syndrome. Cutaneous, immunologic, and nervous system manifestations. Neurol Clin 1987;5:405-426.
146. Sheikh SH, Shaw-Stiffel TA. The gastrointestinal manifestations of Sjögren's syndrome. Am J Gastroenterol 1995;90:9-14.
147. Fox RI, Tornwall J, Maruyama T, Stern M. Evolving concepts of diagnosis, pathogenesis, and therapy of Sjögren's syndrome. Curr Opin Rheumatol 1998;10:446-456.
148. Iwasaki K, Okawa-Takatsuji M, Aotsuka S, Ono T. Detection of anti-SS-A/Ro and anti-SS-B/La antibodies of IgA and IgG isotypes in saliva and sera of patients with Sjögren's syndrome. Nihon Rinsho Meneki Gakkai Kaishi 2003;26:346-354.
149. Smeenk RJ. Ro/SS-A and La/SS-B: autoantigens in Sjögren's syndrome? Clin Rheumatol 1995;14(Suppl 1):11-16.
150. Toker E, Yavuz S, Direskeneli H. Anti-Ro/SSA and anti-La/SSB autoantibodies in the tear fluid of patients with Sjögren's syndrome. Br J Ophthalmol 2004;88:384-387.
151. Font J, Ramos-Casals M, Cervera R, et al. Antineutrophil cytoplasmic antibodies in primary Sjögren's syndrome: prevalence and clinical significance. Br J Rheumatol 1998;37:1287-1291.
152. Baldini C, Giusti L, Ciregia F, et al. Proteomic analysis of saliva: a unique tool to distinguish primary Sjögren's syndrome from secondary Sjögren's syndrome and other sicca syndromes. Arthritis Res Ther 2011;13:R194.
153. Rasmussen A, Ice JA, Li H, et al. Comparison of the American-European Consensus Group Sjögren's syndrome classification criteria to newly proposed American College of Rheumatology criteria in a large, carefully characterised sicca cohort. Ann Rheum Dis 2014;73:31-38.
154. Luciano N, Valentini V, Calabro A, et al. One year in review 2015: Sjögren's syndrome. Clin Exp Rheumatol 2015;33:259-271.
155. Ihrler S, Zietz C, Sendelhofert A, Riederer A, Lohrs U. Lymphoepithelial duct lesions in Sjogren-type sialadenitis. Virchows Arch 1999;434:315-323.
156. Kjorell U, Ostberg Y. Distribution of intermediate filaments and actin microfilaments in parotid autoimmune sialoadenitis of Sjögren syndrome. Histopathology 1984;8:991-1011.
157. Bahler DW, Swerdlow SH. Clonal salivary gland infiltrates associated with myoepithelial sialadenitis (Sjögren's syndrome) begin as nonmalignant antigen-selected expansions. Blood 1998;91:1864-1872.
158. Daniels TE, Cox D, Shiboski CH, et al. Associations between salivary gland histopathologic diagnoses and phenotypic features of Sjögren's syndrome among 1,726 registry participants. Arthritis Rheum 2011;63:2021-2030.
159. Baer AN, Gourin CG, Westra WH, et al. Rare diagnosis of IgG4-related systemic disease by lip biopsy in an international Sjögren syndrome registry. Oral Surg Oral Med Oral Pathol Oral Radiol 2013;115:e34-39.
160. Hyjek E, Smith WJ, Isaacson PG. Primary B-cell lymphoma of salivary glands and its relationship to myoepithelial sialadenitis. Hum Pathol 1988;19:766-776.
161. Abbondanzo SL. Extranodal marginal-zone B-cell lymphoma of the salivary gland. Ann Diagn Pathol 2001;5:246-254.
162. Streubel B, Simonitsch-Klupp I, Mullauer L, et al. Variable frequencies of MALT lymphoma-associated genetic aberrations in MALT lymphomas of different sites. Leukemia 2004;18:1722-1726.
163. Seror R, Bowman SJ, Brito-Zeron P, et al. EULAR Sjögren's syndrome disease activity index (ESSDAI): a user guide. RMD Open 2015;1:e000022.
164. DiGiuseppe JA, Corio RL, Westra WH. Lymphoid infiltrates of the salivary glands: pathology, biology and clinical significance. Curr Opin Oncol 1996;8:232-237.
165. Fox RI. Sjögren's syndrome. Lancet 2005;366:321-331.

166. Sato K, Kawana M, Sato Y, Takahashi S. Malignant lymphoma in the head and neck associated with benign lymphoepithelial lesion of the parotid gland. Auris Nasus Larynx 2002;29:209-214.
167. Quartuccio L, Baldini C, Bartoloni E, et al. Anti-SSA/SSB-negative Sjögren's syndrome shows a lower prevalence of lymphoproliferative manifestations, and a lower risk of lymphoma evolution. Autoimmun Rev 2015;14:1019-1022.
168. Batsakis JG, Bernacki EG, Rice DH, Stebler ME. Malignancy and the benign lymphoepithelial lesion. Laryngoscope 1975;85:389-399.
169. Brauneis J, Laskawi R, Schroder M, Eilts M. [Squamous cell carcinoma in the area of the parotid gland. Metastasis or primary tumor?] HNO 1990;38(8): 292-294. [German]
170. Nagao K, Matsuzaki O, Saiga H, et al. A histopathologic study of benign and malignant lymphoepithelial lesions of the parotid gland. Cancer 1983;52:1044-1052.
171. Wu LY, Cheng J, Lu Y, Zhou ZY, Saku T. [Epstein-Barr virus infection in benign lymphoepithelial lesions with malignant transformation of salivary glands.] Zhonghua Kou Qiang Yi Xue Za Zhi 2004;39:291-293. [Chinese]

IgG4-Related and Chronic Sclerosing Sialadenitis

172. Geyer JT, Ferry JA, Harris NL, et al. Chronic sclerosing sialadenitis (Küttner tumor) is an IgG4-associated disease. Am J Surg Pathol 2010;34:202-210.
173. Kamisawa T, Nakajima H, Egawa N, Funata N, Tsuruta K, Okamoto A. IgG4-related sclerosing disease incorporating sclerosing pancreatitis, cholangitis, sialadenitis and retroperitoneal fibrosis with lymphadenopathy. Pancreatology 2006;6:132-137.
174. Kitagawa S, Zen Y, Harada K, et al. Abundant IgG4-positive plasma cell infiltration characterizes chronic sclerosing sialadenitis (Küttner's tumor). Am J Surg Pathol 2005;29:783-791.
175. Laco J, Ryska A, Celakovsky P, Dolezalova H, Mottl R, Tucek L. Chronic sclerosing sialadenitis as one of the immunoglobulin G4-related diseases: a clinicopathological study of six cases from Central Europe. Histopathology 2011;58:1157-1163.
176. Cheuk W, Chan JK. IgG4-related sclerosing disease: a critical appraisal of an evolving clinicopathologic entity. Adv Anat Pathol 2010;17:303-332.
177. Della-Torre E, Lanzillotta M, Doglioni C. Immunology of IgG4-related disease. Clin Exp Immunol 2015;181:191-206.
178. Strehl JD, Hartmann A, Agaimy A. Numerous IgG4-positive plasma cells are ubiquitous in diverse localised non-specific chronic inflammatory conditions and need to be distinguished from IgG4-related systemic disorders. J Clin Pathol 2011;64:237-243.
179. Cheuk W, Chan JK. Kuttner tumor of the submandibular gland: fine-needle aspiration cytologic findings of seven cases. Am J Clin Pathol 2002;117:103-108.
180. Leon ME, Santosh N, Agarwal A, Teknos TN, Ozer E, Iwenofu OH. Diagnostic challenges in the fine needle aspiration biopsy of chronic sclerosing sialadenitis (Küttner's tumor) in the Context of head and neck malignancy: a series of 4 cases. Head Neck Pathol 2016;10:389-393.
181. Hayashi Y, Moriyama M, Maehara T, et al. A case of mantle cell lymphoma presenting as IgG4-related dacryoadenitis and sialoadenitis, so-called Mikulicz's disease. World J Surg Oncol 2015;13:225.
182. Ohta M, Moriyama M, Goto Y, et al. A case of marginal zone B cell lymphoma mimicking IgG4-related dacryoadenitis and sialoadenitis. World J Surg Oncol 2015;13:67.
183. Gill J, Angelo N, Yeong ML, McIvor N. Salivary duct carcinoma arising in IgG4-related autoimmune disease of the parotid gland. Hum Pathol 2009;40:881-886.
184. Shimo T, Yao M, Takebe Y, et al. A case of adenoid cystic carcinoma associated with IgG4-related disease. Int J Surg Case Rep 2015;10:12-16.
185. Tian W, Yakirevich E, Matoso A, Gnepp DR. IgG4(+) plasma cells in sclerosing variant of mucoepidermoid carcinoma. Am J Surg Pathol 2012;36:973-979.

Sarcoidosis

186. James DG, Sharma OP. Parotid gland sarcoidosis. Sarcoidosis Vasc Diffuse Lung Dis 2000;17:27-32.
187. Darlington P, Tallstedt L, Padyukov L, et al. HLA-DRB1* alleles and symptoms associated with Heerfordt's syndrome in sarcoidosis. Eur Respir J 2011;38:1151-1157.
188. Mandel L, Surattanont F. Bilateral parotid swelling: a review. Oral Surg Oral Med Oral Pathol Oral Radiol Endod 2002;93:221-237.
189. Ramos-Casals M, Brito-Zeron P, Garcia-Carrasco M, Font J. Sarcoidosis or Sjögren syndrome? Clues to defining mimicry or coexistence in 59 cases. Medicine (Baltimore) 2004;83:85-95.
190. Moller DR. Potential etiologic agents in sarcoidosis. Proc Am Thorac Soc 2007;4:465-468.
191. Saidha S, Sotirchos ES, Eckstein C. Etiology of sarcoidosis: does infection play a role? Yale J Biol Med 2012;85:133-141.

192. Aggarwal AP, Jayaram G, Mandal AK. Sarcoidosis diagnosed on fine-needle aspiration cytology of salivary glands: a report of three cases. Diagn Cytopathol 1989;5:289-292.
193. Frable MA, Frable WJ. Fine-needle aspiration biopsy: efficacy in the diagnosis of head and neck sarcoidosis. Laryngoscope 1984;94:1281-1283.
194. Fauci AS, Haynes BF, Katz P, Wolff SM. Wegener's granulomatosis: prospective clinical and therapeutic experience with 85 patients for 21 years. Ann Intern Med 1983;98:76-85.
195. van der Walt JD, Leake J. Granulomatous sialadenitis of the major salivary glands. A clinicopathological study of 57 cases. Histopathology 1987;11:131-144.
196. Judson MA. Advances in the diagnosis and treatment of sarcoidosis. F1000Prime Rep 2014;6:89.
197. Lazar CA, Culver DA. Treatment of sarcoidosis. Semin Respir Crit Care Med 2010;31:501-518.

Tumor-Like Lesions

198. Abrams AM, Melrose RJ, Howell FV. Necrotizing sialometaplasia. A disease simulating malignancy. Cancer 1973;32:130-135.
199. Brannon RB, Fowler CB, Hartman KS. Necrotizing sialometaplasia. A clinicopathologic study of sixty-nine cases and review of the literature. Oral Surg Oral Med Oral Pathol 1991;72:317-325.
200. Fowler CB, Brannon RB. Subacute necrotizing sialadenitis: report of 7 cases and a review of the literature. Oral Surg Oral Med Oral Pathol Oral Radiol Endod 2000;89:600-609.
201. Imbery TA, Edwards PA. Necrotizing sialometaplasia: literature review and case reports. J Am Dent Assoc 1996;127:1087-1092.
202. Peel R. Diseases of the salivary gland. In: Barnes L, ed. Surgical pathology of the head and neck. New York: Marcel-Dekker; 2000??1: 634-690.
203. Maisel RH, Johnston WH, Anderson HA, Cantrell RW. Necrotizing sialometaplasia involving the nasal cavity. Laryngoscope 1977;87:429-434.
204. Romagosa V, Bella MR, Truchero C, Moya J. Necrotizing sialometaplasia (adenometaplasia) of the trachea. Histopathology 1992;21:280-282.
205. Wenig BM. Necrotizing sialometaplasia of the larynx. A report of two cases and a review of the literature. Am J Clin Pathol 1995;103:609-613.
206. Zschoch H. [Mucus gland infarct with squamous epithelial metaplasia in the lung. A rare site of so-called necrotizing sialometaplasia.] Pathologe 1992;13:45-48. [German]
207. Keogh PV, O'Regan E, Toner M, Flint S. Necrotizing sialometaplasia: an unusual bilateral presentation associated with antecedent anaesthesia and lack of response to intralesional steroids. Case report and review of the literature. Br Dent J 2004;196:79-81.
208. Lamey PJ, Lewis MA, Crawford DJ, MacDonald DG. Necrotising sialometaplasia presenting as greater palatine nerve anaesthesia. Int J Oral Maxillofac Surg 1989;18:70-72.
209. Aydin O, Yilmaz T, Ozer F, Sarac S, Sokmensuer C. Necrotizing sialometaplasia of parotid gland: a possible vasculitic cause. Int J Pediatr Otorhinolaryngol 2002;64:171-174.
210. Rye LA, Calhoun NR, Redman RS. Necrotizing sialometaplasia in a patient with Buerger's disease and Raynaud's phenomenon. Oral Surg Oral Med Oral Pathol 1980;49:233-236.
211. Williams RF. Necrotizing sialometaplasia after bronchoscopy. J Oral Surg 1979;37:816-818.
212. Aframian D, Milhem II, Kirsch G, Markitziu A. Necrotizing sialometaplasia after Silastic ring vertical gastroplasty: case report and review of literature. Obes Surg 1995;5:179-182.
213. Schoning H, Emshoff R, Kreczy A. Necrotizing sialometaplasia in two patients with bulimia and chronic vomiting. Int J Oral Maxillofac Surg 1998;27:463-465.
214. Eversole L. Salivary gland pathology. In: Fu Y, Wenig BM, Abemayor E, Wenig BL, eds. Head and neck pathology: with clinical correlations. Philadelphia: Churchill-Livingstone; 2001:242-291.
215. Mohammed BS, Liu Z, Tang W, Eltorky MA. BCL-2, Ki67 and P53 expression in oral necrotizing sialometaplasia and squamous cell carcinoma. Mod Path 2006;19:105A.
216. Castro WH, Drummond SN, Gomez RS. Subacute necrotizing sialadenitis in the buccal mucosa. J Oral Maxillofac Surg 2002;60:1494-1496.
217. Lombardi T, Samson J, Kuffer R. Subacute necrotizing sialadenitis: a form of necrotizing sialometaplasia? Arch Otolaryngol Head Neck Surg 2003;129:972-975.
218. van der Wal JE, Kraaijenhagen HA, van der Waal I. Subacute necrotising sialadenitis: a new entity? Br J Oral Maxillofac Surg 1995;33:302-303.
219. Werning JT, Waterhouse JP, Mooney JW. Subacute necrotizing sialadenitis. Oral Surg Oral Med Oral Pathol 1990;70:756-759.

Extranodal Sinus Histiocytosis with Massive Lymphadenopathy (Rosai-Dorfman Disease)

220. Rosai J, Dorfman RF. Sinus histiocytosis with massive lymphadenopathy. A newly recognized benign clinicopathological entity. Arch Pathol 1969;87:63-70.
221. Rosai J, Dorfman RF. Sinus histiocytosis with massive lymphadenopathy: a pseudolymphomatous benign disorder. Analysis of 34 cases. Cancer 1972;30:1174-1188.

222. Foucar E, Rosai J, Dorfman R. Sinus histiocytosis with massive lymphadenopathy (Rosai-Dorfman disease): review of the entity. Semin Diagn Pathol 1990;7:19-73.
223. Goodnight JW, Wang MB, Sercarz JA, Fu YS. Extranodal Rosai-Dorfman disease of the head and neck. Laryngoscope 1996;106(Pt 1):253-256.
224. Wenig BM, Abbondanzo SL, Childers EL, Kapadia SB, Heffner DR. Extranodal sinus histiocytosis with massive lymphadenopathy (Rosai-Dorfman disease) of the head and neck. Hum Pathol 1993;24:483-492.
225. Juskevicius R, Finley JL. Rosai-Dorfman disease of the parotid gland: cytologic and histopathologic findings with immunohistochemical correlation. Arch Pathol Lab Med 2001;125:1348-1350.
226. Foucar K, Foucar E. The mononuclear phagocyte and immunoregulatory effector (M-PIRE) system: evolving concepts. Semin Diagn Pathol 1990;7:4-18.
227. Shanmugam V, Margolskee E, Kluk M, Giorgadze T, Orazi A. Rosai-Dorfman Disease Harboring an Activating KRAS K117N Missense Mutation. Head Neck Pathol 2016;10:394-399.
228. Delacretaz F, Meuge-Moraw C, Anwar D, Borisch B, Chave JP. Sinus histiocytosis with massive lymphadenopathy (Rosai Dorfman disease) in an HIV-positive patient. Virchows Arch A Pathol Anat Histopathol 1991;419:251-254.
229. Drosos AA, Georgiadis AN, Metafratzi ZM, Voulgari PV, Efremidis SC, Bai M. Sinus histiocytosis with massive lymphadenopathy (Rosai-Dorfman disease) in a patient with primary Sjögren's syndrome. Scand J Rheumatol 2004;33:119-122.
230. Liu L, Perry AM, Cao W, et al. Relationship between Rosai-Dorfman disease and IgG4-related disease: study of 32 cases. Am J Clin Pathol 2013;140:395-402.
231. Menon MP, Evbuomwan MO, Rosai J, Jaffe ES, Pittaluga S. A subset of Rosai-Dorfman disease cases show increased IgG4-positive plasma cells: another red herring or a true association with IgG4-related disease? Histopathology 2014;64:455-459.
232. Zhang X, Hyjek E, Vardiman J. A subset of Rosai-Dorfman disease exhibits features of IgG4-related disease. Am J Clin Pathol 2013;139:622-632.
233. Harley EH. Sinus histiocytosis with massive lymphadenopathy (Rosai-Dorfman disease) in a patient with elevated Epstein-Barr virus titers. J Natl Med Assoc 1991;83:922-924.
234. Luppi M, Barozzi P, Garber R, et al. Expression of human herpesvirus-6 antigens in benign and malignant lymphoproliferative diseases. Am J Pathol 1998;153:815-823.
235. Ortonne N, Fillet AM, Kosuge H, Bagot M, Frances C, Wechsler J. Cutaneous Destombes-Rosai-Dorfman disease: absence of detection of HHV-6 and HHV-8 in skin. J Cutan Pathol 2002;29:113-118.
236. Tsang WY, Yip TT, Chan JK. The Rosai-Dorfman disease histiocytes are not infected by Epstein-Barr virus. Histopathology 1994;25:88-90.
237. Krzemieniecki K, Pawlicki M, Marganska K, Parczewska J. The Rosai-Dorfman syndrome in a 17-year-old woman with transformation into high-grade lymphoma. A rare disease presentation. Ann Oncol 1996;7:977.
238. Weinreb I, Seethala RR, Hunt JL, Chetty R, Dardick I, Perez-Ordoñez B. Intercalated duct lesions of salivary gland: a morphologic spectrum from hyperplasia to adenoma. Am J Surg Pathol 2009;33:1322-1329.
239. Luna MA. Salivary gland hyperplasia. Adv Anat Pathol 2002;9:251-255.
240. Chetty R. Intercalated duct hyperplasia: possible relationship to epithelial-myoepithelial carcinoma and hybrid tumours of salivary gland. Histopathology 2000;37:260-263.
241. Di Palma S. Epithelial-myoepithelial carcinoma with co-existing multifocal intercalated duct hyperplasia of the parotid gland. Histopathology 1994;25:494-496.
242. Mok Y, Pang YH, Teh M, Petersson F. Hybrid intercalated duct lesion of the parotid: diagnostic challenges of a recently described entity with fine-needle aspiration findings. Head Neck Pathol 2016;10:269-274.
243. Montalli VA, Martinez E, Tincani A, et al. Tubular variant of basal cell adenoma shares immunophenotypical features with normal intercalated ducts and is closely related to intercalated duct lesions of salivary gland. Histopathology 2014;64:880-889.

7 EAR AND TEMPORAL BONE

By Dr. Bruce M. Wenig

EMBRYOLOGY, ANATOMY, AND HISTOLOGY

The ear is the sense organ for hearing and balance. The ear has three distinct regions or compartments: the external ear, the middle ear and temporal bone, and the inner ear (fig. 7-1).

Embryology

External Ear. The external ear develops from the first branchial groove. The external auricle (pinna) forms from the fusion of the auricular hillocks or tubercles, a group of mesenchymal tissue swellings from the first and second branchial arches, that lie around the external portion of the first branchial groove (1). The external auditory canal is considered a normal remnant of the first branchial groove. The tympanic membrane forms from the first and second branchial pouches and the first branchial groove (1). The ectoderm of the first branchial groove gives rise to the epithelium on the external side, the endoderm from the first branchial pouch gives rise to the epithelium on the internal side, and the mesoderm of the first and second branchial pouches gives rise to the connective tissue lying between the external and internal epithelia (1).

Middle Ear. The middle ear space develops from an invagination of the first branchial pouch (pharyngotympanic tube) from the primitive pharynx. The eustachian tube and tympanic cavity develop from the endoderm of the first branchial pouch; the malleus and incus develop from the mesoderm of the first branchial arch (Meckel cartilage), and the incus develops from the mesoderm of the second branchial arch (Reichert cartilage) (1).

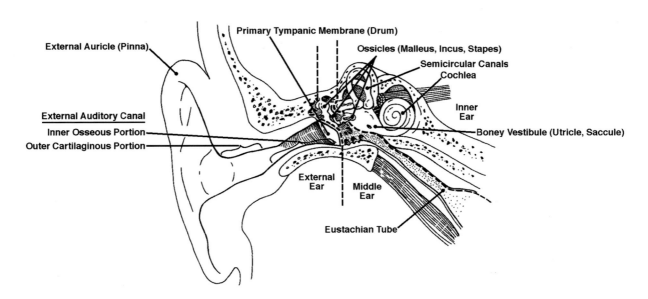

Figure 7-1

ANATOMY

The external (auricle, external auditory canal), middle (eustachian tube, mesotympanum, epitympanum, mastoid), and inner (membranous, osseous labyrinth) ear are the three main divisions and are separated by the dotted lines in this drawing.

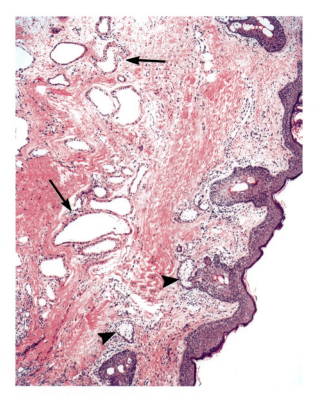

Figure 7-2

EXTERNAL EAR

The auricle is a cutaneous structure histologically composed of keratinizing stratified squamous epithelium (right) with associated cutaneous adnexal structures that include hair follicles (not shown), sebaceous glands (arrowheads), and eccrine sweat glands (arrows).

Inner Ear. The first division of the ear to develop is the inner ear, which appears toward the end of the first month of gestation (1,2). The membranous labyrinth, including the utricle, saccule, three semicircular ducts, cochlear duct, and endolymphatic sac, arises from the placodal thickening of the ectoderm to become a closed otic vesicle (otocyst). The otic vesicle forms from the invagination of the surface ectoderm, located on either side of the neural plate, into the mesenchyme. This invagination eventually loses its connection with the surface ectoderm.

The membranous labyrinth, which is essentially tubular and saccular in turn, is filled with fluid, the endolymph or endolymphatic fluid. The early development of the membranous labyrinth takes place in mesenchyme and subsequently in the cartilage destined to form the petrous portion of the temporal bone. The membranous labyrinth lies in cavities excavated from this mesenchyme or cartilage.

The space lying between the inner surface of the bony wall and the outer surface of the membranous labyrinth is the perilymphatic space. The perilymphatic space develops around the membranous labyrinth by the fusion of mesenchymal spaces to form larger ones surrounding the membranous portion. The bony labyrinth, including the vestibule, semicircular canals, and cochlea, arises from the mesenchyme around the otic vesicle (1–3).

Anatomy

External Ear. The anatomy of the external ear is seen in figure 7-1. The outer portion of the external ear includes the auricle, or pinna, leading into the external auditory canal. The medial limit is the external aspect of the tympanic membrane.

The external auditory canal, or meatus, extends from the concha to its medial limit, which is the external aspect of the tympanic membrane. The lateral portion of its wall consists of cartilage and connective tissue; the medial portion is bone. The cartilaginous part of the external auditory canal constitutes slightly less than half its total length. Inconstant fissures, referred to as the fissures of Santorini, occur in the cartilage; these fissures may transmit infection from the canal to the parotid gland and superficial mastoid regions, or vice versa.

The bony part of the canal is formed by both the tympanic part and the petrous part of the temporal bone. The anterior, inferior, and lower posterior parts of the bony wall are formed by the C-shaped part of the temporal bone, developed from the annulus tympanicus of the fetus. The annulus is incomplete in the posterosuperior part of the wall. In adults, this part of the wall is formed by the squamous and petrous parts of the temporal bone. The anterior and inferior walls of the cartilaginous canal are closely related to the parotid gland. The anterior wall of the bony canal is closely related to the mandibular condyle, the posterior wall to the mastoid air cells, and the medial portion of the superior wall to the epitympanic recess.

The tympanic membrane (ear drum) is situated obliquely at the end of the external auditory canal, sloping medially both from above downward and from behind forward. The tympanic membrane is a fibrous sheet interposed between the external auditory canal and the middle ear cavity. The connective tissue between these two layers consists of radiating fibers attached to the manubrium of the malleus, and are reinforced peripherally by circular fibers. The latter are thickened at the margin of the tympanic membrane to form a fibrocartilaginous ring (annulus fibrocartilaginous) attaching the tympanic membrane to the tympanic sulcus of the temporal bone. In the upper portion of the tympanic membrane, there is a limited area where the connective tissue fibers are lacking; this area is referred to as the pars flaccida, or Shrapnell membrane. In this area, the tympanic portion of the temporal bone is deficient; this gap is referred to as the tympanic incisure, or the notch of Rivinus. The tympanic membrane attaches to the temporal bone. The remainder of the tympanic membrane in which there are intact connective tissue fibers is referred to as the pars tensa.

The outer aspect of the tympanic membrane is concave. The center of the concavity is referred to as the umbo, which is the strong point of attachment of the manubrium of the malleus to the tympanic membrane. The lateral process of the malleus is attached to the anterosuperior portion of the tympanic membrane; from this point of attachment the anterior and posterior mallear folds pass to the cartilaginous annulus and separate the pars flaccida from the pars tensa. In otoscopic examinations of the tympanic membrane, the bright area of light reflection present downward and forward from the umbo is referred to as the "cone of light."

Middle Ear. The middle ear, or tympanic cavity, lies within the temporal bone between the tympanic membrane and the squamous portions of the temporal bone laterally and the petrous portion of the temporal bone surrounding the inner ear medially. The lateral or internal aspect consists of the tympanic membrane and the squamous portion of the temporal bone; the medial aspect is bordered by the petrous portion of the temporal bone; the superior (roof) is delimited by the tegmen tympani, a thin plate of bone that separates the middle ear space from the cranial cavity; the inferior (floor) aspect is bordered by a thin plate of bone separating the tympanic cavity from the superior bulb of the internal jugular vein; the anterior aspect is delimited by a thin plate of bone separating the tympanic cavity from the carotid canal housing the internal carotid artery; and the posterior aspect is delimited by the petrous portion of the temporal bone, which contains the mastoid antrum and mastoid air cells (4–6). The tympanic cavity communicates anteriorly with the nasopharynx by the eustachian (auditory or pharyngotympanic) tube and posteriorly with the mastoid air cells by the aditus and mastoid antrum.

The eustachian tube extends from its tympanic ostium high on the anterior wall of the tympanic cavity to a nasopharyngeal ostium situated posterior to the inferior nasal concha (5). The tube is slightly S-shaped. In the adult, the tympanic ostium is approximately 2.0 to 2.5 cm higher than the nasopharyngeal end; the tube runs downward, medially and anteriorly to the nasopharynx. The length of the tube in adults varies from 31 to 38 mm (7). In infants, the tube is shorter, wider, and more horizontal in its course, and therefore, an easier pathway for infections ascending from the nasopharynx to the tympanic cavity.

The tube is divided into an osseous portion and cartilaginous portion. The osseous portion, or canal, has a bony wall and is the lateral or tympanic third of the tube. The anteromedial two-third portion has a cartilaginous and connective tissue wall, and is referred to as the cartilaginous portion of the tube. The cartilaginous and osseous tubes meet at an obtuse angle.

The contents of the tympanic cavity include the ossicles (malleus, incus, and stapes), ligaments of the ossicles, tendons of the ossicular muscles, eustachian tube, tympanic cavity proper, epitympanic recess, mastoid cavity, and chorda tympani of the facial (VII) nerve. The middle ear as well as the external ear function as conduits for sound from the auditory part of the internal ear. For a more detailed discussion and description of the anatomy of the ear, the reader is referred to additional texts (3).

Inner Ear. The internal (inner) ear, or labyrinth, is embedded within the petrous portion of the temporal bone and comprises the medial portion of the temporal bone adjacent to the cranial cavity (4,6). The inner ear contains the membranous labyrinth, which is surrounded by an osseous layer or bony shell termed the osseous (bony) labyrinth, or otic capsule.

The osseous (bony) labyrinth consists of the vestibular and cochlear capsule. The central portion of the osseous labyrinth cavity is the vestibule, a large ovoid perilymphatic space approximately 4 mm in diameter containing both the saccule and utricle of the membranous labyrinth (4,6). In the floor of the bony vestibule is the elliptical recess for the anterior end of the utricle; anterior and lateral to this is the spherical recess for the saccule. In the lateral wall of the vestibule is the oval window in which the base of the stapes is situated. Through the stapes, the perilymph of the vestibule receives vibrations from the tympanic membrane, and an ossicular chain set up by sound waves reaches the tympanic cavity. Along the medial wall and floor of the vestibule, where it abuts the lateral end of the internal acoustic meatus, are small openings for the entrance of the nerve branches to the vestibular portion of the ear (5).

The bony cochlea, a part of the otic capsule, is a hollowed spiral about two to three fourths turns diminishing from a relatively broad base to a pointed cupula or apex. It is so named because of its resemblance to a snail shell. The base of the cochlea lies against the anteromedial surface of the vestibule and next to the anterior surface of the lateral (blind) end of the internal auditory canal. A central core of bone called the modiolus runs forward from the cochlea but does not reach the cupula. It is around this central core that the spiral channels of the cochlea (perilymphatic and endolymphatic) are arranged. A spiral layer of bone unites the modiolus and the peripheral wall of the bony cochlea and separates successive spiral cavities from each other (4,6). The modiolus is hollow to accommodate the cochlear nerve. The base of the modiolus lies against the lateral end of the internal auditory canal where the cochlear nerve runs.

The vestibular aqueduct extends through the otic capsule from the vestibule to the posterior cranial fossa, transmitting the endolymphatic duct. The terminal end of the vestibular aqueduct is the endolymphatic sac, a dilated area that ends blindly outside the dura (4,6). The cochlear duct opens at one end into the lower end of the scala tympani and at the other end into the subarachnoid cavity (4,6). The issue as to whether the cochlear duct represents an open channel between the subarachnoid space and the perilymphatic space at the lower end of the scala tympani remains controversial (5). A possible role ascribed to the cochlear duct is to serve as part of the pressure-adjusting mechanism of the perilymph in conjunction with the round window (3).

The membranous (otic) labyrinth contains the cochlea, which is the organ of hearing, and the vestibular system, which is the system of balance (equilibrium). The principle components of the membranous labyrinth are the cochlear duct, utricle, saccule, ductus reuniens, semicircular canals with their ampullae, and endolymphatic sac and duct (4,6).

The cochlea is a spiral structure that resembles the shell of a snail, and is composed of the cochlear duct, also known as the scala media, as well as the scala vestibuli and the scala tympani. These three compartments are fluid filled. The cochlear duct, lying between the scala vestibuli and scala tympani, as well as the entire membranous labyrinth, contain endolymph, an intracellular-like fluid containing high potassium and low sodium concentrations. The electrolyte concentration of the endolymph is critical for the normal functioning of the sensory organs. The scala vestibuli and the scala tympani contain perilymph, which is partly a filtration of cerebrospinal fluid (CSF) and partly a filtration from blood vessels of the ear. The CSF communicates directly with the perilymphatic space through the cochlear aqueduct. Perilymphatic fluid resembles the extracellular fluid, with low potassium and high sodium concentrations.

The cochlear duct contains the end organ of hearing known as the organ of Corti. The organ of Corti consists of neurotransmitting hair cells that rest on the basilar membrane. The latter separates the cochlear duct from the scala tympani. The scala tympani lies below the basilar membrane while the scala vestibuli lies above the cochlear duct and is separated from it by Reissner membrane. The scala tympani and scala vestibuli communicate which each other only at the apex, known as the helicotrema. The scala vestibuli and the scala tympani communicate with the middle ear via the oval window and round window, respectively. The cochlear duct connects with the vestibular system via the ductus reuniens located at the saccule. In this way the three semicircular canals that comprise the vestibular system are filled with endolymph.

The vestibular system contains the receptor organs for sense of motion and position. The utricle is an oval-shaped tube lying superior to the saccule in the medial wall of the vestibule. The macule of the utricle is a sensory end organ composed of hair cells and is located in the utricular recess. The three semicircular canals communicate with the utricle via openings formed by the union of the nondilated or nonampullary ends of the superior and posterior canals, termed the commun crus. The dilated or ampullary ends of each semicircular canal contain the neuroepithelium, called the crista ampullaris. The crista is saddle-shaped and packed with specialized mechanoreceptor hair cells. The neural structures of the inner ear, including the 8th cranial nerve (vestibulocochlear) and the 7th cranial nerve (facial) enter the inner ear through the internal auditory canal.

Histology

External Ear. Histologically, the auricle is a cutaneous structure composed of keratinizing, stratified squamous epithelium with associated cutaneous adnexal structures that include hair follicles, sebaceous glands, and eccrine sweat glands (fig. 7-2). The subcutaneous tissue is composed of fibroconnective tissue, fat, and elastic-type fibrocartilage; the latter gives the auricle its structural support.

In addition to the cutaneous adnexal structures, the outer third of the external canal is noteworthy for the presence within the submucosa of modified apocrine glands, called ceruminal glands, which replace the eccrine glands seen in the auricular dermis. Ceruminal glands produce cerumen and are arranged in clusters composed of two cell layers, including inner, or secretory, cells and outer, or myoepithelial, cells. The secretory cells are cuboidal cells with eosinophilic cytoplasm often containing a granular, golden-yellow pigment (cerumen); secretory cells show holocrine (decapitation)-type secretion (fig. 7-3). The myoepithelial cells are flattened cells located peripheral to the secretory cells.

The ear lobe is devoid of cartilage and is replaced by a pad of adipose tissue. The perichondrium is composed of loose vascular connective tissue. Similar to the auricle, the external auditory canal is lined by keratinizing squamous epithelium which runs throughout the canal and covers the external aspect of the tympanic membrane.

In the inner portion of the external auditory canal, ceruminal glands and other adnexal structures are absent. The inner two thirds of the external auditory canal consists of bone rather than cartilage (3). The tympanic membrane has a central bilaminated zone, including lateral, radially arranged and medial, circularly arranged collagenous fibers (figs. 7-4, 7-5). The inner two thirds of the external auditory canal contain bone rather than cartilage. Because adnexal structures are absent, there is close apposition of the epithelium to the subjacent bone.

Middle Ear. The epithelial lining of the tympanic cavity is a single layer of respiratory epithelium composed of flattened to cuboidal epithelial cells (fig. 7-6). Under normal conditions, there are no glandular elements within the middle ear; the presence of glands in the middle ear is abnormal and can be seen as a metaplastic proliferation in association with chronic otitis media (see later in chapter) (3). Further, stratified squamous epithelium is not present in the tympanic cavity under normal conditions nor does squamous metaplasia occur in the middle ear (3). Ciliated pseudostratified columnar epithelium may be found in limited patches among the flattened or cuboidal epithelial cells.

The eustachian (auditory) tube is lined by low ciliated epithelium for much of its length except as it approaches the nasopharyngeal end, where it becomes ciliated pseudostratified columnar epithelium containing goblet cells. The cartilaginous portion also contains seromucinous glands. The eustachian tube contains a lymphoid component, particularly in children, that is referred to as Gerlach tubal tonsil. Reactive hyperplasia of this lymphoid component, particularly in children, may close off the eustachian tube and provide a desirable milieu for otitis media (3). The mucosa of the osseous portion of the eustachian tube is separated from the carotid canal by a thin plate of bone measuring 1 mm in thickness (3). Dehiscence of the carotid canal is fairly frequent (8). The cartilage of the nasopharyngeal portion of the eustachian tube is hyaline type.

The mastoid air cells represent a network of intercommunicating spaces that emanate from

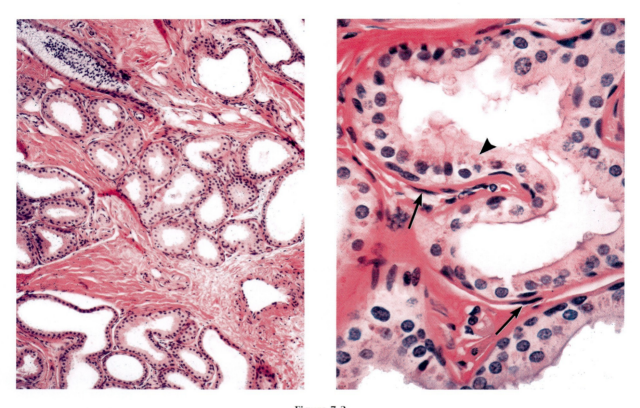

Figure 7-3

EXTERNAL EAR

The outer third of the external auditory canal is noteworthy for the presence of modified apocrine glands, otherwise known as ceruminal glands, which replace the eccrine glands in the auricular dermis.

Left: Ceruminal glands are submucosal and are arranged in clusters or lobules.

Right: At high magnification, ceruminal glands are composed of two cell layers: inner or secretory cells containing intracytoplasmic cerumen appearing as granular, golden-yellow pigmentation (arrowhead) and outer myoepithelial cells appearing as flattened, elongated cells with hyperchromatic nuclei located peripheral to the secretory cells (arrows).

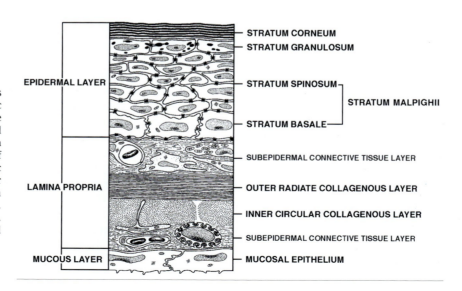

Figure 7-4

PRIMARY TYMPANIC MEMBRANE

A cross section of the pars tensa of the primary tympanic membrane (ear drum) shows the epidermal layer facing the external auditory canal. The pars flaccida (Schrapnell membrane) portion of the drum has a similar histologic makeup minus the outer and inner collagenous layers. (Fig. 1 from Lim DJ. Tympanic membrane. Electron microscopic observation. Part 1. Pars tensa. Acta Otolaryngol 1968;66:182.)

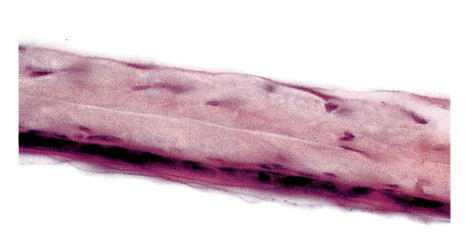

Figure 7-5

PARS TENSA OF TYMPANIC MEMBRANE

The following layers are distinguished from left to right to left: middle ear epithelium, lamina propria, circular arrangement of collagenous fibers (i.e., at right angles to former layer), radial arrangement of collagenous fibers, lamina propria, and stratified squamous epithelium. (Fig. 14.8 from Wenig BM, Michaels L. The ear and temporal bone. In: Mills SE, ed. Histology for pathologists, 4th ed. Philadelphia: Elsevier; 2012:404.)

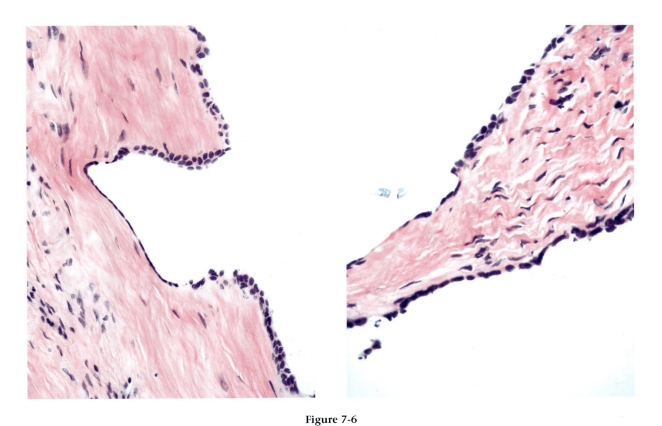

Figure 7-6

EPITHELIUM OF THE MIDDLE EAR

Left, right: The epithelial lining of the tympanic cavity is a single layer of flattened to cuboidal epithelium.

the tympanic cavity (3). Each air cell is lined by flattened to cuboidal epithelium which rests on the periosteum that covers a thin frame of lamellar bone.

The middle ear ossicles develop from cartilage, with a single center of ossification for bone; there is no epiphyseal ossification (3). The persistence of cartilage in each of the ossicles and the bifurcation of the stapes to form the crura with the obturator foramen between them distinguishes the middle ear ossicles from other long bones (3). The head of the stapes is formed of endochondral bone and has a cartilaginous cap at the incudostapedial joint. The crura of the stapes are formed of periosteal bone only. From the middle ear aspect of the stapes footplate to its vestibular surface, the histologic findings include the flattened to cuboidal epithelium of the tympanic cavity, a thin layer of bone, cartilage, and a single flattened (perilymphatic) epithelial cell layer.

The malleus and incus, similar to long bones, have an outer covering of periosteal bone and an inner core of endochondral bone with well-formed haversian systems. The manubrium (handle) of the malleus is predominantly covered by retained cartilage rather than periosteal bone. The entire inner core of the manubrium and the rest of the malleus are composed of endochondral bone. The anterior process is formed in membrane early in fetal life and merges with the malleus after its formation (3). At its superior aspect, the manubrium is separated from the tympanic membrane by a ligament covered by the middle ear epithelium. The short process of the incus has a tip of unossified cartilage.

Both the incudomalleal and incudostapedial joints are diarthrodial. Middle ear epithelium is present on the outer surface of the joint capsule and synovial membrane is present on its inner surface. The joint capsule consists of fibrous tissue with a high elastic fiber content (3). The articular disc, representing the space between the articular ends, is comprised predominantly of fibrocartilage. The articular processes of both the malleus and the incus are covered by cartilage.

The annular ligament binds the cartilaginous edge of the stapes footplate to the cartilaginous rim of the vestibular window (stapediovestibular joint). It is composed of fibrous tissue, with elastic fibers prominent near the ligament surface (9). Cartilage also covers the articular surface of the stapediovestibular joints. The fissula ante fenestrum is the canal linking the middle ear with the vestibule; it lies in the bone just anterior to the stapediovestibular joint and develops as a slit filled with fibrous tissue, often with associated cartilage.

Inner Ear. The complexity of the histology of the inner ear is beyond the scope of this text. The interested reader is referred to other texts that detail the histoanatomy of the inner ear (3,4,6).

CLASSIFICATION

The classification of the non-neoplastic lesions of the ear and temporal bone is listed in Table 7-1.

CONGENITAL ABNORMALITIES

The ear, including the external, middle, and internal ear, is often involved by congenital anomalies. These occur as an isolated defect or in combination with other aural and extra-aural abnormalities, varying from cosmetic defects to complete sensorineural hearing loss. A complete discussion of the developmental defects of the external ear are beyond the scope of this chapter. The interested reader is referred to other texts (10). This section includes the more common developmental abnormalities that the surgical pathologists are likely to be confronted with in daily practice.

Accessory Tragus

Definition. *Accessory tragus* is a duplicated external ear characterized by a pedunculated or polypoid lesion composed of squamous epithelial-lined fibroconnective tissue with centrally situated mature hyaline cartilage. Synonyms include *accessory ear, accessory auricle, supernumerary ear,* and *polyotia*.

Clinical Features. Accessory tragus appears at birth, may be solitary or multiple, unilateral or bilateral, and is located on the skin surface often anterior to the auricle (11). It may clinically be mistaken for a papilloma. Accessory tragus is thought to be related to second branchial arch anomalies; it may occur independent of other congenital anomalies (12), but may occur in association with cleft palate or lip, mandibular hypoplasia, or with other anomalies such as Goldenhar syndrome (oculoauriculovertebral dysplasia) (13–17).

Gross Findings. Accessory tragus is a sessile or pedunculated, soft or cartilaginous, skin-covered nodule or papule (fig. 7-7).

Microscopic Findings. Histologically, accessory tragus recapitulates the normal external auricle and includes skin, cutaneous adnexal structures, and a central core of cartilage (fig. 7-8).

Differential Diagnosis. The differential diagnosis includes squamous papilloma. In contrast to an accessory tragus, squamous papilloma lacks cutaneous adnexal structures and cartilage (18).

Treatment and Prognosis. Simple excision is curative.

Branchial Cleft Anomalies

Definition. *Branchial cleft anomalies* are congenital malformations related to the branchial apparatus. For a more complete discussion, the reader is referred to chapter 4.

Clinical Features. First branchial cleft anomalies typically occur in the area of the external ear and include cysts, sinuses, and fistulas (19). In comparison to second branchial cleft anomalies, first branchial cleft anomalies are uncommon, representing from 1 to 8 percent of all branchial apparatus defects. First branchial cleft anomalies occur in a variety of locations, including preauricular, postauricular, or infra-auricular areas; at the angle of the jaw; associated with the ear lobe; in the external auditory canal; or involving the parotid gland. Involvement of the external auditory canal may result in otalgia or otorrhea. Parotid involvement may result in an intraparotid or periparotid mass that may be mistaken for a parotid gland tumor.

Cysts represent over two thirds (68 percent) of first branchial cleft anomalies (19,20). First branchial cleft cysts appear as solitary lesions without an associated sinus tract. Sinuses and fistulas equally make up the remainder of these lesions. The fistula tract in first branchial cleft anomalies may extend from the skin, over or through the parotid gland, and open in the external auditory canal.

Treatment and Prognosis. Irrespective of the histology, complete surgical excision is the treatment of choice. Inadequate excision results in recurrence and increased risk of infection. Incision and drainage are indicated in cases where abscesses have developed; complete surgical excision must wait until resolution of the infection. Type II anomalies are often intimately associated with the parotid gland and may necessitate a superficial parotidectomy to ensure complete excision.

TUMOR-LIKE LESIONS OF THE EXTERNAL EAR REGION

Keloid

Definition. *Keloid* is a non-neoplastic, dermal, fibroproliferative, exaggerated tissue response to trauma, representing one extreme of the spectrum of reparative reactions of the skin. Keloids are not true neoplasms. The word keloid is derived from the Greek word chele, meaning

---

Table 7-1

CLASSIFICATION OF NON-NEOPLASTIC LESIONS OF THE EAR AND TEMPORAL BONE

External Ear
  Congenital abnormalities
    Accessory tragus
    First branchial cleft anomalies
  Infectious, inflammatory, or tumor-like lesions
    Keloid
    Necrotizing external otitis
    Chondrodermatitis nodularis helicis chronicus
    Idiopathic cystic chondromalacia
    Exostosis
    Synovial chondromatosis
    Kimura disease
  Autoimmune or systemic diseases
    Relapsing polychondritis
    Gout
    Pseudogout

Middle and Inner Ear Including Temporal Bone
  Infectious and Inflammatory
    Otitis media
    Otic or aural polyp
    Cholesteatoma
    Langerhans cell histiocytosis (eosinophilic granuloma)
    Extranodal sinus histiocytosis with massive lymphadenopathy (Rosai-Dorfman disease)
    Heterotopias (central nervous system tissue; salivary gland)
  Autoimmune, degenerative, or systemic disorders
    Otosclerosis
    Granulomatosis with polyangiitis (Wegener granulomatosis)
    Paget disease
    Ménière disease

Developmental and Congenital Anomalies

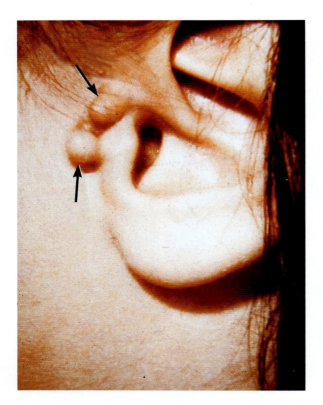
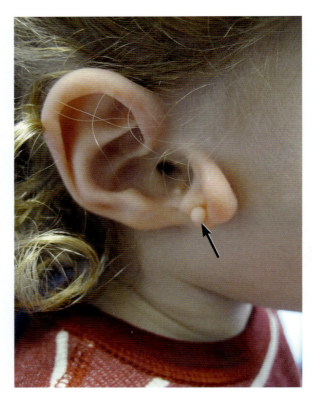

Figure 7-7

ACCESSORY TRAGUS

Left: Preauricular skin-covered papules (arrows) are seen.
Right: Skin-covered papule on the earlobe (arrow). (Courtesy of Dr. J. D. Rosenberg, New York, NY.)

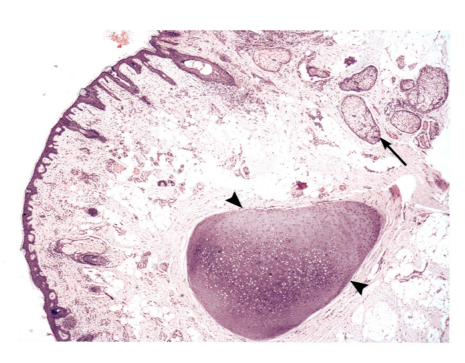

Figure 7-8

ACCESSORY TRAGUS

Histologically, the features of accessory tragi include recapitulation of the normal external auricle, including the presence of keratinizing squamous epithelium; cutaneous adnexal structures including (but not limited to) sebaceous glands (arrow); and a central core of cartilage (arrowheads).

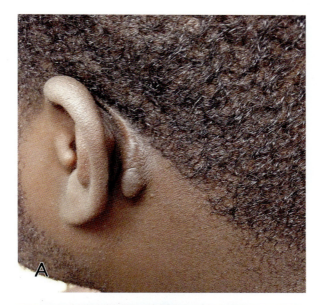

Figure 7-9

KELOID

A: The keloid appears as a polypoid mass variably located postauricular (A), preauricular and postauricular (B), and on the helical rim (C). (A: courtesy of Dr. E. Smouha, New York, NY; B,C: courtesy of Dr. J. D. Rosenberg, New York, NY.)

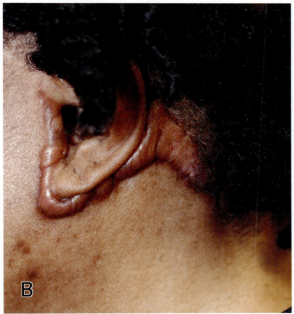

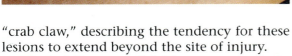

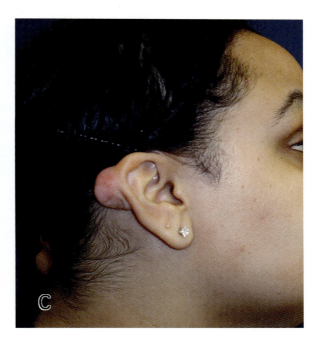

"crab claw," describing the tendency for these lesions to extend beyond the site of injury.

Clinical Features. Keloids occur equally in men and women. They occur at any age, but are most common in young adults under 30 years of age. Keloids most commonly occur in dark skinned people, especially in young black women who have had their ears pierced (21). The most common sites of occurrence are the presternal region, limbs, neck, and face; the latter includes the earlobes and pinna.

Keloids most often are asymptomatic but may be associated with pruritus, paresthesia, and pain (22). They are often associated with a variety of cutaneous injuries, including surgery, ear piercing, BCG vaccinations, injections, burns, lacerations, and insect bites; their development following injury takes from weeks up to a year.

Gross Findings. Keloids are often polypoid in appearance, and covered by thin glistening hairless skin. The size is variable, usually less than 2 cm; however, they can be larger (fig. 7-9).

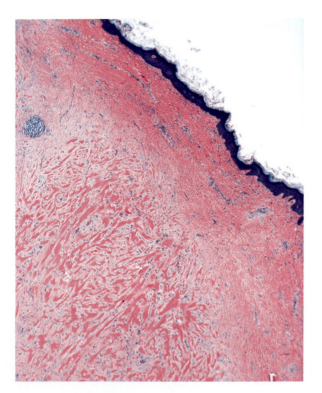 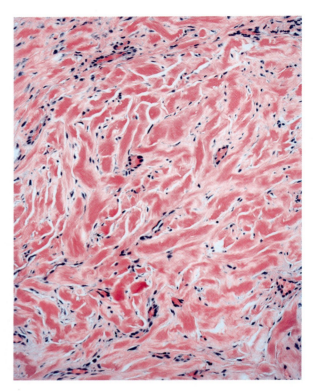

Figure 7-10

KELOID

Left: Irrespective of the location, the histologic features of keloids are similar and characterized by the presence of haphazard fascicles of hyalinized collagen within the dermis; the overlying cutaneous epithelium is thin and devoid of hair follicles.

Right: Higher magnification shows the haphazard fascicles of hyalinized collagen with scattered spindle-shaped fibroblastic cells and limited but identifiable blood vessels.

Microscopic Findings. Keloids consist of haphazardly arranged fascicles of hyalinized collagenous fibers with scattered fibroblasts and myofibroblasts (fig. 7-10). The proliferation is not encapsulated, but blends subtly with the surrounding dermal fibrous tissue; the collagen bundles are often separated by dermal mucosubstances, creating an "edematous" appearance. Keloids are poorly vascularized, with widely scattered dilated blood vessels. The overlying epidermis is thin and atrophic, without dermal adnexal structures.

A foreign body giant cell reaction is uncommon except in patients treated with corticosteroid injection. Pools of amorphous mucin-like material may also be seen following steroid injection.

Differential Diagnosis. The differential diagnosis includes hypertrophic scar, dermatofibroma (DF), and dermatofibrosarcoma protuberans (DFSP). In contrast to keloids, hypertrophic scars lack dense hyalinized collagenous fibers, have more delicate fibrillar collagen, and have a more orderly arrangement of the collagen and fibroblastic cells, often with a parallel orientation to the skin surface. Mature hypertrophic scars generally do not have an abundance of mucosubstances, and therefore have a more compact microscopic appearance (23). Hypertrophic scars usually do not recur following excision while keloids may.

The extremely low cellularity of keloids distinguishes it from DF and DFSP. In contrast to keloids, there is hyperplasia of the overlying epidermis in DFs and DFSPs. Kuo et al. (24) described an unusual variant of DF characterized by keloidal-type changes that they termed keloidal dermatofibroma. Clinically, keloidal DF appears similar to usual DF but is characterized by keloidal-like collagen admixed with elements typically present in DF. In contrast to keloids, DFSP shows immunoreactivity for CD34.

Treatment and Prognosis. Surgical excision is the treatment of choice, although Cheng et al. (25) reported a recurrence rate of 40 percent following simple surgical resection. Intralesional steroid injections alone provide response rates of 50 to 100 percent, with recurrence rates of 5 to 50 percent at 5 years (26,27). Intralesional triamcinolone injections are considered the gold standard for nonsurgical management (28). Intralesional verapamil, independent of or in conjunction with triamcilnone, has shown efficacy in the treatment of keloids (and hypertrophic scars), with flattening of the raised scars and the regaining of normal pigmentation (28). Intralesional cryosurgery has emerged as a safe and effective new treatment which destroys the hypertrophic scar tissue with minimal damage to the skin surface (29).

When surgery is followed by steroid injection or radiation therapy (10 Gy), recurrence rates are consistently below 50 percent (30–33). Intralesional injection of interferon or bleomycin has shown 50 percent reduction in lesion size, and response appears to be limited to the area treated (26,34). Currently, most of the literature supports the use of combination therapy (usually surgery and adjuvant chemotherapy) as the mainstay treatment for keloids (22,35). Transforming growth factor-beta (TGF-β) and platelet-derived growth factor (PDGF) play an integral role in the formation of keloids and the future development of selective inhibitors of TGF-β might produce new therapeutic tools with enhanced efficacy and specificity for their treatment (36,37).

Chondrodermatitis Nodularis Chronicus Helicis

Definition. *Chondrodermatitis nodularis chronicus helicis* (CNCH) is an idiopathic nonneoplastic ulcerative lesion of the auricle. It is also known as *Winkler disease* or *nodule* (38).

Clinical Features. CNCH usually affects late middle-aged and older men, and is uncommon in women (39,40). Patients present with a spontaneously occurring unilateral painful nodule; manipulation of the lesion causes intense pain which eventually prompts patients to seek treatment. CNCH most frequently occurs along the superior portion of the helix; lateral helical, antihelical, and antitragal involvement are also seen. CNCH typically appears as a round, reddish, tender area, usually measuring less than 1 cm in diameter. Many cases are clinically considered to be carcinomas (40).

The etiology of CNCH is not known, but several theories have been suggested, including cold exposure, actinic damage, local trauma, and degenerative change with pressure necrosis. Because the skin of the auricle is thin, with little subcutaneous fat, the area may be unusually sensitive to injury. In addition, the vascular supply to the area is somewhat deficient, with the avascular cartilage depending on the dermal circulation for its sustenance. These anatomic features may predispose the auricle to the development of CNCH. Winkler (38) considered the underlying pathologic event to be a cartilaginous-based process; however, the etiology appears to be linked to a primary cutaneous alteration since the cutaneous changes are more significant and more constant. It is likely that the development of CNCH is multifactorial and includes actinic damage. Upile et al. (41) have suggested that arteriolar narrowing in perichondrium region of the pinna, remote from arterial blood supply (i.e., helix), leads to ischemic changes and death of the metabolically active underlying cartilage, with necrosis and extrusion as a possible cause of the underlying cartilage necrosis that results in CNCH.

Gross Findings. CNCH usually appears as a dome-shaped, discrete nodule with a scale crust covering a central area of ulceration (fig. 7-11). It ranges in diameter from 3 to 18 mm, with an average of 7 mm. Rarely, CNCH may achieve diameters of 2 to 3 cm.

Microscopic Findings. The central portion of the involved epidermis is ulcerated, with the adjacent epithelium showing acanthosis, hyperkeratosis, parakeratosis, and pseudoepitheliomatous hyperplasia (fig. 7-12). The base of the ulcer shows granulation tissue with a pronounced capillary proliferation, edema, fibrinoid necrosis, and an acute or chronic inflammatory cell infiltrate (39). The granulation tissue and inflammatory process usually extend to, and involve, the perichondrium and cartilage (fig. 7-12). Pain is thought to result from this perichondrial involvement. The dermis lacks cutaneous adnexal structures in the area of the lesion, and the vasculature appears telangiectatic. Foci of fibrinoid eosinophilic material or, in some cases, frank necrobiosis of the collagen may be

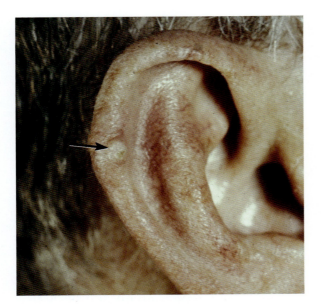

Figure 7-11

CHONDRODERMATITIS NODULARIS CHRONICUS HELICIS

A small discrete nodule is seen along the superior portion of the helix with a central area of ulceration (arrow). The lesion was painful and clinically considered to be carcinoma.

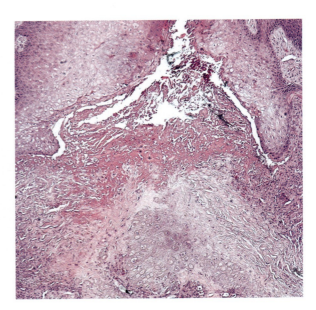

Figure 7-12

CHONDRODERMATITIS NODULARIS CHRONICUS HELICIS

The central portion of the involved epidermis is ulcerated. The base of the ulcer consists of granulation tissue that extends to the subjacent perichondrium and cartilage. Perichondrial involvement is associated with pain. The surface epithelium adjacent to the ulcer shows acanthosis and hyperkeratosis.

present. Occasionally, palisading histiocytes are seen in association with necrobiotic collagen.

The changes in the auricular cartilage deep to the ulcer range from mild perichondritis to variable degenerative changes characterized by edema and loss of chondrocytes, with smudging (i.e., loss of basophilia) and hyalinization of the chondroid matrix. The necrotic material from the dermis, and occasionally even fragments of degenerated cartilage, may protrude into the ulcer crater. Calcification and ossification of the underlying cartilage may be present (42).

Differential Diagnosis. CNCH is frequently misdiagnosed as a cutaneous malignancy, particularly as basal cell carcinoma or squamous cell carcinoma. In 80 percent of CNCHs reviewed by Metzger and Goodman (39), the clinical diagnosis was either a malignant or premalignant lesion. Unfortunately, the same mistake may be perpetuated by microscopic examination, particularly if the epidermal hyperplastic changes are misinterpreted as representing either squamous cell carcinoma or a hypertrophic actinic keratosis. The extensive dermal changes and usually some cartilaginous alterations, along with the well-demarcated nature of the epidermal proliferation and lack of cytologic atypia in the adjacent epidermis, should help in excluding a squamous neoplasm in cases of CNCH.

Treatment and Prognosis. Complete surgical excision, including wedge excision (43) or cartilage excision alone (44), is the treatment of choice and is curative. In a minority of patients, injection of glucocorticoids directly into the lesion is effective in eradicating the lesion. Conservative treatment using pressure-relieving padding has been shown to be effective (45–47). There is no malignant potential.

Idiopathic Cystic Chondromalacia of the Auricular Cartilage

Definition. *Idiopathic cystic chondromalacia* (ICC) of the auricular cartilage is a benign cystic degeneration of the auricular cartilage of unknown etiology. Synonyms include *auricular pseudocyst* or *endochondral pseudocyst*.

Clinical Features. ICC typically occurs in young and middle-aged adult males but may uncommonly occur in woman (48,49). These lesions arise over a period of weeks to years as unilateral, painless swellings of the cartilage without overlying ulceration or erythema. They are occasionally bilateral (50). Although they arise anywhere on the auricle, the scaphoid fossa (80 percent) is the most common site (51). Markedly elevated lactate dehydrogenase (LDH) levels are found in aspirated fluid (52), with a higher percentage of LDH 4 and 5 and a lower percentage of LDH 1 and 2 (53).

Although trauma has been implicated in causing these lesions, there is no definitive connection to a prior traumatic event and the cause for this condition remains unknown. Engel (54), who was the first to describe them in the English literature, believed that these lesions were secondary to repeated minor trauma. He attributed them to the habit of sleeping on hard pillows although he could not substantiate his claim. Others have also believed that these lesions were traumatic in origin, citing the wearing of motorcycle helmets, stereo headphones, or the Italian birthday custom of having one's auricle pulled (48,55,56). Despite these theories, only a few documented cases have a history of preceding trauma (50), including rugby-associated trauma (57). ICCs may arise within a potential plane left during embryonic fusion of the auricular hillocks. Ischemic necrosis of the cartilage or the abnormal release of lysosomal enzymes by chondrocytes may be cofactors (50,58). An inflammatory response has been postulated as crucial to the development of ICC based on the consistent presence of a perivascular inflammatory response (59).

Gross Findings. ICC is a fluid-filled distended mass (fig. 7-13). The excised tissue may include only a fragment of the cyst wall or, less often, a full-thickness excision of the ear. An intact cyst usually contains fluid, which has been described as "olive oil-like" (54). The cyst wall consists of a 1- to 2-mm rim of cartilage. The cyst lining may be a smooth and glistening cartilaginous surface or may consist of roughened rust-colored patches. The cyst is usually an elongated cleft, but multifocal areas of cystic degeneration may be seen.

Microscopic Findings. Histologically, the changes are restricted to the cartilage, within which irregular-shaped cystic areas are seen (fig. 7-14). The cysts lack an epithelial lining, hence the term "pseudocyst," and generally are devoid

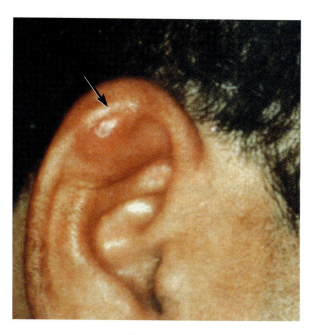

Figure 7-13

IDIOPATHIC CYSTIC CHONDROMALACIA

A painless swelling of the auricular cartilage has intact overlying erythematous skin (arrow).

of content. The cyst is the result of loss of cartilage. The cystic cleft is often centrally placed in the cartilaginous plate, and there may be a rim of fibrous tissue along the inner rim of the cyst. A granulation tissue reaction, composed of fibrovascular tissue and scattered chronic inflammatory cells, may be seen in association with the cysts. In longstanding cases, the fibrous tissue obliterates the cystic space. Some examples of ICC are characterized by a proliferative cartilaginous response, in which a thickened cartilaginous wall develops.

Differential Diagnosis. There may be slight cytologic atypia, however, the orderly nature of the proliferation and the associated central cystic degeneration facilitate the exclusion of malignant neoplasia (49). The differential diagnosis also includes relapsing polychondritis, subperichondrial hematoma, and CNCH.

Treatment and Prognosis. Complete surgical excision without distortion of the underlying cartilaginous framework (surgical deroofing) is the treatment of choice (60–62). Due to the potential for surgical-related deformity, full-thickness resection is not advocated. In addition to

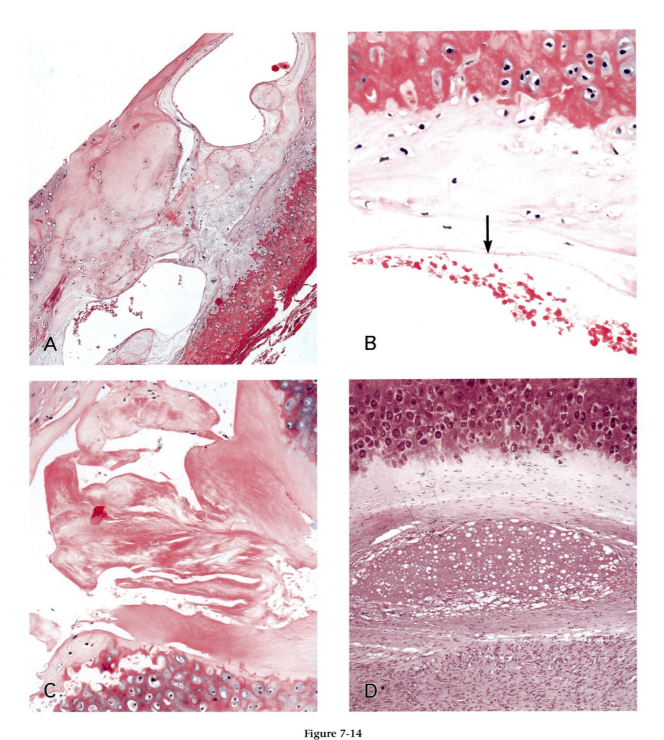

Figure 7-14

IDIOPATHIC CYSTIC CHONDROMALACIA

A: Histologically, idiopathic cystic chondromalacia is characterized by the cystic degeneration of the auricular cartilage. The cysts result in the loss of cartilage.

B: The cysts lack a true epithelial lining (arrow) and thus represent pseudocysts.

C: Along the inner rim of the cyst wall is fibrous tissue.

D: Granulation tissue (bottom) lies adjacent to the cyst.

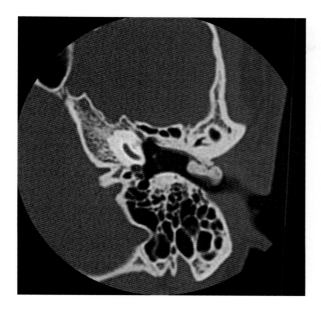 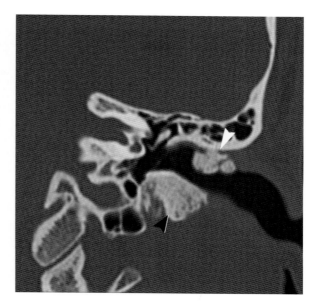

Figure 7-15
EXOSTOSIS OF THE EXTERNAL AUDITORY CANAL
Axial (left) and coronal (right) computerized tomography (CT) images demonstrate a pedunculated mass (arrow) of cortical and trabecular bone occupying the lateral half of the bony external auditory canal. (Courtesy of Dr. A. Khorsandi, New York, NY.)

the obvious cosmetic concerns, longstanding lesions may result in deformity of the ear. Steroid injection alone has been unsuccessful and may result in cartilage deformity. Incision and drainage or curettage has shown variable success. Needle aspiration alone results in rapid reaccumulation of fluid, but when combined with bolster suture compression, long-term follow-up has shown an absence of recurrences (63).

Exostosis

Definition. *Exostosis* is the localized overgrowth of bone. Classically described as a reactive lesion, it consists of a compact proliferation of layers of bone of varied size and appearance, including nodular, mound-like, pedunculated, and flat protuberances, on the surface of a bone. Broad-based lesions are referred to as exostosis while pedunculated lesions are termed *osteomas*. *Surfer ear* is another term for this entity.

Clinical Features. Exostoses usually are multiple and bilateral, broad-based outgrowths of bone arising from the wall of the external auditory canal (64). Most canal exostoses are asymptomatic until they reach a size sufficient to interfere with the normal egress of cerumen and exfoliated skin (64). External auditory canal obstruction may cause recurrent episodes of external otitis, conductive hearing loss, and tinnitus (65). Exostosis of the external auditory canal often occurs in cold water swimmers and surfers, with the highest incidence in Australia and New Zealand (66–68), as well as in white-water kayakers (69,70). Imaging findings include pedunculated overgrowth of bone occupying the lateral half of the bony external auditory canal without aggressive features (fig. 7-15).

Gross Findings. The gross appearance of exostoses are usually better appreciated by the surgeon, as only fragments are available to the pathologist in most cases.

Microscopic Findings. The intact exostosis is a broad-based, mound-like bony proliferation that is similar in color and texture to normal cortical bone (fig. 7-16). The bone is covered by a layer of periosteum with overlying thin skin. The periosteal layers are like the skin of an onion and usually lack a trabecular architecture or bone marrow spaces.

Differential Diagnosis. The chief differential diagnosis is osteoma, which is a much less common lesion in this location. The distinction

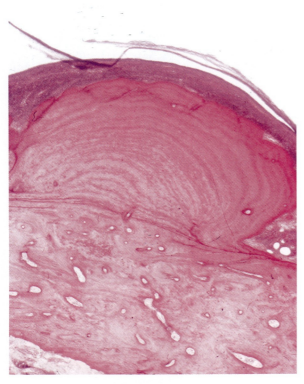

Figure 7-16

EXOSTOSIS OF THE EXTERNAL AUDITORY CANAL

The broad-based, mound-like bony proliferation lacks trabecular architecture or marrow spaces. The periosteal layers resemble the skin of an onion. A layer of periosteum with overlying thin skin covers the bone.

between exostosis and osteoma is determined by the clinical presentation and imaging findings (71). There is controversy regarding the ability to distinguish between the two lesions histologically: some consider the lesions to be histologically different (64,72), while others do not find the microscopic features sufficiently distinctive to be separated (73).

Treatment and Prognosis. Medical treatment resolves the symptomatic external otitis and related hearing loss. For patients who do not respond to medical treatment, transmeatal surgical excision is the treatment of choice (65). Preservation of the canal skin overlying the exostosis limits the amount of exposed surface area and risk of granulation tissue formation with subsequent stenosis. Meticulous postoperative aural hygiene is required until epithelialization is complete.

Synovial Chondromatosis of the Temporomandibular Joint

Definition. *Synovial chondromatosis of the temporomandibular joint* (TMJ) is a reactive process of unknown pathogenesis characterized by the formation of multiple cartilaginous nodules in the synovium; many become detached and float within the joint space. Synonyms include *synovial osteochondromatosis* and *synovial chondrometaplasia* (74).

Clinical Features. TMJ synovial chondromatosis is more common in women and generally occurs in adults. Patients may present with preauricular swelling, limited motion of the TMJ, and deviation of the mandible. Synovial chondromatosis of the TMJ involving the external auditory canal results in an asymptomatic mass lesion (75–80).

The radiographic features include the presence of numerous radiopaque loose bodies within the region of the joint without bone destruction (fig. 7-17) (81). Computerized tomography (CT) scan is excellent to define the bony surfaces of the articular joints but fails to detect loose bodies when these are not yet calcified (82,83). Magnetic resonance imaging (MRI) is considered the gold standard when the diagnosis is suspected since it can visualize loose bodies at early stage and also evaluate disc and eventual extra-articular tissue involvement (fig. 7-17) (82–84). On T2-weighted MRI, signs of low-signal nodules within amorphous iso-intensity signal tissues and signs of low- and intermediate-signal nodules within joint fluids are used to detect loose cartilaginous nodules. This condition occurs in association with pseudogout (calcium pyrophosphate dihydrate deposition disease) on rare occasion (85).

Pathogenesis. Synovial chondromatosis is a condition in which foci of cartilage develop in the synovial membrane of a joint, apparently through metaplasia of the sublining connective tissue of the synovial membrane. Fibroblast growth factor 2 (FGF-2) is expressed in chondrocytes and fibroblast-like cells of the loose bodies, and is believed to be involved in the pathogenesis (86). Transforming growth factor beta 3 (TGF-β3), which is closely related to chondrogenic differentiation, may also participate in the pathogenesis of synovial chondromastosis (87). Recent studies have shown clonal chromosomal alterations

Ear and Temporal Bone

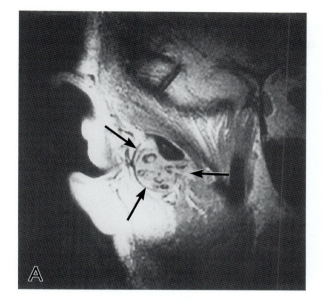
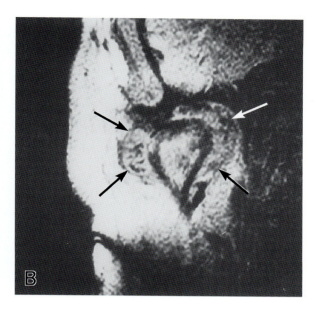
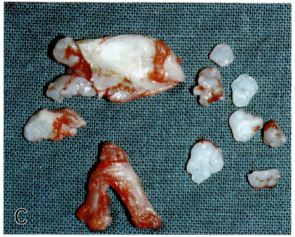
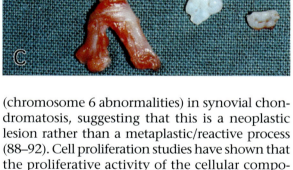

Figure 7-17

SYNOVIAL CHONDROMATOSIS WITH SYNOVIAL BODIES

A: Sagittal image shows expansion of the joint capsule (arrows) with multiple low signal density rounded bodies in the joint.

B: Coronal proton-density magnetic resonance imaging (MRI) shows expansion of the lateral and medial capsule walls (arrows), which indicates a neoplastic intraarticular process with multiple areas of low signal intensity consistent with synovial chondromatosis.

C: Small bodies of cartilage removed from this joint. (Fig. 23-13 from Wenig BM. Atlas of head and neck pathology, 3rd ed. Philadelphia: Elsevier; 2016:1095.)

(chromosome 6 abnormalities) in synovial chondromatosis, suggesting that this is a neoplastic lesion rather than a metaplastic/reactive process (88–92). Cell proliferation studies have shown that the proliferative activity of the cellular composition of synovial chondromatosis is between that of enchondroma and chondrosarcoma (93).

Gross Findings. The synovium may be diffusely studded with innumerable nodules (fig. 7-17). The nodules are polypoid or pedunculated with a delicate stalk, and vary in size from as small as 1 mm to 3 cm. The external surface varies from smooth to convoluted and granular.

Microscopic Findings. Histologically, synovial chondromatosis shows the presence of nodules of cartilage within the synovium and lying loosely in the joint space. The cartilage may appear atypical, with hypercellularity, hyperchromasia, and binucleated chondrocytes (fig. 7-18). There may be increased mitotic activity. Calcification and ossification may be present. There is no increase in proliferation activity as determined by Ki-67 (MIB-1) staining (94).

Differential Diagnosis. The histologic features seen in synovial chondromatosis, including increased cellularity with binucleated chondrocytes, may suggest chondrosarcoma. Correlation with the radiographic appearance is essential to differentiate these lesions. Radiographically, synovial chondromatosis includes the presence of numerous radiopaque loose bodies within the region of the joint.

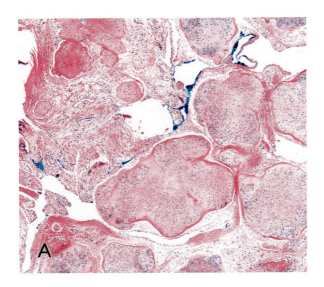
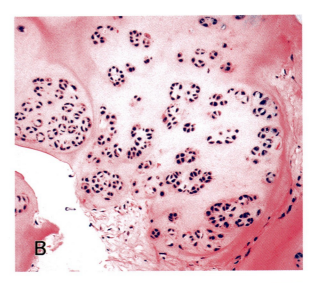
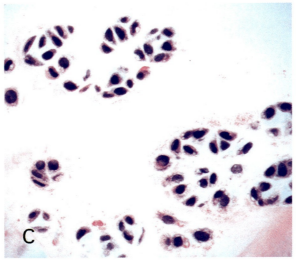
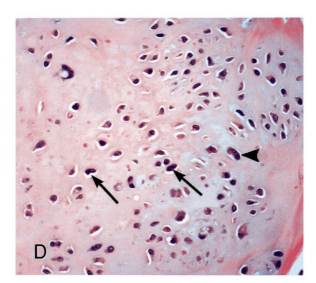
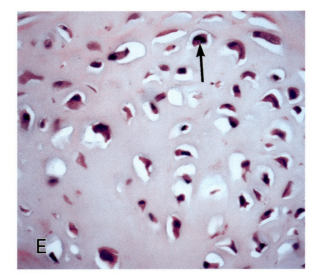

Figure 7-18

SYNOVIAL CHONDROMATOSIS OF THE TEMPOROMANDIBULAR JOINT

A: The excised tissue includes multiple nodular foci of cartilage.

B,C: There is increased cellularity but no significant nuclear pleomorphism or features worrisome for a chondrosarcoma.

D: Another example of synovial chondromatosis with atypical features including increased cellularity with nuclear pleomorphism, hyperchromasia, and binucleated (arrows) and trinucleated (arrowhead) chondrocytes.

E: At higher magnification, there is hypercellularity, nuclear hyperchromasia, pleomorphism, and a binucleated chondrocyte (arrow). Clinical and radiologic correlation is indicated in order to avoid an erroneous diagnosis of a low-grade chondrosarcoma.

Table 7-2

DIFFERENTIATION OF KIMURA DISEASE AND EPITHELIOID HEMANGIOMA

	Kimura Disease	EH (ALHE)[a]
Gender	M>F	M=F or F>M
Peak incidence	2nd to 3rd decade	3rd to 5th decades
Head and neck site	Postauricular, scalp	Periauricular, forehead
Lymphadenopathy	Common	Absent to Rare
Peripheral eosinophilia	>50%	<25%
Location	more deeply situated extending to the subcutaneous fat, fascia, and skeletal muscle	more superficial situated in subcutaneous, dermis
Histology	lymphoid proliferation predominates, vascular component is sparse with minimal epithelioid endothelial changes; numerous eosinophils	nodular vascular proliferation accompanied by a variably dense lymphoid infiltrate rich in eosinophils

[a]EH = epithelioid hemangioma; ALHE = angiolymphoid hyperplasia with eosinophilia.

Treatment and Prognosis. Conservative surgical management is the treatment of choice (76,95). The prognosis is good. The lesion is usually confined to the joint space itself and is easily enucleated. On occasion, the tumor extends beyond the joint capsule into the parotid gland, auditory canal, temporal bone, or even the cranial cavity and skull base (96–100). Reported cases of synovial chondrosarcoma suggest the possibility of malignant transformation (101–103).

Kimura Disease and Epithelioid Hemangioma

Definition. *Epithelioid hemangioma* (EH), also known as *angiolymphoid hyperplasia with eosinophilia* (ALHE), is a controversial lesion with regard to its classification (reactive proliferation or neoplastic process) and its relationship to *Kimura disease*. A reactive etiology, especially secondary to trauma, has been proposed but a neoplastic origin is favored (104). EH is considered to represent the benign end of the spectrum of vascular tumors characterized by epithelioid endothelial cells, many of which are rich in lymphocytes and eosinophils. The malignant end of the spectrum includes epithelioid hemangioendothelioma and epithelioid angiosarcoma.

EH shares features with Kimura disease, but the clinical and histologic differences allow these entities to be separated and considered as distinct clinicopathologic entities (Table 7-2) (105–110).

Clinical Features. Kimura disease primarily occurs in Asians and tends to affect males. It is often associated with regional lymphadenopathy and peripheral eosinophilia; increased serum immunoglobulin E (IgE), proteinuria, and nephrotic syndrome may occur as part of the disease. The lesions in Kimura disease tend to be larger than those of EH and are predominantly subcutaneous nodules with a tendency to occur in locations other than in the head and neck. Kimura disease is usually located much deeper than EH, often extending to the fascia and skeletal muscle. The subcutaneous fat is usually quite fibrotic. The etiology is unknown. The peripheral eosinophilia and elevated serum IgE suggest an immunologic reaction to an unknown stimulus.

EH is a benign angiomatous subcutaneous proliferation with a predilection for the external ear (auricle and external canal), as well as other head and neck sites, including the scalp and forehead (111,112). EH most frequently occurs in the third to fifth decades of life; there is no gender predilection. Symptoms include pruritus and bleeding following scratching. Regional lymphadenopathy and peripheral eosinophilia are uncommon but may be present. A history of trauma elicited in a number of cases, as well as the microscopic impression of vascular damage, and the demonstration of immunoglobulin deposits in the vessels, have lead several observers to favor a reactive or reparative etiology (111–113). Hormonal influences may play a role in some cases, as suggested by the association with pregnancy in some patients and by the age and gender distribution of the disease. Human herpesvirus 8 (HHV8) has not been identified in association with EH.

Figure 7-19
EPITHELIOID HEMANGIOMA (ANGIOLYMPHOID HYPERPLASIA WITH EOSINOPHILIA)

A: This lesion is a dermal, nodular proliferation granulation-like tissue with a patchy inflammatory cell infiltrate that is accompanied by haphazardly arranged, small caliber, irregularly shaped blood vessels.

B: The vascular spaces are lined by plump pleomorphic (epithelioid) endothelial cells with hyperchromatic nuclei. The inflammatory component is characterized by an admixture of mature lymphocytes, numerous eosinophils, and scattered histiocytes.

C: The vascular spaces are lined by plump-appearing (epithelioid) endothelial cells (arrow).

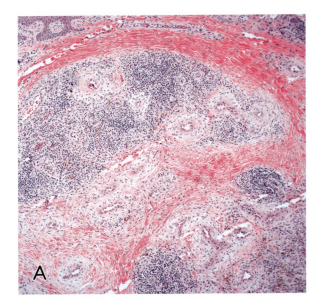

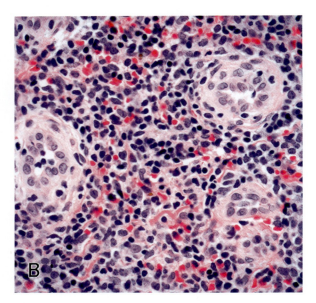

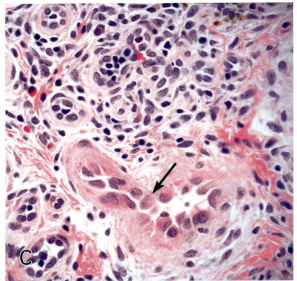

Gross Findings. Grossly, EH is characterized by single or multiple, pink to red-brown indurated cutaneous papules or subcutaneous nodules. These lesions measure from a few millimeters to 1 cm in diameter. Clusters of papules may coalesce to form large plaque-like lesions (111,112).

Microscopic Findings. Histologically, EH is characterized by a nodular vascular proliferation accompanied by a variably dense lymphoid infiltrate rich in eosinophils (fig. 7-19). The process is circumscribed but not encapsulated, and may involve the subcutis, dermis, or both. The vascular component varies in size from capillary to medium-sized arteries and veins. The vascular spaces are lined by plump-appearing (epithelioid) endothelial cells with pleomorphism, hyperchromatic nuclei, copious eosinophilic cytoplasm, and inconspicuous nucleoli (fig. 7-19) (104,107,111). Frequently, the endothelial cells protrude into the vessel lumen in a "hobnail" fashion, creating a cobblestone-like appearance (106). Increased mitotic activity and moderate to marked nuclear pleomorphism is not identified.

The lobular arrangement of the proliferating vessels in EH may be evident, or the distribution of vessels may be haphazard. The vessels vary

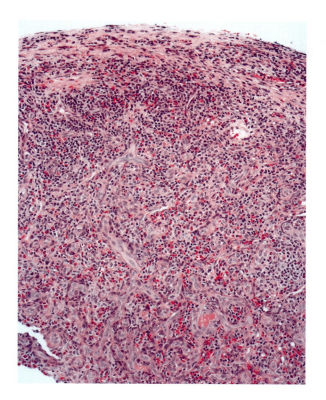 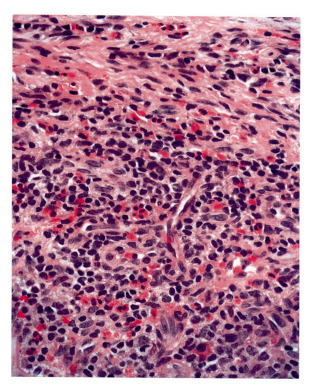

Figure 7-20

KIMURA DISEASE

Left: This lesion was deeply situated in the subcutis, and shows a nodular proliferation of inflammatory cells separated by fibrous tissue.

Right: A mature lymphoid cell proliferation predominates, with admixed eosinophils; the vascular component is sparse, and it lacks the epithelioid endothelial changes seen in angiolymphoid hyperplasia with eosinophilia.

from irregular, poorly canalized thin-walled spaces to rounded, well-formed vessels with thickened walls. In some cases there is evidence of disruption or damage to some of the involved vessels. The origin from a small artery or vein is common but may be dependent on adequate sampling. It is common for the entire lesion to be intravascular (*intravascular EH*) which differs from "conventional" EH by the predominant spindle cell (pericytic) component, predominantly occurring in young to middle-aged adults and presenting as a solitary nodule most often in head and neck or upper limb (114,115). In EH, an inflammatory component surrounds the vascular proliferation and is characterized by an admixture of lymphocytes, histiocytes, and eosinophils; on occasion, eosinophils are few in number or absent.

By immunohistochemical staining, the endothelial cells are reactive for CD31, ERG, and to a lesser extent, CD34. Glucose transporter protein 1 (GLUT1) is negative. Rarely, cytokeratin reactivity is present.

Kimura disease shares many histologic features with EH. In contrast to EH, however, subtle histologic differences are seen. In Kimura disease the lymphoid proliferation predominates and the vascular component is sparse and exhibits minimal epithelioid endothelial changes (fig. 7-20). Eosinophils are always numerous in Kimura disease but may be sparse or even absent in HE. An eosinophilic epithelioid granulomatous reaction or eosinophilic microabscess formation may be identified (116).

Differential Diagnosis. Kimura disease and EH need to be differentiated. Angiosarcoma, also in the differential diagnosis, is a diffusely infiltrative lesion composed of anastomosing vascular channels lined by pleomorphic cells with increased mitotic activity. The characteristic inflammatory infiltrate in Kimura disease and EH is typically not found in angiosarcoma.

Treatment and Prognosis. For Kimura disease and EH, surgical excision or desiccation is the treatment of choice and is curative. Recurrence is occasional. In EH, medical regimens, including intralesional or systemic steroids, have been used with some success in treating symptoms but have not proven to be curative. Investigational protocol of intralesional vincristine, bleomycin, and fluorouracil has not been proven to be of value (117). Malignant transformation or association with malignancy is not reported.

INFECTIOUS DISEASES OF THE EXTERNAL EAR

Necrotizing External Otitis

Definition. *Necrotizing external otitis* (NEO) is a virulent and potentially fatal form of external otitis related to *Pseudomonas aeruginosa* infection. Synonyms include *malignant external otitis* and *necrotizing granulomatous otitis*.

Clinical Features. There is no gender predilection and NEO primarily affects older patients. The typical patient is diabetic (118,119), chronically debilitated, or immunologically deficient (120). NEO, however, may occur in nondebilitated patients (121). NEO originates in the external auditory canal, with the initial symptoms of acute otitis externa. With progression of disease, pain, purulent otorrhea, and swelling occur. If left untreated, the infectious process may extend into the surrounding soft tissue structures (cellulitis), cartilage (chondritis), bone (osteomyelitis), base of skull, and the middle ear space leading to cranial nerve palsies, meningitis, intracranial venous thrombosis, and brain abscess (118,122–124).

Pathogenesis. The pathogenesis of NEO is related to tissue ischemia secondary to an underlying predisposing pathologic state (diabetic angiopathy) and a migratory defect of polymorphonuclear leukocytes related to systemic disease. Host factors that impede the inflammatory response to infection, combined with the destructive devices of *P. aeruginosa*, are thought to be responsible for the lethal potential of NEO (119). The organism, by virtue of its endotoxins and exotoxins, neurotoxins, collagenases, and elastases, is capable of causing rapid extensive

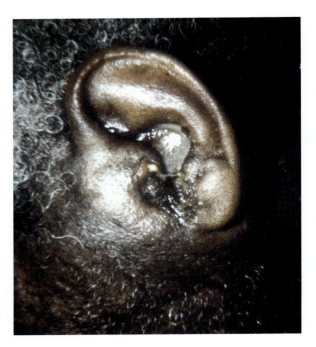

Figure 7-21

NECROTIZING EXTERNAL OTITIS

This diabetic patient complained of aural-related pain. Clinically, purulent otorrhea is present.

tissue necrosis and necrotizing vasculitis, which compound the destruction (119).

Gross Findings. The changes of NEO are most pronounced in the osseous portion of the external canal, where the destructive infection usually begins. In this area, the skin becomes ulcerated, leaving a layer of thick granulation tissue covering the exposed and irregularly eroded bone, usually along the anterior and inferior surfaces of the external auditory canal (125). Necrotic tissue is abundant in fully developed NEO, and may, along with a purulent exudate, obstruct the canal (fig. 7-21).

Microscopic Findings. The histologic appearance of NEO is dominated by surface epithelial ulceration with abundant necrosis, acute and chronic inflammation, and granulation tissue (fig. 7-22). Intact adjacent squamous epithelium may show pseudoepitheliomatous hyperplasia. Marked acute and chronic inflammatory manifestations are seen in the subcutis, and necrotizing vasculitis is commonly present. The bone and cartilage are necrotic, with acute and chronic inflammatory cells massively infiltrating adjacent

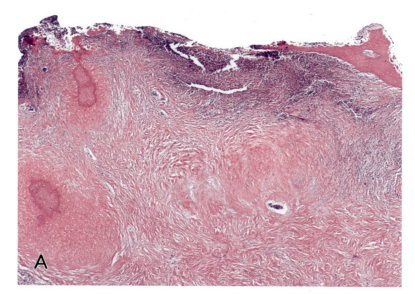

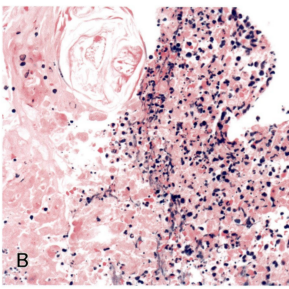
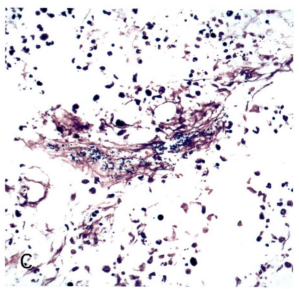

Figure 7-22
NECROTIZING EXTERNAL OTITIS
A: The histologic appearance includes thick, acellular collagen replacing the skin and subcutaneous tissues, with inflammation and necrosis extending within the depth of the tissue to underlying bone (osteomyelitis).
B: Surface ulceration with associated neutrophilic infiltrate.
C: Gram stain shows the presence of numerous Gram-negative bacilli.

viable bone. Sequestration of nonviable bone or cartilage may be seen. The dermis is eventually replaced by acellular collagen.

Special stains for microorganisms show the presence of Gram-negative bacilli easily demonstrated by tissue Gram stain (fig. 7-22). Stains for other microorganisms (e.g., fungus, mycobacteria, protozoa, virus) are usually negative.

Differential Diagnosis. The infectious nature of NEO is usually evident from the clinical course and the histologic findings. The presence of pseudoepitheliomatous hyperplasia (PEH) of the squamous epithelium, with or without an accompanying striking reactive atypia, may suggest a squamous cell carcinoma. Conversely, squamous cell carcinoma, if associated with extensive necrosis, may elude diagnosis by biopsy when only necroinflammatory material, such as present in NEO, is seen. Occasionally, the clinical presentation of squamous cell carcinoma of the external auditory canal closely mimics that of NEO (126,127) or the two diseases occur concurrently (128). In contrast to squamous cell carcinoma, the epithelial proliferation in PEH is cytomorphologically bland and without dysplastic changes.

Treatment and Prognosis. Antibiotic therapy, surgical debridement, and control of diabetes in patients suffering from that disease are the treatments of choice. Cure is achieved with early recognition and aggressive treatment. Combination therapy with intravenous ceftazidime and oral fluoroquinolone remains relevant despite concerns of culture-negative cases and multidrug-resistant *Pseudomonas*. Fungal (aspergillus, others) and polymicrobial temporal bone infections have been reported with increasing frequency (129) and in culture negative or multidrug resistant cases, considerations should be given to causes by organisms other than *P. aeruginosa*. Hyperbaric oxygen therapy may be utilized as an adjunctive modality.

Despite advances in antibiotic treatment, a significant proportion of patients die from this disease. Mortality rates may exceed 75 percent if diagnosis and treatment are delayed (122). Death may result from extensive spread of the infection to adjacent structures including intracranial involvement; involvement of the clivus portends a poorer prognosis (123).

INFECTIOUS AND INFLAMMATORY LESIONS OF THE MIDDLE EAR AND TEMPORAL BONE

Otitis Media

Definition. *Otitis media* is an acute or chronic infectious disease of the middle ear space.

Clinical Features. Otitis media is predominantly, but not exclusively, a childhood disease. Otoscopic examination reveals a hyperemic, opaque, bulging tympanic membrane with limited mobility; purulent otorrhea may be present. Bilateral involvement is common. The middle ear infection is felt to result from infection via the eustachian tube at the time of or following pharyngitis (bacterial or viral).

The most common organisms implicating in causing disease are *Streptococcus pneumoniae* and *Haemophilus influenza*. Uncommonly, otitis media is caused by tuberculosis (130–132); syphilis (133,134); fungi, including *Candida, Mucor, Cryptococcus*, and *Aspergillus* (135); and actinomycosis (136).

The setting for some of these infections, particularly the mycoses, is in patients who are diabetic or debilitated (135). In patients infected with human immunodeficiency virus (HIV) or who have acquired immunodeficiency syndrome (AIDS), *Pneumocystis jiroveci* (formerly *carinii*) is the most common opportunistic organism, usually associated with pneumonia in the immunodeficient host and the most common life-threatening infection in AIDS patients. It is unusual for *P. jiroveci* to cause clinical manifestations outside of the pulmonary system. In the head and neck, *P. jiroveci* infection has involved the external auditory canal and the middle ear (137). The clinical manifestations include ear pain, hypomobility of the tympanic membrane, and otitis media, as well as conductive and sensorineural hearing losses. In this setting, the initial clinical presentation may occur as an aural polyp that by histologic examination shows a characteristic foamy exudate containing the causative organisms (137). The presumed mode of dissemination from the lung to extrapulmonary sites is via vascular channels. Typically, the pulmonary manifestations of pneumocystis infection precede those of extrapulmonary involvement, however, on occasion the diagnosis of AIDS is made following identification of its associated pathology in extrapulmonary locations.

Viruses, including herpes, cytomegalovirus, rubella, rubeola, and mumps, can infect this region. They may result in labyrinthitis and sensorineural hearing deafness (132).

Gross Findings. There are no specific macroscopic features. The tissue specimens usually are received as multiple small fragments of soft to rubbery granulation tissue. If tympanosclerosis is present, then the tissues may be firm to hard, consisting of calcific debris. In general, all of the tissue fragments should be processed for histologic examination.

Microscopic Findings. The histology of otitis media varies and depends on the disease state (138). *Acute otitis media* is virtually never a surgical disease. The inflammatory infiltrate in acute otitis media is predominantly composed of polymorphonuclear leukocytes with a variable admixture of chronic inflammatory cells. *Secretory otitis media* is an effusion behind an intact tympanic membrane; the exudate may be serous, hemorrhagic, fibrinous, mucoid, purulent, or an admixture of types.

Acute otitis media usually heals by resorption by the mucoperiosteum; localized destruction

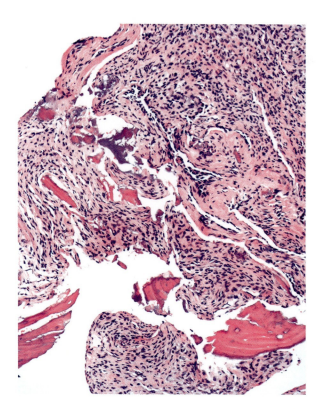 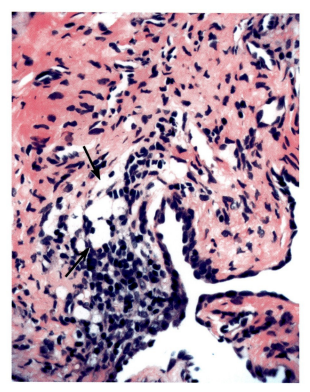

Figure 7-23

CHRONIC OTITIS MEDIA

Left: At low magnification, middle ear epithelium is seen as a thin, flattened to cuboidal epithelial layer lining slit-like spaces, with associated chronic inflammation and fibrosis. Foci of dystrophic mineralization (calcification or ossification) represent the tympanosclerosis often occurring in the setting of recurrent episodes of otitis media.

Right: At higher magnification, chronic inflammation, including mature lymphocytes with admixed foamy histiocytes (arrows), is subjacent to the middle ear epithelium, which appears as flattened to cuboidal cells.

of the middle ear ossicles may occur and granulation tissue may develop, resulting in scar formation. *Fibrosing osteitis,* seen in areas of bone destruction, may result in reactive sclerotic bone. Acute inflammatory cells may be superimposed in *chronic otitis media* (COM).

The histologic changes in COM include a variable amount of chronic inflammatory cells consisting of lymphocytes, histiocytes, plasma cells, and eosinophils, as well as fibrosis. Multinucleated giant cells and foamy histiocytes may be present (fig. 7-23). The low cuboidal epithelium of the middle ear may or may not be seen (fig. 7-23). Glandular metaplasia, a response of the middle ear epithelium to the infectious process, may be present. The glands tend to be more common in nonsuppurative otitis media than in suppurative otitis media. The metaplastic glands are unevenly distributed in the tissue specimens, are variable shaped, and are separated by abundant stromal tissue (fig. 7-24). The glands are lined by columnar to cuboidal epithelium, with or without cilia or goblet cell metaplasia. Glandular secretions may or may not be present, so that the glands may appear empty or contain varying secretions, including thin (serous) or thick (mucoid) fluid. The identification of cilia is confirmatory of middle ear glandular metaplasia and is a feature not found in association with middle ear adenomas (139). In addition to the inflammatory cell infiltrate and glandular metaplasia, other histopathologic findings that usually are seen in association with COM include fibrosis, granulation tissue, calcifications, cholesterol granulomas, and reactive bone formation. Unusual histologic examples of COM include those with a polypoid appearance resulting from the presence of an edematous stroma.

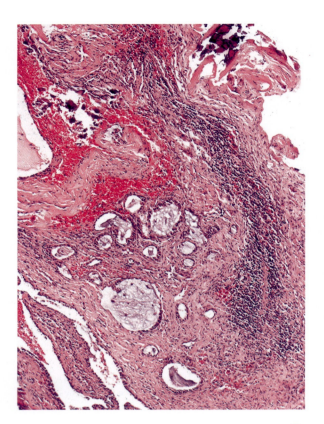 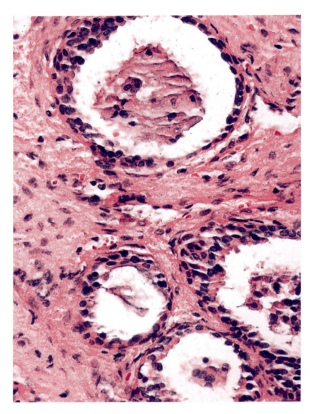

Figure 7-24

CHRONIC OTITIS MEDIA WITH GLANDULAR METAPLASIA

Left: The excised tissue shows a chronic inflammatory cell infiltrate, fibrosis, hemorrhage, foci of calcification (tympanosclerosis), and areas of scattered unevenly distributed metaplastic glandular proliferation; in the lower left of the image are slit-like spaces lined by flattened to cuboidal middle ear epithelial cells.

Right: The glands are lined by a cuboidal to focally columnar epithelium containing serous fluid and surrounding a lymphoplasmacytoid cell infiltrate.

Tympanosclerosis is the dystrophic mineralization (calcification or ossification) of the tympanic membrane or middle ear that is associated with recurrent episodes of otitis media (141). Tympanosclerotic foci may be localized or diffuse, and appear as white nodules or plaques. Histologically, dense "clumps" of mineralized calcified or ossified material or debris are seen within the stromal tissues or in the middle (connective tissue) aspect of the tympanic membrane (fig. 7-25). Tympanosclerosis may cause scarring and ossicular fixation.

Cholesterol granuloma is a foreign body granulomatous response to cholesterol crystals derived from the rupture of red blood cells, with breakdown of the lipid layer of the erythrocyte cell membrane. Cholesterol granulomas arise in the middle ear in any condition in which there is hemorrhage combined with interference in drainage and ventilation of the middle ear space; this results in the otoscopic picture referred to as "blue ear syndrome" (141). The patients may complain of hearing loss and tinnitus. The histology of cholesterol granulomas includes the presence of irregular-shaped, clear spaces surrounded by histiocytes or multinucleated giant cells (foreign body granuloma) (fig. 7-26). Cholesterol granulomas are not related to cholesteatomas but may occur in association with or independent of a cholesteatoma. Tympanosclerosis and cholesterol granulomas may occur independent of otitis media; cholesteatomas may or may not be associated with otitis media.

Differential Diagnosis. The differential diagnosis of the glandular metaplasia seen in otitis media includes a middle ear adenoma (142). The

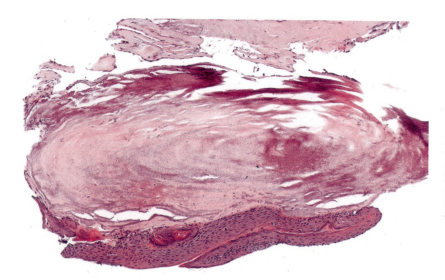

Figure 7-25

TYMPANOSCLEROSIS

Prominent calcification (center) adheres to the tympanic membrane, which is covered on its external (external auditory canal) aspect by keratinizing squamous epithelium (bottom) and on its internal (tympanic cavity) aspect by cuboidal epithelium (top).

haphazard arrangement of the glands and the presence of cilia, occurring in a background of chronic otitis media, should allow for the differentiation of metaplastic from neoplastic glands. The differentiation of chronic otitis media with glandular metaplasia from a middle ear adenoma is generally straightforward. The glandular metaplasia of the surface epithelium resulting from chronic inflammation, however, may be confused with a true gland-forming neoplasm. In middle ear adenomas, the histology is dominated by the presence of a diffuse glandular or solid cell proliferation (fig. 7-27) rather than the haphazard arrangement of the glands in the background of changes of chronic otitis media. A significant number of middle ear adenomas show neuroendocrine features by light microscopy or immunohistochemical staining, engendering nomenclature that includes middle ear adenoma with neuroendocrine differentiation and neuroendocrine adenoma of the middle ear (143). The identification of cilia is confirmatory of middle ear glandular metaplasia and is a feature that is not found in association with middle ear adenomas.

Myospherulosis is an iatrogenically induced pseudomycotic lesion resulting from the interaction of red blood cells and petrolatum-based ointments used after surgery for packing wounds. The myospherules originate from red blood cells that react with the petrolatum or lanolin found in the ointment (144). Typically, prior to the development of a mass, patients had surgery for a variety of disease processes (inflammatory or neoplastic lesions), followed by packing of the area with a petrolatum-based ointment (145).

Chronic otorrhea resulting from myospeherulosis following tympanoplastic has been reported (146–148). Histologically, myospherulosis is characterized by the presence of cysts devoid of an epithelial lining (pseudocysts), embedded within fibrotic tissue, with an associated chronic inflammatory infiltrate composed of lymphocytes, histiocytes, giant cells, and plasma cells (fig. 7-28). The pseudocysts contain round, sac-like structures called "parent bodies" (fig. 7-28); these parent bodies in turn contain numerous spherules or endobodies. Special stains for fungi are invariably negative and assist in differentiating myospherulosis from fungal infections (e.g., rhinosporidiosis, coccidioidomycosis). Treatment is symptomatic.

Malakoplakia, an inflammatory disease that usually involves the genitourinary tract, may occur in the middle ear (149,150). Malakoplakia is derived from Greek and means "soft plaque." The light microscopic features include the presence of solid sheets of histiocytes with slightly granular to vacuolated cytoplasm (so-called Hansemann cells) admixed with inflammatory cells, including lymphocytes, plasma cells, and neutrophils (fig. 7-29). Intracytoplasmic diastase-resistant PAS-positive targetoid basophilic inclusion bodies, termed Michaelis-Gutman bodies, are present within occasional cells. These inclusions, or calcospherites, which

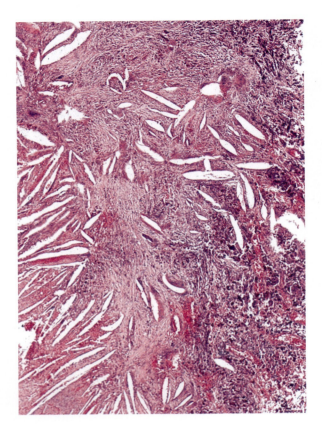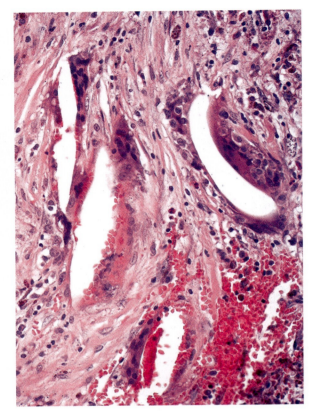

Figure 7-26

CHOLESTEROL GRANULOMA

Left, right: Cholesterol granulomas appear as empty, irregularly shaped clefts or spaces surrounded by histiocytes and multinucleated giant cells. Fresh hemorrhage and hemosiderin pigment are apparent.

Figure 7-27

MIDDLE EAR ADENOMA

In contrast to the glandular metaplasia associated with chronic otitis media, in middle ear adenomas there is a diffuse glandular (and solid) proliferation.

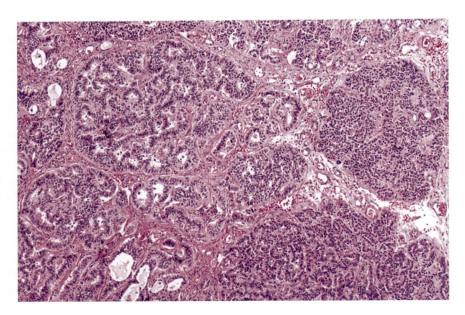

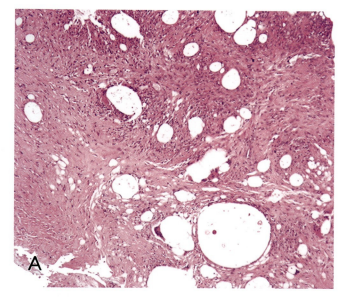

Figure 7-28
MYOSPHERULOSIS

A,B: Myospherulosis is histologically characterized by the presence of cysts devoid of an epithelial lining (pseudocysts) embedded within fibrotic tissue.

C: The pseudocysts contain round, sac-like structures termed "parent bodies" (arrow) that in turn contain numerous spherules or endobodies. Special stains for microorganisms are invariable negative.

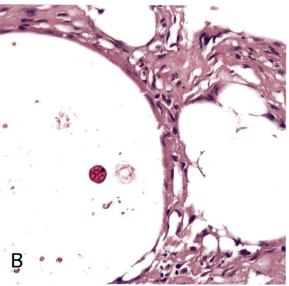
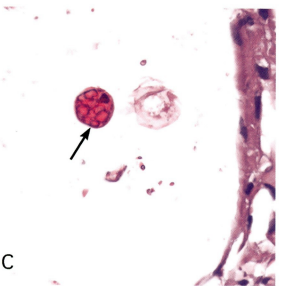

are also seen extracellularly, contain calcium and frequently iron salts, thereby showing reactivity with the von Kossa stain for calcium and Prussian blue stain for iron. Malakoplakia is believed to represent an unusual host response to infection with a variety of organisms and ultrastructurally, phagolysosomes that have ingested breakdown products of bacteria such as *Escherichia coli* have been found.

Treatment and Prognosis. In general, otitis media is managed medically. At times, however, tissue is removed for histopathologic examination. Recurrent infections of the middle ear are common, especially in the pediatric population. In adults, an unresolving otitis media should warrant detailed examination of the nasopharynx in order to rule out the presence of a (malignant) neoplasm (i.e., nasopharyngeal carcinoma). Squamous cell carcinomas of the middle ear typically arise in patients with (longstanding) chronic otitis media. In the antibiotic era, complications associated with otitis media are not generally seen; however, if left unchecked, intratemporal complications (e.g., mastoiditis, petrositis, labyrinthitis, facial nerve paralysis) and intracranial complications

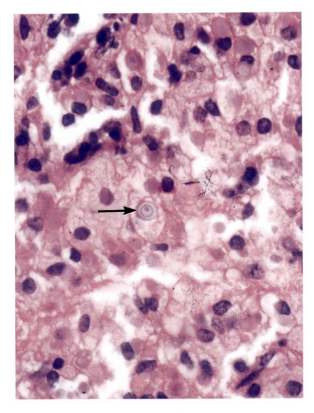

Figure 7-29
MALAKOPLAKIA OF THE MIDDLE EAR
Solid sheets of histiocytes with slightly granular to vacuolated cytoplasm (so-called Hansemann cells) are seen. Intracytoplasmic basophilic inclusion bodies (Michaelis-Gutman bodies) with a targetoid appearance (arrow) are also present.

(e.g., meningitis, lateral sinus thrombophlebitis, brain abscess) may occur (151–156).

Otic (Aural) Polyp

Definition. *Otic (aural) polyp*, also termed *inflammatory polyp*, is an inflammatory polypoid proliferation that originates from the middle ear mucosa as a result of chronic otitis media.

Clinical Features. Otic polyps occur at any age but are most common in children. The symptoms include otorrhea, conductive hearing loss, and a mass protruding from the external auditory canal (157). For large polyps that completely obstruct the external ear, radiographic studies are an invaluable aid in identifying the origin of the polyp. Despite origin from the middle ear, otic polyps may perforate the tympanic membrane and extend into the external auditory canal (158). In this situation, the polyp may appear to be originating from the external auditory canal. In longstanding cases, destruction (partial or complete) of the ossicles may occur (158).

Rarely, otic polyps occur in association with Samter triad/syndrome (159,160), which is characterized by aspirin intolerance, sinonasal polyps, and asthma. In association with Samter triad/syndrome, otic polyps tend to be bilateral and associated with conductive hearing loss, persistent otorrhea, and aural fullness. Otic polyps may represent a secondary immunologic dysfunction and chronic otologic inflammation as a result of Samter triad/syndrome.

Gross Findings. Otic polyps are polypoid, soft to rubbery, tan-white to pink-red lesions.

Microscopic Findings. The polypoid mass is a cellular infiltrate primarily consisting of a chronic inflammatory cell infiltrate, including mature lymphocytes, plasma cells, histiocytes, and eosinophils (fig. 7-30). Russell bodies or Mott cells containing large eosinophilic immunoglobules are seen and are indicative of a benign plasma cell proliferation. Polymorphonuclear leukocytes may be present. The stroma includes granulation tissue that varies in appearance from edematous and richly vascularized to fibrous with a decreased vascular component. Multinucleated giant cells, cholesterol granulomas, and calcific debris (tympanosclerosis) may be present. An overlying epithelium may not be seen but when present, appears as pseudostratified columnar or cuboidal cells with or without cilia. Foci of squamous metaplasia and a glandular metaplastic proliferation may also be seen. Special stains for microorganisms (e.g., fungi, spirochetes, mycobacteria, protozoa, and parasites) are negative but are indicated in order to rule out an infectious etiology.

Differential Diagnosis. In general, the presence of a mixed cell population of chronic inflammatory cells is benign so that a diagnosis of a malignant lymphoproliferative process is not an issue. Rarely, lymphomatous or leukemic involvement of the middle ear and temporal bone occur secondary to systemic disease.

The dense plasma cell component may lead to consideration of a plasmacytoma. While plasma cell dyscrasia may rarely occur in this site, the presence of mature plasma cells, Russell bodies,

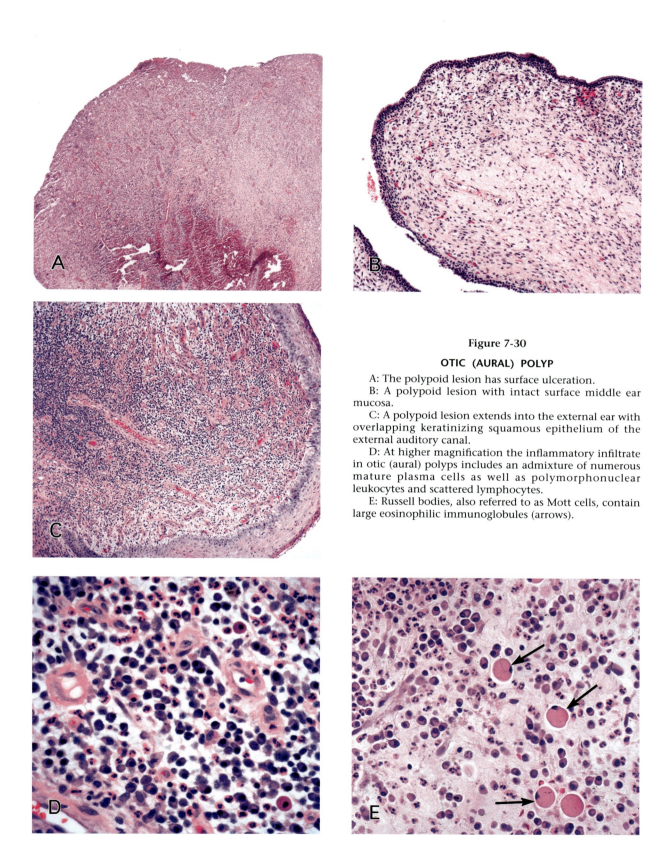

Figure 7-30

OTIC (AURAL) POLYP

A: The polypoid lesion has surface ulceration.

B: A polypoid lesion with intact surface middle ear mucosa.

C: A polypoid lesion extends into the external ear with overlapping keratinizing squamous epithelium of the external auditory canal.

D: At higher magnification the inflammatory infiltrate in otic (aural) polyps includes an admixture of numerous mature plasma cells as well as polymorphonuclear leukocytes and scattered lymphocytes.

E: Russell bodies, also referred to as Mott cells, contain large eosinophilic immunoglobules (arrows).

and polyclonality by immunohistochemistry should preclude a diagnosis of plasmacytoma.

The cellular component in otic polyps may be very dense and may obscure an underlying neoplastic process (e.g., rhabdomyosarcoma, Langerhans cell histiocytosis). If rhabdomyosarcoma is suspected, immunohistochemical stains for desmin, myogenin (MYF-4), and myoglobin assist in diagnosis. Langerhans cells are immunoreactive for S-100 protein, CD1a, and langerin. Other neoplasms that may present as aural polyps are meningioma, malignant melanoma, metastatic renal cell carcinoma, and adenoid cystic carcinoma.

Treatment and Prognosis. In the absence of an infectious etiology, surgical excision is curative.

Cholesteatoma

Definition. *Cholesteatoma* is a pseudoneoplastic lesion of the middle ear characterized by invasive growth and the presence of stratified squamous epithelium that forms a sac-like accumulaton of keratin within the middle ear space. Despite their invasive growth, cholesteatomas are not considered to be true neoplasms.

The term cholesteatoma is a misnomer since it is not a neoplasm and does not contain cholesterol. Other designations include *epidermal cyst* or *epidermal inclusion cyst of the middle ear* (161,162). Perhaps the designation of keratoma would be more accurate but the term cholesteatoma is entrenched in the literature. Cholesteatomas are divided into acquired and congenital types.

Acquired Cholesteatoma. Acquired cholesteatomas is the most common type of cholesteatoma. It is more common in men than in women, and is most common in the third to fourth decades of life. The middle ear space, specifically the upper posterior part of the middle ear space, is the most common site of acquired cholesteatomas (161–163). Most arise in the pars flaccida portion of the tympanic membrane and extend into Prussak space. Prussak space is bordered laterally by the pars flaccida (Schrapnell membrane), medially by the neck of the malleus, superiorly by the attachment of the pars flaccida to the tympanic ring near the scutum, and inferiorly by the lateral or short process of the malleus.

Initially, cholesteatomas may remain clinically silent until extensive invasion of the middle ear space and mastoid occurs. Symptoms include hearing loss, malodorous discharge, and pain and may be associated with a polyp arising in the attic of the middle ear or perforation of the tympanic membrane. Otoscopic examination may reveal the presence of white debris within the middle ear, which is considered diagnostic. Given the localization to Prussak space, most acquired cholesteatomas displace the malleus medially and erode the adjacent bony scutum; from there the mass may extend posteriorly via the epitympanum in the superior incudal space to the posterolateral attic, and then via the aditus ad antrum to the antrum and mastoid air spaces. Radiographic evidence of widening of the aditus is an important diagnostic finding (fig. 7-31).

Acquired cholesteatoma is thought to occur by the migration of squamous epithelium from the external auditory canal or from the external surface of the tympanic membrane into the middle ear. The mechanism by which the epithelium enters the middle ear probably is by a combination of events, including perforation of the tympanic membrane (particularly in its superior aspect, referred to as the pars flaccida or Shrapnell membrane, following an infection) coupled with invagination or retraction of the tympanic membrane into the middle ear as a result of longstanding negative pressure on the membrane secondary to blockage or obstruction of the eustachian tube (164). A decrease in middle ear pressure induces retraction of certain regions of the tympanic membrane in the pars flaccida, pars tensa, or both (164). Retraction pockets are felt to represent the precursors for the development of cholesteatoma (162,165). Dysfunction of the eustachian tube, leading to chronic (recurrent) otitis media, may be a causative factor (164). Other theories by which cholesteatomas are thought to occur include traumatic implantation and squamous metaplasia of the middle ear epithelium.

Congenital Cholesteatoma. Congenital cholesteatoma of the middle ear, also termed *epidermoid* (166) and *epidermoid cyst* (167), exists in the presence of an intact tympanic membrane. It presumably arises from the sequestration of epidermal cells at the time of closure of the neural groove between the third to fifth embryonic week (166). Unlike acquired

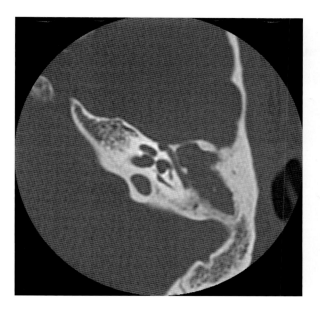
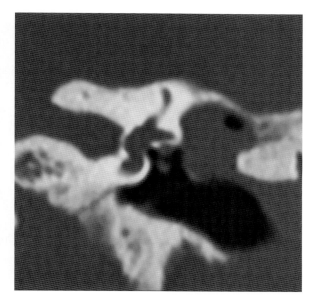

Figure 7-31

CHOLESTEATOMA

Axial (left) and coronal (right) CT images of the left ear demonstrate an expansile lesion involving the left epitympanum with associated erosive changes of the epitympanic ossicular chain and the scutum. (Courtesy of Dr. A. Khorsandi, New York, NY.)

cholesteatomas, congental cholesteatomas are thought to occur in the absence of the chronic otitis media that may result in perforation or retraction of the tympanic membrane (166). Congenital cholesteatomas are found in infants and young children. Most occur in the antero-superior part of the middle ear (166,168). In early lesions, there are no symptoms and lesions are discovered by otoscopic examination; in later lesions, the signs and symptoms may be the same as for acquired cholesteatoma.

Small colonies of epidermoid cells, referred to as epidermoid formations, are found on the lateral anterior-superior surface of the middle ear in the temporal bones after 15 weeks' gestation (169). During the first postpartum year, the epidermoid colonies disappear; however, if the epidermoid cells do not disappear but continue to grow they will become a congenital cholesteatoma.

Gross Findings. Cholesteatoma appears as a cystic, white to pearly white mass of varying size containing creamy or waxy granular material (169).

Microscopic Findings. Irrespective of the location, the histology of cholesteatoma remains the same. The histologic diagnosis is made in the presence of stratified keratinizing squamous epithelium, subepithelial fibroconnective or granulation tissue, and keratin debris (fig. 7-32). The essential diagnostic feature is the keratinizing squamous epithelium; the presence of keratin debris alone is not diagnostic of a cholesteatoma. The keratinizing squamous epithelium is cytologically bland and shows cellular maturation without evidence of dysplasia.

In spite of its benign histology, cholesteatomas are "invasive" and have widespread destructive capabilities (fig. 7-33). The destructive properties result from the mass effect causing pressure erosion of structures surrounding the cholesteatoma, the production of collagenase which has osteodestructive capabilities by its resorption of bony structures, and bone resorption (163). Collagenase is produced by both the squamous epithelial and the fibrous tissue components of the cholesteatoma. This local aggressive behavior is the result of the continuing accumulation of the cholesteatomatous material, with progressive erosion of surrounding structures. Depending on the location and extent of the cholesteatoma, erosion may include the lateral wall of the attic, the middle ear ossicles, the tegmental bone over the attic and antrum,

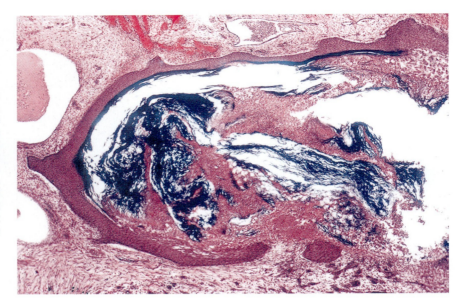

Figure 7-32

CHOLESTEATOMA

The histologic diagnosis of cholesteatoma is based on finding keratinizing squamous epithelium within the middle ear space. The keratinizing squamous epithelium shows cellular maturation and is cytologically bland, lacking dysplastic changes. The presence only of keratin debris without associated epithelium is not considered histologic evidence of cholesteatoma.

and the mastoid cortex (169). Less frequent progression includes erosion of the lateral sinus and jugular bulb, the vestibular and cochlear capsules, the fallopian canal, the dura of the middle and posterior cranial fossa, the semicircular canals, and the facial nerve (164). Sequelae of such erosions may include semicircular canal fistulas, exposed tympanic facial nerve, and brain herniation through the tegmon.

Molecular Genetic Findings. In cholesteatomas there is upregulation of human microRNA-21(HSA-miR-21) concurrent with downregulation of the potent tumor suppressor proteins, PTEN and programmed cell death 4 (170–172). These proteins control aspects of apoptosis, proliferation, invasion, and migration, and represent a model for cholesteatoma proliferation through microRNA dysregulation. Genes induced or upregulated in cholesteatoma include those involved in cell proliferation and differentiation (e.g., calgranulin A, calgranulin B, psoriasin, thymosin beta-10) and genes involved in cell invasion (e.g., cathepsin C, cathepsin D, cathepsin H) (173).

Proliferating cell nuclear antigen (PCNA) and osteoclast stimulating factor-1 (OSF-1), two proteins in the pathogenesis of cholesteatoma related to cellular proliferation and bone destruction, are upregulated (174). The EGFR/PI3K/Akt/cyclinD1 signaling pathway is active in cholesteatoma and may play a role in epithelial hyperproliferation (175). Keratinocyte growth factor (KGF), a mesenchymal cell-derived paracrine growth factor that specifically stimulates epithelial cell proliferation, is present in cholesteatomas (176). Keratinocyte growth factor protein (KGFR) and mRNA are localized in the epithelium in 72 percent of cases. A significant correlation has been reported between KGF/KGFR-positive expression and cholesteatoma recurrence (176).

Angiogenesis and angiogenic growth factors are present in cholesteatoma, and affect the close relationship seen between the density of capillaries, degree of inflammation, and expression of angiogenic factors (177). Angiogenesis enables and supports the sustained migration of keratinocytes into the middle ear cavity and represents a pivotal factor in the destructive behavior of middle ear cholesteatoma (177).

Differential Diagnosis. The histologic diagnosis of cholesteatoma is straightforward in the presence of keratinizing squamous epithelium. In contrast to cholesteatoma, squamous cell carcinoma shows dysplastic or overtly malignant cytologic features, with a prominent desmoplastic stromal response to its infiltrative growth. Cholesteatomas do not transform into squamous cell carcinomas. In an attempt to determine whether cholesteatomas are low-grade squamous carcinomas, Desloge et al. (178) performed DNA analysis on human cholesteatomas to determine whether ploidy abnormalities were

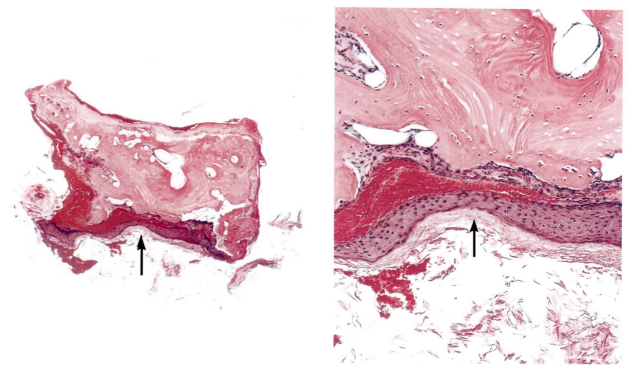

Figure 7-33

CHOLESTEATOMA INVOLVING MIDDLE EAR OSSICLES

Although considered a non-neoplastic process consisting of benign squamous epithelium, cholesteatomas may have infiltrative growth and destructive capability. Depending on the location and extent of the cholesteatoma, erosion may include the lateral wall of the attic, the middle ear ossicles, the tegmental bone over the attic and antrum, and the mastoid cortex. A, B: In these images there is osseous involvement, with the keratinizing squamous epithelium (arrows) diagnostic of a cholesteatoma adherent to bone of the middle ear ossicles.

present. Of 10 cases with interpretable data, 9 were euploid and one was aneuploid. These authors concluded that due to a lack of overt genetic instability, cholesteatomas could not be considered to be malignant neoplasms.

Cholesterol granuloma (see under Chronic Otitis Media) is not synonymous with cholesteatoma. These are different pathologic entities and should not be confused with one another.

Keratosis obturans (KO) results when the normal self-cleaning mechanism of keratin maturation and lateral extrusion from the external auditory canal is defective and keratin debris accumulates deep within the bony aspect of the external auditory canal. Radiologically, KO appears as homogeneous soft tissue filling the external auditory canal, with mild enlargement/widening but without bony erosion (fig. 7-34). The etiology of KO remains unclear. KO occurs most commonly in the first two decades of life and symptoms generally relate to conductive hearing loss due to the keratin plug (179). Pain is a common finding. The keratin debris may exert pressure effects on the bony canal wall, resulting in widening of the external auditory canal, bone remodelling, and inflamed epithelium. The histologic appearance is that of tightly packed keratin squames in a lamellar pattern. The treatment for KO is debridement of the keratin plug. In contrast to KO, external ear canal cholesteatomas generally occur in older individuals, present with otorrhea and unilateral chronic pain, do not produce conductive hearing loss, and are composed histologically of loosely packed, irregularly arranged keratin squames (179).

Treatment and Prognosis. Complete surgical excision of all histologic components of the cholesteatoma is the treatment of choice. If not completely excised, cholesteatomas can have progressive and destructive growth, including

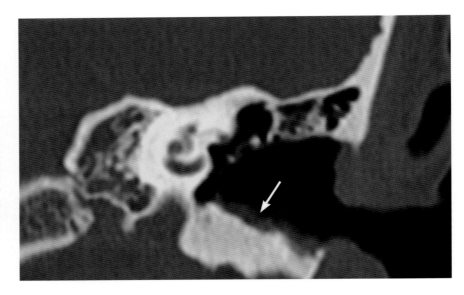

Figure 7-34

KERATOSIS OBTURANS OF THE EXTERNAL AUDITORY CANAL

Coronal CT image demonstrates irregular widening of all the dimensions of the external auditory canal in association with scalloping and remodeling of the cortical bone. Lining the floor of the external auditory canal is a rind of abnormal soft tissue density measuring up to 3 mm (arrow). (Courtesy of Dr. A. Khorsandi, New York, NY.)

widespread bone destruction, which may lead to hearing loss, facial nerve paralysis, labyrnthitis, meningitis, and epidural or brain abscess.

Langerhans Cell Histiocytosis

Definition. *Langerhans cell histiocytosis* (LCH) is a clonal proliferation of Langerhans cells (LCs) occurring as an isolated lesion or as part of a systemic (multifocal) proliferation (180,181). Synonyms include *Langerhans cell (eosinophilic) granulomatosis* (LCG) and *eosinophilic granuloma*. The designation of Langerhans cell histiocytosis has been used to replace the previous nomenclature of the group of diseases termed histiocytosis X, which includes eosinophilic granuloma, Letterer-Siwe syndrome, and Hand-Schüller-Christian disease. Lieberman et al. (182) suggested the designation of Langerhans cell (eosinophilic) granulomatosis to indicate that the LC represents a cellular component of the dendritic cell system rather than a tissue macrophage (histiocyte).

Clinical Features. LCH most commonly occurs in the second and third decades of life, and tends to predilect to males. The lesions are most often osseous based. The most frequently involved osseous sites are in the skull, including the middle ear and temporal bone (183–187). In patients with middle ear and temporal bone involvement, symptoms include aural discharge (otorrhea), swelling of the temporal bone area, otitis media, bone pain, otalgia, loss of hearing, and vertigo. Single or multiple, sharply circumscribed osteolytic lesions are seen radiographically (fig. 7-35).

Microscopic Findings. Histologically, LCH is characterized by a proliferation of LCs, which are arranged in sheets, nests, or clusters. The cells have reniform nuclei characterized by nuclear membrane lobations or indentations (fig. 7-34). The nuclei have vesicular chromatin with inconspicuous to small, centrally located basophilic nucleoli and a moderate amount of eosinophilic cytoplasm. The LCs may show mild pleomorphism and rare mitotic figures. An inflammatory cell infiltrate accompanies the DC and primarily consists of eosinophils. Other inflammatory cells are present, including polymorphonuclear leukocytes, plasma cells, and lymphocytes. Foamy histiocytes and multinucleated giant cells may also be present. These histiocytes may phagocytize mononuclear cells.

LCs are diffusely immunoreactive with S-100 protein and CD1a (fig. 7-34). Langerin, a type II transmembrane C-type lectin associated with the formation of Birbeck granules in LCs, represents a highly selective marker for the lesional cells of LCH (fig. 7-34) (188,189). Langerin immunoreactivity includes a membranous and granular cytoplasmic pattern (fig. 7-34). The foamy histiocytes and multinucleated giant cells are S-100 protein and CD1a negative but react with CD68 (KP1). By electron microscopy, elongated granules, referred to as Langerhans or Birbeck granules, are present within the cytoplasm of the DC (190). *BRAF* (V600E) mutations have been found in LCH

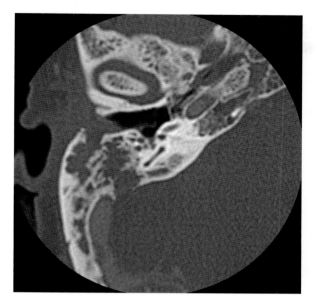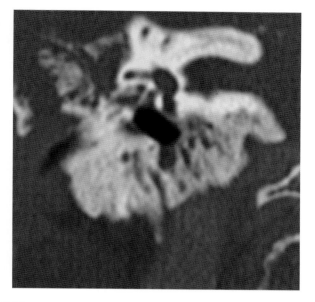

Figure 7-35

LANGERHANS CELL HISTIOCYTOSIS

Axial (left) and coronal (right) images of the temporal bone demonstrate opacification of the mastoid air cell system. Trabecular and cortical osteolysis involves that portion of the mastoid air cell system that is superior and posterior to the lateral aspect of the superior wall of the external auditory canal. (Courtesy of Dr. A. Khorsandi, New York, NY.)

and may provide new opportunities for devising targeted therapy (191,192).

Differential Diagnosis. The histologic differential diagnosis of LCH includes extranodal sinus histiocytosis with massive lymphadenopathy (ESHML), also referred to as Rosai-Dorfman disease, and non-Hodgkin malignant lymphoma. ESHML occasionally involves the ear and temporal bone region (193). The histologic features of ESHML include a polymorphous cellular infiltrate composed of mature lymphocytes, plasma cells, and histiocytes (fig. 7-37). The histiocytes (so-called SHML cells) appear in clusters or cell nests but may be obscured by the nonhistiocytic cell population (particularly the plasma cells). The histiocytic cells are uniform, with mild pleomorphism, and are characterized by round to oval, vesicular to hyperchromatic nuclei, with abundant amphophilic to eosinophilic, granular to foamy to clear cytoplasm (fig. 7-37). The nuclei do not demonstrate nuclear lobation, indentation, or longitudinal grooving as seen in LCs. The histiocytes characteristically demonstrate emperipolesis in which there is phagocytosis of cells, usually lymphocytes but may include plasma cells, erythrocytes, and polymorphonuclear leukocytes (fig. 7-37). Emperipolesis tends to be a less common finding in extranodal sites as compared to nodal-based disease. Similar to LCs, the cells of ESHML are S-100 protein reactive (fig. 7-37) but in contrast to LCs are nonreactive with CD1a and langerin.

Differentiating LCH from a malignant lymphoproliferative disease is usually not problematic by light microscopy. If necessary, immunohistochemical stains help in the differentiation.

Treatment and Prognosis. Treatment options vary depending on the extent of the disease and the severity at onset, and include surgical excision (curettage), radiotherapy, and chemotherapy (used for multifocal or systemic disease) (194–196). The prognosis is very good. Recurrence may be part of a systemic or multifocal process and generally occurs within 6 months of the diagnosis. Failure of a new bone lesion to occur within 1 year of diagnosis is considered a cure. In general, the younger the patient at onset of disease and the more extensive the involvement (multiple sites including bone and viscera), the worse the prognosis.

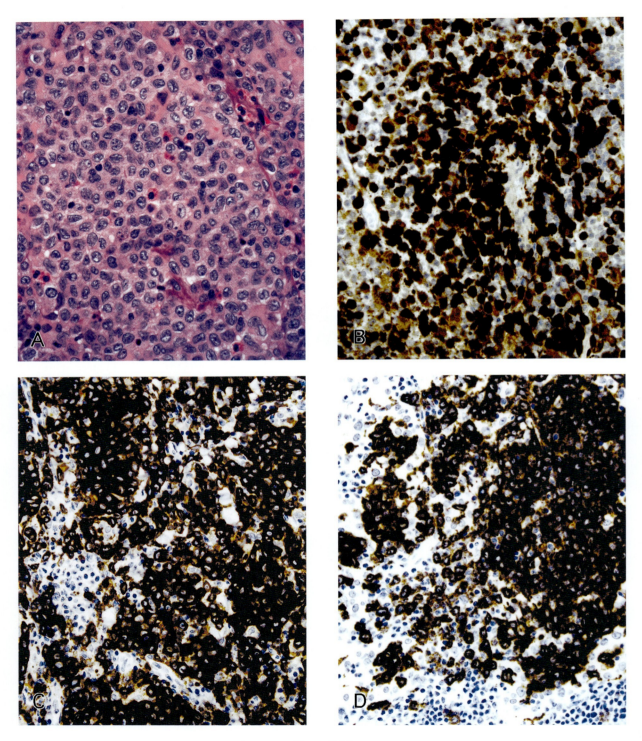

Figure 7-36

LANGERHANS CELL HISTIOCYTOSIS

A: There is a proliferation of Langerhans cells which are cells with reniform nuclei characterized by nuclear membrane lobations or indentations with scattered admixed eosinophils.

B–D: The Langerhans cells are immunoreactive for S-100 protein (B), CD1a (C), and langerin (D).

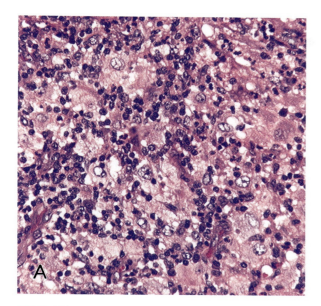
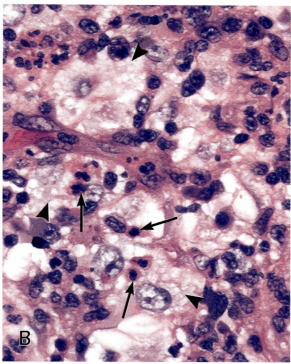
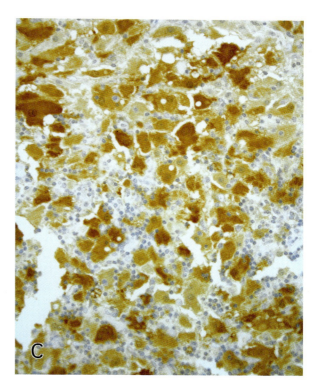

Figure 7-37

EXTRANODAL SINUS HISTIOCYTOSIS WITH MASSIVE LYMPHADENOPATHY (SHML) INVOLVING TEMPORAL BONE

A: At low magnification, there is a polymorphous cellular infiltrate composed of mature lymphocytes, plasma cells, and histiocytes, the latter somewhat obscured by the lymphoplasmacytic cells.

B: The SHML cells have abundant foamy eosinophilic cytoplasm with ill-defined borders (arrowheads). Phagocytized mononuclear cells (emperipolesis) are seen within the cytoplasm of some of the SHML cells (arrows).

C: SHML cells are S-100 protein positive and positive for histiocytic markers including but not limited to CD68 (not shown); SHML is nonreactive for CD1a and langerin.

HETEROTOPIAS OF THE MIDDLE EAR AND MASTOID

Heterotopia, also termed *choristoma* and *ectopia*, is the presence of normal-appearing tissue(s) in an anatomic location in which they normally are not found. Heterotopias that occur in the middle ear include salivary gland tissue and neuroglial tissue. The presence of glial tissue in the middle ear may represent an acquired encephalocele rather than heterotopia.

Middle Ear Salivary Gland Heterotopia

Clinical Features. *Salivary gland choristomas* occur more often in women of a wide age range.

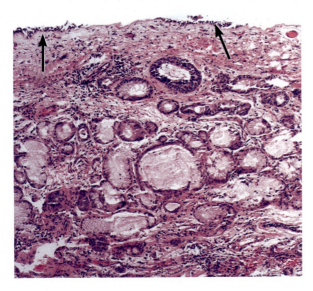

Figure 7-38

HETEROTOPIC SALIVARY GLAND TISSUE

The heterotopic tissue consists of normal-appearing seromucous glands. The mass, which clinically caused conductive hearing loss, was entirely located within the middle ear space with an intact (nonperforated) tympanic membrane. Attenuated to cuboidal middle ear epithelium (arrows) is present overlying the seromucous glands.

Patients present with unilateral conductive hearing loss (197–202). Salivary gland choristomas often arise in conjunction with facial nerve and ossicular chain anomalies (203), explained by a second branchial arch developmental abnormality. Abnormalities of the facial nerve, including bilateral preauricular pits, conchal bands, an ipsilateral facial palsy, and bilateral Mondini-type deformities, may be present.

Gross Findings. Choristoma appears as a lobulated, nonpulsatile soft tissue mass lying in the middle ear space, with an intact tympanic membrane.

Microscopic Findings. The salivary gland tissue includes an admixture of seromucous glands (fig. 7-38), with or without adipose tissue.

Treatment and Prognosis. Conservative surgical removal is the treatment of choice. Choristomas often adhere to a dehiscent facial nerve; if complete surgical resection will compromise the integrity of the facial nerve then incomplete resection is justified. A biopsy for diagnostic purposes, followed by observation, is an alternative to surgical excision. Rarely, salivary gland ectopia may produce a salivary gland neoplastic proliferation (e.g., pleomorphic adenoma) (204).

Middle Ear Neuroglial Heterotopia

True *neuronal heterotopia*, in which isolated neuroglial tissue is located in the middle ear and temporal bone without continuity with the central nervous system, is rare. The more common occurrence is glial-type tissue present within the middle ear/temporal bone in association with an acquired encephalocele.

Acquired Encephalocele

Definition. *Acquired encephalocele* is neuroglial tissue located within the middle ear and mastoid. Synonyms include *ectopic* or *heterotopic CNS tissue*, *brain prolapse*, and *brain herniation*.

Clinical Features. Acquired encephaloceles occur equally in men and women, and although a wide age range is affected, tends to occur in older individuals. Acquired encephaloceles most often occur as an incidental finding in patients requiring surgery for chronic otitis media (205–208). Associated symptoms include unilateral conductive hearing loss, leakage of CNS tissue, and recurrent episodes of meningitis. In patients suspected of having ectopic neuroglial tissue at this site, radiologic imaging (CT, MRI) may identify a defect or connection to the CNS (205,207,209,210).

Pathogenesis. Usually, the presence of CNS tissue within the middle ear and temporal bone region represents an acquired encephalocele, with herniation of the brain into the middle ear and mastoid via compromise of the tegmen, a thin bony shell that separates the middle ear and mastoid cavity from the temporal lobe; the connection to the CNS may not always be identified. The tegmen is compromised or destroyed secondary to trauma, prior surgery, complication of otitis media, or a congenital defect (205,207,208,211,212). Fracture of the temporal bone also results in herniation of the brain into the middle ear and mastoid (213). Some cases appear to occur spontaneously, without known association with an underlying cause or without a history of trauma, tumor, cholesteatoma, or surgery of the mastoid or cranium (214,215).

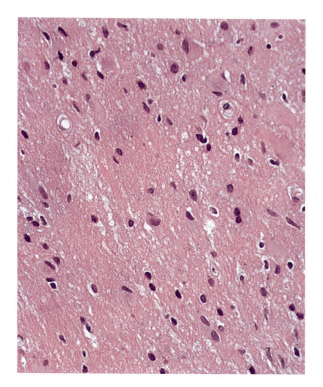 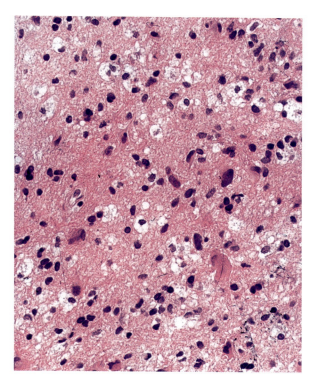

Figure 7-39

ACQUIRED ENCEPHALOCELE

The patient had longstanding chronic otitis media and had undergone several operations. Histologically, the excised tissue includes normal brain, including all cellular components of CNS tissue (left) and reactive alterations of the neuroglial tissue (gliosis) (right). Cases occurring in the setting of chronic otitis media (COM) may include the presence of histologic features of COM such as glandular metaplasia, tympanosclerosis, and fibrosis. Additional histologic findings associated with acquired encephalocele may include the presence of keratinizing squamous epithelium (i.e., cholesteatomas) and cholesterol granuloma formation.

Microscopic Findings. Neuroglial heterotopia consists of a heterogeneous population of cells, including glial cells, histiocytes, and mature lymphocytes (fig. 7-39). Reactive alterations of the neuroglial tissue (gliosis) may be present (fig. 7-39) (211,212), as well as granulation tissue and keratinizing squamous epithelium (cholesteatoma). Meninges are generally not present. The CNS tissue may be associated with findings of other pathologic processes including chronic otitis media and cholesteatoma (keratinizing). Immunohistochemical confirmation of neuroglial tissue includes reactivity with glial fibrillary acidic protein (GFAP).

Differential Diagnosis. In chronic otitis media, a fibrillary stroma is often present, which may simulate the appearance of neurofibrillary matrix. GFAP assists in confirming or excluding neuroglial tissue.

Treatment and Prognosis. Conservative surgical removal is the treatment of choice. Choristomas, however, often adhere to a dehiscent facial nerve. If complete surgical resection will compromise the integrity of the facial nerve then incomplete resection is justified. Biopsy for diagnostic purposes, followed by observation, is an alternative to surgical excision. Potential complications include brain abscess.

AUTOIMMUNE, DEGENERATIVE, AND SYSTEMIC DISEASES

Relapsing Polychondritis

Definition. *Relapsing polychondritis* (RP) is an uncommon, systemic, episodic or relapsing disease characterized by progressive degeneration of cartilaginous structures throughout the body. *Polychondropathia* is another term for this disease.

Clinical Features. RP primarily occurs in whites and affects men and women equally. It occurs at any age, with symptoms most frequently occurring in the fifth to seventh decades of life. RP may affect any cartilage tissue in the body. The auricular cartilage is involved, usually bilaterally, in nearly 90 percent of patients with RP (216–218). The affected ear is erythematous, swollen, and very tender. In advanced cases, there may be distortion of the pinna due to destruction of the cartilage. The overlying skin is not ulcerated. The disease manifestations vary in both severity and frequency of occurrence. Progression of disease may result in "cauliflower" ears and "saddle" nose deformities. Involvement of the audiovestibular system may result in hearing loss (conductive, sensorineural, or mixed) (219). Other cartilaginous sites, as well as noncartilaginous sites of the body, may be involved, causing arthropathy (large and small joints), laryngotracheal and bronchial chondritis, nasal chondritis, cardiovascular complications (valvular insufficiency, aneurysm), ocular manifestations (episcleritis, conjunctivitis, retinopathy), and cutaneous involvement (oral and genital ulcers) (220–222).

RP is defined by three or more of the following: recurrent chondritis of both auricles; nonerosive inflammatory arthritis; chondritis of nasal cartilages; ocular inflammation including conjunctivitis, keratitis, scleritis/episcleritis, and/or uveitis; chondritis of the upper respiratory tract involving the larynx and/or tracheal cartilages; and cochlear and/or vestibular damage manifested by sensorineural hearing loss, tinnitus, and/or vertigo. The diagnosis is confirmed when one or more of the above criteria occur in association with histologic confirmation or by the presence of chondritis in two or more separate anatomic locations with response to steroids or dapsone. Laboratory findings are nonspecific and include elevated erythrocyte sedimentation rate, mild leukocytosis, and normochromic normocytic anemia. Elevated antineutrophil cytoplasmic antibody titers have been reported (223) as have elevated levels of proteinase 3 (224).

Pathogenesis. The etiology of RP has not been clearly elucidated. There is evidence, however, for an autoimmune process. Some patients with RP have other autoimmune disorders, including systemic lupus erythematosus, rheumatoid arthritis, scleroderma, Sjögren syndrome, Reiter syndrome, glomerulonephritis, autoimmune thyroid disease, ulcerative colitis, pernicious anemia, and Raynaud syndrome (217,225). In approximately 30 percent of cases, an association with other diseases, especially systemic vasculitis or myelodysplastic syndrome, is detected (226).

Patients with RP have factors in their serum that react with cartilage (227). These patients have circulating antibodies to type II collagen (228), found only in cartilage with titers reflecting the severity of disease, and immunofluorescent localization of immune complex components at the perichondral-cartilaginous interface (229,230). Patients with RP have immune complexes of immunoglobulins and complement detected in the biopsy specimens taken from inflamed cartilage of involved ears (231). RP is likely a Th1-mediated disease since serum levels of interferon (IFN)-γ, interleukin [IL]-12, and IL-2 parallel changes in disease activity, while the levels of Th2 cytokines do not (232). These findings, coupled with the association of RP with an array of known autoimmune systemic diseases, lend support to an autoimmune etiology. There is no evidence to support either hereditary or familial predisposition.

Gross Findings. RP is characterized by the presence of diffuse redness and swelling of the ear (fig. 7-40).

Microscopic Findings. The histologic findings include perichondrial inflammation, with a mixed infiltrate of lymphocytes, plasma cells, polymorphonuclear leukocytes, and occasional eosinophils, which blurs the interface between the perichondrium and the auricular cartilage (fig. 7-41). There is loss of the usual basophilia in the cartilage, which assumes an eosinophilic appearance with hematoxylin and eosin (H&E) staining. At the advancing edge of the inflammation, there is loss of chondrocytes and destruction of the lacunar architecture. As cartilage is destroyed, it is replaced by tissue and eventually by fibrous tissue. Diffuse granular deposition of IgG and C3 in the perichondrial fibrous tissue may be demonstrated (233).

Differential Diagnosis. The differential diagnosis includes external otitis, acute infectious perichondritis, gout, systemic vasculitides such as granulomatosis with polyangiitis (formerly referred to as Wegener granulomatosis), and rheumatoid arthritis.

Treatment and Prognosis. The treatment of RP depends on the stage. In the acute stage of disease, corticosteroids are utilized. In more advanced stages, immunosuppressive agents may be used. The prognosis is variable and unpredictable, with some patients having a prolonged disease course and others having a more aggressive and fulminant course. The prognosis for patients with respiratory tract involvement is poor (218). Death may occur and is most often the result of respiratory tract or cardiovascular system involvement.

Granulomatosis with Polyangiitis

Definition. *Granulomatosis with polyangiitis* (GPA) is a systemic necrotizing vasculitis that typically involves the kidney, lung, and upper aerodigestive tract. Formerly, this was referred to as *Wegener granulomatosis*. For a more complete discussion, including images, see chapter 1.

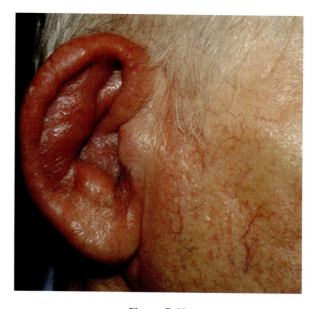

Figure 7-40

RELAPSING POLYCHONDRITIS

The affected ear is diffusely erythematous and swollen. (Courtesy of Dr. E. Smouha, New York, NY.)

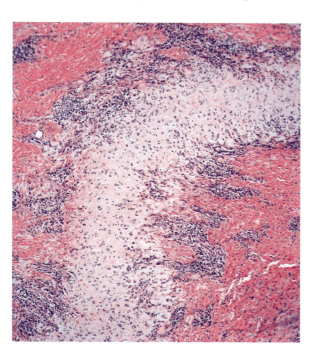 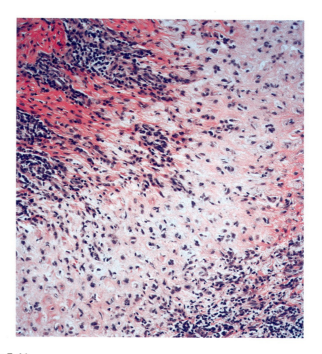

Figure 7-41

RELAPSING POLYCHONDRITIS

Left: The mixed inflammatory infiltrate blurs the interface between the perichondrium and the auricular cartilage. The cartilage has a ragged border with loss of its normal basophilic appearance.

Right: At higher magnification, the inflammatory cell infiltrate includes mature lymphocytes, plasma cells, and neutrophils, obscuring the normal perichondrial-cartilaginous interface as well as within the cartilage (intrachondral).

Clinical Features. Otologic involvement occurs in 20 to 60 percent of patients with GPA (234–239). The most common otologic manifestations are unilateral or bilateral otitis media (serous or suppurative), perforation of the tympanic membrane, and sensorineural hearing loss (234–240). Cutaneous involvement of the external ear results in perforation of the ear lobes and external otitis (235,237,241). Facial palsy may occur as the initial manifestation of disease (236,242–244). The middle ear may be involved secondary to nasopharyngeal and sinonasal disease, via the eustachian tube, or may be directly involved by disease. Antineutrophil cytoplasmic autoantibodies (ANCA) and proteinase 3 (PR3) are elevated in the active phase of GPA (245–247).

Microscopic Findings. The histologic features are similar to those described in the lung, kidney, and upper aerodigestive tract, and include: vasculitis; granulomatous inflammation characterized by scattered multinucleated giant cells rather than the presence of well-formed granulomas; involvement by the giant cells of vessel walls as well as the supporting tissues; and ischemic-type tissue necrosis (referred to as geographic necrosis). Special stains for microorganisms, including GMS and AFB, are negative.

Differential Diagnosis. Other autoimmune or systemic diseases that involve the middle or inner ear include polyarteritis nodosa and rheumatoid arthritis. Polyarteritis nodosa is a necrotizing vasculitis of small and medium-sized muscular arteries. Aural-related symptoms include otitis media with effusion (248). Sensorineural hearing loss may be the initial presentation or may occur after the diagnosis has been established (248). The histologic diagnosis is dependent on the presence of necrotizing vasculitis. Treatment includes corticosteroids and immunosuppressant agents.

The manifestations of rheumatoid arthritis of the audiovestibular system include conductive hearing loss due to involvement of the incudomalleal and incudostapedial articulations (249). High-dose salicylates in combination with steroids and nonsteroidal anti-inflammatory agents is the treatment of choice.

Treatment and Prognosis. For GPA, combined corticosteroid and immunosuppressive therapy may result in long-term remissions and is capable of reversing the hearing loss and facial palsy if the diagnosis can be established and treatment initiated early in the disease course (250).

Tophaceous Gout

Definition. *Tophaceous gout* is a disorder of purine metabolism or renal excretion of uric acid in which there is a precipitation of monosodium urate as deposits (tophi) throughout the body. It is also termed *crystal deposition disease*.

Clinical Features. Nearly 90 percent of cases occur in men, with a peak incidence in these older than 50 years of age (251). One of the more common sites of gouty tophi is the helix of the ear (252). In this location, tophi may present as painful, skin-covered firm nodules (fig. 7-42).

Laboratory findings include an elevated urinary uric acid, leukocytosis, and increased erythrocyte sedimentation rate. Measurement of 24-hour urinary uric acid excretion helps in determining whether uric acid overproduction is a cause of the hyperuricemia (253). In normal body tissues, sodium urate is deposited (tophi) but in urine, with a lower pH, uric acid is precipitated (253).

Pathogenesis. Gout occurs as an inherited or acquired disease (251). Primary gout (90 percent of cases) is an inherited error of metabolism that results from either an enzymatic defect in purine synthesis or a defect in the renal excretion of uric acid. Secondary or acquired gout (10 percent of cases) occurs secondary to disorders that increase the production of uric acid (e.g., leukemias) or decrease excretion of uric acid (e.g., chronic renal failure).

Gross Findings. Gout consists of subcutaneous nodules that appear salmon pink in color. When pressed, gouty tophi exude a chalky white material.

Microscopic Findings. Histologically, gouty tophi are composed of needle-shaped aggregates of urate crystals with a surrounding foreign body giant cell reaction (fig. 7-43). If a diagnosis of gout is suspected, the resected tissue should be fixed in absolute alcohol or any nonaqueous fixative since the urate crystals are water soluble. Over time, mineralization (calcification) and, occasionally, ossification may occur in these sodium urate aggregates.

Differential Diagnosis. Tophaceous gout may share similar clinical features with tophaceous pseudogout (see below). However, radiographic calcification in gouty tophi is uncommon and the identification of the specific positive birefringence of the calcium pyrophosphate crystals of tophaceous pseudogout is the differentiating finding.

Treatment and Prognosis. Treatment is directed toward the systemic disorder. In acute gout, pharmacologic intervention is usually necessary and includes nonsteroidal anti-inflammatory drugs, oral colchicine, and corticosteroids. Anti-IL-1 therapy may also be beneficial in treating acute gout symptoms (254,255).

Tophaceous Pseudogout

Definition. *Tophaceous pseudogout* is the presence of calcium pyrophosphate dihydrate crystal deposition in the synovial fluid of patients who have gout-like symptoms but no sodium urate crystals. The designation of pseudogout was initially coined by McCarty et al. (256). Other

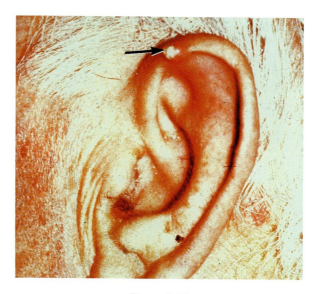

Figure 7-42
GOUTY TOPHUS
A chalky white helical lesion (arrow) is seen.

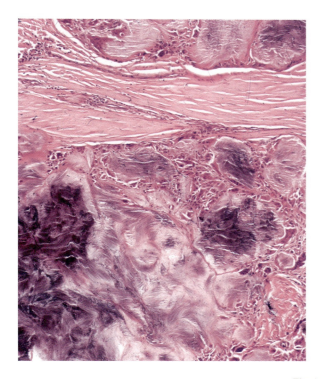 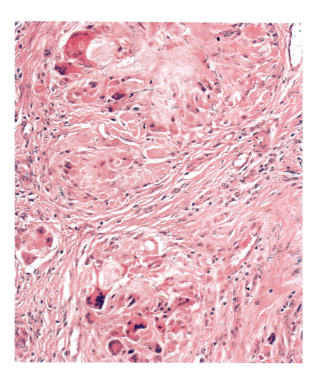

Figure 7-43
GOUTY TOPHUS

Left: Histologically, gout is characterized by the presence of a foreign body giant cell reaction typically surrounding needle-shaped crystals.

Right: In this example, a foreign body giant cell reaction is present but the crystals are not readily identifiable as the tissue was not fixed in absolute alcohol or a nonaqueous fixative.

designations include *tumoral calcium pyrophosphate dihydrate deposition (CPPD) disease* (257), *chondrocalcinosis, pyrophosphate arthropathy,* and more recently, *CPPD crystal deposition disease* (258).

Clinical Features. Tophaceous pseudogout is one of the rarest clinical forms of CPPD crystal deposition disease. It mainly affects middle-aged and elderly patients. There is a female predilection.

The clinical manifestations of CPPD crystal deposition disease vary widely. Most cases are found incidentally and are asymptomatic. Deposition of CPPD commonly occurs in the articular and para-articular joints. The most common location of tophaceous pseudogout is the temporomandibular joint (TMJ) where it may be confused with synovial chondromatosis (257,259). Other sites of involvement include the finger, toe, wrist, hip, cervical spine, shoulder, elbow, and knee.

The most common symptom of tophaceous pseudogout is a painless mass or swelling; involvement of the spine may be associated with neurological disturbances such as progressive myelopathy. Tophaceous pseudogout may present as a calcified soft tissue mass, with or without bone erosion. Awareness of this possible presentation, which is similar to a malignant soft tissue tumor, may assist in avoiding a diagnosis of a sarcoma.

The skeletal distribution of tophaceous pseudogout is different from that of the common forms of CPPD deposition disease in which the knee and wrist are the most frequently affected joints. Radiographic evidence of other joint involvement by CPPD crystal deposition disease is seen in approximately 20 percent of patients. In general, patients with tophaceous pseudogout do not have familial CPPD crystal deposition disease or other associated metabolic disorders. However, mutations in the ANK human gene (*ANKH*) have been shown to cause familial CPPD (260).

Gross Findings. Grossly, tophaceous pseudogout is composed of multiple fragments of friable, tan-white, chalky material.

Microscopic Findings. Histologically, tophaceous pseudogout is characterized by the presence of variably cellular, chondroid tissue within which is crystalline material (fig. 7-44). The crystalline material appears rhomboid or needle shaped, and under polarized light microscopy, the crystals show weak positive birefringence. In decalcified material, the crystals may be lost. A foreign body granulomatous reaction is associated with the crystal deposition. Chondroid metaplasia is often present in and around the areas of CPPD deposition. There is some evidence to indicate that metaplastic chondrocytes play a role in the initial precipitation of CPPD crystals. Synovial chondrometaplasia may be seen in patients with pyrophosphate arthropathy. The metaplastic chondrocytes may show cytologic atypia that could lead to a diagnosis of chondrosarcoma (fig. 7-44). This is particularly true in decalcified sections from which CPPD crystals are lost.

Differential Diagnosis. The differential diagnosis of tophaceous pseudogout includes gout, tumoral calcinosis, synovial chondromatosis, and benign (chondromyxoid fibroma, chondroma, chondroblastoma, and osteochondroma), and malignant (chondrosarcoma, osteosarcoma, and chordoma) tumors (257).

The presence of the crystals (the exact nature of which can be determined by radiographic defraction or electron probe analysis) and a granulomatous response differentiate tophaceous pseudogout from chondrosarcoma (261). Similarly, the presence of birefringent rhomboid to needle-like crystals differentiates tophaceous pseudogout from synovial chondromatosis (257). In decalcified sections, empty outlines of crystals in the chondroid matrix can be seen, although birefringent crystals are not identified directly.

Tophaceous gout may share similar clinical features with tophaceous pseudogout. However, radiographic calcification in gouty tophi is uncommon. The identification of the specific positive birefringent calcium pyrophosphate crystals of tophaceous pseudogout is the differentiating finding.

Tumoral calcinosis may be mistaken for tophaceous pseudogout. Tumoral calcinosis tends to affect patients who are young and black, and often have a family history of tumoral calcinosis with hyperphosphatemia. The calcified material in tumoral calcinosis lacks crystalline structures but is amorphous and granular, and is mainly composed of hydroxyapatite (262).

Treatment and Prognosis. Surgery is the treatment of choice. Recurrence may occur following surgical resection.

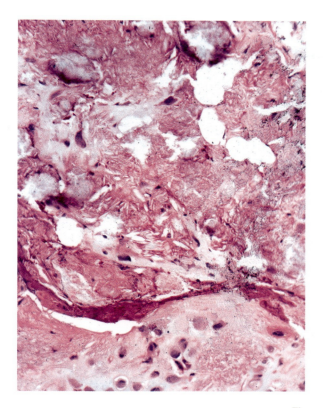 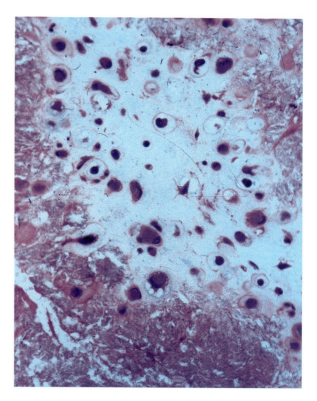

Figure 7-44

TOPHACEOUS PSEUDOGOUT

Left: Variably cellular chondroid tissue within which is identifiable crystalline rhomboid or needle-shaped material (under polarized light microscopy the crystals showed weak positive birefringence, not shown).

Right: Chondroid metaplasia is present, which may show cytologic atypia.

Otosclerosis

Definition. *Otosclerosis* is a disorder of the bony labyrinth and stapedial footplate that exclusively occurs in humans and is of unknown etiology. Otosclerosis means hardening of the ear and is derived from Greek (ous, ear; skleros, hard; osis, condition). Synonyms include *chronic metaplastic ostitis* and *progressive otospongiosis*.

Clinical Features. Otosclerosis affects women more often than men; a family history is present in over 50 percent of cases. The prevalence of otosclerosis varies with race and is highest in Caucasians and lowest in African Americans, Asians, and Native Americans (263). Otosclerosis primarily causes conductive hearing loss that usually begins in the second and third decades of life and is slowly progressive. The extent of the hearing loss directly correlates with the degree of stapedial footplate fixation. Patients with otosclerosis also tend to have vestibular disturbances (264,265). Otosclerosis usually involves both ears (85 percent of cases) (266).

Imaging studies confirm the clinical consideration of otosclerosis. High resolution CT is the modality of choice for evaluating middle and inner ear structures, including labyrinthine windows, stapes foot plate, and cochlear capsule (fig. 7-45) (267).

Pathogenesis. Although many theories regarding the etiology of otosclerosis appear in the literature, the etiology remains unclear (268, 269). Hereditary factors are often cited as among the causes of otosclerosis (263), although the mode of inheritance is still uncertain. A family history is present in over 50 percent of cases. Most epidemiological studies on families with otosclerosis suggest an autosomal dominant mode of inheritance, with reduced penetrance of 25 to 40 percent (263). Genetic linkage studies have demonstrated the presence of six

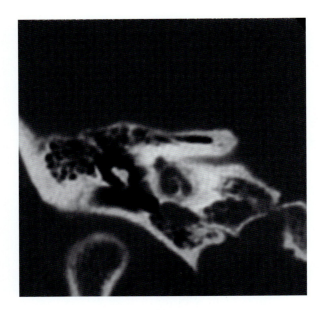

Figure 7-45

OTOSCLEROSIS

Coronal CT image of the right ear demonstrates obliterative otosclerosis involving the lumen of the basal segment of the first turn of the cochlea. (Courtesy of Dr. A. Khorsandi, New York, NY.)

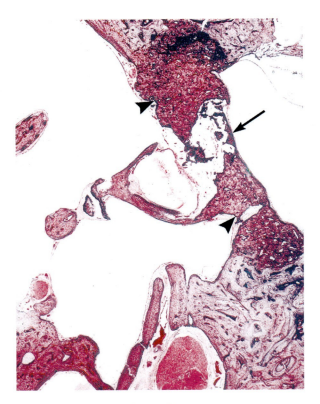

Figure 7-46

OTOSCLEROSIS OF THE STAPEDIAL FOOTPLATE

The densely sclerotic bone (arrowheads) results in fixation of the stapes (arrow). The clinical manifestation resulting from these histopathologic findings is conductive hearing loss.

loci (*OTSC1, OTSC2, OTSC3, OTSC4, OTSC5,* and *OTSC7*) located on chromosomes 15q, 7q, 6p, 16q, 3q, and 6q, respectively, although no causative genes have been identified (270). Disturbed bone metabolism, persistent measles virus infection, autoimmunity, and hormonal and environmental factors also may play contributing roles in the pathogenesis (269).

Based on the invasiveness of the plaques apparently derived from the periosteum of the external layer of the otic capsule (271), some authorities have suggested that otosclerosis is a neoplasm of bone that forms a replica of the external layer otic capsule tissue, (i.e., Volkmann canals and lamellar bone). This is supported by the marked proliferation of osteoblasts and concomitant production of minicanals seen at the advancing edge of the plaques (272).

Microscopic Findings. The initial histologic alteration is resorption of bone around blood vessels. The cellular fibrovascular tissue replaces the resorbed bone, resulting in softening of the bone (otospongiosis). Immature bone is laid down, with continuous active resorption and remodeling. The new bone is rich in ground substance and deficient in collagen but, over time, more mature bone with increased collagen and less ground substance is produced, resulting in densely sclerotic bone. This process most often begins anterior to the oval window and eventually involves the footplate of the stapes (fig. 7-46). Stapedial involvement causes fixation of the stapes and the inability to transmit sound waves, resulting in conductive hearing loss.

While the otosclerotic changes may be seen in a resected stapedial footplate, even when the footplate is removed intact, it may be free of otosclerotic changes because fixation results via pressure on the nonotosclerotic footplate from swelling of the otosclerotic process in the adjacent temporal bone (273). Similar pathologic involvement of the inner ear may produce sensorineural hearing loss.

Differential Diagnosis. The differential diagnosis includes Paget disease of bone (see below).

Treatment and Prognosis. Surgical management of the conductive hearing loss caused by stapes fixation (stapedectomy) is the treatment of choice, with replacement of the fixed stapes by a prosthesis. The resected bone may include the entire stapes, including the footplate, or only the superstructure, which includes the head and crura without the footplate.

Paget Disease of Bone

Definition. *Paget disease of bone* is a chronic progressive disorder of unknown etiology. It is also termed *osteitis deformans*.

Clinical Features. Paget disease is primarily a disease of the axial skeleton. In the head and neck, the skull and temporal bone are involved in approximately 70 percent of cases (274). Other sites of involvement include the external auditory canal, tympanic membrane, eustachian tube, ossicles, oval window, round window, internal auditory canal, cochlea, and endolymphatic sac (274). Paget disease is slightly more common in men than in women. It affects about 3 percent of the population over 40 years of age and as much as 11 percent of the population over 80 years of age (275,276).

The symptoms include hearing loss, tinnitus, and vertigo. The facial nerve is spared. The hearing loss is sensorineural, mixed sensorineural and conductive, and less often, only conductive. Hearing losses are progressive and are due to involvement of the osseous portion of the external auditory canal, involvement of the ossicles, or involvement of the cochlea and labyrinth (277).

Imaging studies confirm the clinical consideration of Paget disease. High resolution CT of the temporal bone may show bone thickening and sclerosis. In the temporal bone, the disease begins at the petrous apex and progresses inferolaterally; with progression, demineralization of the otic capsule may occur. The stapedial footplate may become involved (i.e., thickened), contributing to the (conductive) hearing loss. Frequently, the central skull is also involved.

Pathogenesis. The etiology of Paget disease is unknown but consideration has been given to an infectious (viral) etiology in genetically predisposed individuals (278). Measles virus may play an important role as an environmental factor in the pathogenesis of Paget disease (279). Interleukin-6 (IL-6) is increased in the bone marrow of Paget patients and measles virus nucleocapsid protein (MVNP) induces IL-6 secretion by pagetic osteoclasts (280,281). IL-6 plays a critical role in the development of the pagetic osteoclasts and bone lesions induced by Paget disease, but the mechanisms regulating IL-6 production by MVNP remain unclear. MVNP decreases FOXO3/SIRT1 signaling to enhance the levels of IL-6, which in part mediate the contribution of MVNP to the development of Paget disease.

Microscopic Findings. Paget disease is characterized by three histologic phases. In the first, or osteolytic phase, there is excessive osteoclastic activity resulting in bone resorption. In the second, mixed or combined phase, new bone formation (osteoblastic activity) predominates over bone resorption (osteoclastic activity), with deposition of new bone next to areas of bone resorption. In the third, or osteoblastic phase, there is increased new bone characterized by dense irregular masses showing a mosaic pattern, referred to as cement lines.

Differential Diagnosis. The differential diagnosis includes otosclerosis. Patients with Paget disease have a later age of onset, greater sensorineural hearing loss, enlarging calvaria, and enlargement and tortuosity of the superficial temporal artery and its anterior branches (275), differentiating it from ostosclerosis.

Treatment and Prognosis. Treatment is directed at slowing or preventing progression of disease by suppressing increased bone turnover. Biphosphonates, which act by decreasing the number of osteoclasts with deposition of structurally normal bone as opposed to deposition of less disordered bone deposition, are used. Anti-inflammatory medications are used in relieving bone and joint pain. Hearing loss is permanent and cannot be reversed by medical therapy. Sarcomatous transformation occurs in approximately 1 percent of cases (282) and usually results in an osteosarcoma (283–286). Osteosarcomas arising in Paget disease are highly malignant, with a 4 percent 5-year survival rate (285).

Ménière Disease

Definition. *Ménière disease* is an idiopathic disorder of the inner ear associated with a symptom complex of spontaneous, episodic attacks of vertigo, sensorineural hearing loss, tinnitus, and a sensation of aural fullness. Synonyms include *endolymphatic hydrops, idiopathic endolymphatic hydrops,* and *Lermoyez syndrome.*

Clinical Features. Ménière disease is more common in women than men (287). The peak incidence is in the fifth to seventh decades of life, but it may occur in children as well as in older individuals (ninth and tenth decades). Ménière disease is characterized by a set of symptoms that includes paroxysmal episodes of vertigo that are often accompanied by nausea and vomiting, fluctuating sensorineural hearing loss, tinnitus, and pressure sensation in the ear (288). The striking symptom is the rotary vertigo that is frequently sudden in onset and reaches maximum intensity within a few minutes; this lasts from 1 to several hours and either subsides completely or continues as a sensation of unsteadiness for hours to days.

Pathogenesis. The etiology is uncertain although the incidence of Ménière disease is increased in patients with certain genetically acquired major histocompatibility complexes (MHCs), including HLA B8/DR3 and Cw7, suggesting a possible autoimmune etiology (289–291). Familial occurrence of Ménière disease has been reported (292,293), although the role of genetic inheritance is uncertain.

In Ménière disease, distortion of the membranous labyrinth, defined as changes in the anatomy of the membranous labyrinth, occur as a consequence of the overaccumulation of endolymph (endolymphatic hydrops) and at the expense of the perilymphatic space (288,293,294). Endolymph, which is produced by the stria vascularis in the cochlea and by cells in the vestibular labyrinth, circulates in a radial and longitudinal fashion. In patients with Ménière disease it is believed that there is inadequate absorption of endolymph by the endolymphatic sac (293).

Microscopic Findings. In the early stages of the disease, endolymphatic hydrops primarily involves the cochlear duct and saccule but in the later stages the entire endolymphatic system is involved. Alterations of the membranous labyrinth include dilatation, outpouching, rupture, and collapse. Fistulae (unhealed ruptures) may occur. Severe cytoarchitectural and atrophic changes may occur in the sense organs, with loss of neurons in the cochlea.

Treatment and Prognosis. Medical management is the mainstay of therapy. Therapy is aimed at reduction of symptoms and is therefore empiric and supportive. Optimally, management should resolve the vertigo, tinnitus, and hearing loss. Vertigo is the most debilitating of the symptoms and current management is directed at its relief. Symptomatic therapies include antivertiginous medications, antiemetics, sedatives, antidepressants, and psychiatric management. Other therapy includes prophylaxis via reduction of endolymph accumulation by dietary modification, intermittent dehydration, diuretics, enhancement of the microcirculation of the ear using vasodilators, reduction in immune reactivity using steroids, immunoglobulin and allergy therapy, and intratympanic perfusion of steroids or gentamicin (295). Improvement occurs in 60 to 80 percent of patients (290).

Surgical treatment is reserved for those patients who have failed medical management (approximately 10 percent) and includes endolymphatic sac decompression or mastoid shunt (296). Endolymphatic sac surgery is reported to be effective at controlling vertigo in the short term (>1 year of follow-up) and long term (more than 2 years) in at least 75 percent of the patients with Ménière disease who have failed medical therapy (296).

DEVELOPMENTAL DEFECTS OF THE MIDDLE EAR AND TEMPORAL BONE

There are numerous developmental or congenital anomalies that affect the middle ear and temporal bone. In brief, these include a variety of anatomic variations and anomalies, hereditary deafness that is primarily conductive occurring in syndromes, deafness caused by noxious prenatal influences, first and second branchial arch syndromes, dysplasias of the osseous and membranous cochlea and vestibular labyrinth, and hereditary/genetic sensorineural hearing loss (297,298). Other dysplasias of the external, middle, and inner ear include a combination of hypertelorism, microtia, and clefting, an 18q syndrome.

Anatomic variations and anomalies may involve the facial nerve, jugular bulb, and intratemporal carotid artery. Facial nerve anomalies include congenital bony dehiscence of the facial canal, anatomic variation or anomalies in the course of the facial nerve, mastoid segment anomalies, anatomic variation of the chorda tympani nerve, and abnormal facial artery and vein. Jugular bulb anomalies include superolateral extension of the bulb or superomedial enlargement of the bulb. Abnormalities of the intratemporal carotid artery include aneurysm, aberrant location, abscess and inflammatory necrosis, traumatic lacerations, and atherosclerotic changes.

Hereditary deafness, primarily conductive, occurs with the following: mandibulofacial dysostosis (Treacher-Collins syndrome), acrofacial dysostosis (Nager syndrome), craniofacial dysostosis (Crouzon syndrome), Klippel-Feil syndrome (fused vertebra, short neck, facial asymmetry, visceral abnormalities, deafness), Marfan syndrome (arachnodactyly, ectopia lentis, deafness), and Pierre Robin syndrome (cleft palate, micrognathia, glossoptosis, low set ears, deformed pinna and hearing loss). Other hereditary diseases causing conductive hearing loss include osteoporosis (Albers-Schonberg disease or marble bone disease), otosclerosis, and osteogenesis imperfecta. Deafness caused by noxious prenatal influences (embryopathic atresias) include maternal rubella, birth injuries, hyperbilirubinemia (erythroblastosis fetalis), drugs (including thalidomide, quinine), and cretinism.

First and second branchial arch syndromes include a variety of abnormalities with nonotologic and otologic manifestations. The otologic abnormalities include malformed or absent external ears, atretic external auditory canal, and impaired hearing. The nonotologic features include asymmetric facies, temporomandibular joint and neuromuscular abnormalties, and associated abnormalities of the cardiovascular, renal, and central nervous systems. Goldenhar syndrome, also known as oculoauriculovertebral dysplasia, is a first and second branchial arch syndrome characterized by ear tags, preauricular pits and fissures, epidermoids, lipodermoids, and vertibral column abnormalities.

Of the approximately 2,000 to 3,000 profoundly deaf infants born yearly in the United States, 35 to 50 percent have a defined genetic origin for their hearing impairment. In one third, the hearing loss is syndromal or associated with other anomalies. In adults, approximately 20 percent of sensorineural hearing loss is of genetic etiology. Etiologic factors vary with age. More than 50 percent of early-onset hearing loss is due to genetic factors, of which 60 to 70 percent are autosomal recessive (both parents carry the affected gene and involvement of the offspring is 25 percent), 20 to 30 percent autosomal dominant (one parent carries the affected gene and the incidence of involvement of the offspring is approximately 50 percent), and 2 percent are X-linked. In patients with late-onset hearing loss, approximately 20 percent are due to infections; about 7 percent are due to trauma; 35 percent due to old age, heredity, and noise trauma; and approximately 35 percent are of unknown cause. See Table 7-3 for categories of sensorineural hearing loss.

Dysplasia of the inner ear may be inherited, sporadic, or the result of chromosomal aberrations. Typically, both ears are involved but perhaps not to a similar extent. The classification of dysplasias of the osseous and membranous cochlea and vestibular labyrinth are divided into eight types (see Table 7-4). This subclassification is based on earlier reports detailing the morphologic changes involving the cochlear modiolus, osseous spiral lamina, and contents of the vestibule and endolymphatic sac and duct. The original designations for the dysplasias of the cochlea and vestibular labyrinth in patients with profound congenital hearing loss include: Michel type, Mondini or Mondini-Alexander type, Scheibe type, and Siebenmann-Bing type. The Michel type includes bilateral aplasia of the cochlear and vestibular capsule with bilateral aplasia of the 8th nerve. The Mondini type includes anomalies of the cochlea which may include the presence of a single coil or flattening and underdevelopment. The Scheibe type referred to as cochleo-saccular dysplasia, includes morphologic changes limited to the membranous cochlea and saccule. The utricle and semicircular canals are not involved. Siebenmann-Bing type includes dysplasia of the membranous cochlea and vestibular labyrinth, with a well-formed bony labyrinth (cochlear capsule).

Table 7-3
CATEGORIES OF SENSORINEURAL HEARING LOSS

Autosomal Recessive Hereditary Sensorineural Hearing Loss
    Hereditary recessive sensorineural hearing loss without associated defects (about 50 percent of recessive hereditary deafness), including recessive congenital severe deafness, high-frequency deafness, mid-frequency deafness
    Inborn errors of metabolism and deafness
    Albinism and deafness
    Hurler syndrome (abnormality of mucopolysaccharide metabolism)
    Tay-Sachs disease (ganglioside lipidoses and deafness)
    Wilson disease (hepatolenticular degeneration and deafness)
    Degenerative diseases of the nervous system and deafness: Friedrich ataxia (spinocerebellar ataxia, deafness)
    Congenital heart disease and deafness: Jervell and Lange-Nielsen syndrome (cardiac conduction anomaly, deafness)
    Endocrine system disorders and deafness: Pendred syndrome (nonendemic goiter and deafness)
    Ocular diseases and deafness: Usher syndrome (retinitis pigmentosa, deafness); Cockayne syndrome (retinitis Pigmentosa, mental retardation, dwarfism, retinal atrophy, deafness); Alstrom syndrome (retinitis pigmentosa, Obesity, diabetes mellitus, deafness)

Autosomal Dominant Hereditary Sensorineural Hearing Loss
    Inborn errors of metabolism and deafness; Tietz syndrome (albinism, deafness, abnormality of tyrosine metabolism); Waardenbërg syndrome (partial albinism, deafness, abnormality of tyrosine metabolism); Schafer syndrome (hereditary mental retardation, deafness, abnormality of tyrosine metabolism); hereditary mental retardation, homocystinemia, deafness, abnormality of methionine metabolism); nephropathies and deafness
    Alport syndrome (hereditary nephritis, deafness); Muckle and Well syndrome (hereditary nephritis, urticaria, Amyloidosis, deafness); Herrmann syndrome (hereditary nephritis, mental retardation, epilepsy, diabetes and Dominant nerve deafness); ectodermal defects and deafness; von Recklinghausen disease (vestibular schwannomas [uni-, bilateral] and deafness)

Table 7-4
DYSPLASIAS OF THE OSSEOUS AND MEMBRANOUS COCHLEA AND VESTIBULAR LABYRINTH

Type I:	isolated aplasia or dysplasia of the lateral semicircular canal;
Type II:	type I plus cochlear dysplasia
Type III:	type I plus aplasia or rare club-shaped distension of the vestibule with rudimentary superior or posterior semicircular canals; a normal cochlea is present
Type IV:	aplasia or dysplasia of all 3 semicircular canals plus severe cochlea dysplasia
Type V:	aplasia or dysplasia of all 3 semicircular canals plus normal cochlea
Type VI:	aplasia of all 3 semicircular canals plus cochlea aplasia
Type VII:	normally configured vestibular labyrinth with aplasia of the cochlea
Type VIII:	aplasia of the vestibular labyrinth and cochlea

REFERENCES

Embryology, Anatomy and Histology

1. Moore KL, Persaud TV. Development of ear. In: Moore KL, Persaud TV, eds. The developing human: clinically oriented embryology. Seventh edition. Philadelphia: Saunders, 2003:476-483.
2. Dayal VS, Farkashidy J, Kokshanian A. Embryology of the ear. Can J Otolaryngol 1973;2:136-142.
3. Wenig BM, Michaels L. The ear and temporal bone. In: Mills, SE, ed. Histology for pathologists. Fourth edition. Walters Kluwer: Lippincott Williams and Wilkins; Philadelphia. 2012:399-432.
4. Adams JC, Liberman MC. Anatomy. In: Merchant SN, Nadol Jr JB, eds. Schuknecht's Pathology of the ear, 3rd ed. United Kingdom: McGraw-Hill Education; 2010:53-95.
5. Hollinshead WH: The ear. In: Hollinshead WH, ed. Anatomy for surgeons. 3rd ed. Philadelphia: Harper and Row, 1982:159-221.
6. Nager GT. Anatomy. In: Nager GT, ed. Pathology of the ear and temporal bone. Baltimore: Williams & Wilkins; 1993:3-187.
7. Graves GO, Edwards LF. The Eustachian tube: A review of its descriptive, microscopic, topographic and clinical anatomy. Arch Otolaryngol 1944;39:359-397.
8. Moreano EH, Paparella MM, Zelterman D, Goycoolea MV. Prevalence of carotid canal dehiscence in the human middle ear: a report of 1000 temporal bones. Laryngoscope 1994;104:612-8.
9. Davies DV. A note on the articulations of the auditory ossicles and related structures. J Laryngol Otol 1948;62:533-6.

Congenital Abnormalities

10. Merchant SN. Genetically determined and other degenerative defects. In: Merchant SN, Nadol Jr JB, eds. Schuknecht's pathology of the ear. Third edition. United Kingdom: McGraw-Hill Education. 2010:137-277.
11. Jansen T, Romiti R, Altmeyer P. Accesory tragus: report of two cases and review of the literature. Pediatr Dermatol 2000;17:391-394.
12. Sebben JE. The accessory tragus—no ordinary skin tag. J Dermatol Surg Oncol 1989;15:304-307.
13. Miller TD, Metry D. Multiple accessory tragi as a clue to the diagnosis of the oculo-auriculo-vertebral (Goldenhar) syndrome. J Am Acad Dermatol 2004;50:S11-13.
14. Lam J, Dohil M. Multiple accessory tragi and hemifacial microsomia. Pediatr Dermatol 2007;24:657-658.
15. Mehta B, Nayak C, Savant S, Amladi S. Goldenhar syndrome with unusual features. Indian J Dermatol Venereol Leprol 2008;74:254-256.
16. Rankin JS, Schwartz RA. Accessory tragus: a possible sign of Goldenhar syndrome. Cutis 2011;88:62-64.
17. Gaurkar SP, Gupta KD, Parmar KS, Shah BJ. Goldenhar syndrome: a report of 3 cases. Indian J Dermatol 2013;5:244.
18. Brownstein MH, Wanger N, Helwig EB. Accessory tragi. Arch Dermatol 1971;104:625-631.
19. Olsen KD, Maragos NE, Weiland LH. First branchial cleft anomalies. Laryngoscope 1980;90:423-436.
20. Greenway RE, Hurst L, Fenton NA. An unusual first branchial cleft cyst. J Laryngol 1981;10:219-225.

Keloid

21. Murray JC, Pollack SV, Pinnel SR. Keloids: a review. J Am Acad Dermatol 1981;4:461-470.
22. Trisliana Perdanasari A, Lazzeri D, Su W, et al. Recent developments in the use of intralesional injections keloid treatment. Arch Plast Surg 2014;41:620-629.
23. Blackburn WR, Cosman B. Histologic basis of keloid and hypertrophic scar differentiation. Arch Pathol 1966;82:65-71.
24. Kuo TT, Hu S, Chan HL. Keloidal dermatofibroma: report of 10 cases of a new variant. Am J Surg Pathol 1998;22:564-568.
25. Cheng LH. Keloid of ear lobe. Laryngoscope 1972;82:673-681.
26. Griffith BH, Monroe CW, McKinney P. A follow-up study on the treatment of keloids with triamcinolonec acetonide. Plast Reconstr Surg 1970;46:145-150.
27. Kiil J. Keloids treated with topical injections of triamcinolone acetonide (kenalog). Immediate and long-term results. Scand J Plast Reconstr Surg 1977;11:169-172.
28. Ahuja RB, Chatterjee P. Comparative efficacy of intralesional verapamil hydrochloride and triamcinolone acetonide in hypertrophic scars and keloids. Burns 2014;40:583-588.
29. Har-Shai Y, Brown W, Labbé D, et al. Intralesional cryosurgery for the treatment of hypertrophic scars and keloids following aesthetic surgery: the results of a prospective observational study. Int J Low Extrem Wounds 2008;7:169-175.
30. Escarmant P, Zihmermann S, Amar A, et al. The treatment of 783 keloid scars by iridium 192 interstitial radiation after surgical excision. Int J Radiat Oncol Biol Phys 1993;26:245-257.
31. Sallstrom KO, Larson O, Hedén P, Eriksson G, Glas JE, Ringborg U. Treatment of keloids with surgical excision and postoperative x-ray radiation. Scand J Plast Surg 1989;23:211-215.

32. Stucker FJ, Shaw GY. An approach to management of keloids. Arch Otolaryngol Head Neck Surg 1992;188:63-67.
33. Tang YW. Intra and postoperative steroid injections for keloids and hypertrophic scars. Br J Plast Surg 1992;45:371-373.
34. Larrabee WF Jr, East CA, Jaffe HS, Stephenson C, Peterson KE. Intralesional interferon gamma treatment for keloids and hypertrophic scars. Arch Otolaryngol Head Neck Surg 1990;116:1159-1162.
35. Jones CD, Guiot L, Samy M, Gorman M, Tehrani H. The use of chemotherapeutics for the treatment of keloid scars. Dermatol Reports 2015;7:5880.
36. Abdou AG, Maraee AH, Al-Bara AM, Diab WM. Immunohistochemical expression of TGF-β1 in keloids and hypertrophic scars. Am J Dermatopathol 2011;33:84-91.
37. Tiede S, Ernst N, Bayat A, Paus R, Tronnier V, Zechel C. Basic fibroblast growth factor: a potential new therapeutic tool for the treatment of hypertrophic and keloid scars. Ann Anat 2009;191:33-44.

Chondrodermatitis Nodularis Chronicus Helicis

38. Winkler M. Knötchenformige erkrankung am helix (Chondrodermatitis nodularis chronica helicis). Arch Dermatol Syph 1915;121:278-285.
39. Metzger SA, Goodman ML. Chondrodermatitis helicis: A clinical re-evaluation and pathological review. Laryngoscope 1976;86:1402-1412.
40. Shuman R, Helwig EB. Chondrodermatitis helicis: chondrodermatitis nodularits chronica helciis. Am J Clin Pathol 1954;24:126-144.
41. Upile T, Patel NN, Jerjes W, Singh NU, Sandison A, Michaels L. Advances in the understanding of chondrodermatitis nodularis chronicus helicis: the perichondrial vasculitis theory. Clin Otolaryngol 2009;34:147-150.
42. Goette DK. Chondrodermatitis nodularis chronica helicis: a perforating necrobiotic granuloma. J Am Acad Dermatol 1980;2:148-154.
43. Kitchens GG. Auricular wedge resection and reconstruction. Ear Nose Throat 1989;68:673-683.
44. Lawrence CM. The treatment of chondrodermatitis nodularis with cartilage removal alone. Arch Dermatol 1991;127:530-535.
45. Moncrieff M, Sassoon EM. Effective treatment of chondrodermatitis nodularis chronica helicis using conservative approach. Br J Dermatol 2004 May;150(5):892-894.
46. Sanu A, Koppana R, Snow DG. Management of chondrodermatitis nodularis chronica helicis using a 'doghnut pillow'. J Laryngol Otol 2007;121:1096-1098.
47. Kuen-Spiegl M, Ratzinger G, Sepp N, Fritsch P. Chondrodermatitis nodularis chronica helicis—a conservative therapeutic approach by decompression. J Dtsch Dermatol Ges 2011;9:292-296.

Idiopathic Cystic Chondromalacia of the Auricular Cartilage

48. Hansen JE. Pseudocysts of the auricle in caucasians. Arch Otolaryngol Head Neck Surg 1967;85:13-14.
49. Heffner DK, Hyams VJ. Cystic chondromalacia (endochondral pseudocyst) of the auricle. Arch Pathol Lab Med 1986;110:740-743.
50. Lazar RH, Heffner DK, Huges GB, Hyams VK. Pseudocyst of the auricle: a review of 21 cases. Otolaryngol Head Neck Surg 1986;94:360-361.
51. Kontis TC, Goldstone A, Brown M, Paull G. Pathological quiz case 1: Auricular pseudocyst (benign idiopathic cystic chondromalacia, endochondral pseudocyst, or seroma of the auricle). Arch Otolaryngol Head Neck Surg. 1992;118:1128-1130.
52. Ichioka S, Yamada A, Ueda K, Harii K. Pseudocyst of the auricle: case reports and its biochemical characteristics. Ann Plast Surg 1993;31:471-474.
53. Chen PP, Tsai SM, Wang HM, et al. Lactate dehydrogenase isoenzyme patterns in auricular pseudocyst fluid. J Laryngol Otol 2013;127:479-482.
54. Engel D. Pseudocysts of the auricle in Chinese. Arch Otolaryngol 1966;83:197-202.
55. Borroni G, Brazzelli V, Merlino M. Pseudocyst of the auricle. A birthday ear pull. Br J Dermatol 1991;125:292-294.
56. Grabski WJ, Salasche SJ, McCollough ML, Angeloni VL. Pseudocyst of the auricle associated with trauma. Arch Dermatol 1989;125:528-530.
57. Kallini JR, Cohen PR. Rugby injury-associated pseudocyst of the auricle: report and review of sports-associated dermatoses of the ear. Dermatol Online J 2013;19:11.
58. Saunders MW, Jones NS, Balsitis M. Bilateral auricular pseudocyst: a case report and discussion. J Laryngol Otol 1993;107:39-41.
59. Lim CM, Goh YH, Chao SS, Lim LH, Lim L. Pseudocyst of the auricle: a histologic perspective. Laryngoscope 2004;114:1281-1284.
60. Lim CM, Goh YH, Chao SS, Lynne L. Pseudocyst of the auricle. Laryngoscope 2002;112:2033-2036.
61. Ramadass T, Ayyaswamy G. Pseudocyst of auricle—etiopathogenesis, treatement update and literature review. Indian J Otolaryngol Head Neck Surg 2006;;58:156-159.
62. Patigaroo SA, Mehfooz N, Patigaroo FA, Kirmani MH, Waheed A, Bhat S. Clinical characteristics and comparative study of different modalities of treatment of pseudocyst pinna. Eur Arch Otorhinolaryngol 2012;269:1747-1754.
63. Ophir D, Marshak G. Needle aspiration and pressure sutures for auricular pseudocyst. Plast Reconstr Surg 1991;87:783-784.

Exostosis

64. Nager GT. Osteomas and exostoses. In: Nager GT, ed. Pathology of the ear and temporal bone. Baltimore, Williams & Wilkins, 1993:483-512.
65. Whitaker SR, Cordier A, Kosjakov S, Charbonneau R. Treatment of external auditory canal exostoses. Laryngoscope 1998;108:195-199.
66. Fisher EW, McManus TC. Surgery for external auditory canal exostoses and osteomata. J Laryngol Otol 1994;108:106-110.
67. Kroon DF, Lawson ML, Derkay CS, Hoffmann K, McCook J. Surfer's ear: external auditory exostoses are more prevalent in cold water surfers. Otolaryngol Head Neck Surg 2002;126:499-504.
68. Nakanishi H, Tono T, Kawano H. Incidence of external auditory canal exostoses in competitive surfers in Japan. Otolaryngol Head Neck Surg 2011;145:80-85.
69. Cooper A, Tong R, Neil R, Owens D, Tomkinson A. External auditory canal exostoses in white water kayakers. Br J Sports Med 2010;44:144-147.
70. Moore RD, Schuman TA, Scott TA, Mann SE, Davidson MA, Labadie RF. Exostoses of the external auditory canal in white-water kayakers. Laryngoscope 2010;120:582-590.
71. Carbone PN, Nelson BL. External auditory osteoma. Head Neck Pathol 2012;6:244-246.
72. Graham MD. Osteomas and exostoses of the external auditory canal. A clinical, histopathological, and scanning electron microscopic study. Ann Otol Rhinol Laryngol 1979;88(Pt 1):566-572.
73. Fenton JE, Turner J, Fagan PA. A histopathologic review of temporal bone exostoses and osteomata. Laryngoscope 1996;106(Pt 1):624-628.

Synovial Chondromatosis

74. Villacin AB, Brigham LN, Bullough PG. Primary and secondary synovial chondrometaplasia: histopthologic and clinicoradiologic differences. Hum Pathol 1979;10:439-451.
75. Allias-Montmayeur F, Durroux R, Dodart L, Combelles R. Tumours and pseudotumorous lesions of the temporomandibular joint: a diagnostic challenge. J Laryngol Otol 1997;111:776-781.
76. Bell G, Sharp CW, Fourie LR, Hutchinson D. Conservative surgical management of synovial chondromatosis. Oral Surg Oral Med Oral Pathol Oral Radiol Endod 1997;84:592-593.
77. Psimopoulou M, Karakasis D, Magoudi D, Tzarou V, Eleftheriadis I. Synovial chondromatosis of the temporomandibular joint. Br J Oral Maxillofac Surg 1998;36:317-318.
78. Nussenbaum B, Roland PS, Gilcrease MZ, Odell DS. Extra-articular synovial chondromatosis of the temporomandibular joint: pitfalls in diagnosis. Arch Otolaryngol Head Neck Surg 1999;125:1394-1397.
79. Ardekian L, Faquin W, Troulis MJ, Kaban LB, August M. Synovial chondromatosis of the temporomandibular joint: report and analysis of eleven cases. J Oral Maxillofac Surg 2005;63:941-947.
80. Sink J, Bell B, Mesa H. Synovial chondromatosis of the temporomandibular joint: clinical, cytologic, histologic, radiologic, therapeutic aspects, and differential diagnosis of an uncommon lesion. Oral Surg Oral Med Oral Pathol Oral Radiol 2014:117:e269-274.
81. Deahl ST 2nd, Ruprecht A. Asymptomatic radiographically detected chondrometaplasia in the temporomandibular joint. Oral Surg Oral Med Oral Pathol 1991;72:371-374.
82. Testaverde L, Perrone A, Caporali L, et al. CT and MR findings in synovial chondromatosis of the temporo-mandibular joint: our experience and review of literature. Eur J Radiol 2011;78:414-418.
83. Varol A, Sencimen M, Gulses A, Altug HA, Dumlu A, Kurt B. Diagnostic importance of MRI and CT scans for synovial osteochondromatosis of the temporomandibular joint. Cranio 2011;29:313-317.
84. Wang P, Tian Z, Yang J, Yu Q. Synovial chondromatosis of the temporomandibular joint: MRI findings with pathological comparison. Dentomaxillofac Radiol 2012;41:110-116.
85. Matsumura Y, Nomura J, Nakanishi K, Yanase S, Kato H, Tagawa T. Synovial chondromatosis of the temporomandibular joint with calcium pyrophosphate dihydrate crystal deposition disease (pseudogout). Dentomaxillofac Radiol 2012;41:703-707.
86. Li Y, Cai H, Fang W, et al, Deng M, Long X. Fibroblast growth factor 2 involved in the pathogenesis of synovial chondromatosis of temporomandibular joint. J Oral Pathol Med 2014;43:388-394.
87. Li Y, El Mozen LA, Cai H, et al. Transforming growth factor beta 3 involved in the pathogenesis of synovial chondromatosis of the temporomandibular joint. Sci Rep 20156;5:8843.
88. Buddingh EP, Krallman P, Neff JR, Nelson M, Liu J, Bridge JA. Chromosome 6 abnormalities are recurrent in synovial chondromatosis. Cancer Genet Cytogenet 2003;140:18-22.
89. Mertens F, Jonsson K, Willén H, et al. Chromosome rearrangements in synovial chondromatous lesions. Br J Cancer 1996;74:251-254.
90. Kyriazoglou AI, Rizou H, Dimitriadis E, Arnogiannaki N, Agnantis N, Pandis N. Cytogenetic analysis of a low-grade secondary peripheral chondrosarcoma arising in synovial chondromatosis. In Vivo 2013;27:57-60.
91. Sciot R, Dal Cin P, Bellemans J, Samson I, Van den Berghe H, Van Damme B. Synovial chondromatosis: clonal chromosome changes provide further evidence for a neoplastic disorder. Virchows Arch 1998;433:189-191.

92. Tallini G, Dorfman H, Brys P, et al. Correlation between clinicopathological features and karyotype in 100 cartilaginous and chordoid tumours. A report from the Chromosomes and Morphology (CHAMP) Collaborative Study Group. J Pathol 2002;196:194-203.
93. Davis RI, Foster H, Arthur K, Trewin S, Hamilton PW, Biggart DJ. Cell proliferation studies in primary synovial chondromatosis. J Pathol 1998;184:18-23.
94. Yoshida H, Tsuji K, Oshiro N, Wato M, Morita S. Preliminary report of Ki-67 reactivity in synovial chondromatosis of the temporomandibular joint: an immunohistochemical study. J Craniomaxillofac Surg 2013;41:473-475.
95. Cai XY, Yang C, Chen MJ, et al. Arthroscopic management for synovial chondromatosis of the temporomandibular joint: a retrospective review of 33 cases. J Oral Maxillofac Surg 2012;70:2106-2113.
96. Karlis V, Glickman RS, Zaslow M. Synovial chondromatosis of the temporomandibular joint with intracranial extension. Oral Surg Oral Med Oral Pathol Oral Radiol Endod 1998;86:664-666.
97. Yokota N, Inenaga C, Tokuyama T, Nishizawa S, Miura K, Namba H. Synovial chondromatosis of the temporomandibular joint with intracranial extension. Neurol Med Chir (Tokyo) 2008;48:266-270.
98. Campbell DI, De Silva RK, De Silva H, Sinon SH, Rich AM. Temporomandibular joint synovial chondromatosis with intracranial extension: a review and observations of patient observed for 4 years. J Oral Maxillofac Surg 2011;69:2247-2252.
99. Mupparapu M. Synovial chondromatosis andibular joint with extension to the middle cranial fossa. J Postgrad Med 2005;51:122-124.
100. Pau M, Bicsák T, Reinbacher KE, Feichtinger M, Kärcher H. Surgical treatment of synovial chondromatosis of the temporomandibular joint with erosion of the skull base: a case report and review of the literature. Int J Oral Maxillofac Surg 2014;43:600-605.
101. Davis RI, Hamilton A, Biggart JD. Primary synovial chondromatosis: a clinicopathologic review and assessment of malignant potential. Hum Pathol 1998;29:683-688.
102. Ichikawa T, Miyauchi M, Nikai H, Yoshiga K. Synovial chondrosarcoma arising in the temporomandibular joint. J Oral Maxillofac Surg 1998;56:890-894.
103. Coleman H, Chandraratnam E, Morgan G, Gomes L, Bonar F. Synovial chondrosarcoma arising in synovial chondromatosis of the temporomandibular joint. Head Neck Pathol 2013;7:304-309.

Kimura Disease and Epithelioid Hemangioma

104. Rosai J, Gold J, Landy R. The histiocytoid hemangioma. A unifying concept embracing several previously described entities of skin, soft tissues, large vessels, bone and heart. Hum Pathol 1979;10:707-730.
105. Allen PW, Ramakrishna B, MacCormac LB. The histiocytoid hemangiomas and other controversies. Pathol Ann 1992;27(Pt 2):51-87.
106. Chun SI, Ji HG. Kimura's disease and angiolymphoid hyperplasia with eosinophilia: clinical and histopathologic differences. Am Acad Dermatol 1992;27:954-958.
107. Googe PB, Harris NL, Mihm MC Jr. Kimura's disease and angiolymphoid hyperplasia with eosinophilia: two distinct histopathological entities. J Cutan Pathol 1987;14:263-271.
108. Kuo TT, Shih LY, Chan HL. Kimura's disease: involvement of regional lymph nodes and distinction from angiolymphoid hyperplasia with eosinophilia. Am J Surg Pathol 1988;12:843-854.
109. Tsang WY, Chan JK. The family of epithelioid vascular tumors. Histol Histopathol 1993;8:187-212.
110. Urabe A, Tsuneyoshi M, Enjoji M. Epithelioid hemangioma verses Kimura's disease. A comparative clinicopathologic study. Am J Surg Pathol 1987;11:758-766.
111. Barnes L, Koss W, Nieland ML. Angiolymphoid hyperplasia with eosinophilia: a disease that may be confused with malignancy. Head Neck Surg 1980;2:425-434.
112. Olsen TG, Helwig EB. Angiolymphoid hyperplasia with eosinophilia. A clinicopathologic study of 116 patients. J Am Acad Dermatol 1985;12:781-796.
113. Fetsch JF, Weiss SW. Observations concerning the pathogenesis of epithelioid hemangioma (angiolymphoid hyperplasia). Mod Pathol 1991;4:449-455.
114. Renshaw AA, Rosai J. Benign atypical vascular lesions of the lip. A study of 12 cases. Am J Surg Pathol. 1993;17:557-665.
115. Rosai J, Ackerman LR. Intravenous atypical vascular proliferation. A cutaneous lesion simulating malignant vascular tumors. Arch Dermatol 1974;109:714-717.
116. Hosaka N, Minato T, Yoshida S, et al. Kimura's disease with unusual eosinophilic epithelioid granulomatous reaction: a finding possibly related to eosinophil apoptosis. Hum Pathol 2002;33:561-564.
117. Baum EW, Sams WM Jr, Monheit GD. Angiolymphoid hyperplasia with eosinophilia. The disease and a comparison of treatment modalities. J Dermatol Surg Oncol 1982;8:966-970.

Langerhans Cell Histiocytosis

180. Willman CL. Detection of clonal histiocytes in Langerhans cell histiocytosis: biology and cli6nical significance. Br J Cancer Suppl 1994;23:S29-33.
181. Willman CL, Busque L, Griffith BB, et al. Langerhans' cell histiocytosis (histiocytosis X) —a clonal proliferative disease. N Engl J Med 1994;331:154-160.
182. Lieberman PH, Jones CR, Steinman RM, et al. Langerhans cell (eosinophilic) granulomatosis: A clinicopathologic study encompassing 50 years Am J Surg Pathol 1997;20:519-552.
183. al-Ammar AY, Tewfik TL, Bond M, Schloss MD. Langerhans' cell histiocytosis: paediatric head and neck study. J Otolaryngol 1999;28:266-272.
184. Appling D, Jenkins HA, Patton GA. Eosinophilic granuloma in the temporal bone and skull. Otolaryngol Head Neck Surg 1983;91:358-365.
185. Bayazit Y, Sirikci A, Bayaram M, Kanlikama M, Demir A, Bakir K. Eosinophilic granuloma of the temporal bone. Auris Nasus Larynx 2001;28:99-102.
186. Cochrane LA, Prince M, Clarke K. Langerhans' cell histiocytosis in the paediatric population: presentation and treatment of head and neck manifestations. J Otolaryngol 2003;32:33-37.
187. McCaffrey TV, McDonald TJ. Histiocytosis X of the ear and temporal bone: a review of 22 cases. Laryngoscope 1979;89:1735-1742.
188. Chikwava K, Jaffe R. Langerin (CD207) staining in normal pediatric tissues, reactive lymph nodes, and childhood histiocytic disorders. Pediatr Dev Pathol 2004;7:607-614.
189. Lau SK, Chu PG, Weiss LM. Immunohistochemical expression of Langerin in Langerhans cell histiocytosis and non-Langerhans cell histiocytic disorders. Am J Surg Pathol 2008;32:615-619.
190. Ide F, Iwase T, Saito I, Umemura S, Nakajima T. Immunohistochemical and ultrastructural analysis of the proliferating cells in histiocytosis X. Cancer 1984;53:917-921.
191. Machnicki MM, Stoklosa T. BRAF—a new player in hematological neoplasms. Blood Cells Mol Dis 2014;53:77-83.
192. Rizzo FM, Cives M, Simone V, Silvestris F. New Insights into the molecular pathogenesis of langerhans cell histiocytosis. Oncologist 2014;19:151-163.
193. Wenig BM, Abbondanzo SL, Childers E, Kapadia SB, Heffner DR. Extranodal sinus histiocytosis with massive lymphadenopathy (Rosai-Dorfman disease) of the head and neck. Hum Pathol 1993;24:483-492.
194. Haupt R, Minkov M, Astigarraga I, et al. Langerhans cell histiocytosis (LCH): guidelines for diagnosis, clinical work-up, and treatment for patients till the age of 18 years. Pediatr Blood Cancer 2013;60:175-184.
195. Satter EK, High WA. Langerhans cell histiocytosis: a review of the current recommendations of the Histiocyte Society. Pediatr Dermatol 2008;25:291-295.
196. Wang J, Wu X, Xi ZJ. Langerhans cell histiocytosis of bone in children: a clinicopathologic study of 108 cases. World J Pediatr 2010;6:255-259.

Middle Ear Salivary Gland Heterotopia

197. Amrhein P, Sittel C, Spaich C, et al. [Middle ear salivary gland choristoma related to branchio-oto-renal syndrome diagnosed by array-CGH.] HNO 2014;62:374-377. [German]
198. Bottrill ID, Chawla OP, Ramsay AD. Salivary gland choristoma of the middle ear. J Laryngol Otol 1992;106:630-632.
199. Cannon CR. Salivary gland choristoma of the middle ear. Am J Otol 1980;1:250-251.
200. Fois P, Giannuzzi AL, Paties CT, Falcioni M. Salivary gland choristoma of the middle ear. Ear Nose Throat J 2014;93:458-464.
201. Saeger KL, Gruskin P, Carberry JN. Salivery gland choristoma of the middle ear. Arch Pathol Lab Med 1982;106;39-40.
202. Toros SZ, Egeli E, Kiliçarslan Y, Gümrükçü G, Gökçeer T, Noseri H. Salivary gland choristoma of the middle ear in a child with situs inversus totalis. Auris Nasus Larynx 2010;37:365-368.
203. Kartush JM, Graham MD. Salivary gland choristoma of the middle ear: A case report and review of the literature. Laryngoscope 1984;94:228-230.
204. Saeed YM, Bassis ML. Mixed tumor of the middle ear. A case report. Arch Otolaryngol 1971;93:433-434.

Acquired Encephalocele

205. Aristeui M, Falcioni M, Saleh E, et al. Meningoencephalic herniation into the middle ear: a report of 27 cases. Laryngoscope 1995;105:512-518.
206. Glassock ME 3rd, Dickins JR, Jackson CG, Wiet RJ, Feenstra L. Surgical management of brain tissue herniation into the middle ear and mastoid. Laryngoscope 1979;89:1743-1754.
207. Jackson CG, Pappas DG Jr, Manolidis S, et al. Brain herniation into the middle ear and mastoid: concepts in diagnosis and surgical management. Am J Otol 1997;18:198-205.
208. Mosnier I, Fiky LE, Shahidi A, Sterkers O. Brain herniation and chronic otitis media: diagnosis and surgical management. Clin Otolaryngol Allied Sci 2000;25:385-391.
209. Bowes AK, Wiet RJ, Monsell EM, Hahn YS, O'Connor CA. Brain herniation and space-occupying lesions eroding the tegmen tympani. Laryngoscope 1987;97:1172-1175.

210. Martin N, Sterkers O, Murat M, Hahum N. Brain herniation into the middle ear cavity: MR imaging. Neuroradiology 1989;31;184-186.
211. Gyure KA, Thompson LD, Morrison AL. A clinicopathological study of 15 patients with neuroglial heterotopias and encephaloceles of the middle ear and mastoid region. Laryngoscope 2000;110(Pt 1):1731-1735.
212. Heffner DK. Brain in the middle ear or nasal cavity: heterotopia or encephalocele? Ann Diagn Pathol 2004;8:252-257.
213. Nishiike S, Miyao Y, Gouda S, et al. Brain herniation into the middle ear following temporal bone fracture. Acta Otolaryngol 2005;125:902-905.
214. Alkhalidi H, de Tilly LN, Fenton R, Munoz DG. Spontaneous middle-ear encephalocele: report of two cases and brief review. Clin Neuropathol. 2008;27:357-360.
215. Gray BG, Willinsky RA, Rutka JA, Tator CH. Spontaneous meningocele, a rare middle ear mass. AJNR Am J Neuroradiol 1995;16:203-207.

Relapsing Polychondritis

216. Damiani JM, Levine HL. Relapsing polychondritis—report of ten cases. Laryngoscope 1979;89:929-946.
217. McAdam LP, O'Hanlan MA, Bluestone R, Pearson CM. Relapsing polychondritis: prospective study of 23 patients and a review of the literature. Medicine 1976;55:193-215.
218. Yang H, Peng L, Jian M, Qin L. Clinical analysis of 15 patients with relapsing auricular polychondritis. Eur Arch Otorhinolaryngol 2014;271:473-476.
219. Cody DT, Sones DA. Relapsing polychondritis: Audiovestibular manifestations. Laryngoscope 1971;81:1208-1222.
220. Cantarini L, Vitale A, Brizi MG, et al. Diagnosis and classification of relapsing polychondritis. J Autoimmun 2014;48-49:53-59.
221. McCaffrey TV, McDonald TJ, McCaffrey LA. Head and neck manifestations of relapsing polychondritis: review of 29 cases. Otolaryngol 1978;86(Pt 1):473-478.
222. Yoo JH, Chodosh J, Dana R. Relapsing polychondritis: systemic and ocular manifestations, differential diagnosis, management, and prognosis. Semin Ophthalmol 2011;26:261-269.
223. Mattiassich G, Egger M, Semlitsch G, Rainer F. Occurrence of relapsing polychondritis with a rising cANCA titre in a cANCA-positive systemic and cerebral vasculitis patient. BMJ Case Rep 2013;15:2013.
224. Geffriaud-Ricouard C, Noel LH, Chauveau D, et al. Clinical spectrum associated with ANCA of defined antigen specificities in 98 selected patients. Clin Nephrol 1993;39:125-136.
225. Harisdangkul V, Johnson WW. Association between relapsing polychondritis and systemic lupus erythematosus. South Med J 1994;87:753-757.
226. Lahmer T, Treiber M, von Werder A, et al. Relapsing polychondritis: an autoimmune disease with many faces. Autoimmun Rev 2010;9:540-546.
227. Dolan DL, Lemmon GB Jr, Teitelbaum SL. Relapsing polychondritis. Analytical literature review and studies on pathogenesis. Am J Med 1966;41:285-299.
228. Ebringer R, Rook G, Swana T, Bottazzo GF, Doniach D. Autoantibodies to cartilage and type II collagen in relapsing polychondritis and other rheumatic diseases. Ann Rheum Dis 1981;40:473-479.
229. Helm TN, Valenzuela R, Glanz S, Parker L, Dijkstra J, Bergfeld WF. Relapsing polychondritis: a case diagnosed by direct immunofluorescence and coexisting with pseudocyst of the auricle. J Am Acad Dermatol 1992;26:315-318.
230. Valenzuela R, Cooperrider PA, Gogate P, Deodhar SD, Bergfeld WF. Relapsing polychondritis: immunomicroscopic findings in cartilage of ear biopsy specimens. Hum Pathol 1980;11:19-22.
231. Lang B, Rothenfusser A, Lanchbury JS, et al. Susceptibility to relapsing polychondritis is associated with HLA-DR4. Arthritis Rheum 1993;36:660-664.
232. Arnaud L, Mathian A, Haroche J, Gorochov G, Amoura Z. Pathogenesis of relapsing polychondritis: a 2013 update. Autoimmun Rev 2014;13:90-95.
233. Irani BS, Martin-Hirsch DP, Clark D, Hand DW, Vize CE, Black J. Relapsing polychondritis—a study of four cases. J Laryngol Otol 1992;106:911-914.

Granulomatosis with Polyangiitis

234. Bucolo S, Torre V, Montemagno A, Beatrice F. Wegener's granulomatosis presenting with otologic and neurologic symptoms: clinical and pathological correlations. J Oral Pathol Med 2003;32:438-440.
235. Illum P, Thorling K. Otologic manifestations of Wegener's granulomatosis. Laryngoscope 1982;92:801-804.
236. Kornblut AD, Wolff SM, Fauci AS. Ear disease in patient's with Wegener's granulomatosis. Laryngoscope 1982;92(Pt 1):713-717.
237. McCaffrey TV, McDonald TJ, Facer GW, DeRemee RA. Otologic manifestations of Wegener's granulomatosis. Otolaryngol Head Neck Surg 1980;88:586-593.
238. Srouji IA, Andrews P, Edwards C, Lund VJ. Patterns of presentation and diagnosis of patients with Wegener's granulomatosis: ENT aspects. J Laryngol Otol 2007;121:653-658.

239. Wierzbicka M, Szyfter W, Puszczewicz M, Borucki L, Bartochowska A. Otologic symptoms as initial manifestation of wegener granulomatosis: diagnostic dilemma. Otol Neurotol 2011;32:996-1000.
240. Okamura H, Ohtani I, Anzai T. The hearing loss in Wegener's granulomatosis: relationship between hearing loss and serum ANCA. Auris Nasus Larynx 1992;19:1-6.
241. Fauci AS, Haynes BF, Katz P, Wolff SM. Wegener's granulomatosis: prospective clinical and therapeutic experience with 85 patients for 21 years. Ann Intern Med 1983;98:76-85.
242. Dagum P, Roberson JB Jr. Otologic Wegener's granulomatosis with facial nerve palsy. Ann Otol Rhinol Laryngol 1998;107:555-559.
243. Ferri E, Armato E, Capuzzo P, Cavaleri S, Ianniello F. Early diagnosis of Wegener's granulomatosis presenting with bilateral facial paralysis and bilateral serous otitis media. Auris Nasus Larynx 2007;34:379-382.
244. Maranhão AS, Chen VG, Rossini BA, Testa JR, Penido Nde O. Mastoiditis and facial paralysis as initial manifestations of Wegener's Granulomatosis. Braz J Otorhinolaryngol 2012;78:80-86.
245. Csernok E, Holle J, Hellmich B, et al. Evaluation of capture ELISA for detection of antineutrophil cytoplasmic antibodies directed against proteinase 3 in Wegener's granulomatosis: first results from a multicentre study. Rheumatology 2004:43:174-180.
246. Nolle B, Specks U, Ludemann J, Rohrbach MS, DeRemee RA, Gross WL. Anticytoplasmic autoantibodies: their immunodiagnostic value in Wegener's granulomatosis. Ann Int Med 1989;111:28-40.
247. Specks U, Wheatley CL, McDonald TJ, Rohrbach MS, DeRemee RA. Anticytoplasmic autoantibodies in the diagnosis and follow-up of Wegener's granulomatosis. Mayo Clin Proc 1989;64:28-36.
248. Wolf M, Kronenberg J, Engelberg S, Leventon G. Rapidly progressive hearing loss as a symptom of polyarteritis nodosa. Am J Otolaryngol 1987;8:105-108.
249. Gussen R. Atypical ossicle joint lesions in rheumatoid arthritis with sicca syndrome (Sjögren syndrome). Arch Otolaryngol 1977;103:284-286.
250. McDonald TJ, DeRemee RA. Wegener's granulomatosis. Laryngoscope 1983;93:220-231.

Tophaceous Gout

251. Czerniak B. Tophaceous gout. In: Czerniak B, ed. Dorfman and Czerniak's bone tumors, 2nd ed. Philadelphia: Elsevier; 2016:1420-1421.
252. Chabra I, Singh R. Gouty tophi on the ear: a review. Cutis 2013;92:190-192.
253. Grahame R, Scott JT. Clinical survey of 354 patients with gout. Ann Rheum Dis 1970;29:461-468.
254. Crittenden DB, Pillinger MH. New therapies for gout. Annu Rev Med 2013;64:325-337.
255. Harrold L. New developments in gout. Curr Opin Rheumatol 2013;25:304-309.

Tophaceous Pseudogout

256. McCarty DJ, Hollander JL. Identification of urate crystals in gouty synovial fluid. Ann Intern Med 1961;54:452-460.
257. Ishida T, Dorfman HD, Bullough PG. Tophaceous pseudogout (tumoral calcium pyrophosphate dihydrate crystal deposition disease). Hum Pathol 1995;26:587-593.
258. Vargas A, Teruel J, Trull J, Lopez E, Pont J, Velayos A. Calcium pyrophosphate dihydrate crystal deposition disease presenting as a pseudotumor of the temporomandibular joint. Eur Radiol 1997;7:1452-1453.
259. Zweifel D, Ettlin D, Schuknecht B, Obwegeser J. Tophaceous calcium pyrophosphate dihydrate deposition disease of the temporomandibular joint: the preferential site? J Oral Maxillofac Surg 2012;70:60-67.
260. Abhishek A, Doherty M. Pathophysiology of articular chondrocalcinosis—role of ANKH. Nat Rev Rheumatol 2011;7:96-104.
261. Slater LJ. Distinguishing calcium pyrophosphate dihydrate deposition disease from synovial chondrosarcoma. J Oral Maxillofac Surg 1998;56:693-694.
262. Goldblum JR, Folpe AL, Weiss SW. Tumoral calcinosis. In: Goldblum JR, Folpe AL, Weiss SW, eds. Enzinger & Weiss's soft tissue tumors, 6th ed. Philadelphia: Elsevier; 2014:947-951.

Otosclerosis

263. Nager GT. Otosclerosis. In: Nager GT, ed. Pathology of the ear and temporal bone. Baltimore: Williams & Wilkins; 1993:943-1010.
264. Cody DT, Baker HL Jr. Otosclerosis: vestibular symptoms and senosrineural hearing loss. Ann Otol Rhinol Laryngol 1978;87:778-796.
265. Morales-Garcia C. Cochleo-vestibular involvement in otosclerosis. Acta Otolaryngol 1972;73:484-492.
266. McKenna MJ, Merchant SN. Disorders of bone. In: Merchant SN, Nadol Jr JB, eds. Schuknecht's Pathology of the ear, 3rd ed. United Kingdom: McGraw-Hill Education; 2010:715-771.
267. Purohit B, Hermans R, Op de Beeck K. Imaging in otosclerosis: a pictorial review. Insights Imaging 2014;5:245-252.
268. Ealy M, Smith RJ. The genetics of otosclerosis. Hear Res 2010;266:70-74.

269. Karosi T, Sziklai I. Etiopathogenesis of otosclerosis. Eur Arch Otorhinolaryngol 2010;267:1337-1349.
270. Moumoulidis I, Axon P, Baguley D, Reid E. A review of the genetics of otosclerosis. Clin Otolaryngol 2007;32:239-247.
271. Michaels L, Soucek S. Origin and growth of otosclerosis. Acta Otolaryngol 2011;131:460-468.
272. Michaels L, Soucek S. Atypical mature bone in the otosclerotic otic capsule as the differentiated zone of an invasive osseous neoplasm. Acta Otolaryngol 2014;134:118-123.
273. Wenig BM, Michaels L. The ear and temporal bone. In: Mills, SE, ed. Histology for pathologists. Fourth edition. Philadelphia: Walters Kluwer: Lippincott Williams and Wilkins; 2012:399-432.

Paget Disease

274. Schuknecht HF. Paget's disease. In: Pathology of the ear, 2nd ed. Philadelphia: Lea & Febiger; 1993:379-90.
275. Davies DG. The temporal bone in Paget's disease J Laryngol Otol 1970;84:553-560.
276. Nager GT. Osteitis deformans Paget. In: Nager GT, ed. Pathology of the ear and temporal bone. Baltimore: Williams & Wilkins; 1993:1011-1050.
277. Monsell EM. The mechanism of hearing loss in Paget's disease of bone. Laryngoscope 2004;114: 598-606.
278. Birgerson L, Gustavson K, Stahle J. Familial Meniere's disease: a genetic investigation. Am J Otol 1987;8:323-326.
279. Kurihara N, Hiruma Y, Yamana K, et al. Contributions of the measles virus nucleocapsid gene and the SQSTM1/p62(P392L) mutation to Paget's disease. Cell Metab 2011;13:23-34.
280. Teramachi J, Zhou H, Subler MA, et al. Increased IL-6 Expression in osteoclasts is necessary but not sufficient for the development of Paget's Disease of bone. J Bone Miner Res 2014;29:1456-1465.
281. Wang FM, Sarmasik A, Hiruma Y, et al. Measles virus nucleocapsid protein, a key contributor to Paget's disease, increases IL-6 expression via down-regulation of FoxO3/Sirt1 signaling. Bone 2013;53:269-276.
282. Seitz S, Priemel M, Zustin J, et al. Paget's disease of bone: histologic analysis of 754 patients. J Bone Miner Res 2009;24:62-69.
283. Deyrup AT, Montag AG, Inwards CY, Xu Z, Swee RG, Krishnan Unni K. Sarcomas arising in Paget disease of bone: a clinicopathologic analysis of 70 cases. Arch Pathol Lab Med 2007;131:942-946.
284. Haibach H, Farrell C, Dittrich FJ. Neoplasms arising in Paget's disease of bone: a study of 82 cases. Am J Clin Pathol 1985;83:594-600.
285. Shaylor PJ, Peake D, Grimer RJ, Carter SR, Tillman RM, Spooner D. Paget's osetosarcoma—no cure in sight. Sarcoma 1999;3:191-192
286. Wick MR, McLeod RA, Siegel GP, et al. Sarcomas of bone complicating osteitis deformans (Paget's disease): fifty years' experience. Am J Surg Pathol 1981;5:47-59.

Ménière Disease

287. Murdin L, Schilder AG. Epidemiology of balance symptoms and disorders in the community: a systematic review. Otol Neurotol 2015;36:387-392.
288. Nager GT. Ménière disease. In: Nager GT, ed. Pathology of the ear and temporal bone. Baltimore: Williams & Wilkins; 1993:1213-1228.
289. Morrison AW, Mowbray JF, Williamson R, Sheeka S, Sodha N, Koskinen N. On genetic and environmental factors in Meniere's disease. Am J Otol 1994;15:35-39.
290. Ruckenstein MJ, Rutka JA, Hawke M. The treatment of Meniere's disease: Torok revisited. Laryngoscope 1991;101:211-218.
291. Xenellis J, Morrison AW, McClowskey D, Festenstein H. HLA antigen in the pathogenesis of Meniere's disease. J Laryngol Otol 1986;100:21-24.
292. Birgerson L, Gustavson K, Stahle J. Familial Meniere's disease: a genetic investigation. Am J Otol 1987;8:323-326.
293. Paparella MM. The cause (multifactorial inheritence) and pathogenesis (endolymphatic malabsorption) of Meniere's disease and its symptoms (mechanical and chemical). Acta Otolaryngol (Stockh) 1985;99:445-451.
294. Klis SFL, Buijs J, Smoorenburg GF. Quantification of the relationship between electrophysiologic and morphologic changes in experimental endolymphatic hydrops. Ann Otol Rhinol Laryngol 1990;99:566-570.
295. Hamid M. Medical management of common peripheral vestibular disease. Curr Opin Otolaryngol Head Neck Surg 2010;18:407-412.
296. Sood AJ, Lambert PR, Nguyen SA, Meyer TA. Endolymphatic sac surgery for Ménière disease; a systematic review and meta-analysis. Otol Neurotol 2014;35:1033-1045.

Developmental Defects of the Middle Ear and Temporal Bone

297. Nager GT. Dysplasia of the external and middle ear. In: Pathology of the ear and temporal bone. Baltimore: Williams & Wilkins; 1993:83-118.
298. Nager GT. Dysplasia of the osseous and membranous cochlea and vestibular labyrinth. In: Pathology of the ear and temporal bone. Baltimore: Williams & Wilkins; 1993:119-146.

Index

A

Aberrant rest, 108, 327
    larynx/trachea, 327
    oral cavity, 108
Accessory ear/auricle, 420
Accessory parotid glands, 375
Accessory tragus, 420
Acquired cholesteatoma, 446
Acquired encephalocele, middle ear, 454
Acquired immunodeficiency syndrome, pharynx, 235
    disease classification, 236
    diagnostic criteria, 241
    opportunistic infections, 245
    pathogenesis, 235
    spectrum of disease, 236
    staging, 238
    surveillance case definition, 239, 240
Acquired immunodeficiency syndrome-related parotid cyst, 387
Actinomycosis, 298, 330
    larynx/trachea, 330
    neck, 298
Acute fulminant *Aspergillus* sinusitis, 66
Acute invasive rhinosinusitis, 66
Acute sialadenitis, 386
Adenomatoid hyperplasia, salivary gland, 377
Adenomatous ductal hyperplasia, salivary gland, 401
Adenomatous hyperplasia, salivary gland, 382
Adenocarcinoma, nasal cavity, 34, 38
    differentiation from respiratory epithelial adenomatoid hamartoma, 34; from seromucinous hamartoma, 38
Allergic fungal rhinosinusitis, 61
    clinical features, 62
    definition, 61
    differential diagnosis, 63
    gross findings, 62
    immunohistochemical/histochemical findings, 63
    in situ hybridization, 63
    microscopic findings, 63
    pathogenesis, 62
    treatment and prognosis, 65
Allergic fungal sinusitis, 61
Allergic laryngitis, 334
Allergic rhinosinusitis, 90
Allergic sinonasal aspergillosis, 61
Alveolar ridges, 103
Amalgam tattoo, 170
Amebiasis, 87
Amyloidosis, laryngeal, 347
Anatomy, normal, 1, 6, 103, 207, 263, 319, 324, 369, 414
    ear and temporal bone, 414
        external ear, 414
        inner ear, 415
        middle ear, 415
    larynx, 319
    nasal cavity, 1
        ethmoid sinus, 7
        frontal sinus, 7
        maxillary sinus, 6
        osteomeatal complex, 7
        sphenoid sinus, 7
    neck, 263
        anterior triangle, 263
        cervical lymph nodes, 263
        posterior triangle, 263
    oral cavity and jaw, 103
        alveolar ridges, 103
        buccal mucosa, 103
        floor of mouth, 103
        gingiva, 104
        gnathic bones, 104
        hard palate, 104
        lips, 103
        periodontal ligament, 104
        retromolar trigone, 103
        teeth, 104
        tongue, 104
    paranasal sinuses, 6
    pharynx, 207
        hypopharynx, 208
        nasopharynx, 208
        oropharynx, 207
        parapharyngeal space, 209
    salivary glands, 369
        minor glands and seromucous glands, 371
        parotid gland, 369
        sublingual gland, 370
        submandibular gland, 370
    trachea, 324

Aneurysmal bone cyst, differentiation from central and peripheral giant cell granuloma, 149
Angioedema, larynx, 334
Angiolymphoid hyperplasia with eosinophilia, ear, *see* Epithelioid hemangioma
Angular cheilitis, 117
Antrochoanal polyp, nasal cavity, 22
Aphthous stomatitis, 190
    herpetiform, 191
    major, 191
    minor, 191
Apical cyst, 187
Apical periodontal cyst, 187
Aspergilloma, 65
Aspergillus fungi, 62
Aspergillus mycetoma, 65
Aspirin-exacerbated respiratory disease, 91
Aspirin intolerance, 91
Atrophic rhinosinusitis, 90
Aural polyp, 444
Autoimmune diseases, 189, 335, 455
    ear, 455
    larynx/trachea, 335
    oral cavity, 189

B

Bacillary angiomatosis, 302
Bacteria ball, 82
Bacterial diseases, 76, 120, 248, 331, 438 *see also under individual entities*
    ear, 438
        otitis media, 438
    larynx/trachea, 331
        abscess, retropharyngeal, peritonsillar, laryngeal, 332
        diphtheria, 332
    nasal cavity and paranasal sinuses, 76
        bacterial rhinoscleroma, 76
        mycobacteria, 84
        sinonasal botryomycosis, 83
    oral cavity, 120
        gonorrhea, 121
    pharynx, 248
        gonorrhea, 248
Bacterial sinusitis, 90
Basal cell carcinoma, 184, 401
    differentiation from dentigerous cyst, 184; from intercalated duct lesion, 401
Basal layer hyperplasia, larynx, 354
Benign lymphoepithelial lesion, salivary gland, 390
Black hairy tongue, 174
Blastomycosis, sinonasal, 74
Boeck disease, 396
Botryoid odontogenic cyst, 186
Botryomycosis, sinonasal, 82
Brain prolapse/herniation, middle ear, 454
Branchial anomalies, 264, 421
    ear and temporal bone, 421
    neck, 264
        branchial apparatus and derivatives, 266
        first branchial anomalies, 267
        fourth branchial anomalies, 280
        second branchial anomalies, 269
        third branchial anomalies, 279
Branchial apparatus, 266
Branchial cleft carcinoma, differentiation from second branchial anomalies, 277
Branchial cleft cyst, 267, 271, 421
Bronchial cyst, 287
Bronchogenic cyst, 287
Brown tumor of hyperparathyroidism, differentiation from central and peripheral giant cell granuloma, 149
Buccal mucosa, 103

C

Calcifying fibroblastic granuloma, 134
Candida albicans, 116, 248
Candidiasis, 116, 248, 333
    larynx/trachea, 333
    oral cavity, 116
        chronic hyperplastic candidiasis, 117
        erythematous candidiasis, 116
        mucocutaneous candidiasis, 117
        pseudomembranous candidiasis, 116
    pharynx, 248
Candidosis, 116
Canker sore, 190
Cat scratch disease, 300, 330
    larynx/trachea, 330
    neck, 300
Cemento-osseous dysplasia, 169
    florid, 169
    focal, 169
    periapical, 169
Centers for Disease Control classification for HIV

infection, 237
Central and peripheral giant cell granulomas, 144
   clinical features, 144
     differential diagnosis, 147; differentiation from giant cell tumor of bone, 149; brown tumor of hyperparathyroidism, 149; aneurysmal bone cyst, 149
   microscopic findings, 146
   treatment and prognosis, 152
Central papillary atrophy of the tongue, 117
Cervical lymph nodes, 263
   levels, 264
Cervical thymic cyst, 285
Cervicofacial actinomycosis, 298
Cholesteatoma, middle ear, 446
   acquired cholesteatoma, 446
   congenital cholesteatoma, 446
   definition, 446
   differential diagnosis, 448; differentiation from cholesterol granuloma, 449; from keratosis obturans, 449
   gross and microscopic findings, 447
   molecular genetic findings, 448
   treatment and prognosis, 449
Cholesterol granuloma, differentiation from cholesteatoma, 449
Chondrocalcinosis, ear, 460
Chondrodermatitis nodularis chronicus helicis, 425
Chondroid hamartoma, 40
Chondro-osseous and respiratory epithelial hamartoma, 39
Choristomas, 108, 111, 219, 327, 375, 453
   larynx/trachea, 327
   middle ear, 453
   oral cavity, 108, 111
   pharyngeal, 219
   salivary gland, 375
Chronic fibrosing tonsillitis, 224
Chronic granulomatous rhinosinusitis, 67
Chronic hyperplastic candidiasis, 177
Chronic invasive rhinosinusitis, 67
Chronic metaplastic ostitis, 461
Chronic multifocal candidiasis, 117
Chronic nonautoimmune sialadenitis, 386
Chronic sclerosing sialadenitis, 394
Ciliary dysfunction, 16
Classification of non-neoplastic lesions, 8, 109, 215, 265, 325, 375, 421

   ear and temporal bone, 421
   laryngeal/tracheal, 325
   neck, 265
   oral cavity, 109
   pharynx, 215
   salivary glands, 375
   sinonasal tract, 8
Coccidioidomycosis, sinonasal, 74
Cochlea, 416
Condyloma acuminatum, 122
   oral mucosal condyloma acuminatum, 122
Congenital abnormalities, *see* Developmental lesions
Congenital cholesteatoma, 446
Congenital epulis, 160
Congenital flaccid larynx, 324
Congenital gingival granular cell tumor, 160
Congenital granular cell epulis, 160
Congenital laryngeal stridor, 324
Congenital pleomorphic adenoma, 224
Contact ulcer of larynx, 342
Corditis nodosa, 339
Craniofacial dermoid cyst, 15
Cryptococcosis, sinonasal, 74
Crystal deposition disease, ear, 458
Cystic chondromalacia, idiopathic, of auricular cartilage, 426
Cysts and cystic lesions, 113, 212, 264, 340, 342, 377, 421
   ear and temporal bone, 421
     branchial cleft cysts, 421
   larynx, 340, 342
     oncocytic cystadenoma, 342
     retention cyst, 342
     saccular cyst, 340
   oral cavity, 113
     nasopalatine duct cyst, 114
     oral lymphoepithelial cyst, 113
   neck, 264
     branchial anomalies, 264
     bronchogenic cyst, 287
     cervical thymic cyst, 285
     dermoid cyst, 292
     thyroglossal duct cyst, 280
   pharynx, 212
     Rathke pouch cyst, 215
     Thornwaldt cyst, 216
   salivary glands, 377

lymphoepithelial cyst, 381
mucous retention cyst, 377
mucus extravasation phenomenon, 379
polycystic disease, 382
ranula, 389
salivary duct cyst, 377
Cytomegalovirus, 120, 245
    oral cavity, 120
    pharynx, 245

D

Dental cyst, 187
Dental follicle, differentiation from dentigerous cyst, 180
Dentigerous cyst, 178
    definition and clinical features, 178
    differential diagnosis, 180; differentiation from dental follicle, 180; from odontogenic keratocyst, 182;
        nevoid basal cell carcinoma, 184
    gross and microscopic findings, 180
    treatment and prognosis, 184
Denture stomatosis, 117
Dermoid cyst, 292
Destombes-Rosai-Dorfman disease, 51, 400
    oral cavity and sinuses, 51
    salivary glands, 400
Developmental lesions, 8, 108, 212, 264, 324, 375, 420
    ear and temporal bone, 420, 464
        accessory tragus, 420
        branchial cleft abnormalities, 421
        dysplasias, 466
        sensorineural hearing loss, 466
    larynx, 324
        laryngomalacia, 324
        tracheopathia osteochondroplastica, 325
    nasal cavity and paranasal sinuses, 8
        encephalocele, 11
        heterotopic central nervous system tissue, 8
        nasal dermoid sinus and cyst, 15
        primary ciliary dyskinesia, 16
    neck, 264
        branchial anomalies, 264
        bronchogenic cyst, 287
        cervical thymic cyst, 285
        dermoid cyst, 292
        thyroglossal duct cyst, 280
    oral cavity and jaw, 108
        ectopic thyroid tissue, 109
        exostoses, 112
        Fordyce granules, 108
        heterotopias, 108
        oral choristoma, 111
        tori, 112
    pharynx, 212
    salivary glands, 375
        accessory parotid glands, 375
        adenomatoid hyperplasia, 377
        hamartomas, 377
        salivary gland heterotopia, 375
Diffuse infiltrating lymphocytosis, and HIV salivary gland disease, 388
Diffuse oncocytosis, salivary gland, 382
Diphtheria, 332
Drug-induced fibrous hyperplasia, 153
Drug-related gingival hyperplasia, 153
Dysplasia versus radiation-induced changes, 358
Dysplasia versus reactive epithelial changes, 356

E

Ear and temporal bone, 413
Ectopia, 108, 327, 375, 453
    larynx/trachea, 327
    middle ear, 453
    oral cavity, 108
    salivary gland, 375
Ectopic lingual thyroid, 109
Ectopic thyroid tissue, 109
Embryology, 1, 6, 103, 207, 319, 324, 369, 413
    ear and temporal bone, 413
    larynx, 319
    nasal cavity, 1
    oral cavity and jaw, 103
    paranasal sinuses, 6
    pharynx, 207
    salivary glands, 369
    trachea, 324
Encephalocele, 8, **11**
    clinical features, 12
    definition, 11
    differential diagnosis, 14; differentiation from heterotopic central nervous system tissue, 8
    embryogenesis, 12
    gross findings, 13
    microscopic findings, 14
    treatment and prognosis, 15

Endogenous pigmentations, oral cavity, 172
   melanotic macule, 172
Endolymphatic hydrops, 464
Eosinophilic angiocentric fibrosis, 54
Eosinophilic chronic rhinosinusitis syndrome, 91
Eosinophilic fungal rhinosinusitis, 61
Eosinophilic mucin rhinosinusitis, 61
Epidermal cyst, middle ear, 446
Epidermal inclusion cyst, middle ear, 446
Epidermoid cyst, middle ear, 446
Epidermolysis bullosa, larynx, 360
Epithelial inflammatory or tumor-like processes, oral cavity, 122, *see also under individual entities*
   condyloma acuminatum, 122
   focal epithelial hyperplasia, 124
   inflammatory papillary hyperplasia, 129
   oral hairy leukoplakia, 125
   proliferative verrucous leukoplakia, 132
   pseudoepitheliomatous hyperplasia, 129
   verruca vulgaris, 122
   verruciform xanthoma, 126
Epithelioid angiomatosis, 302
Epithelioid hemangioma, ear, 433
   association with Kimura disease, 433
   definition and clinical features, 433
   differential diagnosis, 435; differentiation from Kimura disease, 435
   gross and microscopic findings, 434
   intravascular epithelioid hemangioma, 435
Epithelioid hemangioma-like vascular proliferation, 302
Epstein-Barr virus, 120, 230
   oral cavity, 120
   pharynx, 230
Epulis fissuratum, 140
Epulis granulomatosa, 157
Epulis gravidarum, 57
Eruption cyst, 185
Erythematous candidiasis, 116
Ethmoid sinus, 7
Eustachian tube, 415
Exogenous pigmentations, oral cavity, 170
   amalgam tattoo, 170
   differentiation from melanoma, 171
   graphite tattoo, 171
Exostoses, 112, 429
   ear, 429
   oral cavity, 112
      buccal exostoses, 112
      palatal exostoses, 112
External ear, 414
Extranodal sinus histiocytosis with massive lymphadenopathy, 51, 400, 451
   nasal cavity and sinuses, 51
      definition and clinical features, 51
      differential diagnosis, 52; differentiation from Langerhans cell histiocytosis, 54, 451; from rhinoscleroma, 54; from hematolymphoid malignancy, 54
      gross and microscopic findings, 52
      pathogenesis, 51
      treatment and prognosis, 54
   salivary glands, 400
Extravasation mucocele, salivary gland, 379

F

Fibrinous laryngotracheobronchitis, 330
Fibroepithelial polyp, 139
Fibromatosis/extraabdominal fibromatosis, oral cavity, differentiation from gingival fibromatosis, 153
Fibro-osseous lesions of craniofacial bones, 161
   cemento-osseous dysplasia, 169
   fibrous dysplasia, 161
Fibrosing lesions, oral, 152
Fibrosing osteitis, 439
Fibrous dysplasia, craniofacial bones, 161
   clinical features, 162
   definition, 161
   differential diagnosis, 163; differentiation from ossifying fibroma, 163; psammomatoid ossifying fibroma, 164
   gross and microscopic findings, 163
   pathogenesis, 162
   treatment and prognosis, 168
   variants, 162
      McCune-Albright syndrome, 162
      monostotic fibrous dysplasia, 162
      polyostotic fibrous dysplasia, 162
Fibrous epulis, 139
Fibrous nodule, 139
First branchial anomalies, 267
   clinical features, 267
   differential diagnosis, 269
   microscopic findings, 268

treatment and prognosis, 269
Florid cemento-osseous dysplasia, 169
Focal cemento-osseous dysplasia, 169
Focal epithelial hyperplasia, oral cavity, 124
Focal fibrous hyperplasia, 139
Follicular cyst, 178
Fordyce granules, 108
Fourth branchial anomalies, 280
Frontal sinus, 7
Fungal diseases, larynx/trachea, 333
Fungal diseases, nasal cavity and paranasal sinuses, 61, *see also under individual entities*
    blastomycosis, coccidiomycosis, cryptococcosis, histoplasmosis, 74
    fungal rhinosinusitis, 61
        acute invasive fungal rhinosinusitis, 66
        allergic fungal rhinosinusitis, 61
        chronic granulomatous rhinosinusitis, 67
        chronic invasive rhinosinusitis, 67
        fungus ball, 65
    rhinosporidiosis, 72
    sinonasal mucormycosis, 69
    sporotrichosis, 74
Fungal rhinosinusitis, 61, *see also under individual entities*
    acute invasive fungal rhinosinusitis, 66
    allergic fungal rhinosinusitis, 61
    chronic granulomatous rhinosinusitis, 67
    chronic invasive rhinosinusitis, 67
    fungus ball, 65
Fungus ball, nasal cavity and paranasal sinuses, 65

G

Giant cell fibroma, 142
Giant cell lesions, oral cavity, 144
    central and peripheral giant cell granuloma, 144, *see also* Central and peripheral giant cell granuloma
Giant cell tumor of bone, differentiation from central and peripheral giant cell granuloma, 149
Gingiva, 104
Gingival fibromatosis, 152
    differential diagnosis, 153; differentiation from fibromatosis/extraabdominal fibromatosis, 153; from myofibroma/myofibromatosis, 155
    general features, 152
    microscopic findings, 153

treatment and prognosis, 155
Glandular hamartoma, 32, 35
Glandular odontogenic cyst, 185
Gnathic bones, 104
Godwin lesion, 390
Gonorrhea, 121, 248
    oral cavity, 121
    pharynx, 248
Granulomatosis with polyangiitis, 40, 189, 335, 457
    ear, 457
    larynx/trachea, 335
        definition and clinical features, 335, 336
        differential diagnosis, 338; differentiation from Churg-Strauss disease, 338; from NK/T-cell lymphoma, 338
        microscopic findings, 337
        treatment and prognosis, 338
    nasal cavity, 40
        clinical features, 41
        definition, 40
        diagnosis, 46
        differential diagnosis, 46; differentiation from NK/T-cell lymphoma, 46; from fungal infection, 46
        gross and microscopic findings, 43
        immunohistochemical findings, 45
        laboratory findings, 42
        pathogenesis, 41
        treatment and prognosis, 48
    oral cavity, 189
Graphite tattoo, 171

H

Hamartomas, 30, 108, 219, 327, 377, *see also under individual entities*
    laryngeal/tracheal hamartomas, 327
    oral cavity hamartomas, 108
    pharyngeal hamartomas, 219
    salivary gland hamartomas, 377
    sinonasal hamartomas, 30
Hard palate, 104
Heerfordt syndrome, 397
Hereditary gingival fibromatosis, 152
Herpes simplex virus, 120, 245
    oral cavity, 120
    pharynx, 245
Heterotopias, 108, 219, 375, 453
    middle ear and mastoid, 453

acquired encephalocele, 454
  neuroglial heterotopia, 454
  salivary gland heterotopia, 453
 oral cavity, 108
 pharynx, 219
 salivary gland, 375
Heterotopic central nervous system tissue, 8, 219
 middle ear, 454
 nasal cavity, 8
  clinical features, 8
  definition, 8
  differential diagnosis, 11; differentiation from encephalocele, 8; from inflammatory polyp, 8; from olfactory neuroblastoma, 8
  gross and microscopic findings, 9
  treatment and prognosis, 11
 pharynx, 219
Heterotopic thyroid tissue, 109
Histioid mycobacteriosis, 297
Histology, normal, 1, 7, 105, 320, 324, 371, 417
 ear and temporal bone, 417
  external ear, 417
  inner ear, 420
  middle ear, 417
 larynx, 320
 nasal cavity, 1
  nasal septum, 3
 oral cavity and jaw, 105
  juxtaoral organ of Chievitz, 106
  lip, 105
  minor salivary glands, 106
  nonepithelial intraepithelial cells, 108
  oral mucosa, 106
  taste buds, 106
  tongue, 106
 paranasal sinuses, 7
 pharynx, 209
  hypopharynx, 212
  oropharynx, 209
  nasopharynx, 212
 salivary glands, 371
  acini, 371
  ducts, 373
  minor salivary glands, 373
  parotid gland, 373
  sublingual gland, 373
  submandibular gland, 373
 trachea, 324

Histoplasmosis, sinonasal, 74
Human immunodeficiency virus, 235, 387
 pharynx, 235
  diagnostic criteria, 241
  disease classification, 236
  lymphoid changes, tonsils, 237
  staging, 238
  surveillance case definition, 239, 240
 salivary gland, 387, *see also* Human immunodeficiency virus salivary gland disease
Human immunodeficiency virus salivary gland disease, 387
 association with diffuse infiltrating lymphocytosis, 388
 definition and clinical features, 387
 gross and microscopic findings, 388
 treatment and prognosis, 390
Human immunodeficiency virus-related diseases, 294, 302
 bacillary angiomatosis, 302
 tuberculosis, neck, 294
Human immunodeficiency virus-related lymphoid changes, tonsils, 237
Human papillomavirus, 119, 235, 331
 larynx/trachea, 331
 oral cavity, 119
 pharynx, 235
Hybrid intercalated duct lesion, 401
Hyperplastic tonsils, 224
Hypopharynx, 208

I

Idiopathic cystic chondromalacia of auricular cartilage, 426
Idiopathic gingival fibromatosis, 152
IgG4-related sialadenitis, 394
 chronic sclerosing sialadenitis, 394
 Mikulicz disease, 394
Immotile cilia syndrome, 16
Immune reconstitution inflammatory syndrome, 294
Immunosialadenitis, 390
Infectious diseases, 61, 116, 224, 292, 328, 386, 436, 438, *see also under individual entities*
 external ear, 436
  necrotizing external otitis, 436
 larynx/trachea, 328
  bacterial diseases, 331
  fungal diseases, 333

granulomatous laryngopharyngitis, 329
protozoal diseases, 334
viral diseases, 330
middle ear and temporal bone, 438
otic polyp, 444
otitis media, 438
nasal cavity and paranasal sinuses, 61
bacterial diseases, 76
fungal diseases, 61
protozoal diseases, 85
viral diseases, 87
neck, 292
actinomycosis, 298
bacillary angiomatosis, 302
cat scratch disease, 300
mycobacterial spindle cell pseudotumor, 297
mycobacterial tuberculosis infection, 292
scrofula, 294
oral cavity, 116
bacteria and spirochetes, 120
fungal diseases, 116
viral diseases, 118
pharynx, 224
acquired immunodeficiency syndrome, 245
bacteria and spirochetes, 248
cytomegalovirus, 245
fungal infections, 248
herpes simplex virus, 245
human immunodeficiency virus diseases, 235
human papillomavirus diseases, 235
infectious mononucleosis, 230
Lemierre disease, 230
measles, 248
peritonsillar abscess, 228
tonsillitis, 224
salivary gland, 386
acute sialadenitis, 386
chronic nonautoimmune sialadenitis, 386
human immunodeficiency virus diseases, 387
viral parotitis, 386
Infectious mononucleosis, 230
definition and clinical features, 230
differential diagnosis, 232
laboratory findings, 231
microscopic findings, 232
pathogenesis, 231
treatment and prognosis, 232
Infectious rhinosinusitis, 90

Inflammatory papillary hyperplasia, 129
Inflammatory polyp, 8, 444
ear, 444
nasal cavity, 8
differentiation from respiratory epithelial adenomatoid hamartoma, 35
Inner ear, 415
Inspissated mucus, 61
Intercalated duct adenoma, differentiation from intercalated duct lesion, 401
Intercalated duct hyperplasia, 401
Intercalated duct lesion, salivary gland, 401
differential diagnosis, 401; differentiation from intercalated duct adenoma, 401; from basal cell adenoma, 401
hybrid intercalated duct lesion, 401
intercalated duct hyperplasia, 401
Intravascular epithelioid hemangioma, 435
Intravascular pyogenic granuloma, 157
Intubation granuloma, 342
Inverted sinonasal papilloma, differentiation from respiratory epithelial adenomatoid hamartoma, 34
Irritation fibroma, 139
definition and clinical features, 139
differential diagnosis, 142
gross and microscopic findings, 140
treatment and prognosis, 142

J

Juxtaoral organ of Chievitz, 106

K

Keloid, ear, 421
Keratoma, vocal cord, 354
Keratosis, larynx, 354
Keratosis obturans, differentiation from cholesteatoma, 449
Kimura disease, 433, 435
association with epithelioid hemangioma, ear, 433
differentiation from epithelioid hemangioma, ear, 435
Klebsiella rhinoscleromatis, 76

L

Langerhans cell histiocytosis, middle ear, 54, 450
definition and clinical features, 450

differential diagnosis, 451; differentiation from extranodal sinus histiocytosis with massive lymphadenopathy, 54, 451; from non-Hodgkin lymphoma, 451
   microscopic findings, 450
   treatment and prognosis, 451
Laryngeal abscess, 332
Laryngeal amyloidosis, 347
Laryngeal cartilages, 322
Laryngocele, 340
Laryngomalacia, 324
Laryngotracheal stenosis, 349
Larynx, 319
Lateral periodontal cyst, 186
Leishmaniasis, 85
Lemierre disease/syndrome, 230
Leprosy, 84
Lermoyez syndrome, 464
Lichen planus, 189
Lingual thyroid, 109
Lip, 103
Lobular capillary hemangioma, 57, 157
   nasal cavity, 57
   oral cavity, 157
Lymphangiomatous polyp of tonsil, 222
Lymphoepithelial cyst, 113, 381
   oral cavity, 113
   salivary gland, 381
Lymphoepithelial sialadenitis, 390
   associated lesions, 390
Lymphoid polyp, tonsil, 222

M

Malakoplakia, differentiation from otitis media, 441
Malignant external otitis, 436
Maxillary sinus, 6
McCune-Albright syndrome, 162
Measles, pharynx, 248
Median anterior maxillary cyst, 114
Median rhomboid glossitis, 117
Melanoma, 170, 174
   differentiation from exogenous pigmentation, oral cavity, 170; from melanotic macule, oral cavity, 174
Melanotic macule, oral cavity, 172
   differentiation from melanoma, 174
Membranous labyrinth, 416
Ménière disease, 463

Mesenchymal lesions, oral cavity, 134, *see also under individual entities*
   giant cell fibroma, 142
   irritation fibroma, 139
   peripheral odontogenic fibroma, 138
   peripheral ossifying fibroma, 134
Metaplasia and hyperplasia, salivary gland, 382
   oncocytic metaplasia, 382
   oncocytosis, 382
   sialadenosis, 385
Microglandular adenosis, 35
Middle ear, 415
Middle ear adenoma, differentiation from otitis media, 440
Mikulicz disease, 394
Minor salivary glands, 371
Moniliasis, 116
Monostotic fibrous dysplasia, 162
Mucocutaneous candidiasis, 117
Mucocutaneous leishmaniasis, 85
Mucormycosis, 69
Mucous membrane pemphigoid, larynx, 360
Mucus extravasation phenomenon, salivary gland, 379
Mulberry turbinate, 25
Mumps, 386
Mycetoma, 65
Mycobacteria, 84, 292, 329
   larynx/trachea, 329
   nasal cavity, 84
   neck, 292
Mycobacteria avium-intracellulare pseudotumor, 297
Mycobacterial pseudotumor, 297
Mycobacterial spindle cell pseudotumor, 297
Mycobacterial tuberculosis infection, neck, 292
Myoepithelial sialadenitis, 390
Myofibroma/myofibromatosis, oral cavity, differentiation from gingival fibromatosis, 155
Myospherulosis, 49, 177, 441
   differentiation from otitis media, 441
   nasal cavity, 49
   oral cavity, 177

N

Nasal cavity, 1
Nasal chondromesenchymal hamartoma, 40
Nasal dermoid sinus and cyst, 15

Nasal hamartoma, 32, 40, *see also* Sinonasal hamartoma
Nasal septum, 3
Nasopalatine duct cyst, 114
Nasopharyngeal angiofibroma, differentiation from pyogenic granuloma, 60
Nasopharyngeal cysts, 212
Nasopharyngeal dermoid/teratoid, 219
Nasopharyngeal hamartomas, 219
　differentiation from teratoma, 219
Nasopharynx, 208
Neck, 263
Necrotizing external otitis, 436
Necrotizing granulomatous otitis, 436
Necrotizing sialometaplasia, 345, 398
　larynx, 345
　salivary glands, 398
　　differential diagnosis, 399
Neisseria gonorrhea, 121, 248
Neuroglial heterotopia, middle ear, 454
NK/T-cell lymphoma, larynx, nasal cavity, differentiation from granulomatosis with poly angiitis, 46, 338
Nodular oncocytic hyperplasia, salivary gland, 382
Nodular oncocytosis, salivary gland, 382
Nonallergic rhinosinusitis with eosinophilia syndrome, 91
Non-Hodgkin lymphoma, differentiation from Langerhans cell histiocytosis, 451
Noninfectious inflammatory and tumor-like processes, 19, 250, 306, 339, 398, *see also under individual entities*
　larynx and trachea, 339
　　angioedema/allergic laryngitis, 334
　　contact ulcer, 342
　　laryngeal amyloidosis, 347
　　laryngocele, 340
　　necrotizing sialometaplasia, 345
　　radiation-associated change, 357
　　reactive epithelial changes, 354
　　rheumatoid nodule, 351
　　saccular cyst, 340
　　sarcoidosis, 335
　　subglottic stenosis, 349
　　Teflon granuloma, 351
　　vocal cord nodules, 339
　nasal cavity and paranasal sinuses, 19
　　eosinophilic angiocentric fibrosis, 54
　　extranodal sinus histiocytosis with massive lymphadenopathy, 51
　　granulomatosis with polyangiitis, 40
　　myospherulosis, 49
　　necrotizing sialometaplasia, 54
　　paranasal sinus mucocele, 27
　　pyogenic granuloma/lobular capillary hemangioma, 57
　　relapsing polychondritis, 56
　　rhinophyma, 55
　　sarcoidosis, 55
　　sinonasal hamartomas, 30
　　　chondro-osseous and respiratory epithelial hamartoma, 39
　　　nasal chondromesenchymal hamartoma, 40
　　　respiratory epithelial adenomatoid hamartoma, 32
　　　seromucinous hamartoma, 35
　　sinonasal inflammatory polyps, 19
　neck, 306
　　sarcoidosis, 306
　pharynx, 250
　　Tangier disease, 250
　salivary gland, 398
　　extranodal sinus histiocytosis with massive lymphadenopathy, 400
　　intercalated duct cyst, 401
　　necrotizing sialometaplasia, 398

O

Odontogenic cysts, 178, *see also under individual entities*
　dentigerous cyst, 178
　eruption cyst, 185
　glandular odontogenic cyst, 185
　lateral periodontal cyst, 186
　periapical cyst, 187
Odontogenic epithelial hamartoma, 138
Odontogenic keratocyst, differentiation from dentigerous cyst, 182
Olfactory neuroblastoma, differentiation from heterotopic central nervous system tissue, 8
Oncocytic cystadenoma, larynx, 342
Oncocytic hyperplasia, salivary gland, 382
Oncocytic metaplasia, salivary gland, 382
　differentiation from oncocytoma, 385; from carcinoma, 385
Oncocytosis, salivary gland, 382

Oral candidiasis, see Candidiasis
Oral cavity and jaw, 103
Oral cavity hamartoma, 108
Oral cavity heterotopia, 108
Oral choristoma, 108, 111
Oral fibrosing lesions, 152
    gingival fibromatosis, 152
    oral submucous fibrosis, 152
Oral lymphoepithelial cyst, 113
Oral hairy leukoplakia, 125, 248
    oral cavity, 125
    pharynx, 248
Oral mucosa, 106
Oral mucosal condyloma acuminatum, 122
Oral submucous fibrosis, 152
Oral thrush, 116
Oropharyngeal histoplasmosis, 248
Oropharynx, 207
Osseous labyrinth, 416
Ossifying fibroid epulis, 134
Ossifying fibroma, craniofacial bones, differentiation from fibrous dysplasia, 163
Osteitis deformans, ear, 463
Osteoma, ear, 429
Osteomeatal complex, 7
Otic polyp, 444
Otitis media, 438
    acute otitis media, 438
    cholesterol granuloma, 440
    chronic otitis media, 439
    differentiation from middle ear adenoma, 440; from myospherulosis, 441; from malakoplakia, 441
    fibrosing osteitis, 439
    secretory otitis media, 438
    tympanosclerosis, 440
Otosclerosis, 461
Ozena, 90

P

Pachyderma laryngis, 354
Paget disease of bone, ear, 463
Papillary thyroid carcinoma, 278, 285
    differentiation from second branchial anomalies, 278; from thyroglossal duct cyst, 285
Paranasal sinuses, 1
Paranasal sinus mucocele, 27
Parapharyngeal space, 209
Parotid gland, 369
Parulis, 157
Pemphigus, larynx, 360
Periapical cemento-osseous dysplasia, 169
Periapical abscess, 188
Periapical cyst, 187
Periapical granuloma, 187
Peripheral fibroameloblastic fibroma, 138
Peripheral fibroma with calcification, 134
Peripheral giant cell granuloma, see Central and peripheral giant cell granuloma
Peripheral odontogenic fibroma, 138
Peripheral ossifying fibroma, 134
    definition and clinical features, 134
    differential diagnosis, 135, 137
    microscopic findings, 135
    treatment and prognosis, 138
Peritonsillar abscess, 228, 332
Pharyngeal bursa, 216
Pharynx, 207
Pigmented lesions, oral cavity, 169
    black hairy tongue, 174
    exogenous pigmentations, 170
    endogenous pigmentations, 172
    myospherulosis, 177
Polychondritis, relapsing, see Relapsing polychondritis
Polychondropathia, ear, 455
Polychondropathy, larynx, 338
Polycystic (dysgenetic) disease, salivary gland, 382
Polyostotic fibrous dysplasia, 162
Polyotia, 420
Post-transplant lymphoproliferative disorder, differentiation from tonsillitis, 228
Pregnancy tumor, 57, 157
Primary ciliary dyskinesia, 16
    clinical features, 17
    definition, 16
    diagnosis, 19
    differential diagnosis, 19
    genetic mutations, 16
    nitric oxide measurements, 17
    pathogenesis, 16
    treatment and prognosis, 19
    ultrastructural findings, 17
Progressive otospongiosis, ear, 461
Proliferative verrucous leukoplakia, 132, 355
    larynx, 355

oral cavity, 132
    differential diagnosis, 134
Protozoal diseases, 85, 334
    larynx/trachea, 334
    nasal cavity and paranasal sinuses, 85
        amebiasis, 87
        mucocutaneous leishmaniasis, 85
Pseudoepitheliomatous hyperplasia, 129, 354
    larynx, 354
    oral cavity, 129
        definition, 129
        clinical features, 130
        differential diagnosis, 132; differentiation from squamous cell carcinoma, 132
        microscopic findings, 130
        treatment and prognosis, 132
Pseudogranuloma, nasal cavity, 25
Pseudolymphangioma, nasal cavity, 25
Pseudomembranous candidiasis, 116
Pseudomonas sp, 82, 436
Punctate parotitis, 390
Pyogenic granuloma of larynx, 342
Pyogenic granuloma/lobular capillary hemangioma, 57, 157
    nasal cavity, 57
        definition and clinical features, 57
        differential diagnosis, 60; differentiation from sinonasal glomangiopericytoma, 60; from nasopharyngeal angiofibroma, 60
        gross and microscopic findings, 58
        pathogenesis, 58
        treatment and prognosis, 61
    oral cavity, 157
        definition and clinical features, 157
        differential diagnosis, 161
        microscopic findings, 158
        pathogenesis, 157
        treatment and prognosis, 161
Pyrophosphate arthropathy, ear, 460

Q

Quinsy, 228

R

Radiation-associated changes, 192, 357
    larynx, 357
        differentiation from dysplasia, 358; from carcinoma, 358

oral cavity, 192
    definition and clinical features, 192
    differential diagnosis, 193
    microscopic findings, 192
Radicular cyst, 187
Ranula, 380
Rathke cleft cyst, 215
Rathke pouch cyst, 215
    definition and clinical features, 215
    microscopic findings, 216
    treatment and prognosis, 216
Reactive epithelial changes, larynx, 354
    basal layer hyperplasia, 354
    differentiation from dysplasia, 356
    keratosis, 354
    pseudoepitheliomatous hyperplasia, 354
    simple hyperplasia, 354
    verrucous hyperplasia, 354
Reinke space edema, 339
Relapsing polychondritis, 56, 338, 455
    ear, 455
    larynx, 338
    nasal cavity, 56
Respiratory epithelial adenomatoid hamartoma, nasal cavity, 32
    definition and clinical features, 32
    differential diagnosis, 34; differentiation from adenocarcinoma, 34; from inverted sinonasal papilloma, 34; from inflammatory polyps, 35
    pathogenesis, 32
    microscopic findings, 32
Retention cyst, larynx, 342
Retention mucocele, salivary gland, 377
Retrocuspid papule, 140
Retropharyngeal abscess, 332
Rheumatoid nodule, 351
Rhinocerebral/rhinoorbitocerebral mucormycosis, 69
Rhinophyma, 55
Rhinoscleroma, 54, 76, 329
    differentiation from extranodal sinus histiocytosis with massive lymphadenopathy, 54
    larynx/trachea, 329
    sinonasal, 76
        definition and clinical features, 76
        differential diagnosis, 82
        immunohistochemical findings, 81
        microscopic findings, 78
        pathogenesis, 78

treatment and prognosis, 82
Rhinosinusitis, 61, 87
    allergic rhinosinusitis, 90
    atrophic rhinosinusitis, 90
    bacterial sinusitis, 90
    definition and clinical features, 87
    differential diagnosis, 89
    fungal, 61, see also Fungal rhinosinusitis
    infectious rhinosinusitis, 90
    microscopic findings, 88
    radiologic findings, 87
    treatment and prognosis, 89
    viral rhinosinusitis, 90
Rhinosporidiosis, 72
Rhinosporidium seeberi, 73
Rhizopus sp, 69
Rosai-Dorfman disease, see Extranodal sinus histiocytosis with massive lymphadenopathy
Rubeola, pharynx, 248

S

Saccular cyst, larynx, 340
Salivary glands, 369
Salivary gland anlage tumor, 224
Salivary gland heterotopia/choristoma, middle ear, 453
Salivary gland hamartoma, 377
Salivary gland heterotopia/ectopia/choristoma, 375
Samter syndrome, 91
Sarcoidosis, 55, 306, 335, 396
    larynx, 335
    nasal cavity, 55
    neck, 306
    salivary gland, 396
        Heerfordt syndrome, 397
Scleroma, 76
Scrofula, neck, 294
Scrofulous gumma, 294
Scrofulous lupus, 76
Second branchial anomalies, 269
    branchial cleft cyst, 271
    clinical features, 269
    differential diagnosis, 273; differentiation from metastatic cystic squamous cell carcinoma, 273; from branchial cleft carcinoma, 277; from papillary thyroid carcinoma, 278
    microscopic findings, 271
    treatment and prognosis, 279

Secondary ciliary dyskinesia, 16
Seromucinous salivary glands, 371
Seromucinous hamartoma, nasal cavity, 35
    differentiation from adenocarcinoma, 38
Sialadenitis, 386
    acute, 386
    chronic, 386
    IgG4-related, 394
    lymphoepithelial, 390
    viral, 386
Sialadenosis, 385
Sialocyst, 377
Sialo-odontogenic cyst, 185
Sialosis, 385
Simple hyperplasia, larynx, 354
Singer nodule, 339
Sinonasal botryomycosis, 83
Sinonasal glomangiopericytoma, differentiation from pyogenic granuloma, 60
Sinonasal hamartomas, 30, see also under *individual entities*
    chondro-osseous and respiratory epithelial hamartomas, 39
    classification, 30
    features of each compared, 30
    granulomatosis with polyangiitis, 40
    myospherulosis, 49
    nasal chondromesenchymal hamartoma, 40
    respiratory epithelial adenomatoid hamartoma, 32
    seromucinous hamartoma, 35
Sinonasal inflammatory polyps, 19
    antrochoanal polyps, 22
    association with other lesions, 22
    definition and clinical features, 19
    differential diagnosis, 26
    gross and microscopic findings, 20
    mulberry turbinate, 25
    pathogenesis, 20
    polyps with atypical stromal cells, 22
    polyps with cystic fibrosis, 25
    polyps with partial infarction, 25
    pseudogranuloma, 25
    pseudolymphangioma, 25
    treatment and prognosis, 27
Sinonasal mucormycosis, 69
    definition and clinical features, 69
    differential diagnosis, 71
    microscopic findings, 71

pathogenesis, 69
treatment and prognosis, 72
Sinusitis, bacterial, 90
Sjogren syndrome, 390
    clinical features, 391
    definition, 390
    diagnostic criteria, 391, 393
    differential diagnosis, 393
    gross and microscopic findings, 391
    laboratory findings, 391
    lip biopsy, 392
    pathogenesis, 391
    treatment and prognosis, 393
Snotoma, 61
Sphenoid sinus, 7
Spindled nontuberculous mycobacteriosis, 297
Spirochetes, 121, 248
Sporotrichosis, nasal cavity, 74
Squamous cell carcinoma, 132, 273
    differentiation from pseudoepitheliomatous hyperplasia, oral cavity, 132; from second branchial anomalies, 273
Subacute necrotizing sialadenitis, 399
Sublingual gland, 370
Subglottic stenosis, 349
Submandibular gland, 370
Supernumerary ear, 420
Surfer ear, 429
Symmetric fibromatosis of the tuberosity, 153
Synovial chondromatosis of temporomandibular joint, 430
Synovial chondrometaplasia, temporomandibular joint, 430
Synovial osteochondromatosis of temporomandibular joint, 430
Syphilis, 121, 248
    oral cavity, 121
    pharynx, 248
Systemic chondromalacia, larynx, 338

T

Tangier disease, 250
Taste buds, 106
Tattoo, 170
Teeth, 104
Teflon granuloma, 351
Teflonoma, 351
Teratoma, differentiation from nasopharyngeal hamartoma, 219
Teratomatous lesions, pharynx, 219
Third branchial anomalies, 279
Thornwaldt bursa, 216
Thornwaldt cyst, 216
Thornwaldt disease, 216
Thrush, *see* Candidiasis
Thyroglossal duct cyst, 280
    associated neoplasms, 285
        papillary thyroid carcinoma, 285
    clinical features, 281
    differential diagnosis, 283
    embryology, 280
    microscopic findings, 282
    treatment and prognosis, 284
Tongue, 104
Tonsillitis, 224
    clinical features, 226
    definition, 224
    differential diagnosis, 227
    microscopic findings, 227
    treatment and prognosis, 227
        post-transplant lymphoproliferative disorder, 228
Tophaceous gout, 458
Tophaceous pseudogout, 459
Tori, oral cavity, 112
    torus mandibularis, 112
    torus palatinus, 112
Trachea, 319
Tracheal stenosis, 349
Tracheopathia osteochondroplastica, 325
Tracheopathia osteoplastica, 325
Traumatic fibroma, 139
Treponemal pallidum, 121
Tumoral calcium pyrophosphate dihydrate deposition disease, ear, 460
Tympanic membrane, 414
Tympanosclerosis, 440

V

Vascular lesions, oral cavity, 157
    congenital epulis, 160
    pyogenic granuloma/lobular capillary hemangioma, 157
Venereal wart/condyloma, oral cavity, 122
Verruca vulgaris, 122
Verruciform xanthoma, 126

definition and clinical features, 126
differential diagnosis, 127
microscopic findings, 127
pathogenesis, 126
treatment and prognosis, 129
Verrucous hyperplasia, larynx, 354
Vestibular system, 417
Viral diseases, 87, 118, 330, 386, *see also under individual entities*
   larynx/trachea, 330
   nasal cavity and paranasal sinuses, 87
   oral cavity, 118
      cytomegalovirus, 120
      Epstein-Barr virus, 120
      herpes virus, 120
      human papillomavirus, 119
   salivary gland, 386
      human immunodeficiency virus diseases, 387
      viral parotitis, 386
Viral parotitis, 386
Viral rhinosinusitis, 90
Vocal cord nodule/polyp, 339

W

Wart, 122
Wegener granulomatosis, *see* Granulomatosis with polyangiitis
Winkler disease/nodule, 425
World Health Organization case definition for HIV infection, 240

Z

Zygomycetes fungi, 69
Zygomycosis, 69